Assisted Reproductive Technology
Accomplishments and New Horizons

This insightful and thought-provoking book describes the many recent advances that have revolutionized reproductive medicine. This rapid transformation is the result of converging and overlapping developments in reproductive biology, molecular biology, and genetics, allied with remarkable developments in new technologies. This book surveys this rapid expansion and looks ahead at the exciting new prospects for the future that stand at the watershed between basic science and clinical application. From oogenesis and spermatogenesis, through to fertilization, embryogenesis and cloning, it looks at state-of-the-art technologies and scientific advances. Subsequent chapters focus on infertility and its diagnosis and treatment using the full armory of assisted reproductive technologies. A concluding section surveys the impact of these developments on the provision, regulation, and financing of reproductive health care in the global community.

This will be essential reading for all practitioners in reproductive medicine: scientists, clinicians and researchers.

Christopher J. De Jonge Professor, Department of Obstetrics and Gynecology, Director of Laboratories, Reproductive Medicine Center, University of Minnesota, Minneapolis, USA.

Christopher L. R. Barratt Professor, Department of Medicine, University of Birmingham Medical School and Birmingham Woman's Hospital, Birmingham, UK.

Assisted Reproductive Technology

Accomplishments and New Horizons

EDITED BY

Christopher J. De Jonge

Reproductive Medical Center,
University of Minnesota,
Minneapolis, USA

Christopher L. R. Barratt

Assisted Conception Unit,
University of Birmingham and
Birmingham Women's Hospital,
Birmingham, UK

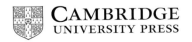

CAMBRIDGE
UNIVERSITY PRESS

PUBLISHED BY THE PRESS SYNDICATE OF THE UNIVERSITY OF CAMBRIDGE
The Pitt Building, Trumpington Street, Cambridge, United Kingdom

CAMBRIDGE UNIVERSITY PRESS
The Edinburgh Building, Cambridge CB2 2RU, UK
40 West 20th Street, New York, NY 10011–4211, USA
477 Williamstown Road, Port Melbourne, VIC 3207, Australia
Ruiz de Alarcón 13, 28014 Madrid, Spain
Dock House, The Waterfront, Cape Town 8001, South Africa

http://www.cambridge.org

First published 2002

Printed in the United Kingdom at the University Press, Cambridge

Typeface Utopia 8½/12 pt.   *System* QuarkXPress®   [SE]

A catalogue record for this book is available from the British Library

Library of Congress Cataloguing in Publication data

Assisted reproductive technology / [edited by] Christopher J. De Jonge, Christopher L. R.
Barratt.
    p.   cm.
Includes bibliographical references and index.
ISBN 0 521 80121 4 (HB: alk. paper)
1. Human reproductive technology.   I. Jonge, Christopher J. De.   II. Barratt, C. L. R.
[DNLM: 1.   Reproduction Techniques.   2.   Embryo Transfer.   3.   Fertilization in Vitro.
4.   Infertility – Diagnosis.   5.   Infertility – Therapy.   WQ 208 A8485 2001]
RG133.5.A786 2001
616.6'9206–dc21   2001043079

ISBN 0 521 80121 4 hardback

2315344x.

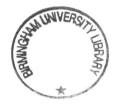

This book is dedicated to our families and in memory of the late Professor Lonnie Russell

Contents

Contributors

Yuksel Agca
Cryobiology Research Institute, The Herman B. Wells Center for Pediatric Research, Riley Hospital for Children, 1044 West Walnut Street, Indianapolis, IN 46202, USA

R. John Aitken
School of Biological and Chemical Sciences, Centre for Life Sciences, University of Newcastle, University Drive, Callaghan, NSW 2308, Australia

Susan M. Avery
Bourn Hall Clinic, Bourn, Cambridge CB3 7TR, UK

Jay Baltz
The Loeb Research Institute, Ottawa Hospital, 725 Parkdale Avenue and Departments of Obstetrics and Gynecology, Division of Reproductive Medicine, and Cellular and Molecular Medicine, University of Ottawa, Ontario K1Y 4E9, Canada

Frank L. Barnes
IVF Labs, L.L.C., 2712 E. Swasont Way, Salt Lake City, UT 84117, USA

Christopher L. R. Barratt
Assisted Conception Unit, University Department of Medicine, Birmingham Women's Hospital, Birmingham B15 2TG, UK

Barry Bavister
Department of Biological Sciences, University of New Orleans, and the Audubon Institute, Center for Research of Endangered Species, 14001 River Road, New Orleans, LA 70131, USA

Peter R. Brinsden
Bourn Hall Clinic, Bourn, Cambridge CB3 7TR, UK

Sandra Ann Carson
Department of Obstetrics and Gynecology, Baylor College of Medicine, 6550 Fannin, Houston, TX, USA

Douglas S. Colvard
Contraceptive Research and Development (CONRAD) Program, Department of Obstetrics and Gynecology, Eastern Virginia Medical School, 601 Colley Avenue, Norfolk, VA 23507, USA

Ian D. Cooke
University of Sheffield, Sheffield S3 7RE, UK

David Cram
Monash IVF and Monash Institute of Reproduction and Development, Melbourne, Australia

John K. Critser
Comparative Medicine Center and College of Veterinary Medicine, 1600 East Rollins Rd, University of Missouri, Columbia, MO 65211, USA

Jim Cummins
Murdoch University, Perth, Western Australia

Christopher De Jonge
Department of Obstetrics and Gynecology and Reproductive Medicine Center, University of Minnesota, 606 24th Avenue South, Minneapolis, MN 55454, USA

David de Kretser
Monash Institute of Reproduction and Development, Melbourne, Australia

Paul Devroey
Center for Reproductive Medicine, University Hospital and Medical School, Dutch-speaking Brussels Free University (Vrije Universiteit Brussel) Brussels, Belgium

Richard P. Dickey
Section of Reproductive Endocrinology and Infertility, Department Obstetrics and Gynecology, Louisiana State University School of Medicine and the Fertility Institute of New Orleans, 6020 Bullard Avenue, New Orleans, LA, USA

Gustavo F. Doncel
Contraceptive Research and Development (CONRAD) Program, Department of Obstetrics and Gynecology, Eastern Virginia Medical School, 601 Colley Avenue, Norfolk, VA 23507, USA

Peter J. Donovan
Kimmel Cancer Center, Thomas Jefferson University, Philadelphia, PA 19107, USA

Nanette R. Elster
Institute for Bioethics, Health Policy and Law, School of Medicine, University of Louisville, Louisville, KY 40202, USA

John D. Gearhart
School of Medicine, Johns Hopkins University, Johns Hopkins Hospital, Baltimore, MD 21287, USA

Michael D. Griswold
Washington State University, Pullman, WA 99164-4660, USA

Kate Hardy
Department of Reproductive Science and Medicine, Institute of Reproductive and Developmental Biology, Imperial College, Hammersmith Hospital, Du Cane Road, London W12 0NN, UK

Laura Hewitson
Pittsburgh Development Center of the Magee Women's Research Institute and the Department of Obstetrics, Gynecology and Reproductive Sciences, University of Pittsburgh, Pittsburgh, PA, USA

Michael K. Holland
Pest Animal Control CRC, GPO Box 284, Canberra, ACT 2601, Australia

Bernard Jégou
GERM-INSERM U.435, Campus de Beaulieu, Université de Rennes I, 35042 Rennes, Bretagne, France

Howard W. Jones Jr.
Eastern Virginia Medical School, Norfolk, VA and Johns Hopkins University School of Medicine, Baltimore, MD, USA

Axel Kamischke
Institute of Reproductive Medicine of the University (WHO Collaborating Centre for Reseach in Human Reproduction), Domagkstr. 11, D-48129, Münster, Germany

Gregory S. Kopf
Contraception Women's Health Research Institute, Wyeth Ayerst Research, PO Box 8299, Philadelphia, PA 19101, USA

Ann M. Lawler
School of Medicine, Johns Hopkins University, Johns Hopkins Hospital, Baltimore, MD 21287, USA

Ellen Matulich
Fertility Institute of New Orleans, 6020 Bullard Avenue, New Orleans, LA, USA

Christine Mauck
Contraceptive Research and Development (CONRAD) Program, Department of Obstetrics and Gynecology, Eastern Virginia Medical School, 601 Colley Avenue, Norfolk, VA 23507, USA

Eileen A. McLaughlin
Pest Animal Control CRC, GPO Box 284, Canberra, ACT 2601, Australia

Shoukhrat Mitalipov
Division of Reproductive Sciences, Oregon Regional Primate Research Center, Beaverton OR, USA

Eberhard Nieschlag
Institute of Reproductive Medicine of the University (WHO Collaborating Centre for Research in Human Reproduction), Domagkstr. 11, D-48129, Münster, Germany

Charles Pineau
GERM-INSERM U.435, Campus de Beaulieu, Université de Rennes I, 35042 Rennes, Bretagne, France

Peter Platteau
Center for Reproductive Medicine, University Hospital and Medical School, Dutch-speaking Brussels Free University (Vrije Universiteit Brussel) Brussels, Belgium

The late Lonnie D. Russell
Formerly of Southern Illinois University School of Medicine, Carbondale, IL 62901, USA

Gerald Schatten
Pittsburgh Development Center of the Magee Women's Research Institute, Pittsburgh PA 15213 and the Department of Obstetrics, Gynecology and Reproductive Sciences, University of Pittsburgh, Pittsburgh, PA, USA

Françoise Shenfield
Reproductive Medicine Unit, University College Hospital and the Royal Free and University College Hospitals Medical School, the London Women's Clinic, Harley Street, London, UK

Cal Simerly
Pittsburgh Development Center of the Magee Women's Research Institute, Pittsburgh PA 15213 and the Department of Obstetrics, Gynecology and Reproductive Sciences, University of Pittsburgh, Pittsburgh, PA, USA

Joe Leigh Simpson
Department of Obstetrics and Gynecology, Baylor College of Medicine, 6550 Fannin, Houston, TX, USA

Jorma Toppari
Department of Pediatrics and Physiology, University of Turku, Turku 20520, Finland

Herman J. Tournaye
Center for Reproductive Medicine, University Hospital and Medical School, Dutch-speaking Brussels Free University (Vrije Universiteit Brussel), Brussels, Belgium

Alexander J. Travis
Center for Research on Reproduction and Women's Health, University of Pennsylvania Medical Center, Biomedical Research Building II/III, 421 Curie Blvd, Philadelphia, PA 19104-6142, USA

Alan Trounson
Centre for Early Human Development, Monash Institute of Reproduction and Development, 27–31 Wright St, Clayton, Victoria 3168, Australia

Jonathan Van Blerkom
Department of Molecular, Cellular and Developmental Biology, University of Colorado, Boulder 80309 and Colorado Reproductive Endocrinology, Rose Medical Center, Denver 80220, CO, USA

André C. Van Steirteghem
Center for Reproductive Medicine, University Hospital and Medical School, Dutch-speaking Brussels Free University (Vrije Universiteit Brussel), Brussels, Belgium

Donna L. Vogel

National Cancer Institute, 31 Center Drive, Bethesda, MD 20892-2440, USA

Don P. Wolf

Division of Reproductive Sciences, Oregon Regional Primate Research Center, Beaverton, OR, USA

Erik J. Woods

Cryobiology Research Institute, The Herman B. Wells Center for Pediatric Research, Riley Hospital for Children, 1044 West Walnut Street, Indianapolis, IN 46202, USA

Lourens J. D. Zaneveld

Program for Topical Prevention of Conception and Disease (TOPCAD), Rush University, Chicago, IL, USA

Foreword

ART: today and beyond

Just think, prior to World War II, it was thought that the genetic message of our species was packaged in 48 chromosomes.

The 1950s saw what might be called the chromosomal revolution. In the early 1950s, I had a telephone call from Lawson Wilkins, Professor of Pediatrics at Johns Hopkins, who said that he had been at a medical meeting where an anatomist had indicated that it was possible to diagnose the sex of a cell and, therefore, of the individual, by examining a nerve cell under the microscope. Specifically, a large percentage of nuclei from females had a small unique granule or body. Lawson said "this was the damnest thing I ever heard." He invited me to attend a meeting that afternoon with Dr. George Streeter, Director of the Carnegie Institute of Embryology, Dr. Carl Hartman, an eminent primatologist at the Institute, and the two of us to discuss this matter and see whether it had any clinical application. The result of this meeting was that it was decided that skin biopsies could be taken from several patients that Dr. Wilkins and I jointly had and who had problems of sexual differentiation. We reasoned that it might be possible, therefore, to make a nuclear sex determination of the individuals and to correlate that with the other criteria of sex identification. The amazing thing was that patients with Turner's syndrome proved to be Barr body negative. Coincidentally, it had been the anatomist, Murray Barr, who had presented the paper that had intrigued Lawson Wilkins' interest. Thus, we were forced to the conclusion that patients with Turner's syndrome must have the Y chromosome.

However, a few years later, in 1956, Tjio and Levan showed that in the human there were but 46 chromosomes. Soon after that, in 1959, Charlie Ford showed that patients with Turner's syndrome did not have XY sex chromosomes but were indeed characterized by having 45 chromosomes and only one sex chromosome, i.e., a single X. This was the same year that Lejeune had shown that patients with mongolism, later called Down syndrome, had an extra chromosome 21. By the end of the 1950s, clinical cytogenetics had become a reality.

On a parallel track, molecular genetics was having its own revolution. In 1953, Watson and Crick brought forth their blockbuster notion of the double helix. As a consequence, the concepts of Mendel, Garrod, and others acquired a molecular basis, with guanine, cytosine, thymine, and adenine becoming household words in homes tuned to the molecular age.

On still another track, another revolution was occurring. Chang, in 1958, using the rabbit, proved that a mammalian egg could be fertilized in vitro and develop into a normal rabbit. Twenty years later, Edwards and Steptoe achieved the first pregnancy in the human by what has come to be known clinically as in vitro fertilization (IVF).

The overall result is that in the early twenty-first century, all three of these revolutions are milling about in the same dish, that is the culture dish of the embryologist, who supervises on a more or less routine basis the union of the sperm and the egg by attractive forces that remain among nature's mysteries.

While the clinician and the embryologist strive to get conditions just right to optimize the process of in vitro fertilization, it has now become possible to examine the chromosomes and indeed the molecular aspects of the genetic message along the way. It seems certain that, by the middle of the twenty-first century, the current diagnostic efforts will seem primitive indeed, but a beginning is being made in a very dynamic and rapidly moving field. It is possible to be comfortable in predicting that in due time therapy for chromosome and molecular abnormalities will be available to improve the human condition. Who could object to that?

Not to be forgotten is the fact that fertilization in vitro, with the gadgets to watch it and examine it along the way, has made all this possible. Furthermore, and most importantly, all these revolutions have taken place within the span of a single generation – clear evidence that we are not dealing with a mature discipline – on the contrary, we seem to be in the midst of an investigative whirlwind.

Therefore, the trinity of chromosomology, the molecular basis of genetics, and clinical IVF requires a "snapshot" from time to time so that all of those involved from the patient, and therefore the public, to the clinician and to the laboratory worker will know where we are and where we might go.

This is the eminently appropriate raison d'être for this snapshot – this book.

Howard W. Jones Jr.

Professor Emeritus, Eastern Virginia Medical School, Norfolk, VA and
Professor Emeritus, Johns Hopkins University School of Medicine, Baltimore, MD, USA

Part I

The gametes: present and future

Spermatogenesis in vitro in mammals

Bernard Jégou[1], Charles Pineau[1], and Jorma Toppari[2]

[1] GERM-INSERM U.435, University of Rennes I, Rennes, France
[2] Department of Pediatrics and Physiology, University of Turku, Finland

Introduction

Since the introduction of the first tissue cultures at the beginning of the twentieth century (embryonic fragments of nervous tissues: Harrison, 1907; fragments of chicken heart: Carrel, 1912), we have been able to study the behavior of animal cells without the complexities and systemic variations that arise in living animals.

Tissue culture has also been used to study testicular function without interference from hormones and to study cultures of isolated cells without the local controls imposed by the neighboring cells with which they normally communicate in situ. This technique was first described by Champy (1920), who maintained the testes on a "culture medium" constituted by a plasma clot as originally proposed by Carrel (1912). Since then, numerous attempts have been made to culture testes, testicular fragments, segments of seminiferous tubules, and dispersed heterogeneous or homogeneous populations of testicular cells, with varying degrees of success. Only a few reviews have been written on the subject (Wolff and Haffen, 1965; Kierszenbaum, 1994). However, because of the renewed interest in the culture of primary testicular explants or cells in mice, rats, and humans, we will review and analyze the data obtained in their historical and biological contexts. In view of the extremely complex cellular organization of the testis and the highly sophisticated mechanisms that control spermatogenesis, this review will begin with a brief overview of the anatomy of the testis, spermato-genesis, and the hormonal and paracrine control of this process.

Anatomy of the testis, spermatogenesis and its control

Although the genetic determination of sex of mammals occurs at fecondation, both sexes are morphologically identical until 12 days postcoitum (dpc) in the mouse, 13.5 dpc in the rat, and until week 7 of gestation in humans. The first recognizable event is the appearance of Sertoli cells in the gonads just after the expression of the sex-determining gene (*SRY*; Magre and Jost, 1980; Orth, 1993; Schmahl et al., 2000). Shortly after entering the genital ridge, the primordial germ cells (PGC), which migrate from the mesoderm, take a male pathway if their genotype is male and if the gonad has a male phenotype (McLaren, 1983). Fetal Sertoli cells aggregate to form the seminiferous cord and eventually enclose the PGC, which are then termed gonocytes. The developing seminiferous cords are rapidly surrounded by a basal lamina in the rat. At about the same time, flat mesenchymal cells become associated with the basal portions of Sertoli cells (Magre and Jost, 1980). In humans, the seminiferous cords become well organized by the end of week 9, and well-organized surrounding peritubular cells are visible by week 18 (Wartenberg, 1989; Orth, 1993). Recognizable Leydig cells appear in the interstitium of the fetal testis after the formation of the seminiferous cords: one to two days postpartum (dpp) in the rat and about 1 week postpartum in humans (Orth, 1993).

Differentiation and organization of the testis

In the adult testis, the seminiferous tubules contain germ cells in various phases of development and nonproliferating Sertoli cells, which are surrounded by peritubular cells. Germ cells, which are continuously renewed, and Sertoli cells, which secrete several hormones and cease to divide during pubertal development, form the seminiferous epithelium. The primary function of the seminiferous tubules is the production of spermatozoa. The convoluted seminiferous tubules of the differentiated gonad are embedded in a connective tissue matrix, called the interstitium, which contains interspersed blood and lymphatic vessels, nerves, fibroblastic cells, macrophages, lymphocytes, rare mast cells, and the Leydig cells. The primary function of the Leydig cells is to produce testosterone.

Spermatogenesis

The complexity of the lining of the seminiferous epithelium is unique (Fawcett, 1975) and, therefore, the complexity of the communication network of cellular activities in the seminiferous tubules is also unique (Jégou, 1993; Gnessi et al., 1997; Jégou et al., 1999). This anatomical and functional communication network is established from the very beginning of the seminiferous cord formation (Pelliniemi et al., 1984; Byskov, 1986; Jégou, 1993; Orth, 1993). The period during which PGC and gonocytes divide is known as prespermatogenesis (Hilscher et al., 1974), whereas the formation of spermatozoa from the most immature germ cells in the postpartum period is called spermatogenesis. Spermatogenesis is classically divided into three phases. In the first, the proliferative or mitotic phase, primitive germ cells, or spermatogonia, replenish their stock and undergo a series of mitotic divisions. Spermatogonia arise from the differentiation of gonocytes after birth (3 dpp in the rat; McGuinness and Orth, 1992). In the second, meiotic phase, the spermatocytes undergo two consecutive

divisions to produce the haploid spermatids. In the third, spermiogenic, phase or spermiogenesis, spermatids metamorphose into spermatozoa. Before any round of spermatogenesis is completed, new spermatogonial divisions are initiated; thus these three phases of spermatogenesis occur simultaneously in the tubules, permitting the production of 100 to 200 million spermatozoa per day in men, and up to several billion according to the mammalian species considered. The overall duration of spermatogenesis is approximately 35 days in the mouse, 50 days in the rat, and 70 days in humans (Courot et al., 1970).

In any given segment of the tubule, several germ cell generations develop simultaneously between the base and the apex of the epithelium. These generations are in close contact with Sertoli cells. The evolution of each generation of germ cell is strictly synchronized. This leads to the formation of defined cell associations. Such associations are known as stages of the seminiferous cycle. The succession of a complete series of stages in a given area of the tubule constitutes the seminiferous epithelial cycle. The duration of the seminiferous epithelial cycle is approximately 9 days in the mouse, 13 days in the rat, and 16 days in humans (Courot et al., 1970). At least four consecutive cycles are required for the complete evolution of a spermatogenic series from the stem spermatogonium to the mature sperm. Fourteen stages have been characterized in the rat (I–XIV; Leblond and Clermont, 1952). Six stages have been identified in humans (I–VI; Clermont, 1963). Unlike most other mammals, including the rat, multiple stages of the cycle can be seen in a single tubular cross-section in humans and a few other primates (Clermont, 1963; Leidl, 1968; Chowdhury and Marshall, 1980). This may be because in most mammalian species the different stages of the seminiferous epithelium cycle follow one another linearly, whereas in a few primates, including humans, a helical pattern may exist (Schulze and Salzbrunn, 1992), thus explaining the mosaic pattern of distribution of the stages of the cycle on each tubular cross-section. However, Johnson (1994) has challenged the existence of complete helically organized spermatogenic waves in humans.

Sertoli cells and the spermatogenic process

Sertoli cells are large cells extending from the innermost layer of the basement membrane that lines the seminiferous tubules towards the lumen. Their cytoplasmic processes envelop the associated germ cells. Because of their position in the seminiferous epithelium, Sertoli cells have the unique ability to communicate with all germ cell generations and with the myoid cells. They can also communicate with the paracrine and endocrine signals originating from both the interstitium and the bloodstream via their bases. Androgen production and Sertoli cell function are controlled by the pituitary hormones luteinizing hormone (LH) and follicle-stimulating hormone (FSH), respectively. Testosterone produced by the action of LH or FSH on the Leydig cells is required for quantitatively and qualitatively normal spermatogenesis (Sharpe, 1994; Weinbauer et al., 2000). The action of these hormones on spermatogenesis is mediated by the Sertoli cells, which express testosterone and FSH receptors, whereas germ cells do not (Jégou, 1992; Weinbauer et al., 2000).

In addition to transducing the hormonal signals, the position of Sertoli cells within the seminiferous tubules allows them to play a key role in the paracrine control of spermatogenesis. Sertoli cells supply each individual germ cell generation, at each stage of testicular development, with the factors needed for their division, differentiation, and metabolism. It is believed that they also assist germ cells in synchronizing their development in the stages of the epithelium cycle, in the transversal axis of the tubule. Furthermore, Sertoli cells and the bridges that interconnect each germ cell generation are key features in the establishment of germ cell synchrony and probably contribute to the maintenance of the wave of spermatogenesis along the longitudinal axis.

On an anatomical basis, Sertoli cells and germ cells communicate via a unique set of structural devices (Russell, 1984; Jégou et al., 1992; Jégou, 1993). During the postnatal development of the testis, the establishment of inter-Sertoli cell tight junctions in the basolateral portion of the cell indicates that Sertoli cells have matured and, therefore, that the meiotic phase of spermatogenesis can proceed. These tight junctions are the major tubular constituent of the blood–testis barrier, which prevents a number of substances present in the testicular blood and lymph vessels from penetrating the seminiferous epithelium. The Sertoli cell barrier divides the seminiferous epithelium into a basal compartment, containing spermatogonia and early primary spermatocytes, and an adluminal compartment, which contains other differentiated primary spermatocytes, secondary spermatocytes, and the various stages of haploid spermatids. The Sertoli cell barrier creates a unique microenvironment that is essential for normal meiosis and spermiogenesis.

Most, if not all, Sertoli cell products assist germ cells through the three phases of spermatogenesis. The tubule fluid is essential for the nutrition of germ cells and for the transport of signals in the transversal axis of the seminiferous epithelium and along the tubule. It is also required for the transport of spermatozoa along the tubules, from the tubules to the rete testis and subsequently to the epididymis (Jégou, 1992).

Although germ cells are under the control of Sertoli cells, they can exert feedback actions on them (Jégou, 1993; Griswold, 1995; Gnessi et al., 1997; Jégou et al., 1999).

The requirement of in vitro spermatogenesis studies

The extremely complex in vivo structural organization of the mammalian testis creates particular difficulties for studying their organization, function, and regulation. This has provided the motivation for developing in vitro systems of spermatogenesis since testicular tissues were first cultured by Champy (1920). The following reasons justify the development of these systems: (i) the necessity to design experiments to determine the role of hormones in spermatogenesis; (ii) the need to study the role of Sertoli cells in the control of spermatogenesis and of putative local regulatory factors on germ cell division, differentiation, and metabolism; (iii) the necessity to study the molecular and cellular mechanisms characterizing and/or controlling each of the different phases of spermatogenesis in normal or pathophysiological contexts; (iv) the generation of germ cells that can repopulate the seminiferous tubules of recipient animals after microinjection; and (v) the production of germ cells and spermatozoa from testicular biopsies from men with spermatogenic arrest to be used for intracytoplasmic sperm injection (ICSI) or elongated spermatid injection (ELSI).

With one, or several, of these goals, the following activities have been developed in this domain: (i) the culture of whole testes, of testicular explants, or of segments of seminiferous tubules; (ii) the culture of mixtures of dissociated testicular cells either for direct use or for transplantation by microinjection into the aspermatogenic seminiferous tubules of recipient animals; (iii) the culture of isolated germ cells purified at particular phases of their development and of spermatogenesis; (iv) the co-culture of purified or unpurified Sertoli cells (primary cultures or cell lines) and germ cells; and (v) the design and culture of immortalized germ cell lines.

In the next section we shall endeavor to describe and to analyze critically the various in vitro systems of spermatogenesis that have been developed and the results generated by these systems.

The culture of testicular tissues

Fetal testis fragments

The differentiation of testes from undifferentiated mouse or rat primordia during in vitro culture has been reported since 1952 (Wolff, 1952; Asayama and Furusawa, 1960, 1961; Byskov and Saxen, 1976; Taketo and Koide, 1981; Agelopoulou et al., 1984; McGuinness and Orth, 1992; Buehr et al., 1993; Olaso et al., 1998). Several key observations have been made using these in vitro systems, particularly in the mouse and rat: (i) cellular mesonephric contribution is required for the establishment of seminiferous

cords (Taketo and Koide, 1981; Buehr et al., 1993); (ii) the proliferation and relocation of gonocytes both begin and continue in culture (McGuinness and Orth, 1992); (iii) Sertoli cells produce bioactive antimüllerian hormone, which induces regression of Müller's duct and is required for germ cell development in neonatal mouse testes (Zhou et al., 1993); (iv) gonocytes spontaneously reenter meiosis in cultured neonatal testes (McGuinness and Orth, 1992); (v) transforming growth factor (TGF) β_1 and β_2 directly increase apoptosis in gonocytes, without changing their mitotic activity during the developmental phases of proliferation (Olaso et al., 1998); and (vi) fetal testicular -β_1 is stimulated significantly by FSH and even more by a combination of LH and FSH (Gautier et al., 1997).

Cell reaggregation experiments in mice showed that the histogenic behavior of germ cells is markedly modified with age. In fact, most germ cells that had been dissociated from fetal testes at 12.5 dpc could be reincorporated into the seminiferous cords, although those dissociated at 14.5 dpc could not. This may be a consequence of changes in Sertoli cell surface properties, which are crucial for their binding to gonocytes when the gonocytes enter their mitotic resting stage (Escalante-Alcalde and Merchant-Larios, 1992).

Finally, only a few spermatocytes developed in vitro when newborn or rats aged one to three days postpartum (dpp) were used (Steinberger, 1967, 1975). This suggests that the differentiation of gonocytes to primitive type spermatogonia is sensitive to culture conditions. This was confirmed by Gelly et al. (1984), who found no differentiation of the germinal elements of the seminiferous tubules from 5 dpp rats after culture for 4 to 12 days.

Postnatal crude testis fragments

In early cultures of postnatal testes or testicular fragments (Champy, 1920; Martinovitch, 1937; Gaillard and Varossieau, 1938, 1940), a plasma clot was used to provide support and a source of nutrients. Therefore, it was not clear whether the spermatogenic cells had developed in vitro or whether they already existed at the onset of culture. Adult testes degenerated on the first day of culture, whereas prepubertal testes survived for eight to nine days (Gaillard and Varossieau, 1940). However, these early attempts were greatly hampered by the lack of objective methods for following cell differentiation.

Trowell (1959) introduced a method in which small tissue fragments were cultured in a chemically defined medium on stainless-steel grids covered with lens paper or with a thin sheet of agar at the liquid–gas interphase. This method was used for long-term cultures of testes from several mammalian species by Steinberger and Steinberger (Steinberger et al., 1964a,b, 1970; Steinberger and Steinberger, 1967; Steinberger, 1967). Tubular architecture, Sertoli cells, and primitive type A spermatogonia could be maintained for six to eight months. Rat spermatocytes survived for three to four weeks, but spermatids only survived for a few days. In an attempt to follow in vitro differentiation, rat preleptotene spermatocytes, which are the most advanced spermatogenic cells replicating DNA, were labeled with [^{3}H]-thymidine and their development was subsequently followed by autoradiography (Steinberger and Steinberger, 1965, 1967, 1970). These cells developed to a late prophase of meiosis, but meiotic divisions and spermiogenesis were never observed (Steinberger and Steinberger, 1970, 1971). Degenerative changes were more prominent in testes from adult animals than in those from prepubertal ones (Steinberger, 1967; Steinberger et al., 1970). This is obviously because of the rapid degeneration of postmeiotic cells in mature testes. Spermatogenic capacity was maintained in vitro for at least seven weeks, because spermatogenesis was completed within 8 to 10 weeks after the cultured fragments had been reimplanted into the testes of adult homologous hosts (Steinberger et al., 1970). Supplementation of the growth medium with vitamins A, C, and E, or glutamine enabled rat primitive type A spermatogonia from prepubertal testes to develop to the pachytene stage of meiosis, but new cell generations did not appear after the first cycle of development (Steinberger and Steinberger, 1966a). Gonadotropins and testosterone did not improve germ cell development (Steinberger et al., 1964c, 1970; Steinberger and Steinberger, 1967).

Spermatogonia from mouse cryptorchid testes could reinitiate meiosis in vitro (Aizawa and Nishimune, 1979). FSH in combination with insulin and transferrin may be able to promote the mitotic activity of type A spermatogonia, although insulin, transferrin, testosterone, dihydrotestosterone, triiodothyronine, dibutyryl 3',5'-cyclic adenosine monophosphate (cAMP), human chorionic gonadotropin, LH, and FSH alone showed no stimulatory effect (Haneji and Nishimune, 1982). Furthermore, retinoids activated cell division in type A spermatogonia and induced their differentiation in vitro (Haneji et al., 1982, 1983a, 1986) whereas FSH had synergistic effects on in vitro spermatogenic cell differentiation when cells were also treated with retinoids or Pedersen type III fetuin (Haneji et al., 1983b, 1984). However, spermatogenic cells that differentiated from cryptorchid adult testis died in the pachytene stage of meiosis (Haneji et al., 1984). On the basis of the numerous studies mentioned above, it has been generally believed that mammalian spermatogenesis cannot be maintained in organ culture beyond the prophase of meiosis (Steinberger, 1975; Setchell, 1978).

However, when rat seminiferous tubular segments from the stages immediately preceding the meiotic divisions were cultured, despite the rapid degeneration of a very large fraction of germ cells, completion of the divisions and early spermiogenesis could be shown (Parvinen et al., 1983). The extent of differentiation was the same with or without the addition of growth factors or hormones (testosterone, FSH). This led to a series of studies by Toppari and collaborators (Toppari et al., 1985, 1986a,b), in which segments of adult rat seminiferous tubules from defined stages of the epithelial cycle were cultured in an attempt to trace the differentiation of spermatogenic cells. The desired stages were isolated by transillumination-assisted microdissection combined with accurate identification of the stages by phase contrast microscopy. Cultures were started at stages II–III, VI, VIII, and XII–XIII of the epithelial cycle and continued for one to seven days in a chemically defined medium. It was found that premeiotic and meiotic phases of spermatogenesis, and the Golgi and cap phases of spermiogenesis, proceeded according to the same time schedule in vitro and in vivo, and the cells differentiated in vitro seemed to be morphologically and functionally normal. However, numerous spermatogenic cells degenerated in culture. The acrosome and maturation phases of spermiogenesis did not occur in vitro. Complete spermiogenesis and better survival of spermatogenic cells in vitro are the main challenges for the development of culture conditions in future.

Spermatogenic cells could be quantified by DNA flow cytometry (Toppari et al., 1985, 1986a). The number of cells obtained at defined stages was consistent with the results of previous morphometric assessments. Different stages had typical DNA histograms, characterized by the location of the hypo–haploid peak caused by the spermatid maturation phase, and by the relative proportions of cells in each DNA class. Secretion of plasminogen activator (PA) was used as a marker of cyclic Sertoli cell function and as an index of local hormone action in seminiferous tubules. The cyclic PA secretion was partially maintained in vitro. FSH was found to stimulate PA activity in stage VIII, but not in stage VI. A combination of FSH, insulin, testosterone, and retinoic acid stimulated both of these stages, whereas testosterone alone had no effect. The results indicated that the effect of FSH was highly stage specific. The seminiferous tubules mainly secreted urokinase-type PA, but tissue-type PA was occasionally found in the culture medium of stage VIII after stimulation by FSH or a combination of FSH, insulin, testosterone, and retinoic acid.

Use of this approach to culture seminiferous tubule fragments at defined stages of the cycle led to the development of a new method to test male germ cell mutagenicity, based on the induction of micronuclei during meiotic divisions in vitro. A model mutagen, adriamycin, caused a dose-dependent increase of micronucleus induction in vitro, at concentrations well below toxic levels (Toppari et al., 1986b). Mixed cultured segments of seminiferous tubules were used in toxicological studies (Allenby et al., 1991) collected at different stages of the cycle from rats that had been exposed to methylmethanesulfonate. Bentley and Working (1988) separated the tubule segments to show that this in vitro system increased the sensitivity of unscheduled DNA synthesis as a function of DNA damage in rat germ cells at different stages of maturity.

Recently, Durand and coworkers reinitiated the use of rat tubular segment cultures for studying spermatogenesis in vitro (Hue et al., 1998; Staub et al., 2000). They used unselected segments, premeiotic rat testes, and a bicameral culture system with a chemically defined medium supplemented with vitamins and hormones, including FSH and testosterone. Furthermore, an unprecedented number of criteria were used to monitor germ cell differentiation: (i) cytological light and electron microscopy immunocytochemical observations; (ii) measurement of genes specifically expressed in pachytene spermatocytes (phosphoprotein p19) and in early spermatids (transition proteins 1 and 2); (iii) ploidy analyses by image analysis; and (iv) the study of the fate of bromodeoxyuridine (BrdU)-labeled leptotene spermatocytes. It was found that, although massive germ cell death was encountered under the relatively long-term culture conditions used (up to three weeks for tubule fragments), a number of pachytene spermatocytes were unequivocally able to differentiate into secondary spermatocytes and then into early spermatids (Hue et al., 1998; Staub et al., 2000). The rate of differentiation of the germ cells observed in these in vitro studies was consistent with the in vivo situation as previously observed by Parvinen et al. (1983) and Toppari et al. (1985).

Most attempts to establish and to study spermatogenesis in vitro were carried out on animals, particularly on rats. As little fresh material is available, few contemporary studies have been carried out on human testes or human testicular fragments. Ghatnekar et al. (1974) used an autoradiographic approach to show that the first meiotic division was completed after 14 days in an organ culture of three human testes at 36°C in a medium supplemented with fetal calf serum (FCS), deproteinized coconut milk, and gonadotropic hormones. Curtis (1981) performed similar cultures without hormones and coconut milk and found labeled diakinetic figures after 10 to 14 days in culture, but did not observe labeled division figures. Heller and Clermont (1963) found that spermatogonia and preleptotene spermatocytes are the only cell types that incorporate [³H]-thymidine in adult human testis, and that preleptotene spermatocytes differentiate to early to mid pachytene spermatocytes after 14 days in vivo. Therefore, it is unlikely that these cells could have reached this stage in that time in vitro, particularly as the workers used an unphysiological temperature of 36 °C (VanDemark and Free, 1970). Seidl and Holstein (1990) cultured human seminiferous tubules that had been mechanically isolated and had the cut edges sealed, at the more favorable temperature of 34.5 °C. In this study, the beneficial influences of FCS, of nerve growth factor (NGF), and of various additional supplements were assessed. The evaluation of the germ cell populations was monitored by [³H]-thymidine labeling combined with light and electron microscopy. It was shown that, in absence of medium supplements, but in presence of 20% FCS, all germ cell types degenerated within three weeks, except dark and pale type A spermatogonia. In the chemically defined medium, only 33.3% of the cross-sections of the tubules cultured for five days without FSH contained labeled germ cells, whereas 83.3% of those from tubules exposed to FCS showed mitotic activity. In these tubules, FCS doubled the number of [³H]-thymidine-labeled germ cells per cross-section. Furthermore, NGF together with FCS had the most beneficial effect on the maintenance of the seminiferous epithelium. NGF action directly maintained a better basal lamina and Sertoli cells integrity.

However, the most spectacular results of human in vitro spermatogenesis were published by Tesarik and coworkers, who used human testicular fragments (Tesarik et al., 1998a,b, 1999, 2000a–c). They reported that in high concentrations of FSH both meiotic and postmeiotic maturation can occur in germ cells collected from testicular biopsies from men with normal spermatogenesis or with maturation arrest after only 24 to 48 hours of culture (it is known that the normal duration of spermatogenesis in humans is approximately 70 days, and that the meiotic prophase and spermiogenesis each last more than three weeks). They also reported that babies have been born following the microinjection of spermatids obtained by in vitro maturation of germ cells from azoospermic patients affected by a spermatogenic maturation arrest (Tesarik et al., 1999). However, the protocols used by this group lacked the prerequisites for an unequivocal demonstration of spermatogenesis in vitro. These studies used insensitive or inappropriate techniques to assess cell viability, to count cells, and to monitor cell differentiation. In the absence of appropriate techniques, we cannot determine whether germ cells really can mature at such an extraordinary velocity (Tesarik et al., 1998a,b). Furthermore, Tesarik et al. (2000b) claimed that other studies on the rat (Parvinen et al., 1983; Le Magueresse-Battistoni et al., 1991; Weiss et al., 1997; Hue et al., 1998) and on humans (Tres et al., 1989) have also shown that meiotic and postmeiotic differentiation events occur more rapidly in vitro than in vivo, although this is not the case (Durand et al., 2001; Jégou et al., 2001). This does not clarify the actual contribution of this group to the development of a culture system to perform human spermatogenesis in vitro.

The culture of testicular cells

Until the recent advances in tissue culture, studies on testicular function had progressively stopped using cultures of testicular fragments and dissected segments of seminiferous tubules, and had concentrated on the development of more sophisticated culture systems, in which Sertoli cells and germ cells were either carefully dispersed in more or less small aggregates or were isolated and purified before being cultured or co-cultured. An attempt was made to develop the tools required to enable better monitoring of the maturation of germ cells and for an analytical study of the interactions between Sertoli cells and germ cells.

Culture of Sertoli cells and of small aggregates of germ cells

Several studies aimed to enrich cell preparations of Sertoli cells and small aggregates of germ cells without breaking their interconnecting junctions and intercellular bridges. Kierszenbaum (1994) reported that the different factors required for successful preparation of Sertoli cell–germ cell co-cultures are: (i) careful enzymatic dissociation to alter the structural interactions between Sertoli cells and germ cells as little as possible; (ii) plating of the aggregates at maximal cell density to keep Sertoli cells in a contact-inhibited state; (iii) the use of a chemically defined medium (serum-free) supplemented with hormones, such as testosterone, dihydrotestosterone, growth hormone, FSH, and growth factors; and (iv) frequent changes of culture medium. Tres and Kierszenbaum (1983) used such a system on prepubertal and pubertal rat testes and showed that in cell reaggregation experiments: (i) germ cells reassociate preferentially with Sertoli cells; (ii) polygonal spermatogonia form long, branched chains of interconnected cells; (iii) that [^{3}H]-thymidine-labeled spermatogonia and preleptotene spermatocytes connected by cytoplasmic bridges have a synchronous S phase; and (iv) labeled preleptotene spermatocytes can progress throughout meiotic prophase stages. They also showed that round spermatids can grow flagella in vitro, but that, although the axoneme of these cells display a typical wave-like motion, the flagella lack outer dense fibers (Tres et al., 1991). The time course of the replacement of the testis-specific histone variants TH2B and H1t in primary spermatocytes in vitro is consistent with that observed in vivo (Smith et al., 1992).

In 1985, Hadley et al. used a reconstituted basement membrane gel to show that some spermatogonia can differentiate to pachytene spermatocytes in a Sertoli cell culture.

Culture of dispersed testicular cells

Primordial germ cells PGC and gonocytes

A few methods have recently been developed that allow the isolation and purification of migratory and postmigratory mouse and rat PGC. Van Dissel-Emiliani et al. (1989) used velocity sedimentation at unit gravity to isolate embryonic gonocytes (70–75% enrichment) from 18 dpc rats. A few years later, De Felici and Pesce (1995a) proposed the use of a PGC-specific TG-1 antibody in combination with immunoaffinity adhesion to plastic plates coated with an anti-mouse IgM secondary antibody for the isolation of migratory PGC from 9.5 to 11.5 dpc mouse embryos and achieved reasonably pure yields. De Felici and Pesce further refined this technique so that the cell sorter MiniMACS magnetic separation system could purify PGC from 10.5 to 13.5 dpc mouse embryos (De Felici and Pesce, 1995b). More recently, van den Ham et al. (1997) adapted a direct immunoseparation technique for the isolation of gonocytes from 18 and 20 dpc rat embryos. This technique used magnetic beads coated with a rat anti-mouse IgM and a monoclonal antibody 4B6.3E10, which specifically reacted with a differentiation antigen on the fetal germ cells.

In a pioneer study, De Felici and McLaren (1983) followed the survival of PGC isolated from 11.5 to 16.5 dpc mouse embryos in single culture using Petri dishes, microtiter plates, or drops under oil. They showed that PGC from embryos at 11.5 and 12.5 dpc could not survive at 37 °C in any of the culture systems used, but that they could survive at 30 °C for at least a week. Interestingly, PGC from 13.5 dpc embryos onwards survived at 37 °C for several days. PGC did not enter meiosis in any culture conditions, but they continued to undergo mitotic proliferation. Several attempts were also made to study the survival and proliferation of freshly isolated PGC/gonocytes in vitro (mouse: De Felici and Dolci, 1989, 1991; Matsui et al., 1991; rat: Li et al., 1997; van Dissel-Emiliani et al., 1993). These attempts yielded a couple of significant observations. The addition of extracellular matrix components (laminin, fibronectin, type I collagen) scarcely improves PGC survival (De Felici and Dolci, 1989), and PGC and gonocytes cannot survive for more than 2 days in vitro (De Felici and Dolci, 1991; Matsui et al., 1991; van Dissel-Emiliani et al., 1993; Li et al., 1997). Mitosis did not resume when gonocytes are cultivated alone (Li et al., 1997). Interestingly, the effects of various compounds on the survival and proliferation of PGC/gonocytes in single culture have been studied (for reviews, see De Felici, 2000; Olaso and Habert, 2000). For example, it has been proposed that stem cell factor and leukemia inhibitory factor (LIF) are survival anti-apoptotic factors for PGC (De Felici and Dolci, 1991; Dolci et al., 1993; De Felici, 2000), whereas TGF-β_1 is required for PGC survival (De Felici and Pesce, 1994a), and that platelet-derived growth factor and estradiol activate gonocyte proliferation (Li et al., 1997). Furthermore, cAMP, pituitary adenylyl cyclase activating polypeptides (PACAPs), and retinoic acid appear to be positive regulators of PGC proliferation (De Felici, 2000). Finally, Di Carlo and De Felici (2000) demonstrated that the formation of germ cell aggregates, which occurs rapidly in culture when dispersed germ cell populations are released from embryonic gonads, and their development are mediated by E-cadherin, depending on the sex of the germ cells.

These studies clearly show that PGC or gonocytes require the environment provided by somatic cells to survive and to differentiate correctly. This highlights the in vivo finding that PGC which do not enter the cords during early development degenerate (Byskov, 1986).

Pubertal and postpubertal germ cells

Morphological analyses showed that primary spermatocytes and round spermatids survived for several days in culture of testicular cell suspensions (Steinberger and Steinberger, 1966b). However, no evidence of cell differentiation was obtained (Steinberger and Steinberger, 1970). Since the mid 1970s, it has been possible to prepare highly purified populations of mammalian germ cells at different stages of development (Grabske et al., 1975; Romrell et al., 1976; Bellvé et al., 1977a,b; Meistrich et al., 1981; Loir and Lanneau, 1982). However, the removal of cells from their normal physiological environment is intrinsically deleterious to all cell types, especially germ cells, which appear to be the least autonomous of all testicular cells in mammals. First, after birth, intact isolates of some germ cells

classes cannot be obtained because of the structural intricacy of Sertoli cells. Second, in isolated culture, germ cell metabolism is greatly altered and the cells cannot survive for more than a few hours or days (Grootegoed et al., 1977, 1989; Jutte et al., 1981, 1982; Le Magueresse and Jégou, 1988; Matsui et al., 1991; Risley and Morse-Gaudio, 1992).

Despite their extreme fragility when isolated from culture, interesting information has been obtained on the behavior of isolated meiotic and postmeiotic germ cells. [^{3}H]-Leucine can be incorporated into isolated germ cells in vitro (Millette and Moulding, 1981), and isolated spermatocytes and early spermatids can synthesize various proteins during short culture periods (Gerton and Millette, 1986). However, it is not known whether these are "physiological" events or whether they reflect a stress response to culture conditions because the cells are known to die massively in these experimental conditions. Early mouse spermatids were able to generate flagella during a 24 hour culture period, but the individual germ cell differentiation was not carefully assessed in this study (Gerton and Millette, 1984). The optimum temperature for germ cell activity (particularly for spermatids) is 34 °C rather than 37 °C (Nakamura et al., 1978, 1984). Lactate and pyruvate are better substrates for spermatocytes and early spermatids in vitro than glucose, which cannot be metabolized (Nakamura et al., 1984). The presence of these two energy-providing substrates in Sertoli cell-conditioned media (Robinson and Fritz, 1981; Jutte et al., 1982; Le Gac et al., 1982, 1983; Mita et al., 1982) may explain the beneficial effect of these media, compared with the nonconditioned media, on pachytene spermatocytes and early spermatids in vitro (Grootegoed et al., 1982).

Recently, 50% of spermatogonia from an 80 dpp piglet were shown to be viable after 30 days when cultured in a potassium-rich medium (Dirami et al., 1999).

However, it is generally accepted that there is no primary culture system available that allows the long-term culture of purified spermatogonia (de Rooij and Russell, 2000) or of other categories of germ cell. Moreover, the annexin V technique showed that a high percentage of rat spermatogonia or pachytene spermatocytes and early spermatids are already apoptotic upon isolation by gradient sedimentation at unit gravity or centrifugal elutriation (these procedures take 4 and 5 hours, respectively) (E. Guillaume, B. Jégou and C. Pineau, unpublished data).

Interestingly, it was recently shown that isolated pachytene spermatocytes from prepubertal rats that had been treated in culture with okadaic acid, a potent phosphatase inhibitor, reach metaphase I arrest within a few hours, unlike the similar process in vivo, which require several days (Handel et al., 1995; Tarsounas et al., 1999). Leptotene/zygotene spermatocytes cannot be activated in this way; therefore, okadaic acid may enable cells to bypass a sensor of meiotic progression that is specific to the pachytene stage, resulting in the rapid degradation of two meiotic-specific proteins SYN1/SCP1 and COR1/SCP3, subsequent desynapsis, and progression to metaphase I. If this system allows the rapid cytological and biochemical analyses of the meiotic events in a "fast forward" mode, as stated by Tarsounas et al. (1999), then it is noteworthy that the spermatocytes were mostly arrested at early metaphase I because of a lack of meiotic spindles. This demonstrates that the germ cells generated after "accelerated" spermatogenesis are very seriously degraded.

Human germ cells also die very quickly in vitro (within 24 to 72 hours) (Aslam and Fishel, 1998). However, flagellar growth occurs in approximately one fifth of human spermatids within 8 hours of culture. It is noteworthy that this growth was essentially unphysiological because it was not coupled to any of the other morphological changes that are normally seen during spermiogenesis in situ. Therefore, instead of being "an excellent way of identifying" viable spermatids, as stated by Aslam and Fishel (1998), this growth should probably be interpreted as an abnormal event connected to spermatid degeneration induced by cell isolation and culture. Consequently, the use of these cells for in vitro fertilization appears to be most risky.

Another group has claimed that extended maturation of human round spermatids in vitro can occur when these cells are co-cultured with Vero cells (Cremades et al., 1999). However, extremely low numbers of germ cells were cultured (2 to 37 depending on the experiment), and an objective method was not used (e.g., [3H]-thymidine or BrdU labeling) to monitor individual cell differentiation. Furthermore, some of the changes occurring during cell degeneration (e.g., changes in the cell shape, flagellar extrusion, or growth) may have been confused with morphological aspects related to spermatid differentiation.

Johnson et al. (1999) performed a very complete comparative morphological study of human germ cells in vitro and in situ within tubules. This allowed the germ cells originating from human isolated seminiferous tubules in vitro to be objectively identified for the first time. The list of distinguishing characteristics of live human germ cells provided by these authors is a very precious tool, both for biologists who will plan future experiments on in vitro spermatogenesis and for technical staff in clinics for the selection of germ cells for in vitro fertilization.

All the in vitro experiments carried out with isolated purified mammalian germ cells in animals and men indicate that their differentiation is particularly dependent on the support of Sertoli cells; this is consistent with the findings of Wolff and Haffen in 1965 (initially quoted by Kierszenbaum, 1994).

The culture of spermatogonia represents a particularly important goal as, if it proves successful, it would allow the study of each step of spermatogenesis in vitro. Furthermore, it has been shown that a heterogeneous mouse testis cell suspension containing stem germ cells could be transplanted, by microinjection into the seminiferous tubules of sterile recipients and totally restore spermatogenesis, even after cryopreservation (Brinster and Avarbock, 1994; Brinster and Zimmermann, 1994). This technique opens up enormous possibilities for the treatment of male sterility, for the protection of endangered species, for engineering genetically manipulated animals, and for determining the origin of arrested spermatogenesis in mutant or mutated experimental animals (for reviews, see Brinster and Nagano, 1998; Johnston et al., 2000; Schlatt et al., 2000).

Following the introduction of this technology, Brinster and coworkers have achieved a number of experimental developments. Crude mouse testicular cells, containing germ stem cells, could be cultured on a feeder layer of STO cells and in a medium containing 10% for four months. When transplanted to busulfan-treated recipient testes, these cells were able to regenerate full spermatogenesis. In contrast, no colonization occurred in absence of the feeder cells, clearly indicating that stem spermatogonia cannot survive or remain functional without somatic assistance (Shinohara et al., 2000). This group also have developed techniques that use a number of cell surface molecules to enrich fractions of mouse spermatogonial stem cells from cryptorchid testes (66-fold). These cells were fractionated by fluorescence-activating cell sorting analysis, based on their light scattering properties (Shinohara et al., 2000).

Several other techniques, which use either sedimentation velocity at unit gravity (Dym et al., 1995) or differential adhesion on plastic dishes coated with lectin (*Datura stramonium*) agglutinin and fractionation on discontinuous Percoll gradient (Morena et al., 1996,) have also been developed to isolate highly purified type A spermatogonia from prepubertal rat testis. Both techniques apparently allow a cell fraction containing up to 85% type A spermatogonia to be recovered. Van Pelt et al. (1996) also proposed a method to isolate synchronized type A spermatogonia from adult vitamin A-deficient rat testes, with a purity of 70–90%. More recently, von Schonfeldt et al. (1999) developed a magnetic cell sorting technique, based on an anti-c-Kit IgG, to enrich highly viable spermatogonia from testes of Djungarian hamster, mouse, and marmoset monkey.

As stated above, the poor viability of mammalian germ cells in culture does not allow their in vitro differentiation to be studied when they are isolated. Consequently, the establishment of immortalized mammalian germ cell lines, capable of in vitro differentiation, would be a major breakthrough. Hofmann and collaborators (1992, 1994, 1995) established an immortalized cell line (GC-1spg) by using the immortalizing properties of the simian virus 40 large tumor antigen (Hofmann et al., 1992). GC-1spg, characterized as a cell line at a stage between type B spermatogonia and primary spermatocyte, were unfortunately unable to differentiate further in vitro, even when co-cultured with immortalized Sertoli cells (Hofmann et al., 1992). More recently, Hofmann et al. (1994) cotransfected primary mouse testicular germ cells with the same simian virus 40 large T antigen gene and the gene coding for a temperature-sensitive (ts) mutant of p53 and established two new germ cell lines (GC-2spd(ts) and GC-3spc(ts)). They then used the property of p53 to abolish the proliferative function of the large T antigen when both molecules are expressed (Fukasawa et al., 1991) and to induce growth arrest at permissive temperatures in the studied cell lines. Both cell lines express the lactate dehydrogenase C_4 and cytochrome c_t isoforms, which are specific for meiotic and postmeiotic germ cells in vivo (Goldberg et al., 1977; Wheat et al., 1977). Moreover, proliferation rates for both cell lines were high at 39 °C, decreased at 37 °C, and were inhibited at 32 °C. Hofmann and coworkers (1994) claimed that at the permissive temperatures of 37 °C and 32 °C only the GC-2spd(ts) line could undergo meiosis and generate haploid cells with an acrosome granule and a flagellar axoneme. This confirms that these cells are early spermatids. However, it was recently reported that GC-2spd(ts) may have become less differentiated and may have lost their postmeiotic potentiality over time (Wolkowicz et al., 1996). Use of DNA flow cytometry to analyze GC-2spd(ts) during 10 days of culture did not detect a peak indicative of the presence of haploid chromosomes. The expression of mRNAs encoding stage-specific proteins (lactate dehydrogenase C4, acrosin, protamine-2, and SP-10) in GC-2spd(ts) was studied by Northern blotting and reverse transcriptase polymerase chain reaction (RT-PCR). These techniques did not reveal the presence of any of these transcripts (Wolkowicz et al., 1996). It is noteworthy that cell lines must be established without the irreversible loss of differentiated properties that is often associated with immortalization. Immortalization generally coincides with an extensive destabilization of the genome (Cerni et al.,

1987; Vogt et al., 1987). Therefore, the immortalization of germinal cells may be incompatible with their entrance into meiosis, for which genomic integrity appears to be essential.

Co-cultures of Sertoli cells and germ cells

Sertoli cells are the physiological nurse cells for germ cells; therefore, much effort has been devoted to the setting-up and development of Sertoli cell cultures. These efforts aimed to characterize Sertoli cells, with particular emphasis on the regulation of spermatogenesis and of the Sertoli cell endocrine function during both fetal (antimüllerian hormone) and postnatal stages (e.g., inhibin production).

A major methodological breakthrough occurred in 1975 when several laboratories developed reproducible protocols for the isolation and culture of Sertoli cells from immature and adult rat testes (Dorrington et al., 1975; Steinberger et al., 1975; Welsh and Wiebe, 1975). Improved protocols now make this possible on a routine basis. The key factors of these protocols are sequential enzymatic digestions and gravity sedimentation of Sertoli cell clusters, plus extensive washes (Skinner and Fritz, 1985; Toebosch et al., 1989). It is important to note that prepubertal animals are generally used as a source of cultured cells and allowed the development of culture systems for the study of spermatogenesis (for reviews, see Russell and Steinberger, 1989; Jégou, 1993).

Because Sertoli cells dedifferentiate when they are cultured and their preparation is tedious, several groups have attempted to establish immortalized Sertoli cell lines. A number of these cell lines are available and are listed in Table 1.1.

The concept of immortalizing Sertoli cells is obviously most interesting, but the cell lines generated only partially conserved the structural and molecular characteristics of the "real" Sertoli cells in situ, and only two cell lines, those used by Hofmann et al. (1992) and 15P-1 used by Rassoulzadegan et al. (1993), have been used to study in vitro spermatogenesis.

De Felici and Siracusa (1985) initially showed that PGC from 12.5 to 15.5 dpc mouse embryos adhere to Sertoli and follicular cells obtained from adult gonads. Since this time, much effort has been made to study PGC/gonocytes survival and proliferation in in vitro systems in which these germ cells are co-cultured on feeder cells. Maekawa and Nishimune (1991) developed a system based on the enzyme-dispersed mouse neonatal testes and demonstrated that germ cells, as well as supporting cells, incorporate [3H]-thymidine and progress through the cell cycle in vitro with no apparent loss of viability after three days of culture. De Felici and Pesce (1994b) subsequently demonstrated that mouse PGC adhere to different cell monolayers, such as STO, TM4, COS, and F9 cells. They suggested that cell–cell interactions are mediated by multiple mechanisms involving Steel factor, c-Kit, carbohydrates, and possibly other unknown factors. The same study showed that (i) Steel factor and LIF prevent PGC death by suppressing apoptosis and are, therefore, survival factors; (ii) dibutyryl cAMP and forskolin, which are known to enhance intracellular levels of cAMP, stimulate PGC proliferation; and (iii) PACAP-27 and PACAP–28 may be physiological activators of adenylyl cyclase in PGC. Co-culture systems have shown that some factors are able, directly or via the co-cultured feeder cells, to modulate the number, proliferation, and/or survival of PGC and/or gonocytes. Such factors can increase (Steel factor: Godin et al., 1991; LIF: Resnick et al., 1992; fibroblast growth factor 2: Resnick et al., 1992, 1998; van Dissel-Emiliani et al., 1996) or decrease (TGF-β_1: Godin and Wylie, 1991) the number of germ cells.

Interestingly, primary cultures of PGC/gonocytes on suitable cell feeder layers, in particular adult or neonatal Sertoli cells, have permitted the survival of germ cells to be studied. They have also allowed cellular processes and structural features that resemble those observed in *vivo* to be established. Gonocytes from 4 to 6 dpc adhere to an underlying neonatal Sertoli cell monolayer and survive for over seven days (Orth and Boehm, 1990). McGuinness and Orth (1992) demonstrated that gonocytes cultured with Sertoli cells can reinitiate mitosis, without added factors. Similarly, Resnick et al. (1992) showed that PGC can proliferate for up to seven days in a feeder-

Table 1.1. Characteristics of established Sertoli cell lines

Name	Permissive temperature	Species	Major Sertoli cell features	Origin	References
TM4[a]	No	Mouse	Transferrin, RBP, PA	Primary testis at 13 days postpartum	Mather, 1980
MSC-1	Yes	Mouse	Transferrin, SGP-2, β-inhibin, β-SGP-1, ABP	Transgenic	Peschon et al., 1992; McGuinness et al., 1994
S14-1	Yes	Mouse	Transferrin, SGP-2	Primary testicular cells	Boekelheide et al., 1993
15P-1 (unpure)	No	Mouse	Steel factor, WT1	Transgenic	Rassoulzadegan et al., 1993
ASC-17D	Yes	Rat	Transferrin, SGP-2	Sexually mature testis	Roberts et al., 1995
SK11 and SK49	No	Mouse	Steel factor, transferrin, SGP-2, α-inhibin, SF-1, GATA-1, RFSH	Transgenic	Walther et al., 1996
SMAT1	No	Mouse	AMH, SF-1	Transgenic	Dutertre et al., 1997
93RS2	Yes	Rat	Transferrin, SGP-2	Prepubertal testis	Jiang et al., 1997
SerW3	No	Rat	Transferrin	Primary testis at 17 days postpartum	Pognan et al., 1997
42 GPA9	No	Mouse	RFSH	Transgenic	Bourdon et al., 1998
MSC-1/RFSH	No	Mouse	RFSH	Transgenic	Eskola et al., 1998
TM4/ABP	No	Mouse	ABP	Original TM4 line	Ducray et al., 1998
45T-1	No	Mouse	Laminin	Transgenic	Szalay et al., 1999

Notes:

RBP, retinol-binding protein; PA, plasminogen activator; SGP, sulfated glycoprotein; WT1, Wilm's tumor 1; AMH, antimüllerian hormone; RFSH, follicle-stimulating hormone receptor; SF-1, steroidogenic factor 1; ABP, androgen-binding protein.

[a] This line is available through the American Type Culture Collection (ATCC; Rockville, MD, USA) and the European Collection of Animal Cell Cultures (ECACC; Valbonne, France).

dependent culture. Interestingly, the presence of an underlying laminin-containing matrix (matrigel) seems to be a prerequisite for the development of cellular extensions by the gonocytes (Orth and McGuinness, 1991). Desmosome-like attachments and gap junctions have also been observed in co-culture. The presence of gap junctions suggests that gonocytes become metabolically coupled to Sertoli cells (Orth and Boehm, 1990) and that diffusible factors can pass between gonocytes and Sertoli cells (Orth and McGuinness, 1991; van Dissel-Emiliani et al., 1993; Orth and Jester, 1995). Furthermore, electron microscopy has shown that quiescent gonocytes isolated from 18 dpc rats, co-cultured with 21–23 dpc Sertoli cells, establish numerous adhesion plaques between the two types of cell (van Dissel-Emiliani et al., 1993). Finally, PGC express several surface molecules that mediate adhesive interactions of PGC with the extracellular matrix, somatic cells and neighboring PGC; these include integrins, E-cadherin, tyrosine kinase receptor c-Kit, and specific types of oligosaccharide (De Felici, 2000; Di Carlo and De Felici, 2000).

Galdieri et al. (1984), Le Gac et al. (1984) and Le Magueresse et al. (1986) developed the first Sertoli–germ cell co-culture systems that used meiotic and postmeiotic germ cells. These authors used "pure" Sertoli cell preparations from prepubertal rat testes (20 dpp) and highly enriched populations of pachytene spermatocytes, early spermatids, and cytoplasts from late spermatids to study the influence of germ cells on the morphology and secretory functions of Sertoli cells (Jégou, 1993; Jégou and Sharpe, 1993). However, this co-culture system was first used to demonstrate that rat pachytene spermatocytes can achieve the meiotic process in vitro in 1991 (Le Magueresse-Battistoni et al., 1991). In this study, germ cell maturation was monitored objectively by use of a purified population of pachytene spermatocytes. Flow cytometry was used to assess the appearance of a haploid peak and to analyze the spermatid-specific protamine-1 mRNA in co-culture extracts. It was demonstrated that under such experimental conditions a low proportion of spermatocytes (10%, mostly advanced in meiosis prophase) could enter meiosis and that, within the seven days the co-culture lasted, differentiation of spermatids could progress to step VII, which is consistent with the corresponding situation in vivo.

A different co-culture system was developed by the Rassoulzadegan and Cuzin group, who established testicular cell lines from transgenic mice expressing the polyoma virus (PyLT) protein in the testis (Paquis-Flucklinger et al., 1993). The 15P-1 cell line, which exhibits several features characteristic of Sertoli cells, was selected because it was claimed that this cell line supported meiotic and postmeiotic differentiation of germ cells collected from four-month-old mice transgenic for bacterial LacZ under the control of the haploid-specific protamine-1 promotor (Rassoulzadegan et al., 1993). This was one of the most astonishing studies ever published on in vitro spermatogenesis from a technical standpoint (the use of different transgenic mice, Sertoli cell lines, flow and image cytometry, light microscropy, thymidine labeling, and PCR) and in terms of the extraordinary results obtained. The 15P-1 cell line was claimed to support meiosis and full spermiogenesis up to the formation of a large number of spermatozoa (43-fold increase) in five days instead of the 35 days required in vivo. The 15P-1 line is not a pure Sertoli cell line as stated in Grandjean et al. (1997) and Rassoulzadegan et al. (1993), as it contains a significant germ cell component (Paquis-Flucklinger et al., 1993). However, our main criticism

of this study is that a very crude mixture of germ cells was added to the 15P-1 cell line; this mixture contained various somatic elements and a large proportion of haploid cells, including spermatozoa. This created a "messy" background in which the appearance of newly generated haploid cells was largely blunted. This problem was not necessarily solved by the use of germ cells expressing the LacZ reporter gene, as non-specific staining can be observed in germ cells from normal mice when exposed to the substrate 5-bromo-4-chloro-3-indolyl-β-D-galactoside (X-Gal) (M. O. Lienard, C. Pineau and B. Jégou, unpublished observations). This is most probably because of the high endogenous β-galactosidase activity in normal mouse testes (Cleutjens et al., 1997). The fact that Rassoulzadegan et al. (1993) observed β-galactosidase accumulation in the testes of 18-day-old mice, although it is generally observed that no or a very low number of spermatids normally exist at this age, and that no sperm cells appeared in the culture when no sperm cells were added (addition of a testicular cell suspension from immature mice), reinforce our conviction that the incredible germ cell proliferation seen in this study is probably largely artefactual. Finally, it is noteworthy that, to the best of our knowledge, seven years after this publication no other laboratory has published similar data using this cell line (or other cell lines), despite the extraordinary interest this new model generated. Despite intensive efforts (some of them in close collaboration with the authors), we were unable to reproduce the data published or to observe any germ cell differentiation when purified mice pachytene spermatocytes were used in the co-culture instead of the crude testicular mixture of cells. It is notable that purified mice pachytene spermatocytes and early spermatids did not adhere well to the 15P-1 cell line, in contrast they adhered well to primary mice Sertoli cells (M. O. Lienard, C. Pineau and B. Jégou, unpublished observations).

Interestingly, when fresh pachytene spermatocytes were co-cultured with the immortalized somatic cells, including Sertoli cells, they were integrated tubule-like structures and some of them could survive for at least seven days (Hofmann et al., 1992).

In a more recent study, rat germ cell differentiation was carefully monitored. Purified germ cells, germ cell-specific complementary DNA probes, and 5-BrdU were co-cultured for 2 weeks with primary Sertoli cells from pubertal rat donors (20 dpp) in a bicameral chamber system (Weiss et al., 1997). These authors demonstrated that, despite massive germ cell death, a proportion of pachytene spermatocytes passed through the meiotic process and developed into early spermatids.

Conclusions

After 80 years of research on in vitro spermatogenesis, which has mobilized the most traditional and modern in vitro technologies (e.g., traditional culture of testicular explants; modern genetically modified testicular cells), and despite the crucial importance of the goals, little progress has been made in this domain. A general rule has arisen: the less the seminiferous tubule architecture is perturbed during tissue/cell preparation(s), the higher the chances are that a modest proportion of germ cells will pass through the different steps of in vitro spermatogenesis. This emphasizes the narrow limits of the technology available in this domain.

Nature resists the in vitro investigation of spermatogenesis because evolution has established an extraordinary interdependency of the cellular constituents of the testis. This interdependency is centered around a highly sophisticated network of anatomical and functional relationships between testicular cells, including the clonal arrangement of the different germ cell generations, the diverse structural and biochemical interconnections between the Sertoli cells themselves, and the connections between Sertoli cells and germ cells. This network is the evolutionary prerequisite for the production of an enormous and continous quantity of spermatozoa by the testes throughout the postpubertal life of mammals. It is estimated that an average human male produces 1500 to 2000 billion spermatozoa in his lifetime.

The most significant results of eight decades of research on in vitro spermatogenesis is the involvement of aspects of the endocrine system in the regulation of spermatogenesis and the determination of the nature of germ cell–Sertoli cell interactions.

There is undoubtedly still a margin for future improvement in this domain that can be used to improve the survival and maturation of germ cells. For example, the recent discovery that germ stem cells can survive for weeks in culture on a feeder layer opens major prospects (Shinohara et al., 2000). The development of this new technique will be invaluable to the scientists working on the germ cell molecular machinery and its control mechanisms. The most crucial objective is to develop further techniques for culturing or immortalizing germ stem cells. These in vitro systems would be useful for heuristic studies and would also allow stem cell multiplication for subsequent transplantation into sterile recipients. This technique would also be an advantage in zootechnology, in particular for the reproduction of high-value domestic animals and endangered mammalian species.

In humans this creates prospects for the treatment of male sterility. The gametes matured in vitro can be injected by germ cell repopulation of empty seminiferous tubules or used for ICSI. However, undertaking such microinjections at the current time would be irresponsible, as the risk of genetic abnormalities occurring in these cells is extremely high because they are immediately oxidized upon removal from their natural cryptic environment in situ, and because of the serious additional degenerative processes they are exposed to during isolation (necrosis and/or apoptosis). Consequently, there is presently no technique that can guarantee that the injected human cells are free from these problems.

Finally, the possibility of culturing spermatogonia automatically opens the way for their genetic manipulation and, therefore, for the generation of transgenic animals, which would be a major breakthrough. In humans, the possibility of genetically modifying germ cells could only be envisaged for the development of gene therapy if the present international ban on germ cell genetic manipulation was lifted. It must still be open to question whether such a move would be desirable.

REFERENCES

Agelopoulou, R., Magre, S., Patsavoudi, E., and Jost, A. (1984). Initial phases of the rat testis differentiation in vitro. *Journal of Embryology and Experimental Morphology*, **83**, 15–31.

Allenby, G., Foster, P.M., and Sharpe, R.M. (1991). Evaluation of changes in the secretion of immunoactive inhibin by adult rat seminiferous tubules in vitro as an indicator of early toxicant action on spermatogenesis. *Fundamentals of Applied Toxicology*, **16**, 710–24.

Asayama, S. and Furusawa, M. (1960). Culture in vitro of prospective gonads and gonad primordia of mouse embryos. *Zoology Magazine*, **69**, 283.

Asayama, S. and Furusawa, M. (1961). Sex differentiation of primordial gonads of the mouse embryo after cultivation in vitro. *Japanese Journal of Experimental Morphology*, **15**, 34–47.

Aslam, I. and Fishel, S. (1998). Short-term in-vitro culture and cryopreservation of spermatogenic cells used for human in-vitro conception. *Human Reproduction*, **13**, 634–8.

Aizawa, S. and Nishimune, Y. (1979). In vitro differentiation of type A spermatogonia in mouse cryptorchid testis. *Journal of Reproduction and Fertility*, **56**, 99–104.

Bellvé, A.R., Cavicchia, J.C., Millette, C.F., O'Brien, D.A., Bhatnagar, Y.M., and Dym, M. (1977a). Spermatogenic cells of the prepubertal mouse: isolation and morphological characterization. *Journal of Cell Biology*, **74**, 68–85.

Bellvé, A.R., Millette, C.F., Bhatnagar, Y.M., and O'Brien, D.A. (1977b). Dissociation of the mouse testis and characterization of isolated spermatogenic cells. *Journal of Histochemistry and Cytochemistry*, **25**, 480–94.

Bentley, K.S. and Working, P.K. (1988). Use of seminiferous tubule segments to study stage specificity of unscheduled DNA synthesis in rat spermatogenic cells. *Environmental Molecular Mutagen*, **12**, 285–97.

Boekelheide, K., Lee, J.W., Hall, S.J., Rhind, N.R., and Zaret, K.S. (1993). A tumorigenic murine Sertoli cell line that is temperature-sensitive for differentiation. *American Journal of Pathology*, **143**, 1159–68.

Bourdon, V., Lablack, A., Abbe, P., Segretain, D., and Pointis, G. (1998). Characterization of a clonal Sertoli cell line using adult PyLT transgenic mice. *Biology of Reproduction*, **58**, 591–9.

Brinster, R.L. and Avarbock, M.R. (1994). Germline transmission of donor haplotype following spermatogonial transplanta-tion. *Proceedings of the National Academy of Sciences USA*, **91**, 11303–7.

Brinster, R.L. and Nagano, M. (1998). Spermatogonial stem cell transplantation, cryopreservation and culture. *Seminars in Cellular and Developmental Biology*, **9**, 401–9.

Brinster, R.L. and Zimmermann, J.W. (1994). Spermatogenesis following male germ-cell transplantation. *Proceedings of the National Academy of Sciences USA*, **91**, 11298–302.

Buehr, M., Gu, S., and McLaren, A. (1993). Mesonephric contribution to testis differentiation in the fetal mouse. *Development*, **117**, 273–81.

Byskov, A.G. (1986). Differentiation of mammalian embryonic gonad. *Physiological Reviews*, **66**, 71–117.

Byskov, A.G. and Saxen, L. (1976). Induction of meiosis in fetal mouse testis in vitro. *Developmental Biology*, **52**, 193–200.

Carrel, A. (1912). On the permanent life of tissues outside the organism. *Journal of Experimental Medicine*, **15**, 516–28.

Cerni, C., Mougneau, E., and Cuzin, F. (1987). Transfer of 'immortalizing' oncogenes into rat fibroblasts induces both high rates of sister chromatid exchange and appearance of abnormal karyotypes. *Experimental Cellular Research*, **8**, 439–46.

Champy, C. (1920). De la méthode de culture des tissus. VI. Le testicule. *Archives of Zoology and Experimental Genetics*, **60**, 461–500.

Chowdhury, A.K. and Marshall, G. (1980). Irregular pattern of spermatogenesis in the baboon (*Papio anubis*) and its possible mechanism. In: *Testicular Development, Structure and Function*, Steinberger, A. and Steinberger, E., eds. Raven Press, New York, pp. 129–37.

Clermont, Y. (1963). The cycle of the seminiferous epithelium in man. *American Journal of Anatomy*, **112**, 35–51.

Cleutjens, K.B., van der Korput, H.A., Ehren-van Eekelen, C.C., et al. (1997). A 6-kb promoter fragment mimics in transgenic mice the prostate-specific and androgen-regulated expression of the endogenous prostate-specific antigen gene in humans. *Molecular Endocrinology*, **11**, 1256–65.

Courot, M., Hochereau-de Reviers, M.T., and Ortavant, R. (1970). Spermatogenesis. In: *The Testis*, Vol. 1, Johnson, A.D., Gomes, W.R. and Vandemark, N.L., eds. Academic Press, New York, pp. 339–432.

Cremades, N., Bernabeu, R., Barros, A., and Sousa, M. (1999). In-vitro maturation of round spermatids using co-culture on Vero cells. *Human Reproduction*, **14**, 1287–93.

Curtis, D. (1981). In vitro differentiation of diakinesis figures in human testis. *Human Genetics*, **59**, 406–11.

De Felici, M. (2000). Regulation of primordial germ cell development in the mouse. *International Journal of Developmental Biology*, **44**, 575–80.

De Felici, M. and Dolci, S. (1989). In vitro adhesion of mouse fetal germ cells to extracellular matrix components. *Cell Differentiation and Development*, **26**, 87–96.

De Felici, M. and Dolci, S. (1991). Leukemia inhibitory factor sustains the survival of mouse primordial germ cells cultured on TM4 feeder layers. *Developmental Biology*, **147**, 281–4.

De Felici, M. and McLaren, A. (1983). In vitro culture of mouse primordial germ cells. *Experimental Cell Research*, **144**, 417–27.

De Felici, M. and Pesce, M. (1994a). Growth factors in mouse primordial germ cell migration and proliferation. *Progress in Growth Factor Research*, **5**, 135–43.

De Felici, M. and Pesce, M. (1994b). Interactions between migratory primordial germ cells and cellular substrates in the mouse. *Ciba Foundation Symposium*, **182**, 140–53.

De Felici, M. and Pesce, M. (1995a). Immunoaffinity purification of migratory mouse primordial germ cells. *Experimental Cell Research*, **216**, 277–9.

De Felici, M. and Pesce, M. (1995b). Purification of mouse primordial germ cells by MiniMACS magnetic separation system. *Developmental Biology*, **170**, 722–5.

De Felici, M. and Siracusa, G. (1985). Adhesiveness of mouse primordial germ cells to follicular and Sertoli cell monolayers. *Journal of Embryology and Experimental Morphology*, **87**, 87–97.

de Rooij, D.G. and Russell, L.D. (2000). All you wanted to know about spermatogonia but were afraid to ask. *Journal of Andrology*, **21**, 776–98.

Di Carlo, A. and De Felici, M. (2000). A role for E-cadherin in mouse primordial germ cell development. *Developmental Biology*, **226**, 209–19.

Dirami, G., Ravindranath, N., Pursel, V., and Dym, M. (1999). Effects of stem cell factor and granulocyte macrophage-colony stimulating factor on survival of porcine type A spermatogonia cultured in KSOM. *Biology of Reproduction*, **61**, 225–30.

Dolci, S., Pesce, M., and De Felici, M. (1993). Combined action of stem cell factor, leukemia inhibitory factor, and cAMP on in vitro proliferation of mouse primordial germ cells. *Molecular Reproduction and Development*, **35**, 134–9.

Dorrington, J.H., Roller, N.F., and Fritz, I.B. (1975). Effects of follicle-stimulating hormone on cultures of Sertoli cell preparations. *Molecular and Cellular Endocrinology*, **3**, 57–70.

Ducray, A., Bloquel, M., Hess, K., Hammond, G.L., Gérard, H., and Gérard, A. (1998). Establishment of a mouse Sertoli cell line producing rat androgen-binding protein (ABP). *Steroids*, **63**, 285–7.

Durand, P., Hue, D., Perrard-Sapori, M.H., and Vigier, M. (2001).

Letter to the editor. *Molecular and Cellular Endocrinology*, **183**, 193.

Dutertre, M., Rey, R., Porteu, A., Josso, N., and Picard, J.Y. (1997). A mouse Sertoli cell line expressing anti-Mullerian hormone and its type II receptor. *Molecular and Cellular Endocrinology*, **136**, 57–65.

Dym, M., Jia, M.C., Dirami, G., et al. (1995). Expression of c-*kit* receptor and its autophosphorylation in immature rat type A spermatogonia. *Biology of Reproduction*, **52**, 8–19.

Escalante-Alcalde, D. and Merchant-Larios, H. (1992). Somatic and germ cell interactions during histogenetic aggregation of mouse fetal testes. *Experimental Cell Research*, **198**, 150–8.

Eskola, V., Ryhanen, P., Savisalo, M., et al. (1998). Stable transfection of the rat follicle-stimulating hormone receptor complementary DNA into an immortalized murine Sertoli cell line. *Molecular and Cellular Endocrinology*, **139**, 143–52.

Fawcett, D.W. (1975). Ultrastructure and function of the Sertoli cell. In: *Handbook of physiology*, Vol. V, Hamilton, D.W. and Greep, R.D., eds. Williams & Wilkins, Baltimore, MD, pp. 21–55.

Fukasawa, K., Sakoulas, G., Pollack, R.E., and Chen, S. (1991). Excess wild-type p53 blocks initiation and maintenance of simian virus 40 transformation. *Molecular and Cellular Biology*, **11**, 3472–83.

Gaillard, P.J. and Varossieau, W.W. (1938). The structure of explants from different stages of development of the testis on cultivation in media obtained from individuals of different ages. *Acta Neerlandica Morphologicae Normalis et Pathologicae*, **1**, 313–27.

Gaillard, P.J. and Varossieau, W.W. (1940). Der einflus des hypophysenvorderlappens auf die morphologische entwicklung des hodens (studiert mit hilfe des kombinierten gewebzühtung in vitro). *Archiv für Experimentelle Zellforschung*, **24**, 141–168.

Galdieri, M., Monaco, L., and Stefanini, M. (1984). Secretion of androgen binding protein by Sertoli cells is influenced by contact with germ cells. *Journal of Andrology*, **5**, 409–15.

Gautier, C., Levacher, C., Saez, J.M., and Habert, R. (1997). Expression and regulation of transforming growth factor beta1 mRNA and protein in rat fetal testis in vitro. *Biochemical and Biophysical Research Communications*, **236**, 135–9.

Gelly, J.-L., Delongeas, J.-L., Barrat, E., Hatier, R., and Grignon G. (1984). In vitro development of seminiferous tubules from immature rat testis: ultrastructural and morphometric studies. *Biology of the Cell*, **50**, 191–4.

Gerton, G.L. and Millette, C.F. (1984). Generation of flagella by cultured mouse spermatids. *Journal of Cell Biology*, **98**, 619–28.

Gerton, G.L. and Millette, C.F. (1986). Stage-specific synthesis and fucosylation of plasma membrane proteins by mouse pachytene spermatocytes and round spermatids in culture. *Biology of Reproduction*, **35**, 1025–35.

Ghatnekar, R., Lima-de-faria, A., Rubin, S., and Menander, K. (1974). Development of human male meiosis in vitro. *Hereditas*, **78**, 265–72.

Gnessi, L., Fabbri, A., and Spera, G. (1997). Gonadal peptides as mediators of development and functional control of the testis: an integrated system with hormones and local environment. *Endocrine Reviews*, **18**, 541–609.

Godin, I. and Wylie, C.C. (1991). TGF beta 1 inhibits proliferation and has a chemotropic effect on mouse primordial germ cells in culture. *Development*, **113**, 1451–7.

Godin, I., Deed, R., Cooke, J., Zsebo, K., Dexter, M., and Wylie, C.C. (1991). Effects of the Steel gene product on mouse primordial germ cells in culture. *Nature*, **352**, 807–9.

Goldberg, E., Sberna, D., Wheat, T.E., Urbanski, G.J., and Margoliash, E. (1977). Cytochrome *c*: immunofluorescent localization of the testis-specific form. *Science*, **196**, 1010–12.

Grabske, R.J., Lake, S., Gledhill, B.L., and Meistrich, M.L. (1975). Centrifugal elutriation: separation of spermatogenic cells on the basis of sedimentation velocity. *Journal of Cellular Physiology*, **86**, 177–89.

Grandjean, V., Sage, J., Ranc, F., Cuzin, F., and Rassoulzadegan, M. (1997). Stage-specific signals in germ line differentiation: control of Sertoli cell phagocytic activity by spermatogenic cells. *Developmental Biology*, **184**, 165–74.

Griswold, M.D. (1995). Interactions between germ cells and Sertoli cells in the testis. *Biology of Reproduction*, **52**, 211–16.

Grootegoed, J.A., Peters, M.J., Mulder, E., Rommerts, F.F., and van der Molen, H.J. (1977). Absence of a nuclear androgen receptor in isolated germinal cells of rat testis. *Molecular and Cellular Endocrinology*, **9**, 159–67.

Grootegoed, J.A., Jutte, N.H.P.M., Jansen, R., Heusdens, F.A., Rommerts, F.F.G., and van der Molen, H.J. (1982). Biochemistry of spermatogenesis. The supporting role of Sertoli cells. In: *Research on Steroids*, Vol. X, *Hormonal Factors in Fertility, Infertility and Contraception* (Proceedings of the Xth Meeting of the International Study Grant for Steroid Hormones), van der Molen, H.J., Klopper, A., Lunenfeld, B., Neves e Castro, M., Sciarra, F., and Vermeulen, A., eds. Excerpta Medica, Roma, pp. 169–83.

Grootegoed, J.A., den Boer, P.J., and Mackenbach, P. (1989). Sertoli cell-germ cell communication. *Annals of the New York Academy of Sciences*, **564**, 232–42.

Hadley, M.A., Byers, S.W., Suarez-Quian, C.A., Kleinman, H.K., and Dym, M. (1985). Extracellular matrix regulates Sertoli cell differentiation, testicular cord formation, and development in vitro. *Journal of Cell Biology*, **101**, 1511–22.

Handel, M.A., Caldwell, K.A., and Wiltshire, T. (1995). Culture of pachytene spermatocytes for analysis of meiosis. *Developmental Genetics*, **16**, 128–39.

Haneji, T. and Nishimune, Y. (1982). Hormones and the differentiation of type A spermatogonia in mouse cryptorchid testes incubated in vitro. *Journal of Endocrinology*, **94**, 43–50.

Haneji, T., Maekawa, M., and Nishimune, Y. (1982). Etinoic acid (vitamin A acid) induces spermatogenesis in adult mouse cryptorchid testes in vitro. *Biochemical and Biophysical Research Communications*, **108**, 1320–4.

Haneji, T., Maekawa, M., and Nishimune, Y. (1983a). Retinoids induce differentiation of type A spermatogonia in vitro: organ culture of mouse cryptorchid testes. *Journal of Nutrition*, **113**, 1119–23.

Haneji, T., Maekawa, M., and Nishimune, Y. (1983b). In vitro differentiation of type A spermatogonia from mouse cryptorchid testes in serum-free media. *Biology of Reproduction*, **28**, 1217–23.

Haneji, T., Maekawa, M., and Nishimune, Y., (1984). Vitamin A and follicle-stimulating hormone synergistically induce differentiation of type A spermatogonia in adult mouse cryptorchid testis in vitro. *Endocrinology*, **114**, 801–5.

Haneji, T., Koide, S.S., Nishimune, Y., and Oota, Y. (1986). Dibutyryl adenosine cyclic monophosphate regulates differentiation of type A spermatogonia with vitamin A in adult mouse cryptorchid testis in vitro. *Endocrinology*, **119**, 2490–6.

Harrison, R.G. (1907). Observations on the living developing nerve fiber. *Proceedings of the Society of Experimental Biology and Medicine*, **4**, 140–3.

Heller, C.G. and Clermont, Y. (1963). Spermatogenesis in man: an estimate of its duration. *Science*, **140**, 185–6.

Hilscher, B., Hilscher, W., Bulthoff-Ohnolz, B., et al. (1974). Kinetics of gametogenesis. I. Comparative histological and autoradiographic studies of oocytes and transitional prospermatogonia during oogenesis and prespermatogenesis. *Cell and Tissue Research*, **154**, 443–70.

Hofmann, M.C., Narisawa, S., Hess, R.A., and Millán, J.L. (1992). Immortalization of germ cells and somatic testicular cells using the SV40 large T antigen. *Experimental Cell Research*, **201**, 417–35.

Hofmann, M.C., Hess, R.A., Goldberg, E., and Millán, J.L. (1994). Immortalized germ cells undergo meiosis in vitro. *Proceedings of the National Academy of Sciences USA*, **91**, 5533–7.

Hofmann, M.C., Abramian, D., and Millán, J.L. (1995). A haploid and a diploid cell cycle coexist in an in vitro immortalized spermatogenic cell line. *Developmental Genetics*, **16**, 119–27.

Hue, D., Staub, C., Perrard-Sapori, M.H., Weiss, M., Nicolle, J.C., Vigier, M., and Durand, P. (1998). Meiotic differentiation of germinal cells in three-week cultures of whole cell population from rat seminiferous tubules. *Biology of Reproduction*, **59**, 379–38.

Jégou, B. (1992). 'The Sertoli cell'. In: *Baillière's Clinical Endocrinology and Metabolism*, Vol. 6, *The Testis*, de Kretser, D.M. ed. Ballière Tindall, London, pp. 273–311.

Jégou, B. (1993). The Sertoli-germ cell communication network in mammals. *International Reviews of Cytology*, **147**, 25–96.

Jégou, B. and Sharpe, R.M. (1993). Paracrine mechanisms in testicular control. In: *The Molecular Biology of the Male Reproductive System*, de Kretser, D., ed. Ch. 8, Academic Press, New York, pp. 271–310.

Jégou, B., Syed, V., Sourdaine, P., et al.(1992). The dialogue between late spermatids and Sertoli cells in vertebrates: a century of research. In: *Spermatogenesis Fertilization–Contraception. Molecular, Cellular and Endocrine Events in Male Reproduction*, Nieschlag E., and Habenicht, U.F., eds., Schering Foundation Series, Springer-Verlag, Berlin, pp. 57–95.

Jégou, B., Pineau, C., and Dupaix, A. (1999). Paracrine control of testis function. In: *Male Reproductive Function*, Wang, C., ed. Endocrine Updates Series, Kluwer Academic, Berlin, pp. 41–64.

Jégou, B., Le Maguéresse-Battistoni, B., and Gérard, N. (2001). Is the in vitro maturation of germ cells accelerated in co-culture with Sertoli cells? *Molecular and Cellular Endocrinology*, **183**, 195.

Jiang, C., Hall, S.J., and Boekelheide, K. (1997). Development and characterization of a prepubertal rat Sertoli cell line, 93RS2. *Journal of Andrology*, **18**, 393–9.

Johnson, L. (1994). A new approach to study the architectural arrangement of spermatogenic stages revealed little evidence of a partial wave along the length of human seminiferous tubules. *Journal of Andrology*, **15**, 435–41.

Johnson, L., Neaves, W.B., Barnard, J.J., Keillor, G.E., Brown, S.W., and Yanagimachi, R. (1999). A comparative morphological study of human germ cells in vitro or in situ within seminiferous tubules. *Biology of Reproduction*, **64**, 927–34.

Johnston, D.S., Russell, L.D., and Griswold, M.D. (2000). Advances in spermatogonial stem cell transplantation. *Reviews in Reproduction*, **5**, 183–8.

Jutte, N.H., Grootegoed, J.A., Rommerts, F.F., and van der Molen, H.J. (1981). Exogenous lactate is essential for metabolic activities in isolated rat spermatocytes and spermatids. *Journal of Reproduction and Fertility*, **62**, 399–405.

Jutte, N.H., Jansen, R., Grootegoed, J.A., Rommerts, F.F., Clausen, O.P., and van der Molen, H.J. (1982). Regulation of survival of rat pachytene spermatocytes by lactate supply from Sertoli cells. *Journal of Reproduction and Fertility*, **65**, 431–8.

Kierszenbaum, A.L. (1994). Mammalian spermatogenesis in vivo and in vitro: a partnership of spermatogenic and somatic cell lineages. *Endocrine Reviews*, **15**, 116–34.

Leblond, C.P. and Clermont, Y. (1952). Definition of the stages of the cycle of the seminiferous epithelium in the rat. *Annals of the New York Academy of Sciences*, **55**, 548–73.

Le Gac, F., Attramadal, H., Horn, R., Tvermyr, M., Frøysa, A., and Hansson V. (1982). Hormone (FSH and isoproterenol) stimulation of lactate/pyruvate secretion by cultured Sertoli cells and maintenance of ATP levels in primary spermatocytes and round spermatids. In: *Miniposters of the Second European Workshop on the Testis*, 11–14 May, 1982. Rotterdam, the Netherlands, Abstract C16.

Le Gac, F., Attramadal, H., Borrebaek, B., et al. (1983). Effects of FSH, isoproterenol, and cyclic AMP on the production of lactate and pyruvate by cultured Sertoli cells. *Archives of Andrology*, **10**, 149–54.

Le Gac, F., Le Maguéresse, B., Loir, M., and Jégou, B. (1984). Influence of enriched pachytene spermatocytes, round spermatids and residual bodies on the Sertoli cell secretory activity in vitro. In: *Proceedings of the 5th Anglo-French Meeting of the Society for the Study of Fertility and Société Française pour l'Etude de la Fertilité*. 7–9 December, Fresnes, p. 22.

Leidl, W. (1968). *Zeitschrift für tierzuchtung und Zuchtungs-biologie*, **84**, 273–89.

Le Maguéresse, B. and Jégou, B. (1988). In vitro effects of germ cells on secretory activity of Sertoli cells recovered from rats of different ages. *Endocrinology*, **122**, 1672–80.

Le Maguéresse, B., Le Gac, F., Loir, M., and Jégou, B. (1986). Stimulation of rat Sertoli cell secretory activity in vitro by germ cells and residual bodies. *Journal of Reproduction and Fertility*, **77**, 489–98.

Le Maguéresse-Battistoni, B., Gérard, N., and Jégou, B. (1991). Pachytene spermatocytes can achieve meiotic process in vitro. *Biochemical and Biophysical Research Communications*, **179**, 1115–21.

Li, H., Papadopoulos, V., Vidic, B., Dym, M., and Culty, M. (1997). Regulation of rat testis gonocyte proliferation by platelet-derived growth factor and estradiol: identification of signaling mechanisms involved. *Endocrinology*, **138**, 1289–98.

Loir, M. and Lanneau, M. (1982). A strategy for an improved separation of mammalian spermatids. *Gamete Research*, **6**, 179–88.

Maekawa, M. and Nishimune, Y. (1991). In-vitro proliferation of germ cells and supporting cells in the neonatal mouse testis. *Cell Tissue Research*, **265**, 551–4.

Magre, S. and Jost, A. (1980). The initial phases of testicular organogenesis in the rat. An electron microscopy study. *Archives d'Anatomie Microscopique et de Morphologie Experimentale*, **69**, 297–318.

Martinovitch, P.N. (1937). Development in vitro of the mammalian gonad. *Nature*, **139**, 413.

Mather, J.P. (1980). Establishment and characterization of two distinct mouse testicular epithelial cell lines. *Biology of Reproduction*, **23**, 243–52.

Matsui, Y., Toksoz, D., Nishikawa, S., et al. (1991). Effect of Steel factor and leukaemia inhibitory factor on murine primordial germ cells in culture. *Nature*, **353**, 750–2.

McGuinness, M.P. and Orth, J.M. (1992). Reinitiation of gonocyte mitosis and movement of gonocytes to the basement membrane in testes of newborn rats in vivo and in vitro. *Anatomical Records*, **233**, 527–37.

McGuinness, M.P., Linder, C.C., Morales, C.R., Heckert, L.L., Pikus, J., and Griswold, M.D. (1994). Relationship of a mouse Sertoli cell line (MSC-1) to normal Sertoli cells. *Biology of Reproduction*, **51**, 116–24.

McLaren, A. (1983). Studies on mouse germ cells inside and outside the gonad. *Journal of Experimental Zoology*, **228**, 167–71.

Meistrich, M.L., Longtin, J., Brock, W.A., Grimes, S.R., Jr., and Mace, M.L. (1981). Purification of rat spermatogenic cells and preliminary biochemical analysis of these cells. *Biology of Reproduction*, **25**, 1065–77.

Millette, C.F. and Moulding, C.T. (1981). Cell surface marker proteins during mouse spermatogenesis: two-dimensional electrophoretic analysis. *Journal of Cell Science*, **48**, 367–82.

Mita, M., Price, J.M., and Hall, P.F. (1982). Stimulation by follicle-stimulating hormone of synthesis of lactate by Sertoli cells from rat testis. *Endocrinology*, **110**, 1535–41.

Morena, A.R., Boitani, C., Pesce, M., De Felici, M., and Stefanini, M. (1996). Isolation of highly purified type A spermatogonia from prepubertal rat testis. *Journal of Andrology*, **17**, 708–17.

Nakamura, M., Romrell, L.J., and Hall, P.F. (1978). The effects of temperature and glucose on protein biosynthesis by immature (round) spermatids from rat testes. *Journal of Cell Biology*, **79**, 1–9.

Nakamura, M., Okinaga, S., and Arai, K. (1984). Metabolism of pachytene primary spermatocytes from rat testes: pyruvate maintenance of adenosine triphosphate level. *Biology of Reproduction*, **30**, 1187–97.

Olaso, R. and Habert, R. (2000). Genetic and cellular analysis of male germ cell development. *Journal of Andrology*, **21**, 497–511.

Olaso, R., Pairault, C., Boulogne, B., Durand, P., and Habert, R. (1998). Transforming growth factor beta1 and beta2 reduce the number of gonocytes by increasing apoptosis. *Endocrinology*, **139**, 733–40.

Orth, J.M. (1993). Cell biology of testicular development in the fetus and neonate. In: *Cell and Molecular Biology of the Testis* Desjardins, C. and Ewing, L.L., eds, Ch. 1. Oxford University Press, New York, pp. 3–42.

Orth, J.M. and Boehm, R. (1990). Functional coupling of neonatal rat Sertoli cells and gonocytes in coculture. *Endocrinology*, **127**, 2812–20.

Orth, J.M. and Jester, W.F. Jr. (1995). NCAM mediates adhesion between gonocytes and Sertoli cells in cocultures from testes of neonatal rats. *Journal of Andrology*, **16**, 389–99.

Orth, J.M. and McGuinness, M.P. (1991). Neonatal gonocytes cocultured with Sertoli cells on a laminin-containing matrix resume mitosis and elongate. *Endocrinology*, **129**, 1119–21.

Paquis-Flucklinger, V., Michiels, J.F., Vidal, F., et al. (1993). Expression in transgenic mice of the large T antigen of polyomavirus induces Sertoli cell tumours and allows the establishment of differentiated cell lines. *Oncogene*, **8**, 2087–94.

Parvinen, M., Wright, W.W., Phillips, D.M., Mather, J.P., Musto, N.A., and Bardin, C.W. (1983). Spermatogenesis in vitro: completion of meiosis and early spermiogenesis. *Endocrinology*, **112**, 1150–2.

Pelliniemi, L.J., Paranko, J., Grund, S.K., Fröjdman, K., Foidart, J.-M., and Lakkala-Paranko, T. (1984). Morphological differentiation of Sertoli cells. In: *Recent Progress in Cellular Endocrinology of the Testis*, Vol. 123, INSERM, pp.121–140.

Peschon, J.J., Behringer, R.R., Cate, R.L., et al. (1992). Directed expression of an oncogene to Sertoli cells in transgenic mice using mullerian inhibiting substance regulatory sequences. *Molecular Endocrinology*, **6**, 1403–11.

Pognan, F., Masson, M.T., Lagelle, F., and Charuel, C. (1997). Establishment of a rat Sertoli cell line that displays the morphological and some of the functional characteristics of the native cell. *Cell Biology and Toxicology*, **13**, 453–63.

Rassoulzadegan, M., Paquis-Flucklinger, V., Bertino, B., et al. (1993). Transmeiotic differentiation of male germ cells in culture. *Cell*, **75**, 997–1006.

Resnick, J.L., Bixler, L.S., Cheng, L., and Donovan, P.J. (1992). Long-term proliferation of mouse primordial germ cells in culture. *Nature*, **359**, 550–1.

Resnick, J.L., Ortiz, M., Keller, J.R., and Donovan, P.J. (1998). Role of fibroblast growth factors and their receptors in mouse primordial germ cell growth. *Biology of Reproduction*, **59**, 1224–9.

Risley, M.S. and Morse-Gaudio, M. (1992). Comparative aspects of spermatogenic cell metabolism and Sertoli cell function in *Xenopus laevis* and mammals. *Journal of Experimental Zoology*, **261**, 185–93.

Roberts, K.P., Banerjee, P.P., Tindall, J.W., and Zirkin, B.R. (1995). Immortalization and characterization of a Sertoli cell line from the adult rat. *Biology of Reproduction*, **53**, 1446–53.

Robinson, R. and Fritz, I.B. (1981). Metabolism of glucose by Sertoli cells in culture. *Biology of Reproduction*, **24**, 1032–41.

Romrell, L.J., Bellvé, A.R., and Fawcett, D.W. (1976). Separation of mouse spermatogenic cells by sedimentation velocity. A morphological characterization. *Developmental Biology*, **49**, 119–31.

Russell, L.D. (1984). Spermiation: the sperm release process: ultrastructural observation and unresolved problems. In: *Ultrastructure of Reproduction: Gametogenesis, Fertilization and Embryogenesis*, Van Blerkom, J. and Motta, P.M., eds. Martinus Nijhoff, Boston, MA, pp. 46–66.

Russell, L.D. and Steinberger, A. (1989). Sertoli cells in culture: views from the perspectives of an in vivoist and an in vitroist. *Biology of Reproduction*, **41**, 571–7.

Schlatt, S., Schepers, A.G., and von Schönfeldt, V. (2000). Germ cell culture, genetic manipulation and transplantation. In: *Testis, Epididymis and Technologies in the Year 2000 (11th European Workshop on Molecular and Cellular Endocrinology of the Testis)*, Jégou, B., Pineau, C., and Saez, J., eds. Workshop Supplement 6. Ernst Schering Research Foundation, Springer-Verlag, Berlin, pp. 69–86.

Schmahl, J., Eicher, E.M., Washburn, L.L., and Capel, B. (2000). Sry induces cell proliferation in the mouse gonad. *Development*, **127**, 65–73.

Schulze, W. and Salzbrunn, A. (1992). Spatial and quantitative aspects of spermatogenic tissue in primates. In: *Spermatogenesis, Fertilization, Contraception*, Nieschlag, E. and Habenicht, U.F., eds. Springer Verlag, Berlin, pp. 267–83.

Seidl, K. and Holstein, A.F. (1990). Organ culture of human seminiferous tubules: a useful tool to study the role of nerve growth factor in the testis. *Cell Tissue Research*, **261**, 539–47.

Setchell, B.P. (ed.) (1978). *The Mammalian Testis*. Paul Elek, London.

Sharpe, R.M. (1994). Regulation of spermatogenesis. In: *The Physiology of Reproduction*, 2nd edn, Knobil, E. and Neill, J.D., eds. Raven Press, New York, pp. 1363–436.

Shinohara, T., Orwig, K.E., Avarbock, M.R., and Brinster, R.L. (2000). From the cover: spermatogonial stem cell enrichment by multiparameter selection of mouse testis cells. *Proceedings of the National Academy of Sciences USA*, **97**, 8346–51.

Skinner, M.K. and Fritz, I.B. (1985). Testicular peritubular cells secrete a protein under androgen control that modulates Sertoli cell functions. *Proceedings of the National Academy of Sciences USA*, **82**, 114–18.

Smith, F.F., Tres, L.L., and Kierszenbaum, A.L. (1992). Expression of testis-specific histone genes during the development of rat spermatogenic cells in vitro. *Developmental Dynamics*, **193**, 49–57.

Staub, C., Hue, D., Nicolle, J.C., Perrard-Sapori, M.H., Segretain, D., and Durand, P. (2000). The whole meiotic process can occur in vitro in untransformed rat spermatogenic cells. *Experimental Cell Research*, **260**, 85–95.

Steinberger, A. (1967). Relationship between the yield of spermatocytes in rat testes-organ culture and age of the donor animal. *Anatomical Records*, **157**, 327.

Steinberger, A. (1975). In vitro techniques for the study of spermatogenesis. In: *Methods in Enzymology*, Vol. 39, Hardman, J.G. and O'Malley, B.W., eds. Academic Press, New York, pp. 283–96.

Steinberger, A. and Steinberger, E. (1965). Differentiation of rat seminiferous epithelium in organ culture. *Journal of Reproduction and Fertility*, **9**, 243–8.

Steinberger, A. and Steinberger, E. (1966a). Stimulatory effect of vitamins and glutamine on the differentiation of germ cells in rat testes organ culture grown in chemically defined media. *Experimental Cell Research*, **44**, 429–35.

Steinberger, A. and Steinberger, E. (1966b). In vitro culture of rat testicular cells. *Experimental Cell Research*, **44**, 443–52.

Steinberger, A. and Steinberger, E. (1967). Factors affecting spermatogenesis in organ cultures of mammalian testes. *Journal of Reproduction and Fertility*, **Suppl. 2**, 117–124.

Steinberger, A. and Steinberger, E. (1970). In vitro growth and development of mammalian testes. In: *The Testis*, Vol. II, Johnson, A.D., Gomes, W.R., and VanDemark, N.L., eds. Academic Press, New York, pp. 363–91.

Steinberger, A. and Steinberger, E. (1971). Replication pattern of Sertoli cell in maturing rat testis in vivo and in organ culture. *Biology of Reproduction*, **4**, 84–7.

Steinberger, E., Steinberger, A., and Perloff, W.H. (1964a). Initiation of spermatogenesis in vitro. *Endocrinology*, **74**, 788–92.

Steinberger, E., Steinberger, A., and Perloff, W.H. (1964b). Studies on growth in organ culture of testicular tissue from rats of various ages. *Anatomical Records*, **148**, 581–9.

Steinberger, A., Steinberger, E., and Perloff, W.H. (1964c). Mammalian testes in organ culture. *Experimental Cell Research*, **36**, 19–27.

Steinberger, E., Steinberger, A., and Ficher, M. (1970). Study of spermatogenesis and steroid metabolism in cultures of mammalian testes. *Recent Progress in Hormone Research*, **26**, 547–88.

Steinberger, A., Heindel, J.J., Lindsey, J.N., Elkington, J.S., Sanborn, B.M., and Steinberger, E. (1975). Isolation and culture of FSH responsive Sertoli cells. *Endocrinology Research Communications*, **2**, 261–72.

Szalay, K., Domonkos, A., Kovacs, J., et al. (1999). 45T-1, an established cell line with characteristics of Sertoli cells, forms organized aggregates in vitro after exposure to tumor necrosis factor alpha. *European Journal of Cell Biology*, **78**, 331–8.

Taketo, T. and Koide, S.S. (1981). In vitro development of testis and ovary from indifferent fetal mouse gonads. *Developmental Biology*, **84**, 61–6.

Tarsounas, M., Pearlman, R.E., and Moens, P.B. (1999). Meiotic activation of rat pachytene spermatocytes with okadaic acid: the behaviour of synaptonemal complex components SYN1/SCP1 and COR1/SCP3. *Journal of Cell Science*, **112**, 423–34.

Tesarik, J., Greco, E., Rienzi, L., et al. (1998a). Differentiation of spermatogenic cells during in-vitro culture of testicular biopsy samples from patients with obstructive azoospermia: effect of recombinant follicle stimulating hormone. *Human Reproduction*, **13**, 2772–81.

Tesarik, J., Guido, M., Mendoza, C., and Greco, E. (1998b). Human spermatogenesis in vitro: respective effects of follicle-stimulating hormone and testosterone on meiosis, spermiogenesis, and Sertoli cell apoptosis. *Journal of Clinical Endocrinology and Metabolism*, **83**, 4467–73.

Tesarik, J., Bahceci, M., Özcan, C., Greco, E., and Mendoza, C. (1999). Restoration of fertility by in vitro spermatogenesis. *Lancet*, **353**, 555–6.

Tesarik, J., Balaban, B., Isiklar, A., et al. (2000a). In-vitro spermatogenesis resumption in men with maturation arrest: relationship with in-vivo blocking stage and serum FSH. *Human Reproduction*, **15**, 1350–4.

Tesarik, J., Mendoza, C., and Greco, E. (2000b). In-vitro maturation of immature human male germ cells. *Molecular and Cellular Endocrinology*, **166**, 45–50.

Tesarik, J., Mendoza, C., Anniballo, R., and Greco, E. (2000c). In-vitro differentiation of germ cells from frozen testicular biopsy specimens. *Human Reproduction*, **15**, 1713–16.

Toebosch, A.M., Robertson, D.M., Klaij, I.A., de Jong, F.H., and Grootegoed, J.A. (1989). Effects of FSH and testosterone on highly purified rat Sertoli cells: inhibin alpha-subunit mRNA expression and inhibin secretion are enhanced by FSH but not by testosterone. *Journal of Endocrinology*, **122**, 757–62.

Toppari, J., Eerola, E., and Parvinen, M. (1985). Flow cytometric DNA analysis of defined stages of rat seminiferous epithelial cycle during in vitro differentiation. *Journal of Andrology*, **6**, 325–33.

Toppari, J., Mali, P., and Eerola, E. (1986a). Rat spermatogenesis in vitro traced by quantitative flow cytometry. *Journal of Histochemistry and Cytochemistry*, **34**, 1029–35.

Toppari, J., Lahdetie, J., Harkonen, P., Eerola, E., and Parvinen, M. (1986b). Mutagen effects on rat seminiferous tubules in vitro: induction of meiotic micronuclei by adriamycin. *Mutation Research*, **171**, 149–56.

Tres, L.L. and Kierszenbaum, A.L. (1983). Viability of rat spermatogenic cells in vitro is facilitated by their coculture with Sertoli cells in serum-free hormone-supplemented medium. *Proceedings of the National Academy of Sciences USA*, **80**, 3377–81.

Tres, L.L., Mesrobian, H.-G., and Abdullah, M. (1989). Human Sertoli–spermatogenic cell cocultures prepared from biopsies of cryptorchid testes performed during orchidopexy. *Journal of Urology (Paris)*, **141**, 1003–9.

Tres, L.L., Smith, F.F., and Kierszenbaum, A.L. (1991). Spermatogenesis in vitro: methodological advances and cellular functional parameters. In: *Reproduction, Growth and Development*, Vol. 71, Negro-Vilar, A. and Perez-Palacios, G., eds. Serono Symposia, Raven Press, New York, pp. 115–25.

Trowell, O.A. (1959). The culture of mature organs in a synthetic medium. *Experimental Cell Research*, **16**, 118–47.

VanDemark, N.L. and Free, M.J. (1970). Temperature effects. In: *The Testis*, Vol. III, Johnson, A.D., Gomes, W.R. and VanDemark, N.L., eds. Academic Press, New York, pp. 233–312.

van den Ham, R., van Pelt, A.M., de Miguel, M.P., Van Kooten, P.J., Walther, N., and van Dissel-Emiliani, F.M. (1997). Immunomagnetic isolation of fetal rat gonocytes. *American Journal of Reproductive Immunology*, **38**, 39–45.

van Dissel-Emiliani, F.M., de Rooij, D.G., and Meistrich, M.L. (1989). Isolation of rat gonocytes by velocity sedimentation at unit gravity. *Journal of Reproduction and Fertility*, **86**, 759–66.

van Dissel-Emiliani, F.M., de Boer-Brouwer, M., Spek, E.R., van der Donk, J.A., and de Rooij, D.G. (1993). Survival and proliferation of rat gonocytes in vitro. *Cell and Tissue Research*, **273**, 141–7.

van Dissel-Emiliani, F.M., de Boer-Brouwer, M., and de Rooij, D.G. (1996). Effect of fibroblast growth factor-2 on Sertoli cells and gonocytes in coculture during the perinatal period. *Endocrinology*, **137**, 647–54.

van Pelt, A.M.M., Morena, A.R., van Dissel-Emiliani, F.M.F., et al. (1996). Isolation of the synchronized A spermatogonia from adult vitamin A-deficient rat testes. *Biology of Reproduction*, **55**, 439–44.

Vogt, M., Lesley, J., Bogenberger, J.M., Haggblom, C., Swift, S., and Haas, M. (1987). The induction of growth factor-independence in murine myelocytes by oncogenes results in monoclonal cell lines and is correlated with cell crisis and karyotypic instability. *Oncogene Research*, **2**, 49–63.

von Schonfeldt, V., Krishnamurthy, H., Foppiani, L., and Schlatt, S. (1999). Magnetic cell sorting is a fast and effective method of enriching viable spermatogonia from Djungarian hamster, mouse, and marmoset monkey testes. *Biology of Reproduction*, **61**, 582–9.

Walther, N., Jansen, M., Ergun, S., Kascheike, B., and Ivell, R. (1996). Sertoli cell lines established from H-2Kb-tsA58 transgenic mice differentially regulate the expression of cell-specific genes. *Experimental Cell Research*, **225**, 411–21.

Wartenberg, H. (1989). Differentiation and development of the testes. In: *The Testis*, 2nd edn, Burger, H. and de Kretser, D., eds. Raven Press, New York, pp. 67–118.

Weinbauer, G.F., Gromoll, J., Simoni, M., and Nieschlag, E. (2000). Physiology of testicular function. In: *Andrology – Male Reproductive Health and Dysfunction*, 2nd edn, Ch. 3, Nieschlag, E. and Behre, H.M., eds. Springer-Verlag, Berlin, pp. 23–87.

Weiss, M., Vigier, M., Hue, D., et al. (1997). Pre- and postmeiotic expression of male germ cell-specific genes throughout 2-week cocultures of rat germinal and Sertoli cells. *Biology of Reproduction*, **57**, 68–76.

Welsh, M.J. and Wiebe, J.P. (1975). Rat sertoli cells: a rapid method for obtaining viable cells. *Endocrinology*, **96**, 618–24.

Wheat, T.E., Hintz, M., Goldberg, E., and Margoliash, E. (1977). Analyses of stage-specific multiple forms of lactate dehydrogenase and of cytochrome *c* during spermatogenesis in the mouse. *Differentiation*, **9**, 37–41.

Wolff, E. (1952). Sur la différenciation sexuelle des gonades de souris explantées in vitro. *Comptes Rendus Hebdomadaires des Seances de l'Academie des Sciences de Paris*, **234**, 1712–14.

Wolff, E. and Haffen, K. (1965). Germ cells and gonads. In: *Cells and Tissues in Culture*, Vol. 2: *Methods, Biology and Physiology*, Willmer E.N., ed. Academic Press, New York, pp. 697–743.

Wolkowicz, M.J., Coonrod, S.M., Reddi, P.P., Millan, J.L., Hofmann, M.C., and Herr, J.C. (1996). Refinement of the differentiated phenotype of the spermatogenic cell line GC-2spd(ts). *Biology of Reproduction*, **55**, 923–32.

Zhou, B., Watts, L.M., and Hutson, J.M. (1993). Germ cell development in neonatal mouse testes in vitro requires mullerian inhibiting substance. *Journal of Urology*, **150**, 613–16.

2

The spermatozoon as a machine: compartmentalized pathways bridge cellular structure and function

Alexander J. Travis and Gregory S. Kopf

Center for Research on Reproduction and Women's Health, University of Pennsylvania, USA

Designing the machine: evolution draws the blueprints

Mammalian spermatozoa have but one purpose: to fertilize an egg. (For the purposes of this chapter and interests of the intended audience, mammalian spermatozoa will be the focus of discussion. In particular, the mouse and human will be used as model systems, with work on other species being cited primarily for comparative purposes or to illustrate evolutionary adaptations.) The absolute necessity for spermatozoa to succeed at this task has resulted in substantial selective pressures. These forces have resulted in one of the most highly differentiated and polarized cell types known, in regard to both structure and division of cellular functions. An understanding of the basic cell biology of these unicellular machines must, therefore, begin with a brief review of the evolutionary forces that molded them.

Spermatozoa have been described as the "microgamete," as opposed to the egg, which is the "macrogamete." Yet how did anisogamy, or this inherent difference in gamete size, evolve? Mathematical models based on the theory of sperm competition, defined as the competition among sperm from different males to fertilize a given egg, dictate that, in species with external fertilization, anisogamy is the evolutionarily stable strategy (Parker, 1982). Even though providing the female gamete with nutrient stores might result in increased zygote survival, it does not pay to have fewer large sperm. Rather, many small sperm increase the odds of fertilizing success for a given male. Despite the development of internal fertilization, anisogamy remains the evolutionarily stable strategy as long as there is some small incidence of sperm competition (females mating with multiple males) (Parker, 1982). For a review of sperm competition, see Birkhead (1996).

The inherent nature of competition requires that there must be some sperm function(s) that is critical in fertilizing success but is variable between individuals or phenotypes. Answering this requirement is the recent observation that motility can determine the outcome of sperm competition *between* males in an in vivo setting (Birkhead et al., 1999). Taken as a whole from models and empirical results, sperm competition theory provides some of the parameters for the construction of this machine; namely that sperm should be small in size relative to the egg, should carry scant provisions for the egg so that the male might instead invest his restricted energy budget in the production of more sperm, and should have relatively high motility.

In addition to the structural design of the machine, evolution has also acted on specific functional components and regulatory pathways. In external fertilizers, it is not only imperative to compete against sperm from the same species, but it is also imperative to ensure a species-specific recognition with the egg on the molecular level to avoid cross-species fertilization. This demand has led to species-specificity of ligands and receptors involved in external fertilization (Swanson and Vacquier, 1998; Vacquier, 1998), a degree of which has been maintained in mammals in proteins of the egg's extracellular matrix, the zona pellucida (ZP), and the poorly characterized receptors on the sperm plasma membrane (Hardy and Garbers, 1994).

The process of making spermatozoa fertilization competent must also be carefully regulated. Indeed, premature acrosomal exocytosis in the male reproductive tract would be highly detrimental because of proteolytic damage to surrounding spermatozoa. Sperm must be maintained in a viable condition until they reach the appropriate environment for fertilization and for a suitable length of time after mating, to coincide with the appearance of the ovulated egg. A process known as "capacitation" describes the maturational changes a sperm must undergo in order to become fertilization competent (Austin, 1951, 1952; Chang, 1951, 1955). This process appears to be synchronized in subpopulations of the ejaculate in a stochastic fashion in order to extend the fertilizable lifespan of the ejaculate (Smith, 1998; Suarez, 1998).

With these parameters and regulatory processes in mind, the highly conserved bipartite structure of mammalian sperm can be appreciated. The sperm head accomplishes the dual purposes of interacting with the female gamete and carrying the male haploid genetic material, whereas the sperm flagellum functions as a specialized cellular motor and is itself subdivided into three regions: the mid-piece, the principal piece, and the end-piece (Fig. 2.1) (Fawcett and Bedford, 1979). Each of these three regions can be distinguished ultrastructurally by the presence of different and, in some cases, unique organelles. The central axoneme is surrounded by cytoskeletal elements known as outer dense fibers in both the mid-piece and principal pieces. Positioned laterally adjacent to the outer dense fibers are either a sheath of mitochondria in the mid-piece or a cytoskeletal element known as the fibrous sheath (FS) in the principal piece. The end-piece marks the distal limit of the FS (Fawcett and Bedford, 1979).

Several restrictions on sperm function stem from their fundamental differences from somatic cells in having scant amounts of cytoplasm and in being transcriptionally and translationally inactive. These adaptations meet the demands of sperm competi-

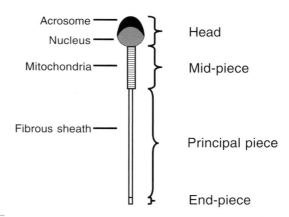

Fig. 2.1. Schematic representation of a mammalian spermatozoon. The sperm head has an exocytotic vesicle, the acrosome, overlying the nucleus. The flagellum is itself divided into three regions: a mid-piece, principal piece, and end-piece. The mid-piece is the sole region of this cell to contain mitochondria. The principal piece accounts for the majority of the flagellum, contains the fibrous sheath, and terminates in a small, distal end-piece.

tion theory by producing a highly streamlined machine devoid of any excess cellular baggage or protein production machinery that is not essential for fertilization. However, these adaptations also constrain the sperm in several ways. The decreased soluble space in sperm is likely to result in a reduced ability to translocate signaling molecules, or metabolic intermediates or substrates, from one region to another. In addition, transcriptional inactivity dictates that sperm cannot make new proteins in response to changing needs as they pass through different regions of the male and female reproductive tracts. To overcome these constraints, we, along with others, have hypothesized that sperm possess compartmentalized metabolic and signaling pathways in specific regions of the cell (Storey and Kayne, 1975; Westhoff and Kamp, 1997; Travis et al., 1998). Efficiency of the machine is improved by having only what is needed, and having it pre-positioned so that it may perform its function where it is needed. Evidence for, and the interrelationships between, these compartmentalized signaling and metabolic pathways will be developed as the major theme of this chapter.

Building the machine: compartmentalized functions require specific protein targeting-events and assembly of macromolecular complexes

It is a well-accepted tenet in the architectural world that form must follow function. In the biological world, a prime example of this is the sperm cell. Spermatozoa comprise several compartments, with each compartment functioning in an independent, yet coordinated fashion. As stated above, sperm undergo several important changes during their life-span. Such changes clearly occur in all these different cellular compartments and necessitate alterations in both metabolism and signal transduction.

For example, sperm maturation during epididymal transit is associated with alterations of the plasma membranes, changes in protein sulfhydryl–disulfide bonding and solubility characteristics, and maturation of signal transduction pathways such that sperm develop progressive motility and the ability to undergo capacitation (Eddy and O'Brien, 1994; Kopf et al., 1999a). Upon entering the female reproductive tract, interactions with the cellular and fluid compartments of this new environment induce sperm capacitation.

Once sperm arrive at the site of fertilization, there are novel interactions between the capacitated sperm's plasma membrane overlying the acrosome, as well as the acrosomal matrix itself, and the ZP (Gerton, 2001; Kim et al., 2001a, b). Such interactions likely involve several sperm-associated binding proteins and/or signaling receptors and specific carbohydrate domains on the ZP (Kopf, 2001). To date, the identity and function of such binding proteins/receptors remains controversial. As a consequence of sperm–ZP interaction, there are a series of signaling events that ultimately lead to acrosomal exocytosis and further interaction with first the ZP and then the egg's plasma membrane (Evans and Kopf, 1998; Evans, 2000). Clearly, these signaling events occur in a spatially discrete compartment

(the head) and must be coordinated in the proper temporal fashion so that fertilization is successful.

Given the fact that sperm do not make new protein, many of these changes in cellular function are likely to be regulated by changes in metabolism, changes in protein structure, and signal transduction resulting in post-translational modifications. Moreover, the fact that these events occur in discrete cellular compartments devoid of any significant cytoplasmic contribution suggests the concerted action of localized multimeric protein complexes that dictate the metabolic state of the compartments as well as signal transduction events that regulate the function of the compartments. Compartmentalized signal transduction and metabolic cascades as they relate to the regulation of somatic cell function are presently very much "in vogue" from a scientific investigative standpoint. Sperm cells likely offer the best system in which to study such compartmentalization of structure and function.

Two examples in sperm of the importance of protein targeting in the establishment and regulation of compartmentalized multimeric complexes/pathways are represented by a germ cell-specific isoform of hexokinase, type 1 (HK1–SC) (Mori et al., 1993; Travis et al., 1998, 1999), and two proteins in the A-kinase anchoring protein (AKAP) family (Carrera et al., 1994; Lin et al., 1995; Johnson et al., 1997; Visconti et al., 1997). An examination of HK1–SC distribution in murine sperm yields a fascinating characteristic; namely, that this one protein targets to three distinct structures: the membranes of the sperm head, the mitochondria of the midpiece, and the FS in the principal piece (Visconti et al., 1996; Travis et al., 1998). In these regions, HK1–SC could be participating in pathways such as glycolysis or the pentose phosphate pathway (PPP), which are critical for both membrane fusion events in the head and motility and signaling in the flagellum. This distribution raises a question of fundamental importance to cell biology: how does one protein target to several disparate cellular structures, given the fact that in somatic cells targeting to at least two of these structures (i.e., membrane and mitochondria) is characterized by organelle-specific targeting motifs?

Indeed, the HK1–SC complementary DNA (cDNA) sequence would predict a protein devoid of a mitochondrial membrane-binding domain (Mori et al., 1993). Characterization of the potential targeting motifs of HK1–SC by heterologous expression of fusion constructs of HK1 with green fluorescent protein in a somatic cell line suggests the importance of both a novel endoplasmic reticulum-targeting motif and the proteolytic processing of a chimeric motif (summarized in Fig. 2.2) (Travis et al., 1999). Knowledge of how such targeting is regulated will be informative with respect to how cellular compartmentalization and the assembly of protein complexes is established during cellular differentiation.

As discussed above with HK1–SC, the targeting of two AKAPs found in male germ cells gives another example of how proteins are localized to discrete compartments. AKAPs are characterized by their ability to anchor the regulatory subunits of protein kinase A (PK-A), thus providing spatial localization of kinase activity to different regions of cells (Pawson and Scott, 1997). Recently, it has been demonstrated that different members of the AKAP family have the ability to bind and anchor other signaling enzymes (e.g., other kinases, phosphatases) and ion channels. Therefore, this family of proteins might provide a scaffold for entire signal transduction complexes acting in local regions of the cell. Although AKAPs have similar properties in regard to the binding of PK-A, the ability to tether other components of a pathway might be the reason why spermatozoa tightly regulate the targeting of specific AKAPs.

For example, S-AKAP 84 (now designated as AKAP1) targets to the mitochondria of the mid-piece of condensing spermatids (Lin et al., 1995), whereas AKAP 82 (now designated as AKAP4) targets to the FS of sperm (Carrera et al., 1994). The targeting of these proteins bears some resemblance to the targeting of HK1–SC. Specifically, S-AKAP 84 targets to the mitochondria by means of an amino-terminal motif (Lin et al., 1995). AKAP 82, by comparison, is initially translated in a "pro" form with an apparent molecular weight of 109 kDa. This form targets to the entire length of the FS, and then proteolytic processing occurs from a proximal to distal direction, leaving the mature 82 kDa protein in place (Johnson et al., 1997).

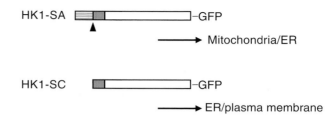

Fig. 2.2. Schematic representation of a potential chimeric mitochondrial/endoplasmic reticulum (ER) targeting motif. HK1-SA and HK1-SC are the predicted protein products of two alternative splice variants of a germ cell-specific type 1 hexokinase. When HK1/green fluorescent protein (GFP) fusion proteins were expressed in a heterologous cell line, the germ cell-specific domain (vertical stripes) shared by both splice variants was necessary and sufficient for targeting to the ER and plasma membrane. However, when the 5′ SA domain (horizontal stripes) was also present, some of the fusion protein was targeted to mitochondria. The possibility of a chimeric targeting motif was strengthened by the additional finding on immunoblots that a population of the recombinant HK1-SA specifically had the SA domain removed by proteolysis, in effect leaving HK1-SC as the mature product. The arrowhead marks the site of proteolysis and underscores that only HK1-SC will be detected if this proteolysis takes place in vivo.

Given the importance of cAMP-mediated events in the regulation of motility, it is likely that the highly regulated targeting of these proteins indicates the presence of signaling complexes critical for the function of the mid-piece and principal piece compartments.

Regulating the function of the machine: compartmentalized signaling pathways coordinate changes in sperm activity

As stated earlier, sperm undergo a variety of changes during their lifespan that contribute to their maturation and ability to fertilize an egg. It is becoming clear that compartmentalized signaling pathways control these different events (Fig. 2.3). In the sperm head, signaling events result in changes that allow the sperm to undergo acrosomal exocytosis. Likewise, capacitation-related signaling pathways in the

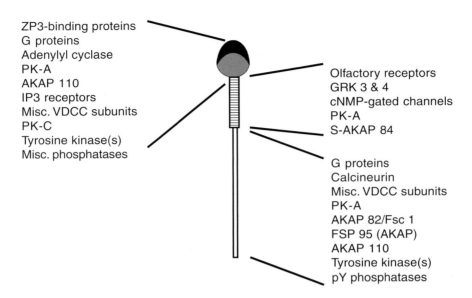

ZP3-binding proteins
G proteins
Adenylyl cyclase
PK-A
AKAP 110
IP3 receptors
Misc. VDCC subunits
PK-C
Tyrosine kinase(s)
Misc. phosphatases

Olfactory receptors
GRK 3 & 4
cNMP-gated channels
PK-A
S-AKAP 84

G proteins
Calcineurin
Misc. VDCC subunits
PK-A
AKAP 82/Fsc 1
FSP 95 (AKAP)
AKAP 110
Tyrosine kinase(s)
pY phosphatases

Fig. 2.3. Compartmentalization of selected signaling molecules. The sperm head contains receptors for the zona pellucida glycoprotein ZP3, heterotrimeric G proteins, adenylyl cyclases, protein kinase A (PK-A), A-kinase anchoring proteins (AKAP 110), various voltage-dependent cation channels (VDCC), protein kinase C (PK-C), and various tyrosine kinases and phosphatases. The mid-piece has been shown to contain olfactory receptors, G protein-related kinases (GRK 3 and 4), cNMP-gated channels, PK-A, and sperm AKAP 84 in condensing spermatids. The principal piece also contains many of the signaling molecules found in other regions, as well as fibrous sheath (FS)-specific AKAPs and calcineurin.

flagellum modulate the changes in flagellar wave-form and beat frequency characteristic of hyperactivation of motility (Si, 1999; Si and Okuno, 1999). Because sperm cannot make new proteins, they must link the changes in these two compartments temporally and spatially through macromolecular movements and/or post-translational modifications of proteins. These types of events are characteristic of the signaling that occurs during capacitation.

Work from several laboratories using in vitro models of capacitation has defined parts of a novel signal transduction pathway, elements of which are summarized below and in various reviews (Kopf et al., 1999a, b). Briefly, it is believed that capacitation is stimulated by several changes occurring at the level of the plasma membrane. These changes include the loss of cholesterol to external acceptor compounds, and the presumed influx of bicarbonate and calcium. Several possible mechanisms have emerged by which these membrane events can be translated into an observed increase in intracellular cAMP, which itself results in increased PK-A activity and downstream protein tyrosine phosphorylation events.

Sperm cell membranes covering both the acrosomal region and the flagellum possess domains that are enriched in cholesterol (Friend, 1982; Pelletier and Friend, 1983; Suzuki and Yanagimachi, 1989; Visconti et al., 1999). In vitro, cholesterol efflux is initiated by cholesterol acceptors such as serum albumin present in the medium. The mechanisms by which cholesterol efflux is initiated at the membrane and by which adsorption to the protein acceptor occurs is still not established (Rothblat et al., 1999). Changes in membrane dynamics could be translated into changes in cellular signaling in a variety of ways, and these different mechanisms are not mutually exclusive. For example, alteration in cholesterol content could influence, either directly or indirectly, the activity of ion transporters and/or signal transduction effector enzymes (Vemuri and Philipson, 1989; Shouffani and Kanner, 1990; Levitan et al., 2000).

Alternatively, the loss of cholesterol could also influence signaling through changes in the distribution/composition of membrane lipid rafts (Pralle et al., 2000; Simons and Ikonen, 2000). Sperm of both sea urchins and mammals have recently been demonstrated to contain membrane fractions with characteristics of lipid rafts (Ohta et al., 2000; A.J. Travis, G.R. Hunnicutt, S.B. Moss, and G.S. Kopf, unpublished observations). The link between changes in membrane dynamics and signaling could be through such raft-associated proteins as caveolins. In addition to being involved themselves in the movement of cholesterol across membranes (Smart et al., 1996; Arakawa et al., 2000), this family of proteins is believed to play a major role in scaffolding specific signaling and metabolic proteins to these subdomains, usually holding them in an inactive state (Okamoto et al., 1998). Because cholesterol is necessary for caveolin to interact with a membrane, the loss of cholesterol from rafts might then cause release and activation of the previously tethered signaling complex. Caveolins have the ability to bind a wide variety of protein kinases, heterotrimeric G proteins, and metabolic enzymes such as phosphofructokinase (for reviews see: Anderson, 1998; Smart et al., 1999; Simons and Toomre, 2000). Because capacitation and acrosomal exocytosis involve such signaling and metabolic components, and because caveolin-1 localizes to the region of the acrosome and to the entire length of the flagellum (A.T. Travis, G.R. Hunnicutt, S.B. Moss, and G.S. Kopf, unpublished observations), this protein is a prime candidate to coordinate these pathways in the sperm. Interestingly, the resultant increase in cAMP triggered by the capacitation-associated signaling pathway may also feed back to effect additional changes in the membranes by increasing lipid disorder through the movement of phospholipids within the membrane bilayer (Gadella and Harrison, 2000; Harrison and Miller, 2000).

Another key protein in the regulation of sperm function is likely to be a novel form of adenylyl cyclase recently found to differ considerably from the classical transmembrane cyclases (Buck et al., 1999; Chen et al., 2000; Sinclair et al., 2000). The most obvious of these differences is reflected in the name of the enzyme, soluble adenylyl cyclase (sAC). Although partly a misnomer in that sAC can associate with particulate organelles (A.J. Travis, G.S. Kopf, L.R. Levin, J. Buck, and S.B. Moss, unpublished observation), this historical name conveys a point critical to the compartmentalization of signaling pathways in sperm: by having an isoform of adenylyl cyclase that can exist in regions other than associated with the plasma membrane, the sperm can produce cAMP locally. Thus, this intracellular second messenger may be produced precisely at the points where it is needed and would not stimulate other nearby pathways as might be the case if cAMP were only produced at the plasma membrane and needed to diffuse throughout the cell.

Other critical differences between sAC and classical cyclases include the sensitivity of sAC activity to physiological levels of bicarbonate and calcium (Chen et al., 2000). This alone makes sAC a potential "linchpin" in sperm function: by coupling its activity to bicarbonate and calcium levels, sAC could in essence be monitoring the extracellular environment for appropriate cues to initiate capacitation. Another topic of great interest in the study of this enzyme is the apparent generation of multiple sAC forms with different activities. Initially translated with an apparent molecular weight of 187 kDa, sAC is believed to be processed to a mature form of 48 kDa (Buck et al., 1999; Chen et al., 2000). More recent work suggests that these two forms arise from alternate splicing (Jaiswal and Conti, 2001). Work done with recombinant proteins suggests that a truncated form approximately equivalent to the 48 kDa processed form has roughly 10-fold the activity of the full-length protein (Buck et al., 1999). Clearly, ongoing studies of sAC function in spermatozoa hold great promise in the elucidation of regulatory signaling pathways in sperm.

Powering the machine: compartmentalized metabolic pathways drive sperm function

All of the functions described thus far, be they in the sperm head or flagellum, require energy, either in

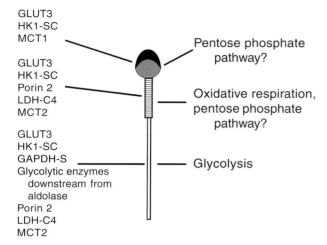

GLUT3
HK1-SC
MCT1 —————

GLUT3
HK1-SC
Porin 2 —————
LDH-C4
MCT2

GLUT3
HK1-SC
GAPDH-S —————
Glycolytic enzymes
   downstream from
   aldolase
Porin 2
LDH-C4
MCT2

Pentose phosphate
pathway?

Oxidative respiration,
pentose phosphate
pathway?

Glycolysis

Fig. 2.4. Compartmentalization of selected metabolic proteins and pathways. Glucose transporter 3 (GLUT3) is present throughout the sperm, as is hexokinase 1–SC (HK1-SC). Glycolytic enzymes such as a germ cell-specific isoform of glyceraldehyde 3-phosphate dehydrogenase (GAPDH-S) are restricted to the principal piece. This pattern suggests that glycolysis is found solely in the principal piece, while an alternative pathway of glucose metabolism, the pentose phosphate pathway, possibly exists in the head and/or mid-piece. The voltage-dependent anion channel porin 1 occurs in the mid-piece, whereas porin 2 occurs in the principal piece. Monocarboxylate transporters 1 and 2 (MCT1 and 2) are found in the head and flagellum, respectively. Coupled with the localization of lactate dehydrogenase (LDH-C4) to the flagellum, these transporters allow the sperm both to recycle NAD⁻ and to utilize lactate for energy.

the form of ATP or as reducing power (e.g. NADPH). Because the sperm is so highly polarized with regard to structure and function, these cells have evolved sophisticated adaptations to provide energy for these functions in the form of compartmentalized and scaffolded metabolic pathways (Fig. 2.4).

The most obvious example of metabolic compartmentalization in spermatozoa is that of oxidative respiration. This pathway occurs in the mitochondria, and these organelles are restricted to the mid-piece of the flagellum. There are significant species-specific adaptations in the enzymatic components of these organelles. For example, species

differences occur in the presence of a malate/aspartate shuttle, L-3-glycerol-phosphate oxidase, acyl CoA L-carnitine transferase, or the ability to oxidize glutamate plus malate; these confer specific functional capabilities to the sperm mitochondria (as discussed by Storey and Kayne (1980)).

Oxidative respiration provides the most efficient generation of ATP in cells, yet the major sites of ATP consumption in sperm are the dynein ATPases found associated with the axoneme throughout the flagellum (Storey and Kayne, 1980; Halangk et al., 1990). How then do the principal piece and end-piece of the flagellum meet their energy needs? In some species such as the sea urchin, a phosphoryl-creatine shuttle functions to transfer high-energy phosphate equivalents from the mitochondria to the principal piece (Tombes and Shapiro, 1985). However, in most mammalian species, this system is either entirely absent or poorly developed (for review see Kaldis et al., 1997). Instead, the sperm of many mammalian species rely on a combination of glycolysis and oxidative respiration for their energy needs.

In much the same way that oxidative respiration is compartmentalized to the mid-piece, it appears that glycolysis is compartmentalized to the FS of the principal piece. This concept was first suggested by the observation of Storey (Storey and Kayne, 1975; Storey, 1980) that glycolytic enzymes downstream from aldolase remain bound to rabbit sperm flagella even after demembranation by incubation in a hypotonic medium. Subsequently, it has been demonstrated that both HK (Mori et al., 1998; Travis et al., 1998) and glyceraldehyde 3-phosphate dehydrogenase (GAPDH) (Westhoff and Kamp, 1997; Bunch et al., 1998) localize to the FS. A similar scaffold arrangement for the enzymes of glycolysis has been demonstrated in skeletal muscle (Arnold and Pette, 1968).

Notions of glycolysis as comprising freely soluble enzymes within the cytosol have been replaced by the recognition that enzymes can function more efficiently when colocalized to specific subcellular structures (Srere, 1987; Clegg, 1992). Indeed, the binding of enzymes such as GAPDH (Tsai et al.,

1982) and HK (Kurokawa et al., 1981) to specific structures has been shown to alter their enzymatic activities. In spermatozoa, the efficiency of the pathway is likely increased by having all the components colocalized to the FS. In addition, scaffolding of the enzymes of glycolysis results in the localized generation of ATP throughout the length of the principal piece, where it can be utilized not only by the dynein ATPases, which power motility, but also by the protein kinases that regulate changes in motility (Travis et al., 1998). This concept will be developed further as links between sperm metabolism and regulation of sperm function are explored below.

Like any engine, the glycolytic pathway must have both a fuel (substrate) and an exhaust (metabolic end-products). For glycolysis, the fuels utilized are simple sugars such as glucose and fructose, the facilitative uptake of which is mediated by a family of transport proteins known as GLUTs, or glucose transporters. The sperm of different species are known to express different GLUT family members, suggesting an important role for these proteins (Burant et al., 1992; Haber et al., 1993; Burant and Davidson, 1994; Urner and Sakkas, 1999b). In particular, the presence of GLUT3 in spermatozoa is intriguing. Because of its low K_m for glucose, this transporter is found in cell types such as macrophages and platelets that experience sudden changes in energy needs following "activation" (Ahmed et al., 1997; Sorbara et al., 1997). Spermatozoa might also be thought of as cells that undergo activation, first acquiring motility in the epididymis and then hyperactivated motility associated with capacitation in the female tract (Fraser and Quinn, 1981; Cooper, 1984). Therefore, the presence of GLUT3 allows sperm a "high-affinity" uptake capability.

Work in several laboratories with sperm of different species has suggested that GLUTs localize to the plasma membrane over the entire length of the flagellum and the sperm head. In the flagellum, therefore GLUTs colocalize with the glycolytic pathway organized in the FS, just beneath the plasma membrane. This colocalization is perfectly designed to channel substrate directly from the transporters to the enzymes of glycolysis, similar to an arrangement found in rod and cone photoreceptor cells of the eye, in which GLUT1 also colocalizes with the glycolytic pathway (Hsu and Molday, 1991). In both circumstances, the arrangement of transporter and metabolic machinery allows for efficient substrate delivery and energy production in specific regions of a highly polarized cell.

The end-products of glycolysis (the "exhaust") must also be considered in sperm design and function. For every molecule of glucose consumed, two molecules each of ATP, pyruvate, NADH, H^+, and water are produced. In this pathway, the presence of NAD^+ is necessary for GAPDH enzyme activity. Therefore, for glycolysis to remain active, the spermatozoa must have a mechanism to replenish the NAD^+. This is accomplished by the conversion of pyruvate into lactate by the enzyme lactate dehydrogenase. This enzyme has a germ cell-specific isoform (Goldberg, 1975), LDH-C4/LDH-X, and an unusual distribution pattern in the matrix of the mitochondria, as well as throughout the principal piece (Burgos et al., 1995). Lactate can thus act as substrate for mitochondrial oxidative phosphorylation in sperm, in contrast to somatic cells. LDH-C4 is also compartmentalized appropriately to recycle NAD^+, allowing continued function of glycolysis.

To avoid intracellular accumulation of lactate, the spermatozoa must also have a mechanism by which they can remove this acid. The family of monocarboxylate transporters (MCTs) allow transport of such molecules across membranes. It is noteworthy that two family members, MCT1 and MCT2, have been identified in hamster spermatozoa, and that at least MCT2 is present in the flagellum (Garcia et al., 1995). Therefore, spermatozoa have different classes of transporter positioned both to deliver fuel to and to remove end-products from glycolysis in the FS. This system is particularly efficient in the flagellum owing to the very high surface area to volume ratio of this compartment; consequently, the ratio of transporters to cytosol volume strongly favors substrate throughput.

The demonstration that HK localizes to the FS was critical for the development of the theory that the entire glycolytic pathway is organized in the FS. Yet as has been noted, this enzyme can also be found associated with the mitochondria of the mid-piece and the membranes of the sperm head. Because GAPDH, the glycolytic enzyme key to ATP production, has not been found in the mid-piece or head (Westhoff and Kamp, 1997; Bunch et al., 1998), the question of the role of HK in these compartments arises. We and others have hypothesized that an alternative pathway of glucose metabolism, the PPP, might be organized in the sperm head and mid-piece to produce reducing power in the form of NADPH (Travis et al., 1998).

Evidence for the importance of this pathway in sperm function has recently been reported. For example, PPP activity has been suggested to be critical for such functions as sperm–egg plasma membrane fusion, and for successful penetration and decondensation of the sperm head (Urner and Sakkas, 1996, 1999a,b). In addition, the PPP might be involved in the production of reduced glutathione to protect sperm membranes and the nuclear material from oxidative stress (Storey et al., 1998). It will be intriguing to see whether future experiments will support the suggestion that sperm have compartmentalized this pathway to the sperm head to provide NADPH for these functions.

The machine in operation from ejaculation to fertilization: the integration of signaling and metabolic pathways

To perform the various tasks required for successful fertilization, the regionalized metabolic and signaling pathways that we have discussed must be able to integrate their functions, both within and between individual compartments. Exploring the relationships between these pathways is a relatively new area of investigation, and we shall, therefore, concentrate first on our own work regarding the integration of glycolysis and signaling events associated with capacitation, and then offer brief speculation on the integration of pathways in other regions of the sperm.

Of the three metabolic substrates (glucose, lactate,

and pyruvate) normally included in media designed to support capacitation in vitro, only glucose is necessary and sufficient to allow the full pattern of protein tyrosine phosphorylation associated with capacitation in murine sperm. As long as glucose is still present, the complete elimination of mitochondrial ATP production by uncouplers and inhibitors of oxidative respiration does not reduce the pattern of protein tyrosine phosphorylation (Travis et al., 2001). As opposed to an indirect effect through metabolism, this effect of glucose on signaling could be a direct action on a signaling molecule such as a phosphodiesterase or an adenylyl cyclase. Precedent for such effects exists for both families of enzymes (e.g., Han et al., 1999). However, a nonmetabolizable analog of glucose, 2-deoxyglucose, fails to support protein tyrosine phosphorylation, suggesting that glucose metabolism is critical for the phosphorylation events (Travis et al., 2001).

These findings suggest a central role for ATP produced by glycolysis (as opposed to oxidative respiration) in supporting not only the dynein ATPase, which power motility, but also the protein kinases believed to regulate motility (Travis et al., 1998, 2001). It should be noted that the lack of a direct signaling effect by glucose pertains solely to the pattern of protein tyrosine phosphorylation in the mouse. A direct effect of glucose on a sperm signaling molecule might still be involved in other aspects of signaling in this or other species, such as bovine spermatozoa in which glucose has dramatically different effects (Parrish et al., 1989; Galantino-Homer et al., 1997).

Consistent with a role for GLUT3 as a transporter in murine spermatozoa, we have shown that low glucose concentrations (10–100 μmol/l) were sufficient for the full pattern of protein tyrosine phosphorylation (Travis et al., 2001). Upon exposure to capacitating conditions, sperm showed an approximate doubling of the equilibrium level of tritiated 2-deoxyglucose they took up (A.J. Travis, G.S. Kopf and S.B. Moss, unpublished observation). Because HK activity in sperm does not appear to be regulated in regard to capacitation (Travis et al., 2001), and sperm size is not known to vary with capacitation, this shift in equilibrium might result from an increase in GLUT activity. This increase might itself reflect an upregulation of individual transporters, or it might reflect the activation of a pool of transporters in a particular sperm compartment. Regardless of the cause of this shift, its presence supports the notion that exposure to the same stimulators of capacitation-associated signaling also influences the uptake of metabolic substrate.

Together, these studies indicate a remarkable symbiosis between metabolism and signaling in the principal piece: instead of metabolism just passively performing housekeeping duties, both metabolic and signaling pathways exert influence over each other. Thus the colocalization of transporters (both GLUTs and MCTs), metabolic enzymes, and signaling molecules in the principal piece is critical for the integrated function of this, the longest section of the sperm flagellum. Possibly organizing these integrated pathways of metabolism and signaling in both the head and flagellum are the membrane rafts enriched in caveolin-1 found in both regions. In the sperm head, caveolin-1 could scaffold the G_i-mediated signaling pathway that regulates acrosomal exocytosis, as well as the PPP required for membrane fusion events. In the flagellum, it could scaffold protein kinases in the proximity of the glycolytic machinery in the FS, and/or scaffold metabolic proteins to the plasma membrane or FS (Fig. 2.5). An understanding of how the integration of these pathways is accomplished at the molecular level will represent a significant leap in our understanding of cellular energetics.

Repairing the machine: implications for assisted reproductive technology

Spermatozoa must perform many steps to fertilize an egg. Changes in cell motility, signal transduction events, cell–extracellular matrix interactions, regulated exocytosis, cell–cell interactions, and membrane fusion events all must be successfully completed for fertilization to take place. Spermatozoa have evolved a highly sophisticated system of compartmentalizing metabolic and sig-

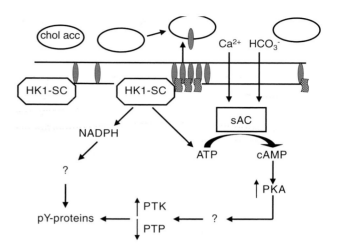

Fig. 2.5. Schematic model integrating metabolic and signaling pathways known to take part in sperm capacitation. Three primary external stimuli have been identified: cholesterol efflux, and calcium and bicarbonate influx. Cholesterol is removed from the plasma membrane by acceptors such as albumin or cyclodextrin (chol acc, cholesterol acceptor). This efflux might be mediated through membrane rafts enriched in cholesterol and caveolin-1 (gray ovals and checked banners, respectively). Caveolins might also tether the signaling and metabolic enzymes to these raft subdomains creating specific transduction super-complexes. Both calcium and bicarbonate have been shown to stimulate soluble adenylyl cyclase (sAC) activity, and this enzyme might represent the connection between these external stimuli and downstream events. cAMP generated by the cyclase could, in turn, stimulate protein kinase A (PKA), which, by either activating other kinases or inactivating phosphatases, would result in the downstream protein tyrosine phosphorylation events. Through glycolysis, hexokinase 1-SC (HK1-SC) could lead to the production of ATP needed both for the cyclase and phosphorylation events or, as has been suggested, could stimulate these events through the pentose phosphate pathway by helping to produce NADPH.

naling pathways to specific regions of the cell so that they may perform these required functions with minimal cellular machinery. This efficiency results in a substantial benefit to the male. Sperm can be generated at minimal energetic cost, allowing the production of vast numbers of gametes, which increases male reproductive success.

However, like any finely tuned machine, a break-down in a specific component may result in loss of function: namely, infertility. Whether in human in vitro fertilization clinics or in food animal industries that rely heavily upon assisted reproduction, diagnosing male infertility has primarily relied upon two criteria, sperm morphology and motility. With improved understanding of the protein targeting necessary for the differentiation of spermatogenic cells into mature spermatozoa, it should be possible to identify the causes of some morphological defects. With improved understanding of the signaling and metabolic processes occurring in the different compartments of spermatozoa, it should be possible to design tests of these pathways to identify previously idiopathic causes of male infertility. Together, these advances will bring clinical investigation of male infertility beyond motility and morphology into actual tests of sperm fertilizing ability. Perhaps even more important than diagnostic applications, advancements in understanding the spermatozoon as a machine might one day also help to correct such defects, if coupled with recent promising advances in in vivo transgenesis and germ cell transplantation (Nagano et al., 2000, 2001).

REFERENCES

Ahmed, N., Kansara, M., and Berridge, M.V. (1997). Acute regulation of glucose transport in a monocyte-macrophage cell line: Glut-3 affinity for glucose is enhanced during the respiratory burst. *Biochemical Journal*, 327, 369–75.

Anderson, R.G.W. (1998). The caveolae membrane system. *Annual Reviews of Biochemistry*, 67, 199–225.

Arakawa, R., Abe-Dohmae, S., Asai, M., Ito, J.I., and Yokoyama, S. (2000). Involvement of caveolin-1 in cholesterol enrichment of high density lipoprotein during its assembly by apolipoprotein and THP-1 cells. *Journal of Lipid Research*, 41, 1952–62.

Arnold, H. and Pette, D. (1968). Binding of glycolytic enzymes to structure proteins of the muscle. *European Journal of Biochemistry*, 6, 163–71.

Austin, C.R. (1951). Observations on the penetration of the sperm into the mammalian egg. *Australian Journal of Scientific Research B*, 4, 581–96.

Austin, C.R. (1952). The 'capacitation' of the mammalian sperm. *Nature* 170, 326.

Birkhead, T.R. (1996). Sperm competition: evolution and mechanisms. *Current Topics in Developmental Biology*, 33, 103–58.

Birkhead, T.R., Martinez, J.G., Burke, T., and Froman, D.P. (1999). Sperm mobility determines the outcome of sperm competition in the domestic fowl. *Proceedings of the Royal Society of London, Series B Biological Science*, 266, 1759–64.

Buck, J., Sinclair, M.L., Schapal, L., Cann, M.J., and Levin, L.R. (1999). Cytosolic adenylyl cyclase defines a unique signaling molecule in mammals. *Proceedings of the National Academy of Sciences USA*, 96, 79–84.

Bunch, D.O., Welch, J.E., Magyar, P.L., Eddy, E.M., and O'Brien, D.A. (1998). Glyceraldehyde 3-phosphate dehydrogenase-S protein distribution during mouse spermatogenesis. *Biology of Reproduction*, 58, 834–41.

Burant, C.F., and Davidson, N.O. (1994). GLUT3 glucose transporter isoform in rat testis: localization, effect of diabetes mellitus, and comparison to human testis. *American Journal of Physiology*, 267, R1488–95.

Burant, C.F., Takeda, J., Brot-Laroche, E., Bell, G.I., and Davidson, N.O. (1992). Fructose transporter in human spermatozoa and small intestine is GLUT 5. *Journal of Biological Chemistry*, 267, 14523–6.

Burgos, C., Maldonado, C., Gerez de Burgos, N.M., Aoki, A., and Blanco, A. (1995). Intracellular localization of the testicular and sperm-specific lactate dehydrogenase isozyme C4 in mice. *Biology of Reproduction*, 53, 84–92.

Carrera, A., Gerton, G.L., and Moss, S.B. (1994). The major fibrous sheath polypeptide of mouse sperm: structural and functional similarities to the A-kinase anchoring proteins. *Developmental Biology*, 165, 272–84.

Chang, M.C. (1951). Fertilizing capacity of spermatozoa deposited into the fallopian tubes. *Nature*, 168, 697–8.

Chang, M.C. (1955). Development of fertilizing capacity of rabbit spermatozoa in the uterus. *Nature*, 175, 1036–7.

Chen, Y., Cann, M.J., Litvin, T.N., et al. (2000). Soluble adenylyl cyclase as an evolutionarily conserved bicarbonate sensor. *Science*, 289, 625–8.

Clegg, J.S. (1992). Cellular infrastructure and metabolic organization. *Current Topics in Cellular Regulation*, 33, 3–14.

Cooper, T.G. (1984). The onset and maintenance of hyperactivated motility of spermatozoa from the mouse. *Gamete Research*, 9, 55–74.

Eddy, E.M., and O'Brien, D.A. (1994). The spermatozoon. In: *The Physiology of Reproduction*, Knobil, E. and Neill, J.D., eds. Raven Press, New York, pp. 29–77.

Evans, J.P. (2000). Getting sperm and egg together: things conserved and things diverged. *Biology of Reproduction*, **63**, 355–60.

Evans, J.P. and Kopf, G.S. (1998). Molecular mechanisms of sperm–egg interactions and egg activation. *Andrologia*, **30**, 297–307.

Fawcett, D.W. and Bedford, J.M. (1979). *The Spermatozoon: Maturation, Motility, Surface Properties and Comparative Aspects*. Urban and Schwarzenberg, New York.

Fraser, L.R. and Quinn, P.J. (1981). A glycolytic product is obligatory for initiation of the sperm acrosome reaction and whiplash motility required for fertilization in the mouse. *Journal of Reproduction and Fertility*, **61**, 25–35.

Friend, D.S. (1982). Plasma-membrane diversity in a highly polarized cell. *Journal of Cell Biology*, **93**, 243–9.

Gadella, B.M. and Harrison, R.A. (2000). The capacitating agent bicarbonate induces protein kinase A-dependent changes in phospholipid transbilayer behavior in the sperm plasma membrane. *Development*, **127**, 2407–20.

Galantino-Homer, H., Visconti, P.E., and Kopf, G.S. (1997). Regulation of protein tyrosine phosphorylation during bovine sperm capacitation by a cyclic adenosine 3′,5′-monophosphate-dependent pathway. *Biology of Reproduction*, **56**, 707–19.

Garcia, C.K., Brown, M.S., Pathak, R.K., and Goldstein, J.L. (1995). cDNA cloning of MCT2, a second monocarboxylate transporter expressed in different cells than MCT1. *Journal of Biological Chemistry*, **270**, 1843–9.

Gerton, G.L. (2001). Function of the sperm acrosome. In: *Fertilization*, Hardy, D.M., ed. Academic Press, New York, pp. 265–302.

Goldberg, E. (1975). Lactate dehydrogenase-X from mouse testes and spermatozoa. *Methods in Enzymology*, **41**, 318–23.

Haber, R.S., Weinstein, S.P., O'Boyle, E., and Morgello, S. (1993). Tissue distribution of the human GLUT 3 glucose transporter. *Endocrinology*, **132**, 2538–43.

Halangk, W., Troger, U., and Bohnensack, R. (1990). Quantification of aerobic energy turnover in epididymal bull spermatozoa. *Biochimica et Biophysica Acta*, **1015**, 243–7.

Han, P., Werber, J., Surana, M., Fleischer, N., and Michaeli, T. (1999). The calcium/calmodulin-dependent phosphodiesterase PDE1C down-regulates glucose-induced insulin secretion. *Journal of Biological Chemistry*, **274**, 22337–44.

Hardy, D.M. and Garbers, D.L. (1994). Species-specific binding of sperm proteins to the extracellular matrix (zona pellucida) of the egg. *Journal of Biological Chemistry*, **269**, 19000–4.

Harrison, R.A. and Miller, N.G. (2000). cAMP-dependent protein kinase control of plasma membrane lipid architecture in boar sperm. *Molecular Reproduction and Development*, **55**, 220–8.

Hsu, S.C. and Molday, R.S. (1991). Glycolytic enzymes and a GLUT-1 glucose transporter in the outer segments of rod and cone photoreceptor cells. *Journal of Biological Chemistry*, **266**, 21745–52.

Jaiswal, B.S. and Conti, M. (2001). Identification and functional analysis of splice variants of the germ cell soluble adenylyl cyclase. *Journal of Biological Chemistry*, **276**, 31698–708.

Johnson, L.R., Foster, J.A., Haig-Ladewig, L., et al. (1997). Assembly of AKAP82, a protein kinase A anchor protein, into the fibrous sheath of mouse sperm. *Developmental Biology*, **192**, 340–50.

Kaldis, P., Kamp, G., Piendl, T., and Wallimann, T. (1997). Functions of creatine kinase isoenzymes in spermatozoa. *Advances in Developmental Biology*, **5**, 275–312.

Kim, K.S., Cha, M.C., and Gerton, G.L. (2001a). Mouse sperm protein sp56 is a component of the acrosomal matrix. *Biology of Reproduction*, **64**, 36–43.

Kim, K.S., Foster, J.A., and Gerton, G.L. (2001b). Differential release of guinea pig sperm acrosomal components during exocytosis. *Biology of Reproduction*, **64**, 148–56.

Kopf, G.S. (2001). Signal transduction mechanisms regulating sperm acrosomal exocytosis. In: *Fertilization*, Hardy, D.M., ed. Academic Press, New York, pp. 181–223.

Kopf, G.S., Ning, X.P., Visconti, P.E., Purdon, M., Galantino-Homer, H., and Fornes, M. (1999a). Signaling mechanisms controlling mammalian sperm fertilization competence and activation. In: *The Male Gamete: From Basic Science to Clinical Applications*, Gagnon, C., ed. Cache River Press, Vienna, IL, pp. 105–18.

Kopf, G.S., Visconti, P.E., and Galantino-Homer, H. (1999b). Capacitation of the mammalian spermatozoon. In: *Advances in Developmental Biochemistry*, Vol. 5, Wassarman, P.M., ed. JAI Press, Stamford, CT, pp. 83–107.

Kurokawa, M., Tokuoka, S., Oda, E., Tsubotani, E., and Ishibashi, S. (1981). Difference in efficiency of function between a mitochondria-bound hexokinase and a non-bound one. *Biochemistry International*, **2**, 645–50.

Levitan, I., Christian, A.E., Tulenko, T.N., and Rothblat, G.H. (2000). Membrane cholesterol content modulates activation of volume-regulated anion current in bovine endothelial cells. *Journal of General Physiology*, **115**, 405–16.

Lin, R.Y., Moss, S.B., and Rubin, C.S. (1995). Characterization of S-AKAP84, a novel developmentally regulated A kinase anchor protein of male germ cells. *Journal of Biological Chemistry*, **270**, 27804–11.

Mori, C., Welch, J.E., Fulcher, K.D., O'Brien, D.A., and Eddy, E.M. (1993). Unique hexokinase messenger ribonucleic acids lacking the porin-binding domain are developmentally expressed in mouse spermatogenic cells. *Biology of Reproduction*, **49**, 191–203.

Mori, C., Nakamura, N., Welch, J. E., et al. (1998). Mouse sper-matogenic cell-specific type 1 hexokinase (mHk1-s) tran-scripts are expressed by alternative splicing from the *mHk1* gene and the HK1–S protein is localized mainly in the sperm tail. *Molecular Reproduction and Development*, **49**, 374–85.

Nagano, M., Shinohara, T., Avarbock, M.R., and Brinster, R.L. (2000). Retrovirus-mediated gene delivery into male germ line stem cells. *FEBS Letters*, **475**, 7–10.

Nagano, M., McCarrey, J.R., and Brinster, R.L. (2001). Primate spermatogonial stem cells colonize mouse testes. *Biology of Reproduction*, **64**, 1409–16.

Ohta, K., Sato, C., Matsuda, T., et al. (2000). Co-localization of receptor and transducer proteins in the glycosphingolipid-enriched, low density, detergent-insoluble membrane frac-tion of sea urchin sperm. *Glycoconjugate Journal*, **17**, 205–14.

Okamoto, T., Schlegel, A., Scherer, P.E., and Lisanti, M.P. (1998). Caveolins, a family of scaffolding proteins for organizing 'pre-assembled signaling complexes' at the plasma membrane. *Journal of Biological Chemistry*, **273**, 5419–22.

Parker, G.A. (1982). Why are there so many tiny sperm? Sperm competition and the maintenance of two sexes. *Journal of Theoretical Biology*, **96**, 281–94.

Parrish, J.J., Susko-Parrish, J.L., and First, N.L. (1989). Capacitation of bovine sperm by heparin: inhibitory effect of glucose and role of intracellular pH. *Biology of Reproduction*, **41**, 683–99.

Pawson, T., and Scott, J.D. (1997). Signaling through scaffold, anchoring, and adaptor proteins. *Science*, **278**, 2075–80.

Pelletier, R.M. and Friend, D.S. (1983). Development of mem-brane differentiations in the guinea pig spermatid during spermiogenesis. *American Journal of Anatomy*, **167**, 119–41.

Pralle, A., Keller, P., Florin, E.L., Simons, K., and Horber, J.K. (2000). Sphingolipid–cholesterol rafts diffuse as small entities in the plasma membrane of mammalian cells. *Journal of Cell Biology*, **148**, 997–1008.

Rothblat, G.H., de la Llera-Moya, M., Atger, V., Kellner-Weibel, G., Williams, D.L., and Phillips, M.C. (1999). Cell cholesterol efflux: integration of old and new observations provides new insights. *Journal of Lipid Research*, **40**, 781–96.

Shouffani, A. and Kanner, B.I. (1990). Cholesterol is required for the reconstruction of the sodium- and chloride-coupled, gamma-aminobutyric acid transporter from rat brain. *Journal of Biological Chemistry*, **265**, 6002–8.

Si, Y. (1999). Hyperactivation of hamster sperm motility by tem-perature-dependent tyrosine phosphorylation of an 80-kDa protein. *Biology of Reproduction*, **61**, 247–52.

Si, Y. and Okuno, M. (1999). Role of tyrosine phosphorylation of flagellar proteins in hamster sperm hyperactivation. *Biology of Reproduction*, **61**, 240–6.

Simons, K. and Ikonen, E. (2000). How cells handle cholesterol. *Science*, **290**, 1721–6.

Simons, K. and Toomre, D. (2000). Lipid rafts and signal trans-duction. *Nature Reviews: Molecular Cell Biology*, **1**, 31–9.

Sinclair, M.L., Wang, X.Y., Mattia, M., et al. (2000). Specific expression of soluble adenylyl cyclase in male germ cells. *Molecular Reproduction and Development*, **56**, 6–11.

Smart, E.J., Ying, Y., Donzell, W.C., and Anderson, R.G.W. (1996). A role for caveolin in transport of cholesterol from endoplas-mic reticulum to plasma membrane. *Journal of Biological Chemistry*, **271**, 29427–35.

Smart, E.J., Graf, G.A., McNiven, M.A., et al. (1999). Caveolins, liquid-ordered domains, and signal transduction. *Molecular Cell Biology*, **19**, 7289–304.

Smith, T.T. (1998). The modulation of sperm function by the ovi-ductal epithelium. *Biology of Reproduction*, **58**, 1102–4.

Sorbara, L.R., Davies-Hill, T.M., Koehler-Stec, E.M., Vannucci, S.J., Horne, M.K., and Simpson, I.A. (1997). Thrombin-induced translocation of GLUT3 glucose transporters in human platelets. *Biochemical Journal*, **328**, 511–16.

Srere, P.A. (1987). Complexes of sequential metabolic enzymes. *Annual Reviews of Biochemistry*, **56**, 89–124.

Storey, B.T. (1980). Strategy of oxidative metabolism in bull sper-matozoa. *Journal of Experimental Zoology*, **212**, 61–7.

Storey, B.T. and Kayne, F.J. (1975). Energy metabolism of sper-matozoa. V. The Embden–Myerhoff pathway of glycolysis: activities of pathway enzymes in hypotonically treated rabbit epididymal spermatozoa. *Fertility and Sterility*, **26**, 1257–65.

Storey, B.T. and Kayne, F.J. (1980). Properties of pyruvate kinase and flagellar ATPase in rabbit spermatozoa: relation to meta-bolic strategy of the sperm cell. *Journal of Experimental Zoology*, **211**, 361–7.

Storey, B.T., Alvarez, J.G., and Thompson, K.A. (1998). Human sperm glutathione reductase activity in situ reveals limitation in the glutathione antioxidant defense system due to supply of NADPH. *Molecular Reproduction and Development*, **49**, 400–7.

Suarez, S.S. (1998). The oviductal sperm reservoir in mammals: mechanisms of formation. *Biology of Reproduction*, **58**, 1105–7.

Suzuki, F. and Yanagimachi, R. (1989). Changes in the distribu-tion of intramembranous particles and filipin-reactive mem-brane sterols during in vitro capacitation of golden hamster spermatozoa. *Gamete Research*, **23**, 335–47.

Swanson, W.J. and Vacquier, V.D. (1998). Concerted evolution in an egg receptor for a rapidly evolving abalone sperm protein. *Science*, **281**, 710–12.

Tombes, R.M. and Shapiro, B.M. (1985). Metabolite channeling: a phosphorylcreatine shuttle to mediate high energy phosphate transport between sperm mitochondria and tail. *Cell*, **41**, 325–34.

Travis, A.J., Foster, J.A., Rosenbaum, N.A., et al. (1998). Targeting of a germ cell-specific type 1 hexokinase lacking a porin-binding domain to the mitochondria as well as to the head and fibrous sheath of murine spermatozoa. *Molecular Biology of the Cell*, **9**, 263–76.

Travis, A.J., Sui, D., Riedel, K.D., et al. (1999). A novel NH(2)-terminal, nonhydrophobic motif targets a male germ cell-specific hexokinase to the endoplasmic reticulum and plasma membrane. *Journal of Biological Chemistry*, **274**, 34467–75.

Travis, A.J., Jorgez, C.J., Merdiushev, T., et al. (2001). Functional relationships between capacitation-dependent cell signaling and compartmentalized metabolic pathways in murine spermatozoa. *Journal of Biological Chemistry*, **276**, 7630–6.

Tsai, I.H., Murthy, S.N., and Steck, T.L. (1982). Effect of red cell membrane binding on the catalytic activity of glyceraldehyde 3-phosphate dehydrogenase. *Journal of Biological Chemistry*, **257**, 1438–42.

Urner, F. and Sakkas, D. (1996). Glucose participates in sperm–oocyte fusion in the mouse. *Biology of Reproduction*, **55**, 917–22.

Urner, F. and Sakkas, D. (1999a). Characterization of glycolysis and pentose phosphate pathway activity during sperm entry into the mouse oocyte. *Biology of Reproduction*, **60**, 973–8.

Urner, F. and Sakkas, D. (1999b). A possible role for the pentose phosphate pathway of spermatozoa in gamete fusion in the mouse. *Biology of Reproduction*, **60**, 733–9.

Vacquier, V.D. (1998). Evolution of gamete recognition proteins. *Science*, **281**, 1995–8.

Vemuri, R. and Philipson, K.D. (1989). Influence of sterols and phospholipids on sarcolemmal and sarcoplasmic reticular cation transporters. *Journal of Biological Chemistry*, **264**, 8680–5.

Visconti, P.E., Ning, X., Fornes, M.W., et al. (1999). Cholesterol efflux-mediated signal transduction in mammalian sperm: cholesterol release signals an increase in protein tyrosine phosphorylation during mouse sperm capacitation. *Developmental Biology*, **214**, 429–43.

Visconti, P.E., Johnson, L., Oyaski, M., et al. (1997). Regulation, localization, and anchoring of protein kinase A subunits during mouse sperm capacitation. *Developmental Biology*, **192**, 351–63.

Visconti, P.E., Olds-Clarke, P., Moss, S.B., et al. (1996). Properties and localization of a tyrosine phosphorylated form of hexokinase in mouse sperm. *Molecular Reproduction and Development*, **43**, 82–93.

Westhoff, D. and Kamp, G. (1997). Glyceraldehyde 3-phosphate dehydrogenase is bound to the fibrous sheath of mammalian spermatozoa. *Journal of Cell Science*, **110**, 1821–9.

3

Attributes of fertile spermatozoa

Christopher De Jonge[1] and Christopher L.R. Barratt[2]

[1]Department of Obstetrics and Gynecology and Reproductive Medicine Center, University of Minnesota, Minneapolis, USA
[2]Department of Medicine, University of Birmingham, Birmingham, UK

Introduction

The process of fertilization can be imagined as an elegant pas de deux: with fertilization success being dependent upon the precise timing and accuracy of a well-choreographed series of steps between male (spermatozoa) and female (oocytes) gametes. Arguably, perhaps the greatest performer in the fertilization process is the spermatozoon. The spermatozoon must *actively* overcome numerous obstacles and undergo many dynamic changes in order to achieve its destiny, while the oocyte assumes a fairly passive role in events leading to and culminating in fertilization. Some of the prefertilization processes that a mammalian spermatozoon must undergo have been revealed only since the mid-1980s, while other aspects still remain somewhat enigmatic.

In 1989, Dr. Rupert Amann published his view of parameters that are requisite for the spermatozoon to be considered as "fertile":

1 Normal structure of vital functional components.
2 Fully functional metabolic pathways for production of sperm motion, maintenance of membrane potentials, ionic microenvironment, pH, or other cellular functions.
3 Motility to penetrate cervix and uterotubal junction, for departure from storage sites, and to contact and penetrate the oocyte and its vestments.
4 Presence of peripheral and/or integral proteins that serve as "survival proteins" to protect the spermatozoa from the hostile environment of the female reproductive tract.
5 Appropriate responses to the microenvironment and stimuli provided by the female reproductive tract.
6 Proteins essential for recognition and binding of the spermatozoon to the zona pellucida and vitelline membrane.
7 Acrosomal enzymes maintained in proenzyme or inhibited form until appropriate time for assisting in oocyte vestment penetration.
8 Fusable plasma and acrosomal membranes.
9 Precise timing in sequence from secondary spermatocyte to cell stage that enters oocyte and forms male pronucleus, the chromosomes of which coalesce with the female pronucleus to produce an embryo with maximum probability of survival. [To the latter we would add: production of an embryo with a structurally and functionally patent genome.]
10 Stable DNA that is capable of decondensation at the appropriate time in the fertilization process.

Today our understanding and appreciation of the significant role that a number of these parameters play in the fertilization process can be viewed, and perhaps naively, as somewhat fundamental, e.g., motility (some strides have been made in the area of sperm kinematics and the reader is encouraged to read the comprehensive review by Mortimer (1997)). However, other "attributes" have been the subject of intensive investigation in the 1990s and they will be the substance of this review. Some of the topics become particularly noteworthy when viewed in light of current technologies used to facilitate fertilization.

The sperm nuclear genome

The multifactorial impact that the paternal genome has on fertilization and parturition has been greatly elaborated on in the past several years.

DNA packaging

First it is helpful to review a model for how DNA is packaged during spermiogenesis. Ward and Coffey (1991) proposed four levels of organization for DNA packaging in the spermatozoon. The first level involves chromosomal anchoring and this refers to the attachment of the DNA to the nuclear annulus. In the second level of organization, DNA loop domains are formed. This occurs as a result of the DNA becoming attached to the newly added nuclear matrix, and in so doing the chromosomes become organized into loops. In the third level of organization, protamines replace histones. The function of the protamines is to condense the DNA into compact doughnuts. The significance of this step will be made apparent below. The fourth and final level of organization involves chromosomal positioning. The chromosomes become organized with their centromeres located in the center of the nucleus and the telomeres at the nuclear periphery. This is significant in that active genes are probably localized to the nuclear center and inactive genes to the periphery.

On the surface, this model appears to be fairly simple. However, closer evaluation reveals that the process of DNA condensation is a very complex one and subject to perturbation that can result in defects. So, how might defects be revealed? First, it is known that sperm with abnormal morphology have decreased fertilizing ability and produce poor quality genomically blocked embryos (Kruger et al., 1986; Awadalla et al., 1987; Ron-El et al., 1991; Janny and Menezo, 1994). Further, it is thought that sperm head morphology alterations are linked to the pro-

portion of DNA packaged by protamines versus histones. The rationale behind this assertion is that space requirements for DNA containment differ depending on whether protamines or histones have been involved in the packaging; histone-packaged DNA requires more space than protamine-packaged DNA. However, adding complexity to the situation are recent data suggesting the lack of a relationship between sperm head morphology and DNA compaction (Lee et al., 1997). These latter data do not diminish the fact that *protamine deposition is critically important to sperm DNA and chromatin stability*. The significance of this becomes apparent when one considers that infertile males are more likely to have chromatin anomalies related to protamine deposition. Further, there is a relationship between under-protamination and damaged sperm DNA (for review see Sakkas et al., 1997).

If the DNA has been damaged during packaging, what impact might this have? Evenson and co-workers (Evenson et al., 1986; Evenson, 1990) have established that there is a distinct relationship between susceptibility of DNA to denaturation (reflective of altered chromatin structure) and the presence of DNA strand breaks measured by both the single-cell electrophoresis (the COMET assay) and terminal transferase-mediated nick and labeling (TUNEL) assays. These investigators have recently found that when more than 30% of sperm contained low pH-inducible DNA denaturation in situ, successful pregnancy was either significantly delayed or did not occur within the span of a year (Evenson et al., 1999). Similar data have been obtained by Spanò and colleagues, who showed that fecundity declines as the percentage of sperm with abnormal chromatin (as measured by sperm chromatin structure assay) increases (Spanò et al., 2000). Larson showed that abnormal chromatin packaging (i.e., when >27% of the sperm showed DNA denaturation) is associated with a failure to achieve successful pregnancies in an in vitro fertilization (IVF) program (Larson et al., 2000). Adding to this are data from Sakkas and colleagues (1997), who found that a high percentage of DNA nicks/strand breaks were correlated with decondensation failure. Therefore, the way in which sperm DNA has been packaged during spermiogenesis will ultimately influence ability to achieve paternity.

Chromosomal abnormalities

The study of sperm chromosome abnormalities has received much attention recently, largely in response to the advent of intracytoplasmic sperm injection (ICSI). There are essentially two classes of abnormality that can be identified: *structural* and *numerical*. Structural abnormalities can loosely be subdivided into deletions, mutations, and translocations. Numerical abnormalities, for present purposes, can simply be classified as aneuploidy. While many examples for each class of chromosome abnormality can be cited, only representative conditions will be presented.

Microdeletions on the variable region of Yq in the *AZF* (azoospermia factor) are probably the most well-known deletions associated with male infertility. Four specific regions (*AZFa, AZFb, AZFc* and *AZFd*) have been identified as areas where deletions are most common (Krausz et al., 2000; Van Landuyt et al., 2000; Liow et al., 2001). As yet there is no clear pathology associated with these deletions although there is a suggestion that larger deletions are associated with a more severe pathology (e.g., complete azoospermia: Silber et al., 1998; Krausz et al., 2000). The incidence of deletions in the Y chromosome in subfertile patients varies widely between studies, the disparity in part being dependent on factors such as screening techniques (and their effectiveness), patient diagnosis, etc. (see Krausz et al., 2000; Liow et al., 2001). In general, however, deletions are present in 2% of potential ICSI candidates (8/402) and 4% of men with azoospermia (9/229) (Van Landuyt et al., 2000).

Point mutations in *AZF* appear to be very rare. For example, only one de novo mutation was found when screening 576 subfertile men for two genes (*USP9Y* (*DFFRY*) and *DBY*) located in the *AZFa* region (Sun et al., 1999). The recent sequencing of the Y chromosome has intensified the search for other, as yet unidentified genes, associated with

spermatogenic defects and this area is likely to see considerable progress in the near future. Because of the severe defects in spermatogenesis that often accompany deletions in *AZF*, few sperm if any are produced and, consequently, the deletions are not usually transmitted; however, sperm from men with deletions in *AZF* can achieve fertilization success at ICSI although the male progeny are likely to carry the deletion (Kent-First et al., 1996; Page et al., 1999). Interestingly, recent data have suggested that, in very specific circumstances, naturally fertile men can harbor large deletions in *AZFc* (Saut et al., 2000). In these cases, the deletion was passed to the sons, who were infertile, suggesting that we still have some way to go before we fully understand the genetics of Y microdeletions.

In addition to microdeletions considerable attention has recently been focused on DNA repeat expansions, for example in the gene for the androgen receptor. Although the data are still somewhat controversial, there appears to be a relationship between the CAG repeat length in this gene and defective spermatogenesis (Dowsing et al., 1999). As ICSI can overcome the potential infertility in some of these men, the concern is whether further elongation of the repeat might occur in future generations; this could result in an increased incidence in neurodegenerative disorders.

Interestingly, a case study of two men with spinocerebellar ataxia type 7 [CAG triplet repeat disease] showed that all the mutant sperm from these men had alleles with very large repeats, so much so that the offspring would likely have a severe form of the disease (Monckton et al., 1999). Perhaps reassuringly, Monckton suggested that the major underrepresentation of such males in the general population probably shows that a large proportion of such alleles may be associated with embryonic lethality. Therefore, spermatozoa with large numbers of CAG repeats may have a significantly reduced fertility potential.

Aneuploidy occurs in cells that do not have an exact multiple of haploid number, for example disomy $(n+1)$ and nullisomy $(n-1)$. In view of a higher incidence of de novo chromosomal abnormalities and sex chromosome aneuploidies in children from ICSI (Bonduelle et al., 1998), specific attention has focused on sperm chromosome abnormalities in subfertile men. FISH (fluorescence in situ hybridization) studies have clearly shown a notably higher incidence of sperm chromosome abnormalities in subfertile men, e.g., severe oligozoospermia (Bernardini et al., 1997; Egozcue et al., 1997, 2000; Vegetti et al., 2000). In addition to these studies, specific patients have also been examined, e.g., those with Klinefelter's syndrome [XXY]. In these men, the testis can produce both normal and abnormal sperm and current data do not allow for accurate predictions of the ratio of abnormal/normal sperm from a blood karyotype, especially when the karyotype shows some degree of mosaicism. In general, men with XXY produce higher numbers of sperm with an abnormal chromosome complement. However, used in conjunction with preimplantation genetic diagnosis (PGD) to screen normal embryos, sperm recovered from the testis of men with complete XXY can produced normal children (Staessen et al., 1996; Ron-El et al., 2000). Current information suggests that in patients with Klinefelter's syndrome FISH analysis of the sperm can provide important information to couples about the possible risks of producing abnormal embryos and should be used as a screening test prior to treatment.

Men with balanced reciprocal translocations have a higher risk of fetal miscarriage and producing chromosomally unbalanced offspring. Although only limited information is available, some of these men can have a normal semen profile but, in general, have a higher incidence of producing chromosomally abnormal sperm (Vegetti et al., 2000). For example, one study on a man with a balanced reciprocal translocation [t(11;22) (g25;q12)] reported that only 36% of the sperm were normal (Van Assche et al., 1999).

Whilst selection against chromosomally abnormal sperm cells does exist, for example at the levels of sperm morphology (Lee et al., 1996) and binding to the zona pellucida (Van Dyk et al., 2000), this is not the case in all situations where abnormal cells can achieve full fertility potential under both natural and assisted conception circumstances.

Imprinting

Imprinting refers to parent-specific differences in the expression of certain genes (Nakao and Sasaki, 1996; Bartolomei and Tilghman, 1997; Mutter, 1997). In other words, the expression level of imprinted genes is dependent on their parental origin. Parental imprinting is the epigenetic marking of certain subregions of the parental genomes in mammals. A paternally imprinted gene is one that has been silenced, thus allowing for expression of the maternally inherited allele.

The exact molecular mechanisms underlying imprinting remain poorly understood (Trasler, 1998; Simon et al., 1999) but allelic-specific methylation has been detected in nearly all imprinted genes. Particularly in the male germ line, the timing of imprinting of individual and groups of genes is also poorly understood (Trasler, 1998; Kerjean et al., 2000). In summary, imprinting is initiated by the erasure of existing imprinting status in primordial germ cells and imprinting is re-established in each generation and before union of sperm and egg. In fact, some evidence from the mouse model indicates that imprinting can occur in the epididymis, postspermiogenesis, as evidenced by changes in methylation of certain genes (Ariel et al., 1994). However, the results from this study remain to be validated.

Imprinted genes are involved in the pathogenesis of several diseases, for example Prader–Willi and Angelman syndromes and various cancers. Osteosarcoma, retinoblastoma, choriocarcinoma, and Wilm's tumors are examples of diseases resulting from paternally imprinted genes.

The impact of and requirement for imprinting for normal embryogenesis and fetal development is dramatically demonstrated in cases of uniparental disomy, i.e., maternal or paternal disomy. Specific examples have been shown using mouse models where maternal disomy (gynogenesis) led to hypertrophy of the inner cell mass and hypotrophy of the extraembryonic tissues and paternal disomy (androgenesis) led to hypertrophy of the extraembryonic tissues. In humans, imprinting is responsible for the failure of monoparental embryos to develop. Specifically, androgenesis leads to the pathological condition called the complete hydatidiform mole. Thus, the paternal genome quantitatively and qualitatively directs invasiveness of placenta.

With the progression of assisted reproductive technology (ART) to use less mature male germ cells for ICSI, one has to question whether the necessary methylation/demethylation processes have occurred that will ultimately contribute to a normal, viable pregnancy. Preliminary data from a small number of children conceived using ejaculated sperm for ICSI indicate no adverse effect on DNA methylation patterns in the 15q11–q13 region (Prader–Willi and Angelman syndromes); however, only nine children were examined where nonejaculated cells were used (Manning et al., 2000). Quite simply, we need more data before we can be confident that imprinting is not adversely modified when using immature germ cells for ICSI. Unfortunately, because we have a relatively poor understanding of the molecular and cellular mechanisms of imprinting, we are a long way from being able to determine experimentally if an individual sperm (or germ cell) has the correct imprinting pattern to form viable conceptions.

The sperm mitochondrial genome

The role of mitochondria in sperm function and, more specifically, in fertilization has legitimately been ascribed as energy generation for the flagella to cause motion. Without sufficient energy production, sperm motion can be retarded or absent, the result being a concomitant decrease in fertilization potential. More recently, however, focus has been directed on the mitochondrial genome and the role it has or may have in sperm function (see review St. John et al., 2000a).

Sperm mitochondrial DNA

All reported human mitochondrial diseases are maternally inherited. This is partly based on the fact that it has not yet been possible to detect paternal mitochondrial DNA (mtDNA) in offspring. Perhaps an explanation for this is that the spermatozoon's mtDNA simply becomes diluted out by maternal mtDNA. The oocyte contains many thousand (>100 000) copies of mtDNA and the spermatozoon contains only about 50–80 copies. That apparently being the case then, how might paternal mtDNA play a role in fertilization and embryonic development?

In contrast to nuclear DNA, mtDNA is highly mutable and readily degradable, and it is transcriptionally competent at the time of oocyte penetration. Higher levels of mtDNA deletions have been detected in the semen of subfertile men (St. John et al., 2001). However, preliminary data from Cummins et al., (1998) have shown that mature and immature sperm mid-pieces disappear sometime between the 4- and 8-cell stage in mouse embryos.

Sperm mtDNA from humans may behave differently. For example, using a highly sensitive nested polymerase chain reaction technique that specifically detects sperm mtDNA, St. John and colleagues (2000b) have the first evidence for the occurrence of paternal mtDNA in defective (polyploid) human embryos. Previously, it had been predicted that sperm mtDNA in mammals is eliminated by the 8-cell stage (Sutovsky et al., 1996). However, results from St. John's study demonstrate the presence of paternal mtDNA up to and past the 8-cell stage. Therefore, their model indicates that paternal mtDNA leakage occurs in defective embryos. If the results are validated in normal human embryos, and to even later stages of embryonic development (e.g., blastocyst), then the consequence of paternal mtDNA leakage could be significant for either the fetus or the offspring, and it could result in an increase in mtDNA disease. There is, therefore, the potential that the use of abnormal sperm in ICSI may facilitate transmission of defective mtDNA (see St. John and De Jonge, 2000).

Finally, some forms of male infertility may be a result of accelerated aging via dysfunctional mitochondria and/or testicular disorders (Cummins et al., 1994). Consequently, an equally pertinent issue regarding sperm mitochondria is the potential impact they may have on nuclear DNA during spermiogenesis when mitochondrial oxidative processes become uncontrollable, the result of which could be irreversible DNA damage (see previous section). This issue requires additional investigation.

The plasma membrane

Studies during the 1990s on the sperm plasma membrane significantly advanced information regarding sperm function and, more specifically, the processes of *capacitation* and the *acrosome reaction*. It is well established that the sperm plasma membrane undergoes changes during passage through the female reproductive tract. Collectively those changes have been called capacitation. Put simply, capacitation can be defined as preparative and requisite changes for acrosomal exocytosis (the acrosome reaction) and fertilization. Recent investigations have yielded data that provide for greater clarity in our understanding of the events and changes that comprise the capacitation and acrosome reaction processes. The following represents some, albeit not all, of the more notable findings.

Lipids

Sperm membranes acquire a large amount of cholesterol from seminal plasma. It has been shown that human sperm incubated in the presence of seminal plasma are insensitive to acrosome reaction stimulation. The purified inhibitory molecule in seminal plasma was identified as cholesterol (Cross, 1996). Albumin, both in vivo and in vitro, acts as a sterol acceptor and induces cholesterol efflux from the sperm plasma membrane (Davis, 1981; Langlais et al., 1988). Commercially available albumin preparations contain lipid transfer protein 1, which is responsible for facilitating cholesterol removal (Ravnik et al., 1993). This molecule has also been found in human follicular fluid (Ravnik et al., 1990).

Capacitation involves the removal of cholesterol from the plasma membrane by albumin and high density lipoproteins present in the uterus and follicular fluid and removal of plasma membrane-bound coating proteins by glycosaminoglycans present in the female reproductive tract. Cholesterol removal results in membrane destabilization, increased membrane fluidity and permeability, and an alteration in the mobility of integral proteins and protein receptors.

Recent data, primarily in the boar, have shown that bicarbonate-induced capacitation results in dramatic changes in the boar sperm plasma membrane (Gadella and Harrison, 2000). Bicarbonate activated the outward translocation of phospholipids (phosphatidylserine, phosphatidylethanolamine, phosphatidylcholine and sphingomyelin), which was accompanied by increased membrane lipid disorder and phospholipid catabolism. These changes were mediated by a cyclic AMP (cAMP)-dependent protein phosphorylation. Gadella and Harrison (2000) suggested that these effects were mediated by a non-specific bidirectional translocase (scramblase) that acted to make the sperm plasma membrane less stable.

The changes that occur in plasma membrane composition and arrangement do not appear to be ubiquitous but rather they appear to be regionally distributed (for review see Flesch and Gadella, 2000). For example, the plasma membrane at the anterior aspect of the sperm head is highly fusogenic whereas the area of plasma membrane at the equatorial region, and the future site of sperm and oolemmal fusion, is less so. A possible reason for this difference is that it has been reported that barriers to membrane protein and lipid lateral diffusion exist at the equatorial region (Arts et al., 1994; Gadella et al., 1995). As an example, the migration of one protein, PH-20, to the equatorial segment may occur, in part, as a result of these barriers (Cowan et al., 1987; Myles et al., 1987; Foster et al., 1994).

Proteins

The dissolution, redistribution, and exposure of some proteins occurs concomitant with or only after capacitation. Some of the proteins function to stabilize the membrane(s) until the appropriate time while others ultimately contribute to membrane loss, i.e., exocytosis.

With such an apparent delicate balance, it is critically important that capacitation and the acrosome reaction occur in a temporal–spatial framework that is conducive to and facilitative of fertilization.

A recently described change that assists in or controls capacitation and that can be related, in part, to cholesterol removal is an increase in phosphorylation on tyrosine residue-containing proteins (Kopf et al., 1995; Carrera et al., 1996; Aitken, 1997; de Lamirande et al., 1997). Tyrosine phosphorylation appears to be regulated by essentially two effector molecules/pathways. The first mechanism for tyrosine phosphorylation involves a change in the oxidation–reduction (redox) state of the cell that is induced by an increase in reactive oxygen species, specifically hydrogen peroxide (Aitken, 1997; Aitken et al., 1998).

The second route for tyrosine phosphorylation increases seems to occur through the activity of cAMP as the effector molecule (Carrera et al., 1996). Rapid progress has been made in elucidating this pathway. For example, recent data from Kopf's laboratory have shown that in mice and humans tyrosine phosphorylation in vitro is dependent on bicarbonate and bovine serum albumin. The latter is proposed to work by removing cholesterol from the plasma membrane and activating cAMP and protein kinase A, with the subsequent stimulation of tyrosine phosphorylation (Osheroff et al., 1999; Visconti et al., 1999a,b). It is unclear exactly how cholesterol activates cAMP but it may have both an indirect effect (via membrane changes associated with efflux) and a direct effect (Kopf et al., 1999). Interestingly, very recently, a soluble mammalian adenylyl cyclase (sAC) has been described which is *directly* activated by bicarbonate (Chen et al., 2000). This sAC, present in spermatozoa, is similar to aden-

ylyl cyclase in cyanobacteria, suggesting a common mechanism for activation. It is not clear if this sAC is responsible for the effects on capacitation in mammalian spermatozoa.

F-actin appears to have a critical dual role in pre-fertilization events. First, actin polymerization occurs during capacitation: binding to and stabilizing the plasma and outer acrosomal membranes, and thereby limiting fusion. Following polymerization, actin binds to the newly tyrosine-phosphorylated molecule phospholipase C. Phospholipase C participates in one or more signal transduction cascades that culminate in the acrosome reaction. However, actin represents the final barrier to fusion and it is not until actin depolymerizes that fusion can occur (Breitbart and Spungin, 1997).

A zona pellucida glycoprotein (ZP3) has been characterized to be a primary ligand for sperm–zona binding and acrosome reaction induction in both the mouse and humans (van Duin et al., 1994; Barratt and Hornby et al., 1995). However, despite knowing the nature of the ligand, the complementary 'receptor' for ZP3 on the spermatozoon remains unknown. A putative ZP3 receptor candidate on human sperm was reported to be a 95 kDa receptor tyrosine kinase (Burks et al., 1995). However, no independent data have been generated to substantiate this candidate. Progress in this area has been painfully slow. Undoubtedly, the major problem has been acquiring enough zona protein (either natural or recombinant) to perform meaningful and comprehensive biochemical experiments. With the paucity of natural product, the focus of attention has been on the production of recombinant ZP3, but purified, biologically active product is still not widely available (see Whitmarsh et al., 1996; Chapman et al., 1998; Harris et al., 1999). Another ZP3 receptor candidate is a lectin that binds mannose-containing ligands (Benoff, 1997). Expression of this receptor is dependent on the time course for capacitation, as capacitation time increases so does receptor expression. The capacitation-dependent localization of the mannose lectin on the sperm plasma membrane overlying the acrosomal cap is consistent with the requirement that a receptor be present in that region in order to coordinate exocytosis. This latter aspect is supported by data demonstrating a correlation between mannose lectin expression and acrosomal status (Benoff, 1997).

Guanine nucleotide-binding proteins (G proteins) are typically involved in communicating the consequence of ligand–receptor binding to an effector molecule to culminate in a cellular response, e.g., exocytosis. There is some evidence for the role of G proteins in communicating the consequence of binding of zona pellucida ligand(s) to receptor(s) on the sperm plasma membrane and induction of the acrosome reaction (Lee et al., 1992; Tesarik et al., 1993; Brandelli et al., 1996; Franken et al., 1996). A G protein-coupled kinase has been reported in association with acrosomal membranes, providing support for the role of G proteins in the acrosome reaction (Sallese et al., 1997). Brandelli and colleagues (1996) reported the involvement of the inhibitory G_i class of protein in the acrosome reaction.

The acrosomal serine glycoproteinase acrosin plays an important role in the fertilization process (e.g., Zaneveld and De Jonge, 1991; Eddy and O'Brien, 1994): (i) acrosin appears to become functional during the acrosome reaction (Tesarik et al., 1988; De Jonge et al., 1989); (ii) active and liberated acrosin has an important role in sperm–oocyte fusion and specifically at the level of zona binding and penetration (Tesarik et al., 1988; Tesarik, 1989); and (iii) it has been shown that residual acrosin remains associated with the outer acrosomal membrane possibly to facilitate sperm binding with the oolemma (Tesarik et al., 1988, 1990).

Acrosin exists in a proenzyme form called proacrosin. Approximately 93% of acrosin exists as proacrosin. Proacrosin has been found localized on the acrosomal membranes and in the acrosomal matrix. However, the latter has not been conclusively proven. The precise in vivo mechanism(s) by which proacrosin (inactive form) is converted to acrosin (active form) is ill defined. One mechanism involves a change in acrosomal pH. Another recent theory implicates the polysulfated binding domain of pro-

acrosin/acrosin as being involved not only in sperm secondary binding during zona pellucida penetration but also in proacrosin activation (Moreno et al., 1998).

To conclude this section on proteins, it is important to mention that a number of signaling pathways have been implicated as having an important role in sperm function, and specifically in association with capacitation and the acrosome reaction.

The following are just a few in a number of elegant reviews on the aforementioned subject(s): Zaneveld et al. (1993), Brucker and Lipford (1995), Aitkin (1997), Breitbart and Spungin (1997) de Lamirande et al. (1997) Benoff (1998), and Kopf et al. (1999).

Ions and channels

The role of ions and ion channels in regulating sperm function has remained somewhat elusive, in part because of the complexities of the cell in question. However, recent advances in molecular cloning, electrophysiogical, and imaging technologies have facilitated new and revealing information (for review see Darszon et al., 1999).

In mammals, specific attention has focused on the pathways of calcium influx during the first stages of the acrosome reaction. In the mouse, hyperpolarization of the sperm plasma membrane, which is concomitant with capacitation, acts to recruit low-voltage activated calcium channels into a closed state prior to interaction with the zona pellucida (Arnoult et al., 1999). Work primarily from Harvey Florman's laboratory and using single cell imaging has shown that the initial response of mouse sperm to zona pellucida is activation of a low-voltage activated T-type calcium channel, leading to a transient rise in calcium ions. This initiates a cascade of events that culminates in the probable activation of store-operated channels to facilitate the necessary changes in calcium levels within the cell for the acrosome reaction (O'Toole et al., 2000).

The molecular identities of these voltage-operated and store-operated channel remains elusive (see Publicover and Barratt, 1999) but studies using antibodies in the rat have identified both low- and high-voltage activated calcium channels located in discrete regional distributions on mature spermatozoa (Westenbroek and Babcock, 1999).

To date only high-voltage activated channels (or hybrids of these) have been detected in human spermatozoa (Goodwin et al., 2000) and the role of the low-voltage forms has yet to be fully investigated, although there is no reason to believe that the human is any different to the mouse.

Recent experiments have focused on the role of store-operated channels in the acrosome reaction (O'Toole et al., 2000). Physiological evidence for these exists in the mouse and pharmacological evidence is available for the human (Rossato et al., 2001) but the regulation/operation of these stores is far from clear. Evidence from other cell types suggests that transient receptor potential (Trp)-like proteins are involved (Birnbaumer et al., 2000; Boulay et al., 1999). Several Trp proteins have been cloned from human testis complementary DNA (cDNA), e.g., TRP6 (Hoffman et al., 1999), that indicates their presence, at least in the testis, but physiological data for their operation in the fully mature human spermatozoon is still awaited. Suffice it to say that spermatozoa are likely to possess a large variety of channels regulating the flow of calcium across the plasma membrane – the nature and operation of which remain to be determined (see Wennemuth et al., 2000).

It's quite remarkable that, in comparison with other cell types, we know so little about calcium signaling in human spermatozoa. Patch clamping studies on mature gametes are unlikely to be fruitful in the near future so we will need to rely on the relatively laborious techniques of molecular cloning, identification and subsequent expression to determine what channels are likely to be active in mature cells and how they are regulated.

Whilst progress in this area will be made, we are unlikely to see, in the near future, the necessary advances that are required to provide an in-depth understanding of how a mature spermatozoon interacts with its ionic environment. This is disappointing, as undoubtedly poor/defective regulation of ions is a cause of subfertility in some men but because our knowledge of the way the cell interacts with its environment is still rudimentary we cannot yet understand the nature of these lesions.

Dynamic interaction of spermatozoa with the human female genital tract

A critical attribute of a fertile spermatozoon is the ability to be transported to the site of fertilization, at the correct time, and in a state of readiness for fertilization. Exactly how this occurs remains a mystery. In contrast to the rapid progress in the field of ART, there have been very few developments in our understanding of sperm transport in the female tract. Extrapolating data from animal studies and using the few human studies that are available, we can gain a sketchy picture of what is happening in this black box (sperm movement from cervix to egg).

The window of sperm transport in the human is not as narrow as once thought as sperm will transcend the female tract and achieve conceptions up to seven days prior to and up to two days after ovulation (Wilcox et al., 1995, 2000; Lenton, et al., 1993; Chauhan et al., 1989).

Not surprisingly, sperm can remain motile within the human female tract for some time; for example, motile sperm have been recovered from the oviduct up to 85 hours after coitus and one report shows sperm remaining in the oviduct 25 days after coitus (Mansour et al., 1993). Therefore, although sperm are, in general, subjected to attack by phagocytes and other processes in the female tract, some, the "selected" minority, can survive in a fertile state for a number of days (see Barratt and Pockley, 1998).

In addition to understanding the physical transport of sperm to the oviduct, the dynamic interactions between the female tract and the spermatozoon are of considerable interest. However, the technical, ethical, and logistical difficulties in performing sperm transport studies in humans have limited progress in this area. The availability of cervical mucus has allowed some understanding of how sperm penetrate (Pandya et al., 1986) and interact. Cervical mucus has a paradoxical effect on spermatozoa. Rapid capacitation is achieved yet sperm within cervical mucus are difficult to activate (e.g., acrosome react in response to physiological agonists – a state of suspended animation (Gould et al., 1984; Zinaman et al., 1989). Presumably, this allows for the availability of sperm for fertilization over a considerable time period and may well function as a putative sperm-storage site.

One proposed mechanism of sperm survival in the female tract is attachment to the oviductal epithelium. Experiments, particularly in pigs and hamsters, suggest that sperm bind in vivo to the oviductal epithelium and are then "activated" by a mechanism as yet unknown to move to the site of fertilization (Smith and Yanagimachi, 1990, 1991; Hunter, 1996). Experiments in hamsters have suggested that achievement of a fully capacitated state is a trigger to detachment from the oviductal epithelium (Smith and Yanagimachi, 1991), supporting the concept that the final stages of capacitation and perhaps the development of hyperactivation take place in the oviduct. Sperm storage in the oviduct, which has been noted in all animals studied to date, is consistent with these observations. Of course we do not know what happens in vivo in the human oviduct, but in vitro experiments with oviductal cells indicate that sperm will bind to the epithelium and that hyperactivation may assist release (Pacey et al., 1995). However, the numerous attempts to locate a sperm reservoir in the human oviduct have been unsuccessful (Williams et al., 1993) suggesting, at least to us, that one does not exist.

While we know little of how a sperm is transported through the female tract, we do know that defective transport is one cause of unexplained infertility (see Mortimer and Templeton, 1982; Templeton and Mortimer, 1982). Such patients are fascinating, as recent experiments in knockout mice have shown that sperm transport to the oviduct can be defective in otherwise healthy animals with good sperm production (and good motility etc.), for example mice knockout for fertilin [Cho et al., 1998] or calmegin [Ikawa et al., 1997]. This is remarkable and allows an insight into possible molecular mechanisms underlying sperm transport while at the same time providing a stimulus for further research into this poorly developed area.

Perhaps the most well-known interaction between the female tract and the spermatozoon is the rapid influx of calcium stimulated by progesterone. This is one of the classical examples of nongenomic signaling (Revelli et al., 1998). Single-cell imaging studies show that progesterone causes a primary transient rise in intracellular calcium levels in approximately 80% of sperm, followed by a secondary rise that is thought to be responsible for the acrosome reaction (Kirkman-Brown et al., 2000). The mechanism(s) of this response are poorly understood and the nature of the progesterone 'receptor' on the sperm plasma membrane remains to be determined. In fact, even the existence of a plasma membrane progesterone receptor in other well-characterized nongenomic systems (e.g., *Xenopus* oocytes) is hotly debated (see discussion in Maller, 2001), with recent data suggesting that a form of the nuclear receptor acts as the cytoplasmic signaling receptor (Bayaa et al., 2000; Tian et al., 2000); that is, the membrane receptor does not exist! This would make sense for spermatozoa with the paucity of cytoplasm and close proximity of the nucleus to the membrane. Whatever the nature and location of the progesterone receptor, the physiological effect is very marked. However, it is still unclear what role, if any, it plays in vivo. One possibility is that progesterone may act at a local level to stimulate hyperactivation to release sperm from the epithelium (see Hunter et al. (1999) for data in pigs); however, this remains to be confirmed in other systems.

Sperm–egg fusion

The process of sperm–egg fusion is only beginning to be understood. However, several features can be identified. The acrosome reaction not only culminates in the release of enzymes but also brings about a remodeling of the plasma membrane. During the acrosome reaction, the plasma and outer acrosomal membranes fuse and the acrosomal matrix disappears. In order for the spermatozoon to maintain a patent enveloping membrane, the inner acrosomal and plasma membranes must fuse. As a result, new sperm membrane proteins become exposed that are likely integral to the success of sperm–egg fusion.

Recent data indicate that sperm–egg fusion is initiated by signal transduction processes involving adhesion molecules in the form of ligands and receptors on both sperm and egg plasma membranes. In fact these molecules are beginning to be characterized and there is significant support for the role of integrins in human sperm–oocyte interactions (Bronson and Fusi, 1996; Allen and Green, 1997; Evans, 2000). Integrins are a class of heterodimeric adhesion receptor molecule that participate in cell-to-cell and cell-to-substratum interactions and are present on essentially all human cells. Further, all mammalian eggs express integrins on their plasma membrane surface.

Integrins that recognize the Arg-Gly-Asp sequence (RGD) have been detected on the plasma membrane of human oocytes. Fibronectin and vitronectin, glycoproteins that contain functional RGD sequences, are present on human spermatozoa (Fusi et al., 1993; Bronson and Fusi, 1996; Snell and White, 1996; Allen and Green, 1997). When oligopeptides specifically designed to block fibronectin or vitronectin receptors were tested on human spermatozoa in a zona-free hamster oocyte assay, it was found that the peptide for blocking cell attachment to fibronectin was without effect while the other peptide, which blocks both fibronectin and vitronectin receptors, inhibited sperm–egg binding. These data suggest that a possible mechanism for sperm–egg adhesion and fusion involves an integrin–vitronectin receptor–ligand interaction (Fusi et al., 1996).

However, the role of the ADAM family (membrane-anchored proteins having a disintegrin and metalloprotease domain; for review see: Evans, 1999; Myles et al., 1999; Primakof and Myles, 2000) in sperm–oocyte interaction in the human is not clearcut. For example, studies from Len Hall have shown that the human sperm surface proteins fertilin α and tMDCII (t metalloproteinase-like, disintegrin-like cystein-rich domain II) are nonfunctional, but are present in many rodents and primates (Frayne et al., 1999; Jury et al., 1998). Interestingly, studies in mice using knockout animals have shown that fertilin α and β, at least in the mouse, are not necessary for membrane fusion (Cho et al., 1998, 2000).

Recent data, in the mouse, have focused on the role of CD9, an integral membrane protein belonging to a family of tetraspan-membrane proteins, which is reported to play a role in cell adhesion (Chen et al., 1999; Miller, et al., 2000). CD9 knockout female mice are normal but fail to undergo sperm–oocyte fusion, demonstrating the importance of CD9 in the fusion process (Kaji et al., 2000; Miyado et al., 2000). This field is rapidly developing and we should have further detailed information on the human in the near future.

Oocyte-activating factor

The spermatozoon is known to be responsible for oocyte activation (Schultz and Kopf, 1995). Activation involves the resumption of meiosis, as evidenced by extrusion of the second polar body, and the release of cortical granules into the perivitelline space. The cortical granules modify zona glycoproteins 2 and 3 on the zona pellucida, resulting in a loss of their ability to stimulate the acrosome reaction and tight binding so as to prevent penetration by supernumerary spermatozoa. This latter event apparently occurs before or simultaneous with the resumption of meiosis. Failure of the oocyte to synthesize or exocytose the cortical granules, and in a timely fashion, will result in polyspermic fertilization and embryodysgenesis.

The first and most notable event postincorporation of spermatozoon into the oocyte is sperm-induced calcium transient fluxes. Calcium is the main intracellular signal responsible for the initiation of oocyte activation. It is important to note that these calcium fluxes occur in series and over time, i.e., calcium oscillations. When only a single transient is induced, either by chemical or mechanical stimulation, the oocyte fails to activate. The precise mechanism(s) by which the spermatozoon induces calcium transients is unknown but there are data that support essentially two models for sperm-induced oocyte activation. The first model involves a ligand–receptor-mediated interaction and the second involves a soluble sperm-derived factor that enters the oocyte at the time of fusion (see Schultz and Kopf, 1995; Parrington, 2001).

Evidence for a receptor-mediated mechanism in oocyte activation comes largely from nonhuman mammalian systems and appears to involve either G protein or tyrosine phosphorylation activation of phospholipase C. This leads to the generation of inositol 1,4,5-trisphosphate, which, in turn, leads to the release of calcium from internal stores. A combination of experimental approaches has validated the participation of each component of this pathway in the stimulation of calcium transients, cortical granule secretion, and zona modifications (see, for example, Schultz and Kopf, 1995).

A second possible mechanism for sperm-induced oocyte activation is gaining credibility, and it can loosely be termed the "soluble sperm factor." It is proposed that during fusion of the plasma membrane with the oocyte membrane, a soluble sperm-derived factor diffuses from the sperm into the egg's cytoplasm, resulting in oocyte activation (e.g., initiation of calcium transients). Microinjection of mammalian sperm extracts has been shown to stimulate egg activation (Stice and Robl, 1990; Swann, 1990).

Recently, it was shown that the injection of a soluble factor from human sperm into human oocytes triggers activation currents (Dale et al., 1996). Interestingly, there appears to be cross-species activity, whereby soluble human sperm extract is able to activate oocytes from a number of nonhuman species. Although the nature of this factor remains to be resolved, recent data have suggested that, at least in mammals, it may be a novel form of phospholipase C (Parrington et al., 1999). In contrast, experiments in sea urchins suggest that nitric oxide synthase and nitric oxide-related bioactivity may act as egg activators (Kuo et al., 2000).

Regardless of which mechanism or collection of mechanisms is ultimately responsible for oocyte activation, the issue remains that at the time of sperm–egg fusion the initiating factor must be appropriately primed and situated to effect the desired response. Therefore, abnormalities in transcription, translation, or any other significant molecular process responsible for producing the oocyte-activating ligand/effector molecule during spermatogenesis and/or spermiogenesis will ultimately render the fertilization event as moot.

The sperm centrosome

During the time course of IVF, the sperm centrosome is orchestrating pronuclear mobilization, syngamy and, ultimately, early cleavage. Most of what is known today about sperm centrosome structure and function has come from the work of Dr. Jerry Schatten and coworkers (for review see Schatten, 1994; Hewitson et al., 1998).

The paternally inherited human sperm centrosome, with the assistance of maternal γ-tubulin, nucleates sperm astral microtubules, unites paternal and maternal genomes, and forms the mitotic spindle. At the time of fertilization, the human sperm centrosome restores the zygotic centrosome, which is the organizing center for microtubules. In doing so, the polarity and three-dimensional structure of the embryo is established.

The significance of the sperm centrosome and its impact on postfertilization events and early embryo development was revealed in a study that investigated oocytes judged to have failed IVF (Asch et al., 1995). Based on immunocytochemistry, these investigators found that approximately 50% of oocytes that "failed" to fertilize had actually started fertilization but for some reason they had arrested at some point during or shortly after sperm penetration. Their results revealed an interesting array of causes, which included (i) egg activation but no sperm incorporation; (ii) arrest after sperm penetration; (iii) no microtubule nucleation; (iv) "silent" polyspermy, in which the number of sperm nuclei within the oocyte are not revealed by counting pronuclear

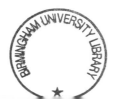

number; (v) sperm aster arrests; (vi) aster growth defect/detachment; and (vii) mitotic arrests.

The above abnormalities arose during the time course of standard IVF. So, the question might be asked: will ICSI help to obviate some of these deleterious events? On the one hand we can probably say, yes. Sperm incorporation problems will be averted. On the other hand, what about postpenetration abnormalities? Preliminary data from rhesus monkey ICSI (Hewitson et al., 1998) indicate that the same types of centrosomal dysfunction occur as were detected in human oocytes. It is hoped that the rhesus model along with new models for assessing centrosomal function (e.g., *Xenopus* oocyte extract) will advance our understanding about centrosomal function and its role in human embryogenesis. In the future, there might even be the potential for centrosome replacement therapy to correct for sperm centrosome-related infertility.

What attributes of spermatozoa are needed for assisted reproduction?

The attributes that we have discussed above primarily relate to those processes that take place during normal, in vivo conception. As the development and use of ART increases, we are slowly learning which functions of a sperm are necessary for the different types of assisted conception. Therefore, the question can be asked: What attributes become redundant when various ARTs are applied?

Because of the limited number of studies and the wide range in patient pathology, it is difficult to detect any deleterious pattern resulting from using germ cells in the extreme case of assisted fertilization, i.e., ICSI. Certainly, many normally requisite in vivo and in vitro functional attributes of the spermatozoon (e.g., motility, capacitation) appear to be irrelevant.

However, when it comes to germ cell maturity there is considerable debate as to what is the least advanced stage (e.g., secondary spermatocyte, spermatid) in germ cell development necessary for full embryonic development and that will lead to a viable fetus. In the human, current consensus is that round spermatid and earlier forms in germ cell development are, in general, lacking the appropriate components necessary for full embryo development. Later forms in germ cell development (e.g., elongating/elongated spermatid stage) do have more of "the right stuff" that contributes to normal embryogenesis and successful parturition (Ghazzawi et al., 1999; Sousa et al., 1999; Silber et al., 2000). Therefore, achievement of the haploid state is, at present, a necessary attribute regardless of the type of ART being applied. If one compares the outcome from ICSI using sperm from patients with nonobstructive and obstructive azoospermia, it is apparent that the progression of pregnancy is adversely affected in the former category of men, suggesting compromised germ cell functional development (for review see Tournaye et al., 1999). Further, the same holds true for ICSI using ejaculated cells and where manifestations of defective spermatogenesis exist (triple defects in semen analysis), the consequence being a significantly higher association with intrauterine death (Aytoz et al., 1998). Therefore, although ICSI can produce viable conceptions there does appear to be a subgroup of men with germ cell functional abnormalities that cannot be compensated for even by sperm injection into the egg cytoplasm.

In the aforementioned examples, one can speculate that one or more dysfunctional molecular processes, as yet undetectable using current methods for semen analysis, occurring during and/or after spermatogenesis and/or spermiogenesis contributed to an inviable pregnancy. Experiments in mammals, such as knockout mice, are providing basic information as to which genes are necessary to achieve fertility but we are still a long way from being able to predict, accurately, which men will or will not achieve success with ICSI (see, for example, Larson et al., 2000).

With the advent of ICSI, significantly reduced fertilization success and fertilization failure at IVF is unusual; however, cases do exist. In contrast to ICSI, unassisted IVF requires motile spermatozoa that can bind to and successfully penetrate the zona pellucida and oolemma. For example, Liu and Baker have studied IVF fertilization failure defects in men with normal semen parameters. In a large proportion of these, the spermatozoa were unable either to bind to or to penetrate the zona pellucida (termed, defective zona-induced acrosome reaction; Liu and Baker, 2000). Although fertilization can be facilitated by ICSI, it remains unclear for these men where in germ cell development the lesion(s) developed and the precise nature of the cellular/molecular dysfunction(s) in the mature spermatozoa. Therefore, sperm from these individuals may serve as a good experimental tool to study at least one attribute required for successful unassisted IVF.

Intrauterine insemination (IUI) is a very effective treatment for mild male factor infertility, so much so that it is often recommended as a first-line treatment (Goverde et al., 2000). In comparison with the natural situation (normal coitus), it is difficult to characterize what attributes a spermatozoon can be lacking yet still achieve success in IUI. For example, the availability of more eggs and achievement of a better synchrony between ovulation and insemination (review Cohlen et al., 2000) are positively associated with increased success. In addition, insemination of greater than approximately 1 million motile spermatozoa into the uterus leads to significantly higher pregnancy rates (Dickey et al., 1999; review Tomlinson et al., 1999). Consequently, a minimum number of cells must be inseminated. Although detailed comparative data are not available on how many sperm are in the uterus under normal circumstances, it appears that IUI delivers significantly higher numbers than would be delivered through normal coitus (Williams et al., 1993; Ripps et al., 1994). In addition, recent data show that IUI success is dependent on maintenance of sperm motility over a 24-hour period (Branigan et al., 1999). However, it can be questioned whether this is any different to the normal situation. Except in the very few cases with cervical hostility, the simple act of placement of spermatozoa in the uterus is unlikely to confer any significant advantage to the spermatozoa, and several studies have shown that, providing success rates for intracervical insemination are high, there is no advantage in natural cycle IUI (for review

see O'Brien and Vandekerckhove, 2000). In summary, the attributes that are unnecessary for a spermatozoon for IUI, compared with natural conception, remain unidentified. However, it is likely that the simple insemination of higher numbers of motile spermatozoa is a primary factor governing success.

Conclusions

This update chapter was not intended to be an exhaustive and intensive review of all the outstanding andrology research that has occurred in the last decade or so. The intent was to highlight certain critical "attributes of the fertile spermatozoon" that have previously been underrepresented or that are recently novel. Each of the attributes has been deemed to play a crucial role in the fertilization process, whether it be at the beginning (e.g., capacitation and acrosome reaction), middle (fusion and oocyte activation), or end (syngamy). We feel that these discoveries, while originating in the basic science laboratory, will ultimately take their place, in one form or another, in the full spectrum of diagnostic tests offered in the clinical andrology laboratory.

REFERENCES

Aitken, R.J. (1997). Molecular mechanisms regulating human sperm function. *Molecular Human Reproduction*, **3**, 169–73.

Aitken, R.J., Harkiss, D., Knox, W., Paterson, M., and Irvine, D.S. (1998). A novel signal transduction cascade in capacitating human spermatozoa characterised by a redox-regulated, cAMP-mediated induction of tyrosine phosphorylation. *Journal of Cell Science*, **111**, 645–56.

Allen, C.A. and Green, D.P. (1997). The mammalian acrosome reaction: gateway to sperm fusion with the oocyte? *Bioessays*, **19**, 241–7.

Amann, R.P. (1989). Can the fertility potential of a seminal sample be predicted accurately? *Journal of Andrology*, **10**, 89–98.

Ariel, M., Cedar, H., and McCarrey, J. (1994). Developmental changes in methylation of spermatogenesis-specific genes include reprogramming in the epididymis. *Nature Genetics*, **7**, 59–63.

Arnoult, C., Kazam, I.G., Visconti, P.E., Kopf, G.S., Villaz, M., and Florman, H.M. (1999). Control of the low voltage-activated calcium channel of mouse sperm by egg ZP3 and by membrane hyperpolarization during capacitation. *Proceedings of the National Academy of Sciences USA*, **96**, 6757–62.

Arts, E., Jager, S., and Hoekstra, D. (1994). Evidence for the existence of lipid-diffusion barriers in the equatorial segment of human spermatozoa. *Biochemical Journal*, **304**, 211–18.

Asch, R., Simerly, C., Ord, T., Ord, V.A., and Schatten, G. (1995). The stages at which fertilization arrests in humans: defective sperm centrosome and sperm asters as causes of human infertility. *Human Reproduction*, **10**, 1897–906.

Awadalla, S.G., Friedman, C.I., Schmidt, G., Chin, N., and Kim, M.H. (1987). In vitro fertilization and embryo transfer as a treatment for male factor infertility. *Fertility and Sterility*, **47**, 807–11.

Aytoz, Carnus, M., Tournaye, H., Bonduelle, M., Van Steirteghem, A., and Devroey, A. (1998). Outcome of pregnancies after intracytoplasmic sperm injection and the effect of sperm origin and quality on this outcome. *Fertility and Sterility*, **70**, 500–5.

Barratt, C.L.R. and Hornby, D.P. (1995). Induction of the human acrosome reaction by rhuZP3. In: *Human Sperm Acrosome Reaction*, Fenichel, P. and Parinaud, J., eds. Colloque INSERM, John Libby Eurotext, Montrouge, France, pp. 105–22.

Barratt, C.L.R. and Pockley, G.A. (1998). New perspectives on immunorecognition of gametes and embryos: sperm survival in the female reproductive tract: presence of immunosuppression or absence of recognition? *Molecular Human Reproduction*, **4**, 309–17.

Bartolomei, M.S. and Tilghman, S.M. (1997). Genomic imprinting in mammals. *Annual Review of Genetics*, **31**, 493–525.

Bayaa, M., Booth, R.A., Sheng, Y., and Liu, X.J. (2000). The classical progesterone receptor mediates *Xenopus* oocyte maturation through a nongenomic mechanism. *Proceedings of the National Academy of Sciences USA*, **97**, 12607–12.

Benoff, S. (1997). Carbohydrates and fertilization: an overview. *Molecular Human Reproduction*, **3**, 599–637.

Benoff, S. (1998). Voltage dependent calcium channels in mammalian spermatozoa. *Frontiers in Bioscience*, **3**, d1220–40.

Bernardini, L., Martini, E., Geraedts, G.P.M., et al. (1997). Comparison of gonosomal aneuploidy in spermatozoa of normal fertile men and those with severe male factor detected by in-situ hybridization. *Molecular Human Reproduction*, **3**, 431–8.

Birnbaumer, L., Boulay, G., Brown, D., et al. (2000). Mechanism of capacitative Ca^{2+} entry (CCE): interaction between IP3 receptor and TRP links the internal calcium storage compartment to plasma membrane CCE channels. *Recent Progress in Hormone Research*, **55**, 127–61.

Bonduelle, M., Aytoz, A., Van Assche, E., Devroey, P., Liebaers, I., and Van Steirteghem, A. (1998). Incidence of chromosomal aberrations in children born after assisted reproduction through intracytoplasmic sperm injection. *Human Reproduction*, **13**, 781–2.

Boulay, G., Brown, D.M., Qin, N., et al. (1999). Modulation of Ca^{2+} entry by polypeptides of the inositol 1,4,5-trisphosphate receptor (IP3R) that bind transient receptor potential (TRP): evidence for roles of TRP and IP3R in store depletion-activated Ca^{2+} entry. *Proceedings of the National Academy of Sciences USA*, **96**, 14955–60.

Brandelli, A., Miranda, P.V., and Tezon, J.G. (1996). Voltage-dependent calcium channels and G_i regulatory protein mediate the human sperm acrosomal exocytosis induced by *N*-acetylglucosaminyl/mannosyl neoglycoproteins. *Journal of Andrology*, **17**, 522–9.

Branigan, E.F., Estes, M.A., and Muller, C.H. (1999). Advanced semen analysis: a simple screening test to predict intrauterine insemination success. *Fertility and Sterility*, **71**, 547–51.

Breitbart, H. and Spungin, B. (1997). The biochemistry of the acrosome reaction. *Molecular Human Reproduction*, **3**, 195–202.

Bronson, R. A. and Fusi, F. M. (1996). Integrins and human reproduction. *Molecular Human Reproduction*, **2**, 153–68.

Brucker, C. and Lipford, G.B. (1995) The human sperm acrosome reaction: physiology and regulatory mechanisms: an update. *Human Reproduction Update*, **1**, 51–62.

Burks, D.J., Carballada, R., Moore, H.D.M., and Saling, P.M. (1995). Interaction of a tyrosine kinase from human sperm with the zona pellucida at fertilization. *Science*, **269**, 83–6.

Carrera, A., Moos, J., Gerton, G.L., Tesarik, J., Kopf, G.S., and Moss, S.B. (1996). Regulation of protein tyrosine phosphorylation in human sperm by a calcium/calmodulin dependent mechanism: identification of A kinase anchor proteins as major substrates for tyrosine phosphorylation. *Developmental Biology*, **180**, 284–96.

Chapman, N.R., Kessopoulou, E., Andrews, P.D., Hornby, D.P., and Barratt, C.L.R. (1998). The polypeptide backbone of recombinant human zona pellucida glycoprotein 3 initiates acrosomal exocytosis in human spermatozoa *in vitro*. *Biochemical Journal*, **330**, 839–45.

Chauhan, M., Barratt, C.L.R., Cooke, S., and Cooke, I.D. (1989). Differences in the fertility of donor insemination recipients – a study to provide prognostic guidelines as to the success and outcome. *Fertility and Sterility*, **51**, 815–19.

Chen, M.S., Tung, K.S.K., Coonrod, S.A., et al. (1999). Role of the integrin-associated protein CD9 in binding between sperm

ADAM 2 and the egg integrin $\alpha6\beta1$: implications for murine fertilization. *Proceedings of the National Academy of Sciences USA*, **96**, 11830–5.

Chen, Y., Cann, M.J., Litvin, T.N., et al. (2000). Soluble adenylyl cyclase as an evolutionarily conserved bicarbonate sensor. *Science*, **289**, 625–8.

Cho, C., Bunch, D.O., Faure, J.E., et al. (1998). Fertilization defects in sperm from mice lacking fertilin beta. *Science*, **281**, 1857–9.

Cho, C., Ge, H., Branciforte, D., Primakoff, P., and Myles, D.G. (2000). Analysis of mouse fertilin in wild-type and fertilin $\beta-$ sperm: evidence for C-terminal modification, α/β dimerization, and lack of essential role of fertilin α in sperm–egg fusion. *Developmental Biology*, **222**, 289–95.

Cohlen, B.J., Vandekerckhove, P., te Velde, E.R., and Habbema, J.D.F. (2000). Timed intercourse versus intra-uterine insemination with or without ovarian hyperstimulation for subfertility in men (Cochrane Review). In: *The Cochrane Library*, Vol. 4. Update Software, Oxford.

Cowan, A.E., Myles, D., and Koppel, D. (1987). Lateral diffusion of the PH-20 protein on guinea pig sperm: evidence that barriers to diffusion maintain plasma membrane domains in mammalian sperm. *Journal of Cell Biology*, **104**, 917–23.

Cross, N.L. (1996). Human seminal plasma prevents sperm from becoming acrosomally responsive to the agonist, progesterone: cholesterol is the major inhibitor. *Biology of Reproduction*, **54**, 138–45.

Cummins, J.M., Jequier, A.M., and Kan, R. (1994). Molecular biology of human male infertility – links with aging, mitochondrial genetics, and oxidative stress? *Molecular Reproduction and Development*, **37**, 345–62.

Cummins, J.M., Wakayama, T., and Yanagimachi, R. (1998). Fate of microinjected spermatid mitochondria in the mouse oocyte and embryo. *Zygote*, **6**, 213–22.

Dale, B., Fortunato, A., Monfrecola, V., and Tosti, E. (1996). A soluble sperm factor gates calcium-activated potassium channels in human oocytes. *Journal of Assisted Reproduction and Genetics*, **13**, 573–7.

Darszon, A., Labarca, P., Nishigaki, T., and Espinosa, F. (1999). Ion channels in sperm physiology. *Physiological Reviews*, **79**, 481–510.

Davis, B.K. (1981). Timing of fertilization in mammals: sperm cholesterol/phospholipid ratio as a determinant of the capacitation interval. *Proceedings of the National Academy of Sciences USA*, **78**, 7560–4.

De Jonge, C.J., Mack, S.R., and Zaneveld, L.J.D. (1989). Inhibition of the human sperm acrosome reaction by proteinase inhibitors. *Gamete Research*, **23**, 387–97.

de Lamirande, E., Leclerc, P., and Gagnon, C. (1997). Capacitation as a regulatory event that primes spermatozoa for the acrosome reaction and fertilization. *Molecular Human Reproduction*, **3**, 175–94.

Dickey, R.P., Pyrzak, R., Lu, P.Y., Taylor, S.N., and Rye, P.H. (1999). Comparison of the sperm quality necessary for successful intrauterine insemination with World Health Organization threshold values for normal sperm. *Fertility and Sterility*, **71**, 684–9.

Dowsing, A.T., Yong, E.L., Clark, M., McLachlan, R.I., de Kretser, D.M., and Trounson, A.O. (1999). Linkage between male infertility and trinucleotide repeat expansion in the androgen-receptor gene. *Lancet*, **354**, 640–3.

Eddy, E.M. and O'Brien, D.A. (1994). The spermatozoon. In: *The Physiology of Reproduction*, Vol. 1, Knobil, E. and Neill, J., eds. Raven Press, New York, p. 29–77.

Egozcue, J., Blanco, J., and Vidal, F. (1997). Chromosome studies in human sperm nuclei using fluorescence in-situ hybridization (FISH). *Human Reproduction Update*, 3, 441–52.

Egozcue, S., Blanco, J., Vendrell, J.M., et al. (2000). Human male infertility: chromosome anomalies, meiotic disorders, abnormal spermatozoa and recurrent abortion. *Human Reproduction Update*, **6**, 93–105.

Evans, J.P. (1999). Sperm disintegrins, egg integrins, and other cell adhesion molecules of mammalian gamete plasma membrane interactions. *Frontiers in Bioscience*, **4**, d114–31.

Evans, J.P. (2000). Getting sperm and egg together: things conserved and things diverged. *Biology of Reproduction*, **63**, 355–60.

Evenson, D.P. (1990). Flow cytometric analysis of male germ cell quality. *Methods in Cell Biology*, **33**, 401–10.

Evenson, D.P., Darzynkiewicz, Z., Jost, L., Janka, F., and Ballachey, B. (1986). Changes in accessibility of DNA to various fluorochromes during spermatogenesis. *Cytometry*, **7**, 45–53.

Evenson, D.P., Jost, L.K., Marshall, D., et al. (1999). Utility of the sperm chromatin structure assay as a diagnostic and prognostic tool in the human fertility clinic. *Human Reproduction*, **14**, 1039–49.

Flesch, F.M. and Gadella, B.M. (2000). Dynamics of the mammalian sperm plasma membrane in the process of fertilization. *Biochimica et Biophysica Acta*, **1469**, 197–235.

Foster, J.A., Klotz, K., Flickinger, C.J., et al. (1994). Human SP-10: acrosomal distribution, processing, and fate after the acrosome reaction. *Biology of Reproduction*, **51**, 1222–31.

Franken, D.R., Morales, P.J., and Habenicht, U.F. (1996). Inhibition of G protein in human sperm and its influence on acrosome reaction and zona pellucida binding. *Fertility and Sterility*, **66**, 1009–11.

Frayne, J., Dimsey, E.A. Jury, J.A., and Hall, L. (1999). Transcripts encoding the sperm surface protein tMDCII are non-functional in the human. *Biochemical Journal*, **341** (pt 3), 771–5.

Fusi, F.M., Vignali, M., Gailit, J., and Bronson, R.A. (1993). Mammalian oocytes exhibit specific recognition of the RGD (Arg-Gly-Asp) tripeptide and express oolemmal integrins. *Molecular Reproduction and Development*, **36**, 212–19.

Fusi, F.M., Bernocchi, N., Ferrari, A., and Bronson, RA. (1996). Is vitronectin the velcro that binds the gametes together? *Molecular Human Reproduction*, **2**, 859–66.

Gadella, B.M. and Harrison, R.A.P. (2000). The capacitating agent bicarbonate induces protein kinase A-dependent changes in phospholipid transbilayer behavior in the sperm plasma membrane. *Development*, **127**, 2407–20.

Gadella, B.M., Lopes-Cardozo, M., van Golde, L.M.G., Colenbrander, B., and Gadella, T.W.J., Jr. (1995). Glycolipid migration from the apical to the equatorial subdomains of the sperm head plasma membrane precedes the acrosome reaction. Evidence for a primary capacitation event in boar spermatozoa. *Journal of Cell Science*, **108**, 935–46.

Ghazzawi, I.M., Alhasani, S., Taher, M., and Souso, S. (1999). Reproductive capacity of round spermatids compared with mature spermatozoa in a population of azoospermic men. *Human Reproduction*, **14**, 736–40.

Goodwin, L.O., Karabinus, D.S., Pergolizzi, R.G., and Benoff, S. (2000). L-type voltage-dependent calcium channel α-1C subunit mRNA is present in ejaculated human spermatozoa. *Molecular Human Reproduction*, **6**, 127–36.

Gould, J.E., Overstreet, J.W., and Hanson, F.W. (1984). Assessment of human sperm function after recovery from the female reproductive tract. *Biology of Reproduction*, **31**, 888–94.

Goverde, A.J., McDonnell, J., Vermeiden, J.P., Schats, R., Rutten, F.F., and Schoemaker, J. (2000). Intrauterine insemination or in-vitro fertilisation in idiopathic subfertility and male subfertility: a randomised trial and cost-effectiveness analysis. *Lancet*, **355**, 13–18.

Harris, J.D., Seid, C.A., Fontenot, G.K., and Liu, H.F. (1999). Expression and purification of recombinant human zona pellucida proteins. *Protein Expression and Purification*, **16**, 293–307.

Hewitson, L., Simerly, C., Takahashi, D., and Schatten G. (1998). The role of the sperm centrosome during human fertilization and embryonic development: implications for intracytoplasmic sperm injection and other sophisticated ART strategies. In: *Modern ART in the 2000s: Andrology in the Nineties*, Ombelet, W., Bosmans, E., Vandeput, H., Vereecken, A., Renier, M., and Hoomans, E., eds. Parthenon, Lancaster, UK, pp. 139–56.

Hoffman, T., Obukhov, A.G., Schaefer, M., Harteneck, C.,

Gudermann, T., and Schultz, G. (1999). Direct activation of human TRPC6 and TRPC3 channels by diacylglycerol. *Nature*, **397**, 259–63.

Hunter, R.H. (1996). Ovarian control of very low sperm/egg ratios at the commencement of mammalian fertilisation to avoid polyspermy. *Molecular Reproduction and Development*, **44**, 417–22.

Hunter, R.H., Petersen, H.H., and Greve, T. (1999). Ovarian follicular fluid, progesterone and Ca^{2+} ion influences on sperm release from the fallopian tube reservoir. *Molecular Reproduction and Development*, **54**, 283–91.

Ikawa, M., Wada, I., Kominami, K., et al. (1997). The putative chaperone calmegin is required for sperm fertility. *Nature*, **387**, 607–11.

Janny, L. and Menezo, Y.J.R. (1994). Evidence for a strong paternal effect on human preimplantation embryo development and blastocyst formation. *Molecular Reproduction and Development*, **38**, 36–42.

Jury, J.A., Frayne, J., and Hall, L. (1998). Sequence analysis of a variety of primate fertilin alpha genes: evidence for non-functional genes in the gorilla and man. *Molecular Reproduction and Development*, **51**, 92–7.

Kaji, K., Oda, S., Shikano, T., et al. (2000). The gamete fusion process is defective in eggs of Cd9-deficient mice. *Nature Genetics*, **24**, 279–82.

Kent-First, M.G., Kol, S., Muallem, A., et al. (1996). The incidence and possible relevance of Y-linked microdeletions in babies born after intracytoplasmic sperm injection and their infertile fathers. *Molecular Human Reproduction*, **2**, 943–50.

Kerjean, A., Dupont, J., Vasseur, C., et al. (2000). Establishment of the paternal methylation imprint of the human *H19* and *MEST/PEG1* genes during spermatogenesis. *Human Molecular Genetics*, **14**, 2183–7.

Kirkman-Brown, J.C., Bray, C., Stewart, P.M., Barratt, C.L., and Publicover, S.J. (2000). Biphasic elevation of [Ca(2+)](i) in individual human spermatozoa exposed to progesterone. *Developmental Biology*, **222**, 326–35.

Kopf, G.S., Visconti, P.E., Moos, J., Galantino-Homer, H., and Ning, X.P. (1995). Integration of tyrosine kinase- and G-protein-mediated signal transduction pathways in the regulation of mammalian sperm function. In: *Human Sperm Acrosome Reaction*, Fenichel, P., and Parinaud, J., eds. S. Colloque INSERM, John Libbey Eurotext, p. 191.

Kopf, G.S., Ning, X.P., Visconti, P.E., Purdon, M., Galnatino-Homer, H., and Fornés, M. (1999). Signaling mechanisms controlling mammalian sperm fertilization competence and activation. In: *The Male Gamete: From Basic Science to Clinical Applications*, Gagnon, C., ed. Cache River Press, Vienna, IL, pp. 105–18.

Krausz, C., Quintana-Murci, L., and McElreavey, K. (2000). Prognostic value of Y deletion analysis. What is the clinical prognostic value of Y chromosome microdeletion analysis? *Human Reproduction*, **15**, 1431–4.

Kruger, T.F., Menkveld, R., Stander, F.S.H., et al. (1986). Sperm morphologic features as a prognostic factor in in vitro fertilization. *Fertility and Sterility*, **46**, 1118–23.

Kuo, R.C., Baxter, G.T., Thompson, S.H., et al. (2000). NO is necessary and sufficient for egg activation at fertilization. *Nature*, **406**, 633–6

Langlais, J., Kan, F.W.K., Granger, L., Raymond, L., Bleau, G., and Roberts, K.D. (1988). Identification of sterol acceptors that stimulate cholesterol efflux from human spermatozoa during in vitro capacitation. *Gamete Research*, **20**, 185–201.

Larson, K.L., De Jonge, C.J., Barnes, A.M., Jost, L.K., and Evenson, D.P. (2000). Sperm chromatin structure assay parameters as predictors of failed pregnancy following assisted reproductive techniques. *Human Reproduction*, **15**, 1717–22.

Lee, J.D., Kamiguchi, Y., and Yanagimachi, R. (1996). Analysis of chromosome constitution of human spermatozoa with normal and aberrant head morphologies after injection into mouse oocytes. *Human Reproduction*, **11**, 1942–6.

Lee, J.D., Allen, M.J., and Balhorn, R. (1997). Atomic force analysis of chromatin volumes in human sperm with head-shape abnormalities. *Biology of Reproduction*, **56**, 42–9.

Lee, M.A., Check, L.H., and Kopf, G.S. (1992). Guanine nucleotide-binding regulatory protein in human sperm mediates acrosomal exocytosis induced by the human zona pellucida. *Molecular Reproduction and Development*, **31**, 78–86.

Lenton, E.A. (1993). In: *Donor Insemination*, Barratt, C.L.R. and Cooke, I.D., eds. Cambridge University Press, Cambridge, UK, pp. 97–110.

Liow, S.L., Yong, E.L., and Ng, S.C. (2001). Prognostic value of Y deletion analysis. How reliable is the outcome of Y deletion analysis in providing a sound prognosis? *Human Reproduction*, **16**, 9–12.

Liu, D.Y. and Baker, H.W.G. (2000) Defective sperm-zona pellucida interaction: a major cause of failure of fertilization in clinical in-vitro fertilization. *Human Reproduction* **15**, 702–8.

Maller, J.L. (2001). The elusive progesterone receptor in *Xenopus* oocytes. *Proceedings of the National Academy of Sciences USA*, **98**, 8–10.

Manning, M., Lissens, W., Bonduelle, M., Camus, M., De Rijcke, M., Liebaers, I., and Van Steirteghem, A. (2000). Study of DNA-methylation patterns at chromosome 15q11–q13 in children born after ICSI reveals no imprinting defects. *Molecular Human Reproduction*, **6**, 1049–53.

Mansour, R.T., Aboulghar, M.A., Serour, G.I., Abbas, A.M.,

Ramzy, A.M., and Rizk, B. (1993). In vivo survival of spermatozoa in the human fallopian tube for 25 days: a case report. *Journal of Assisted Reproduction and Genetics*, **10**, 379–80.

Miller, B.J., Georges-Labouesse, E., Primakoff, P., and Myles, D.G. (2000). Normal fertilization occurs with eggs lacking the integrin alpha6beta1 and is CD9-dependent. *Journal of Cell Biology*, **149**, 1289–96.

Miyado, K., Yamada, G., Yamada, S., et al. (2000). Requirement of CD9 on the egg plasma membrane for fertilization. *Science*, **287**, 321–4.

Monckton, D.G., Cayuela, M.L., Gould, F.K., Brock, G.J., Silva, R., and Ashizawa, T. (1999). Very large (CAG) (n) DNA repeat expansions in the sperm of two spinocerebellar ataxia type 7 males. *Human Molecular Genetics*, **8**, 2473–8.

Moreno, R.D., Sepulveda, M.S., de Ioannes, A., and Barros, C. (1998). The polysulphate binding domain of human proacrosin/acrosin is involved in both the enzyme activation and spermatozoa-zona pellucida interaction. *Zygote*, **6**, 75–83.

Mortimer, D. and Templeton, A.A. (1982). Sperm transport in the human female reproductive tract in relation to semen analysis characteristics and the time of ovulation. *Journal of Reproduction and Fertility*, **64**, 401–8.

Mortimer, S.T. (1997). A critical review of the physiological importance and analysis of sperm movement in mammals. *Human Reproduction Update*, **3**, 403–39.

Mutter, G.L. (1997). Role of imprinting in abnormal human development. *Mutation Research*, **396**, 141–7.

Myles, D.G., Koppel, D.E., Cowan, A.E., Phelps, B.M., and Primakoff, P. (1987). Rearrangement of sperm surface antigens prior to fertilization. *Annals of the New York Academy of Sciences*, **513**, 262–73.

Myles, D.G., Cho, C., Yuan, R., and Primakoff, P. (1999). A current model for the role of ADAMS and integrins in sperm–egg membrane binding and fusion in mammals. In: *The Male Gamete: From Basic Science to Clinical Applications*, Gagnon, C., ed. Cache River Press, Vienna, IL, pp. 249–55.

Nakao, M. and Sasaki, H. (1996). Genomic imprinting: significance in development and diseases and the molecular mechanisms. *Journal of Biochemistry*, **120**, 467–73.

O'Brien, P. and Vandekerckhove, P. (2000). Intra-uterine versus cervical insemination of donor sperm for subfertility (Cochrane Review). In: *The Cochrane Library*, Vol. 4. Update Software, Oxford.

Osheroff, J.E., Visconti, P.E., Valenzuela, J.P., Travis, A.J., Alvarez, J., and Kopf, G.S. (1999). Regulation of human sperm capacitation by a cholesterol efflux-stimulated signal transduction pathway leading to protein kinase A-mediated up-regulation of protein tyrosine phosphorylation. *Molecular Human Reproduction*, **5**, 1017–26.

O'Toole, C.M., Arnoult, C., Darszon, A., Steinhardt, R.A., and Florman, H.M. (2000). Ca(2+) entry through store-operated channels in mouse sperm is initiated by egg ZP3 and drives the acrosome reaction. *Molecular Biology of the Cell*, **11**, 1571–84.

Pacey, A.A., Davies, N., Warren, M.A., Barratt, C.L., and Cooke, I.D. (1995). Hyperactivation may assist human spermatozoa to detach from intimate association with the endosalpinx. *Human Reproduction*, **10**, 2603–9.

Page, D.C., Silber, S., and Brown, L.G. (1999). Men with infertility caused by AZFc deletion can produce sons by intracytoplasmic sperm injection, but are likely to transmit the deletion and infertility. *Human Reproduction*, **14**, 1722–6.

Pandya, I.J., Mortimer, D., and Sawers, R.S. (1986). A standardized approach for evaluating the penetration of human spermatozoa into cervical mucus in vitro. *Fertility and Sterility*, **45**, 357–65.

Parrington, J. (2001). Does a soluble sperm factor trigger calcium release in the egg at fertilization? *Journal of Andrology*, **22**, 1–11.

Parrington, J., Jones, K.T., Lai, A., and Swann, K. (1999). The soluble sperm factor that causes Ca^{2+} release from sea-urchin (*Lytechinus pictus*) egg homogenates also triggers Ca^{2+} oscillations after injection into mouse eggs. *Biochemical Journal*, **341**, 1–4.

Primakoff, P. and Myles, D.G. (2000). The ADAM gene family: surface proteins with adhesion and protease activity. *Trends in Genetics*, **16**, 83–7.

Publicover, S.J. and Barratt, C.L.R. (1999). Voltage operated Ca^{2+} channels and the acrosome reaction: which channels are present and what do they do? *Human Reproduction*, **4**, 873–9.

Ravnik, S.E., Zarutskie, P.W., and Muller, C.H. (1990). Lipid transfer activity in human follicular fluid: relation to human sperm capacitation. *Journal of Andrology*, **11**, 216–6.

Ravnik, S.E., Albers, J.J., and Muller, C.H. (1993). A novel view of albumin-supported sperm capacitation: role of lipid transfer protein-I. *Fertility and Sterility*, **59**, 629–38.

Revelli, A., Massobrio, M., and Tesarik, J. (1998). Non-genomic actions of steroid hormones in reproductive tissues. *Endocrine Reviews*, **19**, 3–17.

Ripps, B.A., Minhas, B.S., Carson, S.A., and Buster, J.E. (1994). Intrauterine insemination in fertile women delivers larger numbers of sperm to the peritoneal fluid than intracervical insemination. *Fertility and Sterility*, **61**, 398–400.

Ron-El, R., Nachum, H., Herman, A., Golan, A., Caspi, E., and Soffer, Y. (1991). Delayed fertilization and poor embryonic development associated with impaired semen quality. *Fertility and Sterility*, **55**, 338–44.

Ron-El, R., Strassburger, D., Gelman-Kohan, S., Friedler, S., Raziel, A., and Appelman, Z. (2000). A 47, XXY fetus conceived after ICSI of spermatozoa from a patient with non-mosaic Klinefelter's syndrome. *Human Reproduction*, **15**, 1804–6.

Rossato, M., Di Virgilio, F., Rizzuto, R., Galeazzi, C., and Foresta, C. (2001). Intracellular calcium store depletion and acrosome reaction in human spermatozoa: role of calcium and plasma membrane potential. *Molecular Human Reproduction*, **7**, 119–28.

Sakkas, D., Bianchi, P.G., Manicardi, G., Bizzaro, D., and Bianchi, U. (1997). Chromatin packaging anomalies and DNA damage in human sperm: their possible implications in the treatment of male factor infertility. In: *Genetics of Human Male Fertility*, Barratt, C., De Jonge, C.J., Mortimer, D., and Parinaud, J., eds. Editions E.D.K., Paris, pp. 205–21.

Sallese, M., Mariggio, S., Collodel, G., et al. (1997). G protein-coupled receptor kinase GRK4. Molecular analysis of the four isoforms and ultrastructural localization in spermatozoa and germinal cells. *Journal of Biological Chemistry*, **11**, 10188–95.

Saut, N., Terriou, P., Navarro, A., Lévy, N., and Mitchell, M.J. (2000). The human Y chromosome genes *BPY2*, *CDY1* and *DAZ* are not essential for sustained fertility. *Molecular Human Reproduction*, **6**, 789–93.

Schatten, G. (1994). The centrosome and its mode of inheritance: the reduction of the centrosome during gametogenesis and its restoration during fertilization. *Developmental Biology*, **165**, 299–335.

Schultz, R.M. and Kopf, G.S. (1995). Molecular basis of mammalian egg activation. *Current Topics in Developmental Biology*, **30**, 21–62.

Silber, S.J., Alagappan, R., Brown, L.G., and Page, D.C (1998). Y chromosome deletions in azoospermic and severely oligozoospermic men undergoing intracytoplasmic sperm injection after testicular sperm extraction. *Human Reproduction*, **13**, 3332–7.

Silber, S.J., Johnson, L., Verheyen, G., and Van Steirteghem, A. (2000). Round spermatid injection. *Fertility and Sterility*, **73**, 897–900.

Simon, I., Tenzen, T., Reubinoff, B.E., Hillman, D., McCarrey, J.R., and Cedar, H. (1999). Asynchronous replication of imprinted genes is established in the gametes and maintained during development. *Nature*, **401**, 929–32.

Smith, T.T. and Yanagimachi, R. (1990). The viability of hamster spermatozoa stored in the isthmus of the oviduct: the importance of sperm-epithelium contact for sperm survival. *Biology of Reproduction*, **42**, 450–7.

Smith, T.T. and Yanagimachi, R. (1991). Attachment and release of spermatozoa from the caudal isthmus of the hamster oviduct. *Journal of Reproduction and Fertility*, **91**, 567–73.

Snell, W.J. and White, J.M. (1996). The molecules of mammalian fertilization. *Cell*, **85**, 629–37.

Sousa, M., Barros, A., Takahashi, K., Oliveria, C., Silva, J., and Tesarik, J. (1999) Clinical efficacy of spermatid conception: analysis using a new spermatid classification scheme. *Human Reproduction* **14**, 1279–86.

Spanò, M., Bonde, J.P., Hjøllund, H.I., and The Danish First Pregnancy Planner Study Team (2000). Sperm chromatin damage impairs human fertility. *Fertility and Sterility*, **73**, 43–50.

St. John, J.C. and De Jonge, C.J. (2000). A hypothesis for transmission of paternal mitochondrial DNA. *Reproductive Medicine Review*, **8**, 73–85.

St. John, J.C., Sakkas, D., and Barratt, C.L.R. (2000a). A role for mitochondrial DNA and sperm survival. *Journal of Andrology*, **21**, 189–99.

St. John, J., Sakkas, D., Dimitriadi, K., et al. (2000b). Failure of elimination of paternal mitochondrial DNA in abnormal embryos. *Lancet*, **355**, 200.

St. John, J.C., Jokhi, R.P., and Barratt, C.L. (2001). Men with oligoasthenoteratozoospermia harbour higher numbers of multiple mitochondrial DNA deletions in their spermatozoa, but individual deletions are not indicative of overall aetiology. *Molecular Human Reproduction*, **7**, 103–11.

Staessen, C., Coonen, E., Van Assche, E., et al. (1996). Preimplementation diagnosis for X and Y normality in embryos from three Klinefelter patients. *Human Reproduction*, **11**, 1650–3.

Stice, S. and Robl, J. (1990). Activation of mammalian oocytes by a factor obtained from rabbit sperm. *Molecular Reproduction and Development*, **25**, 272–80.

Sun, C., Skaletsky, H., Birren, B., et al. (1999). An azoospermic man with a de novo point mutation in the Y-chromosomal gene USP9Y. *Nature Genetics*, **23**, 429–32.

Sutovsky, P., Navara, C.S., and Schatten, G. (1996). Fate of the sperm mitochondria, and the incorporation, conversion, and disassembly of the sperm tail structures during bovine fertilization. *Biology of Reproduction*, **55**, 1195–205.

Swann, K. (1990). A cytosolic sperm factor stimulates repetitive calcium increases and mimics fertilization in hamster eggs. *Development*, **110**, 1295–302.

Templeton, A.A. and Mortimer, D. (1982). The development of a clinical test of sperm migration to the site of fertilisation. *Fertility and Sterility*, **37**, 410–15.

Tesarik, J. (1989). Appropriate timing of the acrosome reaction is a major requirement for the fertilizing spermatozoon. *Human Reproduction*, **4**, 957–61.

Tesarik, J., Drahorad, J., and Peknicova, J. (1988). Subcellular immunochemical localization of acrosin in human spermatozoa during the acrosome reaction and the zona pellucida penetration. *Fertility and Sterility*, **50**, 133–41.

Tesarik, J., Drahorad, J., Testart, J., and Mendoza C. (1990). Acrosin activation follows its surface exposure and precedes membrane fusion in human sperm acrosome reaction. *Development*, **110**, 391–400.

Tesarik, J., Carreras, A., and Mendoza, C. (1993). Differential sensitivity of progesterone- and zona pellucida-induced acrosome reactions to pertussis toxin. *Molecular Reproduction and Development*, **34**, 183–9.

Tian, J., Kim, S., Heilig, E., and Ruderman, J.V. (2000). Identification of XPR-1, a progesterone receptor required for *Xenopus* oocyte activation. *Proceedings of the National Academy of Sciences USA*, **97**, 14358–63.

Tomlinson, M.J., Kessopoulou, E., and Barratt, C.L.R. (1999). Predictive clinical value of traditional semen parameters. *Journal of Andrology*, **20**, 588–93.

Tournaye, H., Merdad, T., Silber, S., et al. (1999). No differences in outcome after intracytoplasmic sperm injection with fresh or with frozen-thawed epididymal spermatozoa. *Human Reproduction*, **14**, 90–5.

Trasler, J.M. (1998). Origin and roles of genomic methylation patterns in male germ cells. *Seminars in Cell and Developmental Biology*, **9**, 467–74.

Van Assche, E., Staessen, C., Vegetti, W., et al. (1999). Preimplementation genetic diagnosis and sperm analysis by fluorescence in-situ hybridization for the most common reciprocal translocation t(11;22). *Molecular Human Reproduction*, **5**, 682–90.

van Duin, M., Ploman, J.E.M., De Breet, I.T.M., et al. (1994). Recombinant human zona pellucida protein ZP3 produced by Chinese hamster ovary cells induces the human sperm acrosome reaction and promotes sperm-egg fusion. *Biology of Reproduction*, **51**, 607–17.

Van Dyk, Q., Lanzendorf, S., Kolm, P., Hodgen, G.D., and Mahony, M.C. (2000). Incidence of aneuploid spermatozoa from subfertile men: selected with motility versus hemizonabound. *Human Reproduction*, **15**, 1529–36.

Van Landuyt, L., Lissens, W., Stouffs, K., Tournaye, H., Liebaers, I., and Van Steirteghem, A. (2000). Validation of a simple Yq deletion screening programme in an ICSI candidate population. *Molecular Human Reproduction*, **6**, 291–7.

Vegetti, W., Van Assche, E., Frias, A., et al. (2000). Correlation between semen parameters and sperm aneuploidy rates investigated by fluorescence in-situ hybridization in infertile men. *Human Reproduction*, **15**, 351–65.

Visconti, P.E., Ning, X., Fornés, M.W., et al. (1999a). Cholesterol efflux-mediated signal transduction in mammalian sperm: cholesterol release signals an increase in protein tyrosine phosphorylation during mouse sperm capacitation. *Developmental Biology*, **214**, 429–43.

Visconti, P.E., Stewart-Savage, J., Blasco, A., et al. (1999b). Roles of bicarbonate, cAMP, and protein tyrosine phosphorylation on capacitation and the spontaneous acrosome reaction of hamster sperm. *Biology of Reproduction*, **61**, 76–84.

Ward, W.S. and Coffey, D.S. (1991). DNA packaging and organization in mammalian spermatozoa: comparison with somatic cells (review). *Biology of Reproduction*, **44**, 569–74.

Wennemuth, G., Westenbroek, R.E., Xu, T., Hille, B., and Babcock, D.F. (2000). CaV2.2 and CaV2.3 (N-and R-type) Ca^{2+} channels in depolarization-evoke entry of Ca^{2+} into mouse sperm. *Journal of Biological Chemistry*, **275**, 21210–17.

Westenbroek, R.E. and Babcock, D.F. (1999). Discrete regional distributions suggest diverse functional roles of calcium channel alpha1 subunits in sperm. *Developmental Biology*, **207**, 457–69.

Whitmarsh, A.J., Woolnough, M.J., Moore, H.D.M., Hornby, D.P., and Barratt, C.L.R. (1996). Biological activity of recombinant human ZP3 produced in vitro: potential for a sperm function test. *Molecular Human Reproduction*, **2**, 911–19.

Wilcox, A.J., Weinberg, C.R., and Baird, D.D. (1995). Timing of sexual intercourse in relation to ovulation. *New England Journal of Medicine*, **333**, 1517–21.

Wilcox, A.J., Dunson, D., and Baird, D.D. (2000). The timing of the "fertile window" in the menstrual cycle: day specific estimates from a prospective study. *British Medical Journal*, **321**, 1259–62.

Williams, M., Hill, C.J., Scudamore, I., Dunphy, B., Cooke, I.D., and Barratt, C.L. (1993). Sperm numbers and distribution within the human fallopian tube around ovulation. *Human Reproduction*, **8**, 2019–26.

Zaneveld, L.J.D. and De Jonge, C.J. (1991). Mammalian sperm acrosomal enzymes and the acrosome reaction. In: *A Comparative Overview of Mammalian Fertilization*, Dunbar, B.S. and O'Rand, M.G., eds. Plenum Press, New York, p. 63–79.

Zaneveld, L.J.D., Anderson, R.A., Mack, S.R., and De Jonge, C.J. (1993). Mechanism and control of the human sperm acrosome reaction. *Human Reproduction* **8**, 2006–8.

Zinaman, M., Drobnis, E.Z., Morales, P., et al. (1989). The physiology of sperm recovered from the human cervix: acrosomal status and response to inducers of the acrosome reaction. *Biology of Reproduction*, **41**, 790–7.

4

In vitro oogenesis

Frank L. Barnes

IVF Laboratory, L.L.C., Salt Lake City, Utah, USA

Introduction

Oogenesis is the term used to describe the complete biology of female germ cell growth and development. However, the term as it applies to the treatment of infertility shall describe the period of growth from the meiotic prophase-arrested oocyte of the primary follicle to the fully grown oocyte at metaphase II of meiotic arrest of the ovulated follicle. The need for this discussion regarding in vitro oogenesis starts with our desire to treat disease. Women confronted with life-threatening cancers may be additionally challenged with the concern that current therapies, both chemical and operative, can reduce or conclude their fertility. Schemes once believed to be too futuristic for medical application have moved from experimental modeling in laboratory and livestock animals to the brink of potential patient treatment modalities (Eppig and Schroeder, 1989; Cha et al., 1991; Looney et al., 1994; Trounson et al., 1994; Baird et al., 1999; Newton et al., 1999). Some of these possibilities are also fraught with problems, as reintroduction of disease can be a possibility (Shaw et al., 1996). In vitro oogenesis could electively prolong the fertile life of a woman; a young woman can cryopreserve ovarian tissue and utilize her germ cells later in life when, in vivo, their biological potential would have diminished. In vitro oocyte maturation (IVM), the final stages of in vitro oogenesis, could open up additional uses of this base technology. Controlled ovarian hyperstimulation (COH) in the treatment of infertility could become less a requirement and more of a choice. Immature oocyte collection (IOC) and IVM may not be dependent on COH to provide sufficient numbers of oocytes capable of totipotent development. This choice is attractive to potential oocyte donors, to fertile women whose male partners suffer from infertility, and to those patients that have significant risk of ovarian hyperstimulation syndrome. Therefore, the need exists to move oogenesis into the laboratory.

In vitro growth of follicles and oocytes

Young women challenged with malignant disease and faced with oophorectomy or chemotherapy may chose to have their ovarian cortical tissue frozen. Frozen ovarian cortical tissue can provide two avenues for prolonging fertility in these patients. Frozen thawed tissue may be regrafted to the patient and subsequent ovarian function restored. This approach has been applied in sheep with limited success (Baird et al., 1999). Unfortunately, experiments in mice have demonstrated that if cancer cells are present in the cryopreserved tissue reintroduction of disease is possible (Shaw et al., 1996). This concern could be alleviated if frozen, thawed primary follicles with their enclosed oocytes could be grown in vitro.

Methods for isolating primary follicles have been developed. The dense fibrous stroma of the human ovary creates an additional barrier to follicle isolation not encountered in laboratory animals. Manual isolation of follicles is difficult, tedious, time consuming, and does not lend itself to the recovery of large numbers of preantral follicles. Enzymatic digestion with collagenase has proven to be a satisfactory methodology in laboratory animals and can be successful in large mammals like ewes and women (Roy and Treacy, 1993; Newton et al., 1999). The difficulties with this methodology are the incubation period, the temperature conditions, and the concentration of enzyme required to break down stromal tissue. Roy and Treacy (1993) overcame this problem by adding an initial incubation period of 1 hour at 37°C followed by 36 hours of incubation at 4°C. The subsequent chilled incubation was partially quenched with bovine serum albumin. Metabolic substrate support for the preantral follicles was provided with minimum essential medium (Dulbecco's MEM). Their rationale was that cellular metabolism would be maintained at this reduced incubation temperature and stromal breakdown could occur sufficient to recover large populations of preantral follicles (Roy and Treacy, 1993). Newton and coworkers (1999) selected the ewe as a model to examine freeze–thaw survival of ovarian cortical tissue followed by enzymatic digestion, isolation, and culture. The ewe was selected because the ovine ovary contains fibrous ovarian stroma similar to that in women. Their experiments demonstrated that sheep primary follicles could survive cryopreservation, thawing, and isolation with a 1 hour collagenase digestion at 37°C followed by 3 hours of manual dissection at room temperature. Presumably, small primary follicles ($<190\,\mu$m) were able to survive cryopreservation but could not sustain the insult from enzymatic digestion and, as a consequence, degenerated in culture. Primary follicles larger than $190\,\mu$m faired somewhat better (Newton et al., 1999).

Some of the difficulties in establishing an in vitro culture system are providing substrate, growth factors, and conditions suitable for the different cell types involved. Such studies tend to favor either folliculogenesis or oogenesis. Parameters such as granulosa cell proliferation, steroid production, and follicle antrum formation predominate in folliculogenesis studies. Oocyte growth and meiotic, fertilization, and developmental competencies dominate in oogenesis studies. In recognizing this dilemma,

investigators have developed culture systems that allow the maintenance of the three-dimensional structure of the primary follicle (Roy and Greenwald, 1985; Torrence et al., 1989). Torrence and coworkers (1989) utilized a double collagen gel matrix in the culture of mouse preantral follicles. They reported that in this culture system normal growth of the follicle and the oocyte could occur without evidence of limited gas and metabolic diffusion. Roy and Treacy (1993) utilized an agar sandwich to culture human preantral follicles recovered from women 16 to 32 years of age. They observed that class II primary follicles were able to progress to antral follicles; follicle-stimulating hormone (FSH) was required to stimulate estradiol synthesis and granulosa cell proliferation and to prevent oocyte atresia. Unfortunately, no measurement of oocyte growth was made. As expected, the number of follicles recovered was dependent on the age of patient (Roy and Treacy, 1993).

A gel matrix may only be required for specific follicle size populations. More recent studies in mice and sheep have demonstrated that collagenase-digested ovaries can yield preantral follicles that, when cultured in a multiwell plate, grow and develop an atrum leading to significant oocyte growth (Boland et al., 1993; Spears et al., 1994, 1996; Johnson et al., 1995; Newton et al., 1999). In mice, this has led to oocytes achieving meiotic and developmental competence (Boland et al., 1993; Spears et al., 1994, 1996; Johnson et al., 1995). Follicles grown in 96-well flat-bottomed microtiter plates in α-MEM supplemented with transferrin, human FSH, and 5% mouse serum can ovulate oocytes in response to luteinizing hormone; after fertilization and transfer into pseudopregnant recipients, these oocytes produce viable offspring. It should be noted that follicles in these experiments were derived from mice aged 22 to 32 days (Boland et al., 1993; Spears et al., 1994). A similar approach has been used on cryopreserved and thawed cortical tissue from prepubertal sheep (Newton et al., 1999). Preantral follicles $\geq190\,\mu$m in size were able to grow to antral formation and demonstrate a concomitant increase in oocyte growth. Interestingly, this culture system was unable to support growth of smaller follicles. The authors noted that small preantral follicles lost their three-dimensional structure and appeared to be more sensitive to enzymatic digestion and isolation. This study indicates that three-dimensional structure can be maintained in vitro without a gel matrix although this may be dependent upon follicle size, stage and species.

Eppig and coworkers have shown that an intact follicle is not a requirement for oocyte growth and acquisition of developmental competence (Eppig and Schroeder, 1989; Eppig et al., 1996; Eppig and O'Brien, 1996, 1998). Utilizing 12-day-old mice as oocyte donors, they have isolated cumulus oocyte complexes (COC) by collagenase digestion (Eppig and Schroeder, 1989). These complexes will attach to collagen-impregnated membranes or serum-coated plates. With care not to dislodge the COC from the substrate, oocytes can grow for up to 10 days and achieve a size comparable to those of 18-day-old mice (Eppig and Schroeder, 1989). Oocytes grown in this fashion can be induced to mature and, following fertilization, give rise to viable offspring. The medium used in this system is MEM supplemented with 5% serum (fetal calf) and, in some instances, insulin, selenium and transferrin. FSH was not beneficial for oocyte growth or the acquisition of developmental competence but was required for in vitro meiotic maturation (Eppig and Schroeder, 1989; Eppig and O'Brien, 1996, 1998).

With only limited information available for women, the aforementioned studies present an optimistic view for the future of in vitro oogenesis for the treatment of infertility. Ovarian cortical tissue can successfully be cryopreserved and thawed with at least some preantral follicle categories maintaining viability. Enzymatic digestion can be used in conjunction with manual dissection to isolate efficiently preantral follicles of different sizes and stages. The requirement to use collagen or agar matrix to maintain three-dimensional follicle structure may be dependent on the follicle category and species being investigated. An intact follicular environment may not be necessary, as the culture of COC on collagen-impregnated membranes can produce developmentally competent oocytes. MEM can be use for basic cellular support. Supplements may include transferrin, serum, and pyruvate. The requirement for FSH for granulosa proliferation and oocyte health appears to be species dependent. The protocols discussed can lead to the birth of viable offspring in laboratory animals, but this has not yet been realized in larger mammals.

Current strategies in human in vitro maturation

The final events of in vitro oogenesis are the resumption of meiosis leading to germinal vesicle breakdown, the first meiotic reduction division, and arrest at metaphase II. In mammals, this final step proceeds spontaneously when immature oocytes are removed from antral follicles (Pincus and Enzmann, 1935; Edwards, 1965). The final requirements for the acquisition of developmental competence are as yet undefined because the implantation rate of embryos derived from human IVM oocytes has been low. It is, therefore, important to review the details involved with immature oocyte collection and IVM oocyte.

Cha and coworkers (1991) were the first to define and describe procedures for human oocyte IVM that could lead to pregnancy and birth. In their original work, oocytes were recovered from patients undergoing gynecological surgery and subsequently donated to their in vitro fertilization (IVF) program. When performed in situ, antral follicles were aspirated using a 21 gauge needle attached to a syringe containing media supplemented with 10% fetal cord serum. When oophorectomy was performed, oocytes were recovered by repeatedly slicing and subsequently rinsing the cortical tissue. This process yields two to three times more oocytes than follicle aspiration.

Trounson et al. (1994) were the first to use ultrasound-guided follicle aspiration for the recovery of human immature oocytes. In cooperation with Cook® IVF, they developed a needle with a thicker wall and shorter bevel for increased rigidity. The increased rigidity was required to penetrate the ovarian cortical stroma of patients with polycystic ovarian syndrome; the shortened bevel allowed the entire lumen of the needle to be inside the antral cavity of small follicles. The aspiration pressure used at oocyte collection was reduced to half that used in standard IVF (7.5 kPa versus 15 kPa). Lowered aspiration pressure is believed to reduce the amount of granulosa cells that are stripped from the oocyte during aspiration. Aspirates were recovered in Hepes-buffered HTF (human tubule fluid) medium supplemented with heparin. COCs were isolated by filtration through an EM-Con embryo-concentrating filter (Immuno Systems, Spring Valley, WI, USA). Fresh medium was used to rinse away red blood cells and other debris then the filter retentant was poured into a 100 mm dish for COC isolation using a dissecting microscope. This collection and isolation protocol has been used extensively and successfully in other laboratories (Trounson et al., 1994).

The rinse medium used to recover immature oocytes has varied between studies. Hams F-10, or Hams F-10 supplemented with 0.2% human serum albumin or heparin, has been used in protocols that have consistently produced pregnancies (Cha et al., 1991, 2000; Mikkelsen et al., 1999, 2000). Hepes-buffered HTF and phosphate-buffered saline, similarly supplemented, have been used in protocols with more inconsistent results and fewer reported pregnancies (Trounson et al., 1994; Barnes et al., 1995, 1996; Russell et al., 1997; Suikkari et al., 2000). Interestingly, physiological saline supplemented with heparin has been used in the protocol described by Chian et al. (2000), who have reported a clinical pregnancy rate of 38.5%.

Granulosa cells are the basic support system of the oocyte. Their maintenance and health are critical to oocyte development and maturation. In preliminary experiments using bovine granulosa cells in serum free culture, TCM (tissue culture medium) 199 performed better in maintaining viability compared with a large number of commercially available media. Based on this information, Barnes et al. (1999) used TCM 199 in their maturation protocol that led to the birth of a healthy child following IVM, intracytoplasmic sperm injection, blastocyst development and assisted hatching. Since that publication, TCM 199 has been used in nearly every human IVM protocol published.

Protein supplementation has varied slightly; the use of 10–20% patient or fetal calf serum (bovine spongiform encephalopathy free), 3% synthetic serum substitute or 0.4–0.5% human serum albumin has been reported (Cha et al., 1991; Trounson et al., 1994; Barnes et al., 1995, 1996; Russell et al., 1997; Chian et al., 2000; Suikkari et al., 2000). Gonadotropin concentrations have remained relatively unchanged since the original studies (Trounson et al., 1994). Human recombinant FSH is added at a concentration of 0.075 IU/ml and human chorionic gonadotropin at a concentration of 0.5 IU/ml (Trounson et al., 1994). Recently, Cha et al. (2000) have used gonadotropin from pregnant mares' serum at a concentration of 10 IU/ml and human chorionic gonadotropin at a concentration of 10 IU/ml. Pyruvate is included at a concentration of 0.27–0.33 mmol/l (Cha et al., 1991; Trounson et al., 1994; Barnes et al., 1995, 1996; Russell et al., 1997; Chian et al., 2000; Suikkari et al., 2000). These supplements and the concentrations described have been part of some of the most consistent IVM protocols published.

Estradiol is another common component of maturation medium. The role of estradiol as a supplement is unclear, as good-quality embryos can be produced from IVM oocytes cultured in unsupplemented media (Chian et al., 2000). Estradiol is easily absorbed into the oil overlay of microdrop culture systems. Cumulus granulosa cells produce estradiol when fetal calf serum and FSH are present in the culture medium (Chian et al., 1999). This suggests that estradiol may not be required as a supplement. Epidermal growth factor is emerging as a potential additive to the human IVM system. Its addition alone has been reported to increase the frequency of oocytes maturing to metaphase II, fertilizing, and forming blastocysts (Gomez et al., 1993; Goud et al., 1998; Cobo et al., 1999). The study by Cobo et al. (1999) demonstrating 56% blastocyst formation from IVM oocytes rivals that in standard IVF programs.

IVM protocols are remarkably similar across most studies. Unfortunately, significant differences exist between laboratories in their ability to produce pregnancies consistently. From this observation, it must be determined if the IVM procedure assists in the acquisition of oocyte developmental competence beyond the period of early cleavage and possibly beyond blastocyst development. With the current understanding, IVM may only provide the signal that allows the expression of the developmental potential inherent within the oocyte.

How COCs are processed between egg retrieval and culture, the follicle size from which they are derived, and their stage of growth (growing or atretic) relative to the dominant follicle can all have a dramatic impact on their ability to produce totipotent embryos (Sorensen and Wassarman, 1976; Tsuji et al., 1985; Eppig et al., 1992; Pavlok et al., 1992; Schramm et al., 1993; Blondin and Sirard, 1995; Blondin et al., 1996, 1997a; Moor and Trounson, 1997; Salamone et al., 1999). In cattle, where IOC and IVM are successfully used for the production of embryos from infertile and genetically valuable animals, these variables have been sufficiently characterized (Blondin and Sirard, 1995; Blondin et al., 1996, 1997a; Salamone et al., 1999). Oocytes acquire the competencies to mature, fertilize, and develop into totipotent embryos in a sequential manner. COCs derived from relatively large follicles have superior developmental potential to those from smaller follicles (Sorensen and Wassarman, 1976; Tsuji et al., 1985; Schramm et al., 1993; Eppig et al., 1992; Pavlok et al., 1992; Moor and Trounson, 1997). Within a cohort of follicles, one becomes dominant and the remaining follicles become atretic. If rescued in a timely manner, oocytes from small or large atretic follicles often exhibit surprising developmental potential (Pavlok et al., 1992; Blondin and Sirard, 1995; Moor and Trounson, 1997; Salamone et al., 1999). This points to two very interesting phenomena: (i) there is a transition period concomitant with the emergence of a dominant follicle when cohort follicles have significant developmental potential; and (ii) the initiation of the atretic process allows the expression of developmental competence if the in vitro conditions allow (Blondin and Sirard, 1995; Moor and Trounson, 1997). The duration of this period and the follicle size when competence can be expressed is species specific.

In cattle IOC programs, the dominant follicle (follicles 5 mm or greater) is removed prior to initiating stimulation for one to three days. Cows are then coasted (no additional exogenous gonadotropin administration) for 48 hours prior to IOC followed by IVM, IVF, and in vitro culture (Looney et al., 1994; Blondin et al., 1997b; Sirard et al., 1999). This protocol successfully increases the number of oocytes demonstrating advanced developmental potential. The optimum time of the bovine transition period is 48 hours, a period when follicles are being starved of exogenous FSH and initiating the very early stages of atresia (Sirard et al., 1999).

Definition of this transition period in humans is starting to emerge. Cobo et al. (1999) found that oocytes recovered from follicles prior to emergence of a dominant follicle demonstrated a higher frequency of blastocyst development. The period of dominance occurs when the lead follicle reaches 10 mm. That dominance occurs when the lead follicle reaches 10 mm in size has also been confirmed biochemically. In retrospective analysis, Mikkelsen et al. found that, for oocytes recovered when the lead follicle reached 10 mm, estradiol increased 100% over the value at day 3 and inhibin A increased by 80%; in addition, subsequent pregnancy rates were better (33% per transfer) (Mikkelsen et al., 1999, 2000). These biochemical measurements indicate selection of a dominant follicle and, as these authors stated, "implies that the oocytes selected for IVM . . . were obtained from follicles destined to go into atresia" (Mikkelsen et al., 2000). These studies suggest that an undefined transition period exists for the cohort follicles at the time of emergence of the dominant follicle and this can be visually accessed by ultrasound when the lead follicle achieves 10 mm in diameter.

Chian and co-authors have recently reported pregnancies following the treatment of patients with unstimulated polycystic ovarian syndrome with hCG 36 hours before IOC and IVM (Chian et al.,

2000). They have found that hCG priming of these patients can improve the developmental competence of the recovered oocytes, leading to improved maturation rates and higher pregnancy rates (38.5% per egg retrieval). The mechanism of action of hCG priming is unclear but may involve more than one pathway. It is currently not clear whether the human cumulus granulosa contains receptors for luteinizing hormone; hCG does not elicit a cumulus mucification of small follicles in vivo (less than 12 mm, personal observation). The positive effect of hCG may be derived from communication initiating at the level of the theca interstitial cells progressing to the granulosa syncytium. Potential effects include androgenation of the follicle, which is associated with atresia; alteration of oocyte metabolism through increases in glutamine, glycolytic activity, and mitochondrial glucose oxidation within cumulus cell enclosed oocytes; and/or direct signaling of the granulosa to differentiate (Colonna et al., 1989; Cecconi et al., 1991; Zuelke and Brackett, 1992, 1993). All of the events described could occur independently or together in the absence of cumulus expansion. The 36 hour time interval between hCG priming and IOC and IVM may be a more precise measurement of the transition period between the initiation of the atretic process and acquisition of developmental competence, as discussed in the preceding paragraph.

The seemingly different approaches by the different groups do appear to have a common theme (Cobo et al., 1999; Mikkelson et al., 1999, 2000; Chian et al., 2000). The COCs can be stimulated by a variety of stimuli that force them into the next stage of differentiation. This differentiation pathway may be shared regardless of whether the cumulus oocyte complex is destined to ovulate or degenerate. This event may occur with the selection of the dominant follicle and the artificial initiation of atresia in the cohort.

Eggbert and large offspring syndrome

Eggbert was a mouse produced from an oocyte that had been produced completely in vitro (Eppig and O'Brien, 1996, 1998). The egg that produced Eggbert was first grown within the isolated ovary from a newborn mouse in an organ culture dish for eight days. Oocyte-granulosa cell complexes were then isolated and cultured for an additional 14 days on a collagen-impregnated membrane. Eggbert, at an early age, began to display poor health, obesity, and nervousness. Upon his death, the pathology report indicated that he had lymphosarcoma of the small intestine, hyperplasia of islets of Langerhans, focal areas of lipidosis of the liver, and his brain displayed hydrocephaly. While these anomalies may occur in other male mice at Eggbert's age (14 months), Eggbert demonstrated these problems before he was 12 months old. This observation was alarming enough for the investigators to bring his condition to light (Eppig and O'Brien, 1998).

When sheep and cattle embryos are produced in vitro there are a number of abnormalities observed. These include, among many others, large size at birth, limb contractures, cardiac abnormalities, exencephaly, and neonatal respiratory distress (Willadsen et al., 1991; Walker et al., 1992; Lane and Gardner, 1994; Wilson et al., 1995; Sinclair et al., 1999). Initially, it was believed that these abnormalities were unique to embryo cloning protocols, as this was the first large-scale production of embryos that were allowed to go to term in livestock improvement programs. As research in this area developed, it was discovered that in vitro production, including IVM, IVF, and in vitro culture in the absence of embryo cloning, could cause the same abnormalities (Walker et al., 1992; Sinclair et al., 1999).

There are two possible reasons for these abnormalities: serum-born growth factors and imprinting. Growth factors, as their name implies, stimulate cellular growth. It is speculated that premature exposure to some growth factors may initiate a cascade of precocious differentiation. In mice, insulin-like growth factor II and its receptor are imprinted differentially (Rappolee et al., 1992). Insulin-like growth factor II has been shown to stimulate cell proliferation in early preimplantation mouse embryos, presenting a model whereby embryo growth can be modified through imprinted genes (Rappolee et al., 1992; Chaillet et al., 1991). It can be further postulated that the changing maternal or paternal imprint, at the time of in vitro gametogenesis or embryogenesis, may lead to changes in gene expression, rendering some embryos more susceptible to available growth factors or substrates. This, in turn, may lead to abnormal growth and development. These examples indicate that in vitro culture can have profound consequences on growth and development.

Conclusions

Ovarian cortical tissue can successfully be cryopreserved and thawed. Enzymatic digestion can efficiently be used in conjunction with manual dissection to isolate preantral follicles of different sizes and stages. Culture conditions have been defined in laboratory animals that can yield oocytes that are competent to produce limited post fertilization development in vitro.

In vivo grown oocytes can be matured in vitro and give rise to embryos that are competent to produce viable offspring. The successful outcome of oocyte IVM is dependent on the stage of follicle differentiation when the oocyte is recovered. The COC can be stimulated by a variety of stimuli that force them into the next stage of differentiation. This differentiation pathway may be common regardless of whether the COC is destined to ovulate or to degenerate, and this event may occur with the selection of the dominant follicle and the artificial initiation of atresia in the cohort.

There has been one animal born (Eggbert) from complete in vitro oogenesis (Eppig and O'Brien, 1998). His life appears to have been challenged with several problems. Livestock animals produced by in vitro culture are also plagued with structural and metabolic problems. These well-documented disorders of offspring produced in vitro demand that we carefully investigate and understand subsequent development before we apply these technologies to the treatment of human infertility.

REFERENCES

Baird, D.T., Webb, R., Campbell, B.K., Harkness, L.M., and Gosden, R.G. (1999). Long-term ovarian function in sheep after ovariectomy and transplantation of autografts stored at −196 °C. *Endocrinology*, **140**, 462–71.

Barnes, F.L., Crombie, A., Gardner, D.K., et al. (1995). Blastocyst development and birth after in vitro maturation of human primary oocytes, intracytoplasmic sperm injection and assisted hatching. *Human Reproduction*, **10**, 3243–7.

Barnes, F.L., Kausche, A., Tiglias, J., Wood, C., Wilton, A., and Trounson, A.O. (1996). Production of embryos from in vitro matured primary human oocytes. *Fertility and Sterility*, **65**, 1151–6.

Blondin, P. and Sirard, M.A. (1995). Oocyte and follicular morphology as determining characteristics for developmental competence in bovine oocytes. *Molecular Reproduction and Development*, **41**, 54–62.

Blondin, P., Guilbault, L.A., and Sirard, M.A. (1996). Superovulation can reduce the developmental competence of bovine embryos. *Theriogenology*, **46**, 1191–203.

Blondin, P., Guilbault, L.A., and Sirard, M.A. (1997a). In vitro production of bovine embryos: developmental competence is acquired before maturation. *Theriogenology*, **47**, 1061–75.

Blondin, P., Guilbault, L.A., and Sirard, M.A. (1997b). The time interval between FSH-P administration and slaughter can influence the developmental competence of beer heifer oocytes. *Theriogenology*, **48**, 803–13.

Boland, N.I., Humpherson, D.G., Leese, H.J., and Gosden, R.G. (1993). Pattern of lactate production and steroidogenesis during growth and maturation of mouse ovarian follicles in vitro. *Biology of Reproduction*, **48**, 798–806.

Cecconi, S., Tatone, C., Buccione, R., Mangia, F., and Colonna, R. (1991). Granulosa cell–oocyte interactions: the phosphorylation of specific proteins in mouse oocytes at the germinal vesicle stage is dependent upon the differentiative state of companion somatic cells. *Journal of Experimental Zoology*, **258**, 249–54.

Cha, K.Y., Koo, J.J., Ko, J.J., Choi, D.H., Han, S.Y., and Yoon, T.K. (1991). Pregnancy after in vitro fertilization of human follicular oocytes collected from non-stimulated cycles, their culture in vitro and their transfer in a donor oocyte program. *Fertility and Sterility*, **55**, 109–13.

Cha, K.Y., Han, S.Y., Chung, H.M., et al. (2000). Pregnancies and deliveries after in vitro maturation culture followed by in vitro fertilization and embryo transfer without stimulation in women with polycystic ovary syndrome. *Fertility and Sterility*, **73**, 978–83.

Chaillet, J.R., Vogt, T.F., Beier, D.R., and Leder, P. (1991). Parental-specific methylation of an imprinted transgene is established during gametogenesis and progressively changes during embryogenesis. *Cell*, **66**, 77–83.

Chian, R.C., Ao, A., Clarke, H.J., Tulandi, T., and Tan, S.L. (1999). Production of steroids from human cumulus cells treated with different concentrations of gonadotropins during culture in vitro. *Fertility and Sterility*, **71**, 61–6.

Chian, R.C., Buckett, W.M., Tulandi, T., et al. (2000). Prospective randomized study of human chorionic gonadotropin priming before immature oocyte retrieval from unstimulated women with polycystic ovarian syndrome. *Human Reproduction*, **15**, 165–70.

Cobo, A.C., Requena, A., Neuspiller, F., et al. (1999). Maturation in vitro of human oocytes from unstimulated cycles: selection of the optimal day for ovum retrieval based on follicular size. *Human Reproduction*, **14**, 1864–8.

Colonna, R., Cecconi, S., Tatone, C., Mangia, F., and Buccione, R. (1989). Somatic cell–oocyte interactions in mouse oogenesis: stage-specific regulation of mouse oocyte protein phosphorylation by granulosa cells. *Developmental Biology*, **33**, 305–8.

Edwards, R.G. (1965). Maturation in vitro of mouse, sheep, cow, pig, rhesus monkey and human ovarian oocytes. *Nature*, **102**, 493–7.

Eppig, J.J. and O'Brien, M.J. (1996). Development in vitro of mouse oocytes from primordial follicles. *Biology of Reproduction*, **54**, 197–207.

Eppig, J.J. and O'Brien, M.J. (1998). Comparison of preimplantation developmental competence after mouse oocyte growth and development in vitro and in vivo. *Theriogenology*, **49**, 415–22.

Eppig, J.J. and Schroeder, A.C. (1989). Capacity of mouse oocytes from preantral follicles to undergo embryogenesis and development to live young after growth, maturation, and fertilization in vitro. *Biology of Reproduction*, **41**, 268–79.

Eppig, J.J., Schroeder, A.C., and O'Brien, M.J. (1992). Developmental capacity of mouse oocytes matured in vitro: effects of gonadotrophic stimulation, follicular origin and oocyte size. *Journal of Reproduction and Fertility*, **95**, 119–27.

Eppig, J.J., O'Brien, M., and Wigglesworth, K. (1996). Mammalian oocyte growth and development in vitro. *Molecular Reproduction and Development*, **44**, 260–73.

Gomez, E., Tarin, J.J., and Pellicer, A. (1993). Oocyte maturation in humans: the role of gonadotropins and growth factors. *Fertility and Sterility*, **60**, 40–6.

Goud, P.T., Goud, A.P., Qian, C., et al. (1998). In-vitro maturation of human germinal vesicle stage oocytes: role of cumulus cells and epidermal growth factor in the culture medium. *Human Reproduction*, **13**, 1638–44.

Johnson, L.D., Albertini, D.F., McGinnis, L.K., and Biggers, J.D. (1995). Chromatin organization, meiotic status and meiotic competence acquisition in mouse oocytes from cultured ovarian follicles. *Journal of Reproduction and Fertility*, **104**, 277–84.

Lane, M. and Gardner, D.K. (1994). Increase in postimplantation development of cultured mouse embryos by amino acids and induction of fetal retardation and exencephaly by ammonium ions. *Journal of Reproduction and Fertility*, **102**, 305–12.

Looney, C.R., Lindsay, B.R., Gonseth, C.L., and Johnson, D.L. (1994). Commercial aspects of oocyte retrieval and in vitro fertilization (IVF) for embryo production in the problem cow. *Theriogenology*, **41**, 67–72.

Mikkelsen, A., Smith, S., and Lindenberg, S. (1999). In-vitro maturation of human oocytes from regularly menstruating women may be successful without follicle stimulating hormone priming. *Human Reproduction*, **14**, 1847–51.

Mikkelsen, A., Smith, S., and Lindenberg, S. (2000). Impact of oestradiol and inhibin A concentrations on pregnancy rate in in vitro oocyte maturation. *Human Reproduction*, **15**, 1685–90.

Moor, R.M. and Trounson, A.O. (1977). Hormonal and follicular factors affecting maturation of sheep oocytes in vitro and their subsequent developmental capacity. *Journal of Reproduction and Fertility*, **49**, 101–9.

Newton, H., Picton, H., and Gosden, R.G. (1999). In vitro growth of oocyte–granulosa cell complexes isolated from cryopreserved ovine tissue. *Journal of Reproduction and Fertility*, **115**, 141–50.

Pavlok, A., Lucas-Hahn, A., and Niemann, H. (1992). Fertilization and development competence of bovine oocytes derived from different categories of antral follicles. *Molecular Reproduction and Development*, **31**, 63–7.

Pincus, G. and Enzmann, E.V. (1935). The comparative behavior of mammalian eggs in vivo and in vitro. I. The activation of ovarian eggs. *Journal of Experimental Medicine*, **62**, 655–75.

Rappolee, D.A., Sturm, K.S., Behrendtsen, O., Schultz, G.A., Pedersen, R.A., and Werb, Z. (1992). Insulin-like growth factor II acts through an endogenous growth pathway regulated by imprinting in early mouse embryos. *Genes and Development*, **6**, 939–52.

Roy, S.K. and Greenwald, G.S. (1985). An enzymatic method for dissociation of intact follicles from the hamster ovary: histological and quantitative aspects. *Biology of Reproduction*, **32**, 203–15.

Roy, S.K. and Treacy, B.J. (1993). Isolation and long-term culture of human preantral follicles. *Fertility and Sterility*, **59**, 783–90.

Russell, J.B., Knezevich, K.M., Fabian, K.F., et al. (1997). Unstimulated immature oocyte retrieval: early versus midfollicular endometrial priming. *Fertility and Sterility*, **67**, 616–20.

Salamone, D.F., Adams, G.P., and Mapletoft, R.J. (1999). Changes in the cumulus–oocyte complex of subordinate follicles relative to follicular wave status in cattle. *Theriogenology*, **52**, 549–61.

Schramm, R.D., Tennier, M.T., Boatman, D.E., and Bavister, B.D. (1993). Chromatin configurations and meiotic competence of oocytes are related to follicular diameter in nonstimulated rhesus monkeys. *Biology of Reproduction*, **48**, 349–56.

Shaw, J.M., Bowles, J., Koopman, P., Wood, E.C., and Trounson, A.O. (1996). Fresh and cryopreserved ovarian tissue samples from donors with lymphoma transmit the cancer to graft recipients. *Human Reproduction*, **11**, 1668–73.

Sinclair, K.D., McEvoy, T.G., Maxfield, E.K., et al. (1999). Aberrant fetal growth and development after *in vitro* culture of sheep zygotes. *Journal of Reproduction and Fertility*, **116**, 177–86.

Sirard, M.A., Picard, L., et al. (1999). The time interval between FSH aspiration and ovarian aspiration influences the development of cattle oocytes. *Theriogenology*, **51**, 699–709.

Sorensen, R.A. and Wassarman, P.M. (1976). Relationship between growth and meiotic maturation of the mouse oocyte. *Developmental Biology*, **50**, 531–6.

Spears, N., Boland, N.I., Murray, A.A., and Gosden, R.G. (1994). Mouse oocytes derived from in vitro grown primary ovarian follicles are fertile. *Human Reproduction*, **9**, 527–32.

Spears, N., de Bruin, J.P., and Gosden, R.G. (1996). The establishment of follicular dominance in co-cultured mouse ovarian follicles. *Journal of Reproduction and Fertility*, **106**, 1–6.

Suikkari, A.M., Tulppala, M., Tuuri, T., Hovatta, O., and Barnes, F. (2000). Luteal phase start of low-dose FSH priming of follicles results in an efficient recovery, maturation and fertilization of immature human oocytes. *Human Reproduction*, **15**, 747–51.

Torrence, C., Telfer, E., and Gosden, R.G. (1989). Qualitative study of the development of isolated mouse preantral follicles in collagen gel culture. *Journal of Reproduction Fertility*, **87**, 367–74.

Trounson, A.O., Wood, C., and Kausche, A. (1994). In vitro maturation and the fertilization and development competence of oocytes recovered from untreated polycystic ovarian patients. *Fertility and Sterility*, **62**, 353–62.

Tsuji, K., Masanori, S., and Nakano, R. (1985). Relationship between human oocyte maturation and different follicular sizes. *Biology of Reproduction*, **32**, 413–17.

Walker, S.K., Heard, T.M., and Seamark R.F. (1992). In vitro culture of sheep embryos without co-culture: success and perspectives. *Theriogenology*, **37**, 111–26.

Willadsen, S.M., Janzen, R.E., McAlister, R.J., Shea, B.F., Hamilton, G., and McDermond (1991). The viability of late morula and blastocysts produced by nuclear transplantation in cattle. *Theriogenology*, **35**, 161–70.

Wilson, J.M., Williams, J.D., Bondioli, K.R., Looney, C.R., Westhusin, M.E., and McCalla, D.F. (1995). Comparison of birth weight and growth characteristics of bovine calves produced by nuclear transfer (cloning), embryo transfer and natural mating. *Animal Reproduction Science*, **38**, 73–8.

Zuelke, K.A. and Brackett, B.G. (1992). Effects of luteinizing hormone on glucose metabolism in cumulus-enclosed bovine oocytes matured in vitro. *Endocrinology*, **131**, 2690–6.

Zuelke, K.A. and Brackett, B.G. (1993). Increased glutamine metabolism in bovine cumulus cell-enclosed and denuded oocytes after in vitro maturation with luteinizing hormone. *Biology of Reproduction*, **48**, 815–20.

5

The oocyte as a machine

Kate Hardy

Department of Reproductive Science and Medicine, Imperial College, London, UK

Introduction

Most individual functions in the human body are carried out by a relatively large number of cells performing the same task. By contrast, the oocyte is one single cell that has to fulfill a vital (reproductive) role on its own. A woman will ovulate only 400 or so oocytes during her lifetime, and less than half of these ovulations will occur at a time when she may wish to become pregnant. Considering that a woman is born with around one million oocytes, the majority of which die before and during oocyte growth and maturation, an immense reproductive responsibility is invested in the tiny proportion of oocytes that are selected to ovulate. Defects in these cells will have profound consequences, such as fertilization failure, failure to undergo cell cleavage, developmental arrest, implantation failure or miscarriage. Less than 15% of embryos transferred to the uterus following in vitro fertilization (IVF) will give rise to a baby. This, together with the high incidence of chromosomal abnormalities, underlines the vulnerability and uncertainty of the reproductive process in humans.

The tasks that an oocyte has to perform to accomplish its role successfully are extensive. First, it must be capable of ovulation and survival in the environment of the fallopian tube. Second, it must have the capacity to be fertilized: to admit one and only one sperm, and then to remodel and process the sperm's nuclear material along with its own in a coherent manner to produce the normal diploid complement of the new individual. Finally, since the embryonic genome is not switched on until after the first few cleavage divisions, the oocyte must provide practically all of the developing embryo's cellular machinery, RNA, and protein stores to support development during this period.

The fact that a single cell can reliably perform all of these functions is remarkable and suggests that there must be careful control and coordination of the various processes occurring within the oocyte. It is, therefore, not unreasonable to think of it as an incredibly tiny but sophisticated piece of machinery. Furthermore, it must be amazingly robust since it may lie dormant for up to 50 years, through such major perturbations as puberty or pregnancy, before becoming active.

The aim of this chapter is to review current knowledge about the functioning and regulation of this wonderful machine, focusing on the period of growth, development, and maturation up until the time of ovulation. It turns out that, despite its importance, our understanding of the factors controlling oocyte maturation remains largely incomplete. However, one fact that is well established is that the oocyte's functioning is intimately tied up with its surrounding follicle cells: neither can develop successfully without the other. It is, therefore, perhaps more appropriate to consider the whole follicle as a single functional unit, and this chapter should perhaps have been entitled "The follicle as a machine."

Malfunctions of this machine during oocyte maturation can lead to embryonic loss or infertility. Little is known about the precise causes of such mal-

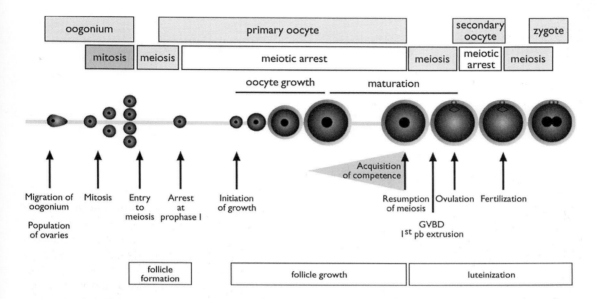

Fig. 5.1. A summary of oogenesis showing oocyte growth and maturation. GVBD, germinal vesicle breakdown; pb, polar body.

functions or about the conditions necessary to generate a "good quality" viable oocyte. A key requirement appears to be that essential hormone and growth factor signals be coordinated at the appropriate time to induce the cellular changes that are required for nuclear and cytoplasmic maturation. A detailed understanding of how human oogenesis and folliculogenesis produces healthy or defective oocytes is a major challenge for the future of assisted reproduction technology.

Folliculogenesis and oocyte growth

During human fetal life, the developing ovaries become populated with primordial germ cells (oogonia), which divide rapidly by mitosis. From the end of the first trimester these oogonia can enter meiosis, whereupon they are termed oocytes (Fig. 5.1). Some oogonia do not enter meiosis until a few weeks before birth. After this time, no new oocytes are produced. At midgestation it is estimated that there are about 7 million germ cells, but this number declines dramatically during late gestation as the majority of oocytes die. Therefore, a human female is born with all the oocytes that she will ever have (approximately one to two million); none of which can ever be replaced (Gosden, 1995).

Upon entering meiosis, oocytes progress to the first prophase, where they arrest. Remarkably, they can remain arrested for up to 50 years until they start growing (Fig. 5.1). It is not known precisely how the oocyte is held in meiotic and growth arrest. When the oocyte enters meiosis it is small (approximately 30 μm in diameter) and becomes enclosed by a single layer of squamous "pregranulosa" cells on a basement membrane. This unit, known as the primordial follicle (Fig. 5.2), resides in the ovarian cortex and is seen in the human fetus from about 22 weeks of gestation. The stimulus that initiates growth of the primordial follicle also remains unknown. Most follicles in women of all ages are at the primordial stage, although the total number declines with age (Gosden, 1995; Faddy, 2000).

From before birth, throughout later childhood, puberty, pregnancy and lactation, there is continual recruitment of small numbers of primordial follicles to start folliculogenesis. This is a lengthy process taking up to six months (Gougeon, 1996), during

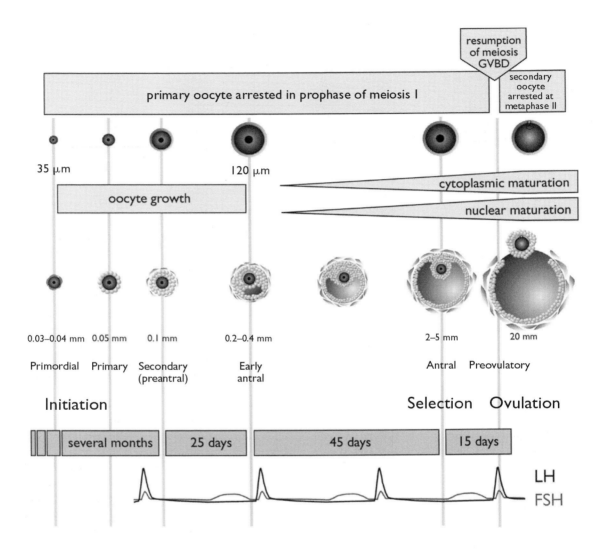

Fig. 5.2. A summary of the relationship between oocyte growth and maturation, the stages of follicle development and the cyclical hormone changes occurring between the primordial and pre-ovulatory stages of folliculogenesis. GVBD, germinal vesicle breakdown; LH, luteinizing hormone; FSH, follicle-stimulating hormone.

which the follicle grows and differentiates (Fig. 5.2). Initiation of growth is thought to be largely gonadotropin independent and continues until the supply of primordial follicles is virtually exhausted, just after the menopause (Gosden, 1995). During the early stages of growth, with the formation of a primary follicle, the granulosa cells become cuboidal in shape and undergo cell division (Fig. 5.2). Subsequently, multiple layers of granulosa cells surround the oocyte. When the follicle reaches the secondary stage, with two or more layers of granulosa cells, a layer of theca cells differentiates from the surrounding stroma around the follicle, and the oocyte lays down a glycoprotein-rich zona pellucida (Fig. 5.2). When there are several layers of granulosa

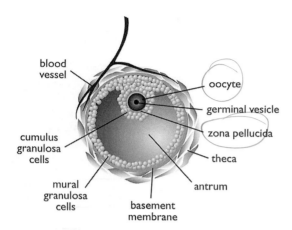

Fig. 5.3. Structure of the follicle.

blood vessel
oocyte
germinal vesicle
zona pellucida
cumulus granulosa cells
theca
mural granulosa cells
antrum
basement membrane

cells and the oocyte is fully grown, a fluid-filled cavity (the antrum) appears and starts expanding (Figs. 5.2 and 5.3). The interior of the growing follicle is avascular (Fig. 5.3), and extensive intercellular communication becomes established throughout the follicle via gap junctions (Anderson and Albertini, 1976). Granulosa cells communicate with each other and also extend processes through the zona pellucida that contact the oolemma and allow direct gap junction communication with the oocyte.

During human preantral development, the oocyte itself is growing, undergoing a 60-fold increase in volume, until it reaches its mature size of about 120 μm in diameter (Figs. 5.1 and 5.2) (Gougeon, 1996). While the oocyte is growing, it is both transcriptionally and translationally very active, with production of large amounts of RNA. A mature mouse oocyte contains 200-fold more RNA and 50- to 60-fold more protein than an average somatic cell (Wassarman and Kinloch, 1992). Most of this is not for immediate use but is stored to maintain the oocyte and early embryo through maturation, fertilization, and early cleavage, before activation of the embryonic genome, which occurs at the 4- to 8-cell stage in the human (Braude et al., 1988; Tesařík et al., 1988). The poly(A) tail carried by mRNA promotes initiation of translation, and in the oocyte different species of RNA are polyadenylated to different

degrees. Some, such as those for actin and globin, have long poly-A tails of approximately 150 adenine residues and are for immediate use. Others have shorter poly-A tails of less than 90 adenine residues, are not immediately translated, and are for long-term storage (Bachvarova, 1992). mRNA is sequestered in the form of ribonucleoprotein particles, which affords protection from degradation until release for translation. Active transcription ceases when meiosis resumes prior to ovulation.

While the oocyte is growing, there are also changes in organelle morphology, distribution, and number, which reflect increasing metabolism and synthesis of macromolecules. The nucleus grows, becomes large and pale, and is known as a germinal vesicle. The nucleus becomes indented and there is an increase in the number of pores in the nuclear membrane. The nucleolus also enlarges, with a change in fine structure from a fibrillogranular network to a dense, uniform fibrillar mass, indicative of intense RNA synthesis. Mitochondria grow and replicate, and their structure changes from elongated mitochondria with numerous transverse cristae to round or oval vacuolated mitochondria with arched and concentrically arranged cristae. During oocyte growth, mitochondria are closely associated with endoplasmic reticulum. The Golgi apparatus also undergoes dramatic ultrastructural changes from flattened stacks of arched lamellae to increased numbers of swollen stacked lamellae associated with vacuoles, granules, and lipid vesicles. These changes are associated with processing of secreted proteins, such as those that make up the zona pellucida (which appears from the secondary follicle onwards) and cortical granules. The zona pellucida is secreted by the oocyte, becoming progressively denser and thicker as growth continues. Cortical granules first appear during oocyte growth and their contents are exocytosed at the time of fertilization to alter the structure of the zona pellucida and prevent polyspermy. The number of ribosomes increases. In general, organelles migrate towards the periphery of the cell (Wassarman, 1996).

Follicular development from the stage of antrum formation to ovulation is subject to endocrine control, predominantly by follicle-stimulating hormone (FSH). In the later stages of follicle growth, the rate of cell division in the granulosa population slows down. These cells start to differentiate and become steroidogenic, utilizing theca-derived androgen to produce increasing amounts of estradiol.

Preantral follicle growth in the human occurs over a period of several menstrual cycles (Fig. 5.2). At the beginning of each cycle, a group of about 6–11 small antral follicles are selected for further growth (Gougeon, 1996). During the next two weeks, one follicle of the group will become dominant and is the one destined to ovulate. The rest of the group become atretic and die by apoptosis (Gougeon, 1996; Morita and Tilly, 1999). The dominant follicle is responsible for about 95% of circulating estradiol levels in the late follicular phase. When it has reached about 10 mm in diameter, its granulosa cells acquire receptors to luteinizing hormone (LH). This represents a further marker of differentiation and heralds their ability to produce estradiol and progesterone in response to LH in the late follicular phase. The preovulatory follicle, which is approximately 20 mm in diameter, consists of a pseudostratified layer of mural granulosa cells surrounding the fluid-filled antrum. The fully grown primary oocyte, surrounded by several layers of cumulus cells, is acentrically placed within the antrum and attached to the mural granulosa by a stalk of granulosa cells (Fig. 5.3).

Oocyte maturation

Cell–cell communication between somatic cells and the oocyte is crucial for follicle development and oocyte maturation. The two cell types are connected via gap junctions (Anderson and Albertini, 1976), which allow the transfer of nutrients, metabolic precursors, and regulatory substances between cumulus cells and the oocyte (Eppig, 1991). Gap junction communication is maintained until around the time when meiotic maturation resumes, when cellular processes are withdrawn. Paracrine signaling within the follicle and possibly between follicles is also crucial to the maturation process.

The oocyte is incapable of resuming meiosis until it is fully grown, around the time of follicular antrum formation in the mouse (Sorensen and Wassarman, 1976). However, in vivo, the oocyte is maintained in meiotic arrest until the follicle itself is fully grown. There is strong evidence that cyclic AMP (cAMP) and other purines are involved in the maintenance of this cell cycle arrest (Eppig, 1989). In vivo, mammalian oocytes resume meiosis after the mid-cycle surge of LH (if they are in a dominant follicle) (Fig. 5.1). Since oocytes do not have receptors for LH, the signal to resume meiosis must be mediated by the granulosa cells. It is still not precisely understood how LH induces oocyte maturation, but there are two hypotheses. The first is that LH causes the degradation of gap junctions between the oocyte and cumulus cells, preventing transmission of meiosis-arresting substances. Evidence for this includes the observation that meiosis does resume when cumulus-enclosed oocytes are physically removed and dissociated from the follicle (Pincus and Enzmann, 1935; Edwards, 1965). Furthermore, changes in phosphorylation state and reduction in expression of the gap junction protein connexin 43 occur in isolated rat follicles following exposure to LH, suggesting mechanisms by which cell–cell communication can be interrupted (Granot and Dekel, 1994). The second hypothesis is that LH induces a meiosis-inducing substance that is passed into the oocyte via the gap junctions. In this context, it has been shown that LH stimulation produces an increase in intracellular calcium in mouse cumulus cells, followed closely by a similar rise in the oocyte (Eppig, 1991; Mattioli and Barboni, 2000).

With the resumption of meiosis, organelles are redistributed and the oocyte undergoes the extensive nuclear and cytoplasmic rearrangements that accompany breakdown of the germinal vesicle (GVBD) and polar body extrusion. Following GVBD, the chromosomes condense and then align at the metaphase equator of the first meiotic spindle. The spindle migrates to the cell cortex and metaphase I is completed with extrusion of the first polar body (containing one of each pair of homologous chromosomes). The chromosomes immediately align at the equator of the second metaphase spindle (Simerly et al., 1995). During this time, the previously tightly packed cumulus and corona cells become mucified and expand. The oocyte (now termed a secondary oocyte) is ovulated whilst proceeding to metaphase II of meiosis, where it arrests again and is only stimulated to complete meiosis at fertilization (Fig. 5.1).

In the mouse, follicle size largely correlates with developmental potential (Eppig et al., 1992), with a progressive stepwise attainment of competence to resume meiosis, undergo fertilization, complete meiosis, and begin embryogenesis. Oocytes isolated from growing early antral follicles are able to undergo GVBD but not progress to metaphase I (Sorensen and Wassarman, 1976). Oocytes from such follicles are almost invariably incapable of being fertilized, while oocytes isolated from larger antral follicles can reach metaphase II and, upon fertilization, cleave to the 2-cell stage. Oocytes from fully grown antral follicles are able to reach the blastocyst stage following fertilization (Eppig et al., 1992; Eppig, 1992). In the human, the potential for the oocyte to undergo GVBD is coincident with the time of antrum formation (Gosden and Bownes, 1995).

In addition to a strong correlation between follicle size and developmental potential, there also appears to be a link between oocyte size (cytoplasmic volume) and potential. This demonstrates that, in addition to interactions between the oocyte and the surrounding somatic cells, there are interactions between the oocyte cytoplasm and its nucleus. In an elegant study, mouse oocytes were bisected so that they contained half, a third, a quarter or trace amounts of cytoplasmic volume (Fulka et al., 1998). These manipulated oocytes were cultured in vitro while GVBD and first polar body extrusion were monitored. As the amount of cytoplasm was reduced, GVBD was increasingly delayed and the incidence of first polar body extrusion was decreased. Oocytes with a minimal amount of cytoplasm rarely underwent GVBD (Fulka et al., 1998). This reflects changes in the nucleus–cytoplasmic ratio as the oocyte grows in vivo, with the associated

steady increase in the acquisition of competence to complete meiosis.

To summarize, human oocyte growth and maturation is a lengthy and complex cellular process taking up to six months. It involves major remodeling of both the nucleus and the cytoskeleton. Furthermore, it encompasses meiosis up to metaphase II; cytoplasmic growth, organelle production and redistribution, stable RNA production to support early embryonic cleavage, nuclear maturation (the acquisition of competence to resume meiosis), and cytoplasmic maturation (with the acquisition of competence for sperm head penetration, decondensation of chromatin, and embryogenesis). Finally, at completion of the maturation process, the oocyte becomes capable of being fertilized and undergoing embryogenesis.

The follicle as a machine

As discussed above, it is now becoming increasingly clear from studies in other mammalian species that the oocyte and the granulosa cells form a mutually interdependent unit (Eppig, 1991). If efficient intercellular communication between the two cell types is disrupted, the unit can no longer function. The oocyte needs the follicle to be able to survive and grow, and the follicle needs the oocyte to maintain its structural integrity and function. Cumulus-free oocytes isolated at midgrowth stages and cultured on a monolayer of granulosa cells do not grow, while cumulus-enclosed oocytes (COC; with intact gap junction communication) do grow and mature in vitro (Eppig, 1977). Only granulosa cells can support oocytes in this way: fibroblasts in gap junction communication with zona-free oocytes support survival but not growth (Buccione et al., 1987). However, growth can be achieved by allowing direct association with preantral granulosa cells (Herlands and Schultz, 1984; Buccione et al., 1987). Granulosa cells can also affect the phosphorylation of oocyte proteins (Colonna et al., 1989) and, as already described, maintain the oocyte in meiotic arrest. Removal of fully grown oocytes, either naked or as

COC, from the follicular environment causes them to resume meiosis (Pincus and Enzmann, 1935; Edwards, 1965). However, if these COC are cultured in contact with mural granulosa cells, meiotic arrest is maintained (Tsafriri and Channing, 1975).

Conversely, follicles do not form in the absence of oocytes. This is apparent in vivo in germ cell-deficient mice and in women with Turner's syndrome, where the germ cells degenerate and follicles fail to form. It is now also clear that various specialized functions of cumulus cells are dependent on the presence of the oocyte. The impact of the oocyte on granulosa cell function can be elegantly demonstrated using a microneedle to pierce and destroy the oocyte within the intact COC in vitro (Buccione et al., 1990). The zona pellucida and three-dimensional structure of the cumulus cells remain intact. Using this approach, it can be shown that the oocyte regulates granulosa cell proliferation (Vanderhyden et al., 1992), steroidogenesis (Vanderhyden et al., 1993), deposition of extracellular matrix (Buccione et al., 1990), and hyaluronic acid synthesis (Salustri et al., 1993). Furthermore, it has been shown that the presence of the oocyte results in downregulation of LH receptor expression in the cumulus mass, but not the mural granulosa cells, of the preovulatory follicle (Eppig et al., 1997). It has also been shown that mice lacking growth differentiation factor 9 (GDF-9) were infertile, with no follicles more advanced than the primordial and primary stages (Dong et al., 1996). It has been suggested that GDF-9 is the oocyte-secreted factor that regulates granulosa cell function. Addition of exogenous recombinant GDF-9 to cultured granulosa cells suppresses LH receptor expression and induces proteins involved in steroidogenesis and hyaluronic acid synthesis. Furthermore, it stimulates cumulus expansion in vitro (Matzuk, 2000). Other proteins produced by the oocyte that may play a role in early folliculogenesis include retinoblastoma protein (Bukovsky et al., 1995) and MYC protein, both of which show strong expression in the oocyte, but not the granulosa cells, of the primordial follicle (Li et al., 1994). It has been suggested that retinoblastoma protein expression in the oocyte nucleolus is associated with production of an inhibitor of cell proliferation. With both retinoblastoma protein and MYC protein, oocyte expression declined and granulosa cell expression increased as follicles grew.

The importance of gap junctions in oocyte growth and maintenance in meiotic arrest has already been alluded to. Gap junctions that are formed by connexin proteins allow the passage of nutrients and signaling molecules, such as cAMP, between cells. Transgenic knockouts of connexin genes have strengthened the evidence that gap junction communication is critical for folliculogenesis and oocyte maturation. In cultured neonatal ovaries from mice homozygous for a null mutation in *Gja1* (encoding connexin 43), folliculogenesis could not proceed beyond the primary stage, showing that this gap junction protein is essential for folliculogenesis (Juneja et al., 1999). Connexin 43 has also been found in the granulosa cells of human follicles (C. Wright, D. L. Becker and K. Hardy, unpublished data). Furthermore, mice deficient in connexin-37 lack preovulatory follicles and oocyte development is arrested before meiotic competence is achieved (Simon et al., 1997).

Studies of mice carrying mutations at the white spotting (*W*) or Steel (*Sl*) locus, which have defects in germ cell development, have shown that the cytokine Kit ligand (or stem cell factor, encoded at the steel locus) and its transmembrane receptor c-Kit (encoded at the *W* locus) are important in early folliculogenesis. Oocytes in mice lacking the c-Kit/Kit ligand pathway fail to develop beyond the primordial stage (Kuroda et al., 1988), suggesting that kit ligand, expressed by granulosa cells in primordial follicles, may be involved in the initiation of oocyte growth via the c-Kit receptor present on the oocyte.

The maturing follicle is responsive to hormones, producing steroids and growth factors, creating a specialized microenvironment for oocyte maturation. Growth factors that have been detected in early follicles include members of the insulin-like growth factor family (Gougeon, 1996; Adashi, 1998) and the transforming growth factor family (Gougeon, 1996). As folliculogenesis occurs over a number of menstrual cycles, the follicle is exposed to a continually changing hormonal environment during growth (Fig. 5.2). Furthermore, the follicular cells are themselves changing: initially dividing, then differentiating.

Defects in oogenesis

Oocyte growth and maturation appears to be vulnerable to disruption by environmental insults, nutritional imbalances, or hormonal disturbance, and these may lead to chromosomal anomalies or embryo loss (Albertini, 1992; Moor et al., 1998). Hormonal protocols used to induce the growth of multiple follicles in patients undergoing IVF may impinge upon the maturation process and thus affect subsequent development. The superovulation regimen can affect embryo metabolism and blastocyst cell number (Hardy et al., 1995) and the concentrations of key regulatory enzymes of carbohydrate metabolism (Yazigi et al., 1993). Studies on the in vitro maturation (IVM) of oocytes from a variety of other species have provided further evidence that the environment of the maturing oocyte is important in later embryonic development. The type of culture medium used for IVM of oocytes affected blastocyst formation and postimplantation development in the mouse (van de Sandt et al., 1990) and blastocyst formation and health in the cow (Rose and Bavister, 1992; Rose-Hellekant et al., 1998; Watson et al., 2000). In vitro maturation of human oocytes aspirated from small follicles of 2–10 mm in diameter is possible with a high degree of success, and these oocytes are capable of being fertilized. However, embryonic development is compromised and the numbers of babies born following transfer of these embryos is very low, in the order of 1 or 2% (Cha and Chian, 1998), although results are improving.

The majority of spontaneous miscarriages in humans are caused by chromosomal abnormalities (Boué et al., 1985) that can be traced to abnormalities originating during meiosis in the oocyte. It is not known why the incidence of these abnormalities is so high in the human, although it is possible that the follicular environment may play a role in their etiology. What is certain is that defects in spindle assembly and function will increase the risk of errors in chromosome balance arising during meiosis. Spindle microtubules are extremely sensitive to cellular environment, chemicals, and temperature (Pickering et al., 1990; Albertini, 1992). Furthermore, Van Blerkom (1996) has shown that follicles with a low dissolved oxygen content tended to give rise to oocytes with a low pH (below 7.1) and a high incidence of scattered chromosomes (Van Blerkom, 1996).

Nuclear and chromosomal abnormalities can also arise after fertilization, during mitosis, resulting in mosaic embryos (Hardy et al., 1993; Munné et al., 1995; Handyside and Delhanty, 1997). Such abnormalities could be the result of defective oocyte maturation, with the spindle or cytoskeleton being disorganized or deficient in the oocyte and early embryo. As a result, accurate meiosis, mitosis, and cytokinesis could be impaired, giving rise to nuclear and chromosomal abnormalities in some cells.

The environment during oogenesis and preimplantation development can also affect postimplantation and even postnatal development. In domestic species, in vitro culture of embryos, particularly after IVM, leads to a high proportion of fetuses with "large offspring syndrome" (reviewed in Young et al., 1998). They are characterized by being abnormally heavy at birth. Such fetuses have an increased abortion rate and an increased length of gestation; phenotypic abnormalities are not infrequent. While it has been demonstrated that it is possible to mature oocytes from primordial and preantral follicles in the mouse, very few liveborn young have been produced (Spears et al., 1994; Eppig and O'Brien, 1996). The mouse (Eggbert) derived from an IVM primordial follicle developed liver and neurological defects and became excessively obese.

Taken together, these studies provide powerful evidence that the environment in which the oocyte matures (i.e., the follicular environment) has a significant effect on both preimplantation and postimplantation embryo development.

Conclusions

Our understanding, and ability to control the development of the follicle and the enclosed oocyte are still at a very crude level. Although the experiments described above have identified crucial components, key questions remain unanswered. What triggers entry of oocytes into meiosis? Precisely how is meiotic arrest maintained for up to 50 years? What controls initiation of follicular growth, supplying a steady trickle of growing follicles? What causes the high incidence of chromosomal abnormalities that arise during meiosis, leading to developmental arrest and miscarriage? Answers to these questions are essential if we wish to develop techniques for in vitro culture, growth and maturation of healthy and developmentally viable oocytes from preantral stages. This would have important therapeutic applications. Defining the culture conditions necessary to support normal folliculogenesis and oocyte maturation would provide a powerful new approach for understanding the factors that regulate normal growth and development of a viable oocyte. It would also help us to understand the causes of many abnormalities of oogenesis and ovulation occurring in vivo.

Unfortunately, currently IVM remains a challenge in any mammalian species. First, a successful technique must provide a milieu that reflects the changing environment to which the follicle is exposed, without damaging the oocyte. Second, the culture system needs to sustain a lengthy period of maturation and the increasing size of the follicle. Finally, support is needed for the complex cellular changes taking place in the follicular cells and in the oocyte and, in particular, the major nuclear and cytoskeletal changes involved in meiosis. It is only through the skillful combination of these factors that it will prove possible to produce an oocyte that is healthy and developmentally competent.

REFERENCES

Adashi, E.Y. (1998). The IGF family and folliculogenesis. *Journal of Reproductive Immunology*, **39**, 13–19.

Albertini, D.F. (1992). Cytoplasmic microtubular dynamics and chromatin organization during mammalian oogenesis and oocyte maturation. *Mutation Research*, **296**, 57–68.

Anderson, E. and Albertini, D.F. (1976). Gap junctions between the oocyte and companion follicle cells in the mammalian ovary. *Journal of Cell Biology*, **71**, 680–6.

Bachvarova, R.F. (1992). A maternal tail of poly(A): the long and the short of it. *Cell*, **69**, 895–7.

Boué, A., Boué, J., and Gropp, A. (1985). Cytogenetics of pregnancy wastage. *Advances in Human Genetics*, **14**, 1–57.

Braude, P., Bolton, V., and Moore, S. (1988). Human gene expression first occurs between the four- and eight-cell stages of preimplantation development. *Nature*, **332**, 459–61.

Buccione, R., Cecconi, S., Tatone, C., Mangia, F., and Colonna, R. (1987). Follicle cell regulation of mammalian oocyte growth. *Journal of Experimental Zoology*, **242**, 351–4.

Buccione, R., Vanderhyden, B.C., Caron, P.J., and Eppig, J.J. (1990). FSH-induced expansion of the mouse cumulus oophorus in vitro is dependent upon a specific factor(s) secreted by the oocyte. *Developmental Biology*, **138**, 16–25.

Bukovsky, A., Caudle, M.R., Keenan, J.A., Wimalasena, J., Foster, J.S., and Van Meter, S.E. (1995). Quantitative evaluation of the cell cycle-related retinoblastoma protein and localization of Thy-1 differentiation protein and macrophages during follicular development and atresia, and in human corpora lutea. *Biology of Reproduction*, **52**, 776–92.

Cha, K.-Y. and Chian, R.C. (1998). Maturation in vitro of immature human oocytes for clinical use. *Human Reproduction Update*, **4**, 103–20.

Colonna, R., Cecconi, S., Tatone, C., Mangia, F., and Buccione, R. (1989). Somatic cell–oocyte interactions in mouse oogenesis: stage-specific regulation of mouse oocyte protein phosphorylation by granulosa cells. *Developmental Biology*, **133**, 305–8.

Dong, J., Albertini, D.F., Nishimori, K., Kumar, T.R., Lu, N., and Matzuk, M.M. (1996). Growth differentiation factor-9 is required during early ovarian folliculogenesis. *Nature*, **383**, 531–5.

Edwards, R.G. (1965). Maturation in vitro of mouse, sheep, cow, pig, rhesus monkey and human ovarian oocytes. *Nature*, **208**, 349–51.

Eppig, J.J. (1977). Mouse oocyte development in vitro with various culture systems. *Developmental Biology*, **60**, 371–88.

Eppig, J.J. (1989). The participation of cyclic adenosine monophosphate (cAMP) in the regulation of meiotic maturation of oocytes in the laboratory mouse. *Journal of Reproduction and Fertility*, **38**(Suppl), 3–8.

Eppig, J.J. (1991). Intercommunication between mammalian oocytes and companion somatic cells. *Bioessays*, **13**, 569–74.

Eppig, J.J. (1992). Growth and development of mammalian

oocytes in vitro. *Archives in Pathology Laboratory Medicine*, **116**, 379–82.

Eppig, J.J. and O'Brien, M.J. (1996). Development in vitro of mouse oocytes from primordial follicles. *Biology of Reproduction*, **54**, 197–207.

Eppig, J.J., Schroeder, A.C., and O'Brien, M.J. (1992). Developmental capacity of mouse oocytes matured in vitro: effects of gonadotrophic stimulation, follicular origin and oocyte size. *Journal of Reproduction and Fertility*, **95**, 119–27.

Eppig, J.J., Wigglesworth, K., Pendola, F., and Hirao, Y. (1997). Murine oocytes suppress expression of luteinizing hormone receptor messenger ribonucleic acid by granulosa cells. *Biology Reproduction*, **56**, 976–84.

Faddy, M.J. (2000). Follicle dynamics during ovarian ageing. *Molecular and Cellular Endocrinology*, **163**, 43–8.

Fulka, J., Jr., First, N.L., and Moor, R.M. (1998). Nuclear and cytoplasmic determinants involved in the regulation of mammalian oocyte maturation. *Molecular Human Reproduction*, **4**, 41–9.

Gosden, R. (1995). Ovulation 1: oocyte development throughout life. In: *Gametes – The Oocyte*, Grudzinkas, J. and Yovich, J., eds. Cambridge University Press, Cambridge, UK, pp. 119–49.

Gosden, R. and Bownes, M. (1995). Molecular and cellular aspects of oocyte development. In: *Gametes – The Oocyte*, Grudzinkas, J. and Yovich, J., eds. Cambridge University Press, Cambridge, UK, pp. 23–53.

Gougeon, A. (1996). Regulation of ovarian follicular development in primates: facts and hypotheses. *Endocrine Reviews*, **17**, 121–154.

Granot, I. and Dekel, N. (1994). Phosphorylation and expression of connexin-43 ovarian gap junction protein are regulated by luteinizing hormone. *Journal of Biological Chemistry*, **269**, 30502–9.

Handyside, A. and Delhanty, J. (1997). Preimplantation genetic diagnosis: strategies and surprises. *Trends in Genetics*, **13**, 270–5.

Hardy, K., Winston, R.M., and Handyside, A.H. (1993). Binucleate blastomeres in preimplantation human embryos in vitro: failure of cytokinesis during early cleavage. *Journal of Reproduction and Fertility*, **98**, 549–58.

Hardy, K., Robinson, F.M., Paraschos, T., Wicks, R., Franks, S., and Winston, R.M. (1995). Normal development and metabolic activity of preimplantation embryos in vitro from patients with polycystic ovaries. *Human Reproduction*, **10**, 2125–35.

Herlands, R.L. and Schultz, R.M. (1984). Regulation of mouse oocyte growth: probable nutritional role for intercellular communication between follicle cells and oocytes in oocyte growth. *Journal of Experimental Zoology*, **229**, 317–25.

Juneja, S.C., Barr, K.J., Enders, G.C., and Kidder, G.M. (1999). Defects in the germ line and gonads of mice lacking connexin43. *Biology of Reproduction*, **60**, 1263–70.

Kuroda, H., Terada, N., Nakayama, H., Matsumoto, K., and Kitamura, Y. (1988). Infertility due to growth arrest of ovarian follicles in Sl/Slt mice. *Developmental Biology*, **126**, 71–9.

Li, S., Maruo, T., Ladines-Llave, C.A., Kondo, H., and Mochizuki, M. (1994). Stage-limited expression of Myc oncoprotein in the human ovary during follicular growth, regression and atresia. *Endocrine Journal*, **41**, 83–92.

Mattioli, M. and Barboni, B. (2000). Signal transduction mechanism for LH in the cumulus–oocyte complex. *Molecular and Cellular Endocrinology*, **161**, 19–23.

Matzuk, M.M. (2000). Revelations of ovarian follicle biology from gene knockout mice [in process citation]. *Molecular and Cellular Endocrinology*, **163**, 61–6.

Moor, R.M., Dai, Y., Lee, C., and Fulka, J., Jr. (1998). Oocyte maturation and embryonic failure. *Human Reproduction Update*, **4**, 223–36.

Morita, Y. and Tilly, J.L. (1999). Oocyte apoptosis: like sand through an hourglass. *Developmental Biology*, **213**, 1–17.

Munné, S., Alikani, M., Tomkin, G., Grifo, J., and Cohen, J. (1995). Embryo morphology, developmental rates, and maternal age are correlated with chromosome abnormalities. *Fertility and Sterility*, **64**, 382–91.

Pickering, S.J., Braude, P.R., Johnson, M.H., Cant, A., and Currie, J. (1990). Transient cooling to room temperature can cause irreversible disruption of the meiotic spindle in the human oocyte. *Fertility and Sterility*, **54**, 102–8.

Pincus, G.P. and Enzmann, E.V. (1935). The comparative behaviour of mammalian eggs in vivo and in vitro. I. The activation of ovarian eggs. *Journal of Experimental Medicine*, **62**, 665–75.

Rose, T.A. and Bavister, B.D. (1992). Effect of oocyte maturation medium on in vitro development of in vitro fertilized bovine embryos. *Molecular Reproduction and Development*, **31**, 72–7.

Rose-Hellekant, T.A., Libersky-Williamson, E.A., and Bavister, B.D. (1998). Energy substrates and amino acids provided during in vitro maturation of bovine oocytes alter acquisition of developmental competence. *Zygote*, **6**, 285–94.

Salustri, A., Hascall, V.C., Camaioni, A., and Yanagishita, M. (1993). Oocyte–granulosa interactions. In: *The Ovary*, Adashi, E.Y. and Leung, P.C.K., eds. Raven Press, New York, pp. 209–25.

Simerly, C., Navara, C., Wu, G.-J., and Schatten, G. (1995). Cytoskeletal organization and dynamics in mammalian oocytes during maturation and fertilization. In: *Gametes – The Oocyte*, Grudzinkas, J. and Yovich, J., eds. Cambridge University Press, Cambridge, UK, pp. 54–94.

Simon, A.M., Goodenough, D.A., Li, E., and Paul, D.L. (1997).

Female infertility in mice lacking connexin 37. *Nature*, **385**, 525–9.

Sorensen, R.A. and Wassarman, P.M. (1976). Relationship between growth and meiotic maturation of the mouse oocyte. *Developmental Biology*, **50**, 531–6.

Spears, N., Boland, N.I., Murray, A.A., and Gosden, R.G. (1994). Mouse oocytes derived from in vitro grown primary ovarian follicles are fertile. *Human Reproduction*, **9**, 527–32.

Tesarík, J., Kopecny, V., Plachot, M., and Mandelbaum, J. (1988). Early morphological signs of embryonic genome expression in human preimplantation development as revealed by quantitative electron microscopy. *Developmental Biology*, **128**, 15–20.

Tsafriri, A. and Channing, C.P. (1975). An inhibitory influence of granulosa cells and follicular fluid upon porcine oocyte meiosis in vitro. *Endocrinology*, **96**, 922–7.

Van Blerkom, J. (1996). The influence of intrinsic and extrinsic factors on the developmental potential and chromosomal normality of the human oocyte. *Journal of the Society for Gynecologic Investigations*, **3**, 3–11.

van de Sandt, J.J., Schroeder, A.C., and Eppig, J.J. (1990). Culture media for mouse oocyte maturation affect subsequent embryonic development. *Molecular Reproduction and Development*, **25**, 164–71.

Vanderhyden, B.C., Telfer, E.E., and Eppig, J.J. (1992). Mouse oocytes promote proliferation of granulosa cells from preantral and antral follicles in vitro. *Biology of Reproduction*, **46**, 1196–204.

Vanderhyden, B.C., Cohen, J.N., and Morley, P. (1993). Mouse oocytes regulate granulosa cell steroidogenesis. *Endocrinology*, **133**, 423–6.

Wassarman, P.M. (1996). Oogenesis. In: *Reproductive Endocrinology, Surgery and Technology*, Adashi, E.Y., Rock, J.A., and Rosenwaks, Z., eds. Lippincott-Raven, Philadelphia, PA, pp. 342–57.

Wassarman, P.M. and Kinloch, R.A. (1992). Gene expression during oogenesis in mice. *Mutation Research*, **296**, 3–15.

Watson, A.J., De Sousa, P., Caveney, A., et al. (2000). Impact of bovine oocyte maturation media on oocyte transcript levels, blastocyst development, cell number, and apoptosis. *Biology of Reproduction*, **62**, 355–64.

Yazigi, R.A., Chi, M.M., Mastrogiannis, D.S., Strickler, R.C., Yang, V.C., and Lowry, O.H. (1993). Enzyme activities and maturation in unstimulated and exogenous gonadotropin-stimulated human oocytes. *American Journal of Physiology*, **264**, C951–5.

Young, L.E., Sinclair, K.D., and Wilmut, I. (1998). Large offspring syndrome in cattle and sheep. *Reviews in Reproduction*, **3**, 155–63.

6

Follicular influences on oocyte and embryo competence

Jonathan Van Blerkom

Department of Molecular, Cellular and Developmental Biology, University of Colorado,
at Boulder and Colorado Reproductive Endocrinology, Rose Medical Center, Denver, USA

Introduction

Despite tens of thousands of in vitro fertilization (IVF) procedures performed in the nearly a quarter of century following the birth of the first human conceived in vitro (Steptoe and Edwards, 1978), our understanding of the origins and fundamental causes of early developmental failure in our species remains largely unknown. We do know, however, that lethal chromosomal defects are often detectable in mature oocytes and preimplantation stage embryos, but we do not fully understand the underlying causes of these abnormalties. We know that within and between cohorts, embryos with different rates of cell division, patterns and extents of fragmentation, and abilities to develop progressively to the blastocyst are common occurrences during the two to six days of culture, which is the interval between insemination and transfer currently used in clinical IVF. Based on outcome, we know that appearance at the light microscopic level is often a poor indictor of competence, as witnessed by failure or singleton implantation after the transfer of multiple cleavage or blastocyst stage-appropriate embryos with equivalent and normal morphological characteristics. Consequently, research directed at the basic causes of differential competence in oocytes and early embryos is a fundamental aspect of clinical IVF, and one that should be designed to provide new and understandable criteria by which the likelihood of pregnancy can be assessed for each patient.

Recent studies have correlated outcome with follicular biology, and there is a growing consensus that specific characteristics of perifollicular blood flow determined for each follicle by color pulsed Doppler ultrasonography may identify oocytes that result in developmentally incompetent embryos, even if the oocytes are morphologically normal and stage-appropriate at the time of transfer. Current findings, which indicate the existence of a developmentally significant relationship between perifollicular blood flow and competence for the corresponding oocyte, form the basis of this review. Relevance in infertility treatment is discussed with respect to how this relationship is detected, and whether it has clinical applications in (i) predicting the likelihood that competent oocytes will occur during a specific natural or stimulated cycle and (ii) identifying specific embryos within cohorts that are the most likely to implant and develop progressively through gestation to birth. Many of the experimental results and clinical findings described in this chapter come from very recent studies. Therefore, the regulatory mechanisms discussed that involve this aspect of follicular biology should be considered speculative and viewed in the context of an emerging area of research in human reproductive biology and medicine. Nevertheless, the current research enterprises engaged in the study of oocyte and embryo competence and follicular blood flow, angiogenesis, and growth factor expression have already contributed new insights into follicular function and dysfunction, and findings which suggest that this line of investigation will indeed be clinically relevant in the diagnosis and treatment of infertility.

Perifollicular blood flow indices: predictors of embryo competence?

The ability to predict developmental competence within cohorts of cultured human embryos and select for transfer or cryopreservation only those with the highest potential to implant and develop through gestation has been one of the foremost challenges in clinical IVF. Outcome from IVF demonstrates that each human embryo has a unique developmental potential (for review see Edwards, 1986; Van Blerkom, 1994), and this fact is most evident during the cleavage stages where some proportion of embryos arrest cell division, fragment, or progress in culture in a manner that is stage-inappropriate with respect to cell number. Reliance on morphological characteristics of early human embryos, such as estimates of cellular volume lost by fragmentation and rates of cell division, is used routinely in the IVF laboratory for embryo selection/deselection on day 2 or 3 (Hoover et al., 1995; Gerris et al., 1999). However, the accuracy of these indicators is often called into question owing to normal gestations resulting from embryos that are "slow-developing" or exhibit certain patterns of fragmentation (Alikani et al., 1999; Antczak and Van Blerkom, 1999). Indeed, developmental arrest of intact embryos during culture, and implantation failure or a singleton gestation after transfer of multiple embryos, can be difficult to explain when all transferred embryos exhibited equivalent and normal morphology during cleavage, and hormonal levels and ultrasonographic measurements of the endometrium indicate a receptive uterus.

Studies of human preovulatory follicles demonstrate that each has unique cell biological, biochemical, and physiological characteristics. Attempts to relate competence in stimulated cycles with these characteristics have included determinations of the concentrations of growth factors, cytokines, steroid hormones (and other macromolecules) (Nayudu et al., 1987, 1989a,b; Klein et al., 1996). However, while these analyses confirm that the intrafollicular environment is highly complex, they have yet to provided a clear set of biochemical markers that unambiguously distinguish one follicle from another with

respect to developmental potential for the corresponding oocyte. At the cellular level, follicle-specific differences in the level of granulosa cell apoptosis (Oosterhuis et al., 1998) may provide some indication of "follicular health," and follicle-specific patterns of cumulus cell attachment and proliferation in vitro have been related to the implantation potential of the oocyte formerly associated with these cells (Gregory et al., 1994). With the exception of cumulus cell behavior, which can be readily assessed in the IVF laboratory, measurements of apoptosis in mural granulosa cells and quantification of specific regulatory factors require expertise and equipment that are not routinely available and have a predictive value that remains to be demonstrated clinically.

In contrast, recent findings suggest that measurement of perifollicular blood flow performed during routine ultrasonographic measurements of follicular growth by color Doppler ultrasonography may provide a noninvasive method to obtain clinically relevant insights into the normality of the corresponding oocyte, and a biological context for the differential competence of embryos that occur in both natural menstrual cycles and in IVF with controlled ovarian hyperstimulation (Fig. 6.1, color plate). In clinical IVF, the number of developing follicles in stimulated cycles is typically monitored by conventional ultrasonography, which, in experienced hands, can provide detailed information on follicle-specific growth rates, diameter, and apparent antral fluid volume. While these findings are used in routine practice to determine when follicular development may be optimal for ovulation induction, they have yet to provide specific indications of potential differences between oocytes that may be predictive of competence. The introduction of color pulsed Doppler ultrasonography to evaluate blood flow within the ovary is a recent development in reproductive medicine that has been applied to the assessment of perifollicular circulation in stimulated cycles.

Histological analyses demonstrate that each follicle is normally associated with a perifollicular capillary bed (Suzuki et al., 1998). Figure 6.2c is an electron microscopic image of an apparently normal preovulatory follicle showing the proximity of capil-

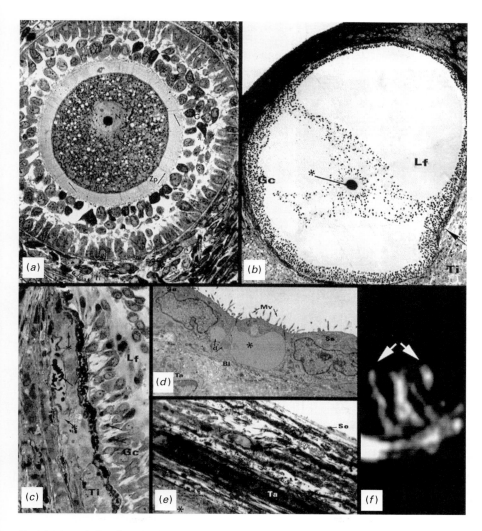

Fig. 6.2. Transmission electron microscopic images of ovarian follicles. (*a–e*) Images of rabbit ovarian follicles. (*a*) This is primary follicle showing transzonal (arrows, Zp) coronal cell processes and granulosa cells on the follicle wall. (*b*) A fully grown, preovulatory follicle showing the centrally located oocyte (asterisk) surrounded by granulosa cells (Gc) within the follicular fluid or liquor folliculi (Lf). The theca interna (Ti) is indicated by an arrow. (*c*) The theca interna (Ti) is shown at higher magnification. Note the proximity to the follicular wall of small vessels containing red blood cells (asterisks). (*d*) During the preovulatory phase in several mammals, leakage of antral fluid through the tunicia albugina (Ta) passes through the basement membrane and accumulates between cells forming the apical superficial epithelium (Se) of the ovary (asterisks) (BL, basal lamina; Mv, microvilli). (*e*) The superficial cells slough off at the follicular apex exposing the underlying connective tissue during the latter phase of the periovulatory stage. (*f*) A power angiographic image of a portion of a type A human follicle examined immediately preceding aspiration. The arrows indicate the follicular apex that is largely devoid of vessels. Magnifications for *a–e*: ×600, ×80, ×750, ×4900 and ×9500, respectively. (Parts *a–e* from Van Blerkom and Motta, 1979.)

laries to the follicular wall. However, several studies have suggested that it is the degree of expansion, the rate of blood flow, or both, through this microvascular network during follicular growth or preovulatory development that is a critical determinant of the normality of the intrafollicular environment and competence for the corresponding oocyte. Evidence for this notion has come from color pulsed Doppler ultrasonographic monitoring of follicles during the follicular and preovulatory phases. Collins et al. (1991) used transvaginal ultrasonography with color flow mapping to study intrafollicular morphology and blood flow in a single patient during a natural cycle. Their results, which indicated an increase in blood flow velocity and detectable blood vessels at the time of the rise in luteinizing hormone (LH), led to the suggestion that follicular angiogenesis is an essential process that may be clinically applicable in the prediction of ovulation and could be used to evaluate the probability of pregnancy. In a follow-up study involving 11 patients, Campbell et al. (1993) confirmed that color Doppler imaging performed over the periovulatory period could identify the leading preovulatory follicle in natural cycles by virtue of a marked increase in peak systolic velocity (PSV). For 27 patients undergoing controlled ovarian hyperstimulation for IVF, Nargund et al. (1996a,b) reported a significant correlation between perifollicular blood flow characteristics detectable by Doppler ultrasonography immediately preceding aspiration, whether an oocyte was recovered after fertilization, and the quality of the resulting embryo during early cleavage. Oocytes tended not to be recovered from follicles without detectable blood flow, and poor embryo morphology was associated with such follicles when PSV was $<10\,cm/s$. In contrast, high frequencies of oocyte recovery and morphologically normal embryos were obtained from follicles with PSV values $>10\,cm/s$. Zaidi et al. (1995) measured perifollicular blood flow in a patient with spontaneous luteinized unruptured follicle syndrome and reported that growth during the follicular phase was slower than typical for normal ovulatory cycles (approximately 2 mm/day). In addition, while perifollicular PSV values rose slightly during onset of the LH surge, after the surge they dropped to levels associated with the follicular phase. These investigators suggested that an apparent increase in blood flow following the LH rise is not necessarily associated with follicular rupture and the release of an oocyte, and that the relatively poor blood flow indices associated with the spontaneous luteinized unruptured follicle syndrome may reflect a primary granulosa cell abnormality in which luteinization was incomplete and subsequent vascularization was abnormal. The absence of a recoverable oocyte from follicles with no detectable blood flow or failure to rupture in the presence of measurable blood flow indicates that granulosa cell function in these follicles may be abnormal and possibly defective in the regulation perifollicular capillary expansion. Taken together, these findings provided the first clinically relevant indications that quantitative measurements of perifollicular blood flow indices may be correlated with follicular and oocyte competence and, for stimulated cycles, that very different perifollicular blood flow characteristics occur between follicles in the same ovary that under conventional ultrasonography may have a similar size and appearance.

The study of Chui et al. (1997) was among the first to correlate perifollicular vascularity in gonadotropin-stimulated ovaries with outcome after embryo transfer on day 2. Each of 38 patients underwent a single transvaginal power Doppler ultrasound scan on the day of follicular aspiration, and the vascularity of individual follicles was graded F1 to F4 on the basis of the percentage of the follicular circumference in which most flow was identified from a single cross-sectional slice. According to this grading, F1 corresponded to follicles in which blood flow was detected in $<25\%$ of the circumference, F2 corresponded to 26–50%; F3 to 51–75%, and F4 to 76–100%. Although described as preliminary, the findings demonstrated that vascularity grading was independent of follicular size ($>16\,mm$), number of oocytes aspirated, fertilization rate, and number and quality of embryos transferred on day 2. However, all pregnancies occurred with embryos that originated from F3 or F4 follicles, with pregnancies resulting in livebirths confined to those embryos obtained from F4 follicles. The pregnancy rate for embryos derived from F4 follicles was 61.5%. These results indicate that oocytes are recoverable from F1- and F2-type follicles, but the absence of a chemically detectable implantation after transfer of such embryos on day 2 strongly suggests that oocyte developmental competence is severely compromised if preovulatory maturation occurs in follicles with absent or poor blood flow indices.

Several recent studies have confirmed the notion that perifollicular vascularity, detectable by Doppler ultrasonography on the day of ovulation induction with human chorionic gonadotropin (hCG) and oocyte competence, demonstrated by outcome after embryo transfer, are related. Bahl et al. (1999) examined 1285 follicles from 200 patients undergoing controlled ovarian hyperstimulation and IVF. With the F1–F4 grading system, 64% were classified as F3 or F4 and 36% as F1 or F2. For individual follicles and their corresponding oocytes, when oocytes from follicles at stages F1 to F4 were compared after IVF, fertilization rates were significantly lower and the frequency of polyspermy, presumably the result of dispermic penetration, was significantly higher for oocytes derived from F1/F2 follicles. However, no correlation was found between vascular grade and embryo morphology on day 2. When outcome after the transfer of specific embryos from follicles of known grade was evaluated, pregnancy rates from F3 and F4 follicles were significantly higher (34.7%) than with embryos from F1 or F2 follicles (7.3%).

Coulam et al. (1999) correlated quantitative and qualitative indices of perifollicular vascularity for 106 patients considered to be at risk of failure owing to advanced reproductive age (>37 years), a history of poor response to gonadotropin stimulation, or multiple failed IVF cycles. A vascularity-grading scheme similar to the one described by Chui et al. (1997) was combined with measurement of follicle-specific PSV by pulsed Doppler spectral analysis on the day of ovulation induction for 565 follicles. Oocyte competence was related to clinical pregnancy outcome after uterine transfer on day 3 (72 hours after retrieval). The results demonstrated a direct relationship between establishment of a clinical pregnancy and vascularity grade and associated follicular blood flow, expressed by PSV values. All pregnancies occurred in women with F3 or F4 follicles and 91% occurred with follicular PSV > 10 cm/s at the time of hCG administration. These authors concluded that this PSV value represented a threshold level predictive of pregnancy in a high-risk population of patients undergoing IVF. However, while the specificity of this index was relatively low (36%), the results were consistent with the findings of Nargund et al. (1996b), who reported that the probability of producing an embryo with high implantation potential was about 75% if it was derived from a follicle PSV value of > 10 cm/s. Coulam et al. (1999) concluded that women who had at least one follicle with a PSV value > 10 cm/s had a significantly higher pregnancy rate than women with a maximum follicular PSV < 10 cm/s. Indeed, for high-risk patients with fewer than four follicles measured at ovulation induction, 33% (three of nine) became pregnant in that cycle if at least one F3/F4 follicle had a PSV at or above the threshold level. These findings indicate that perifollicular vascularity, determined qualitatively by ultrasonographic imaging or quantitatively by PSV determination, or both, has predictive value in assessing relative oocyte and embryo competence when applied to the analysis of individual follicles.

Intrafollicular physiology and perifollicular blood flow

The correlation between competence and perifollicular blood flow supports a general conclusion about outcome in clinical IVF that has remained relatively constant during its 22-year history, namely, that each oocyte and embryo has a unique developmental potential and, as recently applied to blood flow determinations, that specific cellular and biochemical characteristics of each follicle may profoundly influence the developmental competence of the corresponding oocyte and resulting embryo. The studies of Chui et al. (1997) and Bahl et al. (1999) found no apparent relationship between embryo morphology on day 2 and vascular grade at follicular aspiration. Nargund et al. (1996a,b) reported that high-grade or so-called 'top quality' embryos (Gerris et al., 1999), identified at the early cleavage stages by morphology and normality of cell divisions, were not only the most likely to implant but were most often derived from follicles with PSV values of > 10 cm/s. A similar finding was reported by Van Blerkom et al. (1997), who examined vascular indices for over 1000 follicles prior to ovulation induction and, for the corresponding oocytes, embryo development in vitro after IVF. For this study, perifollicular vascularity was assessed quantitatively and qualitatively by color pulsed Doppler ultrasonography with measurements taken at several different sites through each follicle. For each follicle, the maximum (PSV) and mean blood flow velocities were determined on the day of ovulation induction, and the apparent dissolved oxygen content of follicular fluid from each follicle was measured with an oxygen electrode at aspiration. Van Blerkom et al. (1997) grouped follicles into three classes according to the dissolved oxygen content measured in follicular fluid at aspiration: < 1.5%, 1.5–2.5%, and > 3%. The results indicated no significant correlation between follicular dissolved oxygen content and the frequency of maturation to metaphase II (MII) or fertilization rates after insemination in vitro. However, a high proportion of metaphase II oocytes with cytoplasmic defects clearly detectable by routine light microscopy originated from follicles with dissolved oxygen contents of < 1.5%. In the same respect, the majority of embryos that were multinucleated at the 2-cell stage and the mononucleated embryos that on day 2.5 were stage-inappropriate (slow developing or arrested), or classified as poor quality owing to excessive fragmentation, largely originated from follicles with dissolved oxygen contents < 1.5%. In contrast, the majority of high-quality, normal-appearing, stage-appropriate cleavage-stage embryos originated from follicles with oxygen contents > 3%.

Although the aforementioned findings tend to suggest that the dissolved oxygen content of follicular fluid in fully grown, preovulatory follicles may be related to oocyte and embryo developmental competence, in clinical practice, determinations of oxygen content during ovum retrieval are problematic, if not impractical. Because of time and logistical constraints associated with oocyte identification and isolation from aspirated fluids, which are usually examined by decanting aspirates into a large-surfaced cultured dish under laminar airflow, changes in atmospheric content may occur and measured levels may not accurately reflect the intra-follicular condition. The accuracy of atmospheric measurements also relies on the 'purity' of the aspirate and clear documentation of derivation from a specific follicle. These factors can be difficult to manage during ovum retrievals from the multiple closely spaced antral follicles generally produced by gonadotropin stimulation in IVF cycles. The occurrence of significant red blood cell contamination, mixing of fluids between follicles, and the need to 'rinse' follicles with physiological solutions when the oocyte is not present in the initial aspirate may also contribute to imprecision in dissolved oxygen determinations, as may the inability to clear the aspiration needle and tubing between follicular punctures. In routine practice, use of an oxygen electrode is impractical owing to frequent calibration checks and the necessity of maintaining sterility if the probe is placed directly in the aspirate prior to the removal of the oocyte.

In order to eliminate some of the factors that may influence the accuracy of oxygen determinations of follicular fluid, Huey et al. (1999) collected an initial portion of the follicular fluid of 80 follicles by gentle aspiration into vacuum-sealed tubes. After disconnecting the tube, and with the aspiration needle remaining in the follicle, the residual fluid was withdrawn into a second tube. Atmospheric content of follicles was determined with a clinical blood gas analyzer from a small sample ($32\,\mu$l) of the initial aspirate. Values for dissolved oxygen in follicular fluid determined for 80 the follicles in which an initial portion of the aspirate was taken were between < 1.5 and > 3.6%. This range is comparable to the one reported by Van Blerkom et al. (1997) for

1000 whole aspirates analyzed with an oxygen electrode. Van Blerkom et al. (1997) noted that the dissolved oxygen content of follicular fluid derived from follicles of equivalent diameters and volumes on the same and different ovaries could not be predicted by conventional ultrasonographic imaging. A similar finding was reported by Huey et al. (1999), who described a high within-patient variance (57.6%) for follicular fluid oxygen content.

The notion that intrafollicular oxygen content and perifollicular blood flow may be related was suggested by Narglund et al. (1996b). This possibility was investigated for over 1000 follicles by Van Blerkom et al. (1997), who found that follicular fluid oxygen content was associated with perifollicular blood flow indices determined by color pulsed Doppler spectral analysis and imaging. In general, follicles with little or no detectable blood flow were at the low range of dissolved oxygen contents (<1.5%) while those with high PSV and clearly detectable circumferential flow were at the high end (>3.0%). In this study, follicles were classified as types A, B or C according to ultrasonographic findings made on the day of ovulation induction, approximately 14 hours prior to the administration of hCG. The average dissolved oxygen content (±0.2%) of type A, B and C follicles was 4.2%, 1.7%, and 2.4%, respectively. The highest rates of perifollicular blood flow among cohorts of follicles of comparable size were detected in type A follicles; type B follicles had the poorest flow rates, with no detectable flow observed for more than half of these follicles. Type C follicles were intermediate between A and B, with relatively intense flow located at different foci along the follicular circumference. Representative examples of types A, B and C follicles with corresponding spectral analysis of blood flow observed by color pulsed Doppler imaging are shown in Fig. 6.1a–f (color plate). A finding common to both the study of Van Blerkom et al. (1997) and other studies (Chui et al., 1997; Bahl et al., 1999) is that adjacent follicles with the same diameter on the day of ovulation induction by conventional ultrasonography often exhibit very different degrees of perifollicular blood flow when color Doppler ultrasonography is applied. To-date, the collective findings of clinical studies of perifollicular blood flow in gonadotropin-stimulated cycles indicate that for most patients undergoing IVF, the majority of fully grown follicles apparently fail to develop an expanded vasculature, as indicated by absent or diminished blood flow.

In a preliminary study, Stranger et al. (1999) scanned 652 follicles in stimulated and unstimulated cycles for perifollicular blood flow, beginning when follicles were approximately 5 mm and continuing until the day of ovulation induction. From repeated power color Doppler monitoring over several days, the findings demonstrated no change in blood flow rates for vascularized follicles; for those with no detectable flow, an abrupt onset of flow was not observed during the latter portion of the follicular phase. The results showed that apparent follicular vascularization detectable by Doppler ultrasonography during the early growth stage was rare in follicles <10 mm and was detectable in about 35% of all follicles >10 mm in diameter. However, on the day of ovulation induction, when follicles within cohorts were considered fully grown, only 44% of follicles over 19 mm in diameter had demonstrable flow. This finding is consistent with observations from other studies, which indicate, for most patients undergoing controlled ovarian hyperstimulation, that less than half of the fully grown follicles have detectable perifollicular blood flow at the end of the follicular phase. If confirmed, the study of Stranger et al. (1999) is of particular relevance in clinical treatments of infertility because it suggests a similar situation may prevail in unstimulated cycles, especially those cycles involving intrauterine insemination after ovulation induction. Several investigators have noted that for some infertility patients, and women of advanced reproductive age in particular, perifollicular blood flow was undetectable in all stage-appropriate, fully grown follicles; for other patients, the very few follicles with measurable flow were confined to one ovary (J. Stranger and L. Gregory, personal communication). It would appear that each follicle is unique with respect to the level of blood flow in its associated capillary bed and that the rate of antrum expansion or apparent follicular volume and diameter on the day of ovulation induction are unrelated to the degree or rate of perifollicular blood flow as determined by color Doppler imaging or spectral analysis. However, it does appear that the average level of oxygenation detected in follicular fluid aspirates after ovulation induction may be related to perifollicular blood flow rates on the day of ovulation induction.

The findings of Huey et al. (1999) are in contrast to the notion that follicle-specific blood flow rates and levels of oxygenation in follicular fluid are related. At approximately 12–14 hours after an ovulatory dose of hCG, the following perifollicular blood flow indices were obtained for 82 selected follicles: pulsatility index, which measures the systolic to diastolic differential of the velocity pulse, the resistance index (systolic velocity minus the diastolic velocity divided by systolic velocity), the ratio of systolic to diastolic velocities (see Fig. 18.6, p. 287 for explanation of these indices), and PSV. Ovum retrieval occurred 34–36 hours after hCG, at which time the oxygen content of a portion of the aspirate was determined. The findings indicated a negative correlation between perifollicular blood flow indices measured about 24 hours earlier and the dissolved oxygen content in aspirates, which ranged from approximately 1.3% to approximately 3.6%. The different findings reported by Huey et al. (1999) and Van Blerkom et al. (1997) may be related to the methodology used for dissolved oxygen determination or may have a physiological basis related to when blood flow indices were measured in these two studies. For example, changes in blood flow patterns and rates after ovulation induction may result from a deterioration of the vasculature at the follicular apex associated with degeneration of connective tissue and loss of the corresponding ovarian superficial epithelium. Electron microscopic observations of apical portions of preovulatory follicles in animal systems demonstrate significant pooling of blood (hemostasis) and capillary deterioration (e.g., Fig. 6.2e; for review see Van Blerkom and Motta, 1979). The image shown in Fig. 6.2f is a representative power angiographic image of a human follicle classified as well-vascularized prior to ovulation induc-

tion (type A or F4). Loss of vascularity at the follicular apex resulting in an ultrasonographic 'dark zone' (arrows in Fig. 6.2f) was a characteristic feature of preovulatory type A follicles (J. Van Blerkom, unpublished). Therefore, blood flow values obtained after ovulation induction and their relationship to intrafollicular oxygenation may (see below) or may not be representative of the pre-hCG condition. At present, however, the extent to which oxygenation of the follicular fluid is related to perifollicular vascularity and blood flow rates will need to be determined by additional studies.

Perifollicular blood flow indices and outcome

A current consensus of opinion indicates that developmental competence for each embryo, as demonstrated by outcome in IVF cycles, may in large measure be established while an oocyte is still resident in the growing or preovulatory follicle (Nayudu et al., 1987; Chui et al., 1997; Van Blerkom, 1997; Huey et al., 1999). The relationship between outcome and follicle-specific perifollicular blood flow has been examined by correlating the fate of specific transferred embryo(s) with blood flow indices of the corresponding follicle measured on the day of ovulation induction. In routine practice, these correlations can be very difficult to perform, especially when relatively large numbers of follicles have been recruited by gonadotropin stimulation into the growth and ovulatory pathway. Usually, it is practical to follow the in vitro development and post-transfer fate of specific embryos and their follicles of origin when each ovary had developed about six fully grown follicles. In these instances, cartoons or maps of follicles on each ovary are made from Doppler ultrasonographic images and matched to images obtained at the time of follicular aspiration, which is performed under transvaginal ultrasonographic guidance. Outcome reports indicate a significant and positive correlation between embryo implantation potential with day 2 and 3 transfers (4- to 10-cell stage) and the level of perifollicular blood flow measured on the day of ovulation induction. The findings reported by Chui et al. (1997), Van

Blerkom (1997), Bahl et al. (1999), Coulam et al. (1999) and Stranger et al. (1999) are consistent insofar as indicating that embryos with the highest potential to implant and to progress to birth develop from oocytes that originate from follicles with PSV values >10 cm/s and that correlate with type A and F4 follicles as described by Van Blerkom et al. (1997) and Chui et al. (1997), respectively. Both Van Blerkom (1997) and Bahl et al. (1999) reported no pregnancies occurred after transfer of normal-appearing cleavage stage embryos that originated from type B or F1 follicles, i.e., those for which no perifollicular blood flow could be detected. Both studies reported significantly reduced pregnancy rates with embryos that originated from follicles with blood flow classified as focal or diminished, i.e., type C or F2 follicles. Outcome results described by Coulam et al. (1999) for 106 patients undergoing IVF indicated that all pregnancies occurred in women with follicles of F3 or F4 blood flow.

Most studies that correlate specific embryos with specific follicles report pregnancy rates in excess of 50% after the transfer of two or three embryos derived from follicles with high blood flow. This common finding also clearly demonstrates that not all putative 'high-grade' embryos from these follicles are capable of progressive development and, in the absence of serial maternal serum hCG measurements after transfer, it is impossible to know whether demise was pre- or peri-implantation. In addition, it is not known whether transfer of competent embryos to an unreceptive uterus may have contributed to these failures. However, there does appear to be a developmentally significant relationship between embryo competence and the vascular/blood flow characteristics of the follicle from which the oocyte was derived. This apparent relationship is also indicated by the work of Huey et al. (1999), who correlated follicle-specific Doppler ultrasound indices after ovulation induction with embryo cell number on day 3. These investigators reported that certain lower Doppler indices were indicative of poor blood flow in the perifollicular microvasculature and were significantly and negatively correlated with the cleavage status of day 3 embryos (stage-appropriate cell numbers) but not

their morphology. A similar finding was described by Van Blerkom et al. (1997), who reported that after culture for 60 hours, the number of stage-appropriate embryos derived from follicles with good blood flow characteristics was approximately twice that observed for embryos derived from under-oxygenated follicles with poor Doppler flow indices. Although outcome was not assessed after day 3 transfer of morphologically comparable embryos originating from follicles with different blood flow characteristics, Huey et al. (1999) concluded that Doppler analysis may have only moderate predictive power for the selection of embryos with the highest implantation potential. At present, clinical use of Doppler ultrasonography may be most applicable in assessing in stimulated cycles the relative proportion of follicles produced that have high or poor flow, and using this information to distinguish between follicles that may be the least and the most likely to produce competent oocytes.

Perifollicular blood flow and oocyte developmental competence

While current findings indicate that the unique developmental potential of each oocyte is also follicle specific, it is unknown how the degree of expansion of the microvasculature or increased rates of perifollicular blood flow are associated with competence for the oocyte. Differences in dissolved oxygen content of follicular fluids, which we have correlated with Doppler imaging and spectral analysis of blood flow (Van Blerkom et al., 1997), on the day of ovulation induction, if confirmed, may provide new insights into biochemical and physiological differences between follicles that promote or compromise oocyte competence. The notion that the degree of expansion of the perifollicular vasculature may be related both to oxygen tension within the follicle and to the oocyte/embryo competence was first proposed by Gaulden (1992), who suggested underoxygenation in poorly vascularized follicles as a possible cause of trisomy 21 and other chromosomal defects in human oocytes. According to this hypothesis, inadequate vascularization during antral expansion results in an intrafollicular oxygen deficit that approaches an anoxic condition. In this circumstance, biochemical and metabolic activities for the oocyte, and proliferation and normal function for the granulosa, may be perturbed or abnormal. Gaulden (1992) suggested that underoxygenation may have metabolic consequences for the immature oocyte associated with a lowering of intracellular pH, a slight reduction in which, she proposed, could adversely influence the normality of metaphase spindle microtubular polymerization, organization, or movement. Defects in spindle organization or microtubular kinetics could result in monosomic and trisomic oocytes through failed chromosomal capture, premature detachment from the spindle, or malsegregation. While this hypothesis was primarily intended to explain the higher frequencies of chromosomal disorders associated with advanced reproductive age in women, it may also apply to younger women where controlled ovarian hyperstimulation forces the recruitment and growth of supraphysiological numbers of follicles.

Precise measurements of oxygen levels within follicular fluid are fundamentally flawed because they are derived from aspirates produced during ovum recovery and, regardless of the method of analysis, the values obtained (even if reflective of the preovulatory state) probably represent an average of the level that may actually be present. However, these averages may be developmentally relevant, especially when at the low range. Gosden and Byatt-Smith (1986) suggested that the diffusion of oxygen across the follicular wall may establish a dissolved oxygen gradient within the follicular fluid. Uptake of diffused oxygen would be expected to be highest in the mural granulosa at the follicular wall where these cells require oxygen for steroidogenesis (Zoller and Weisz, 1979; Gosden and Byatt-Smith, 1986). Although antral volume increases progressively during follicular growth through transudation from thecal vessels, the apparent absence of a mechanism that can generate intrafollicular turbulence suggests that the pool of follicular fluid may be a relative static one. Consequently, dissolved oxygen levels across this pool may follow predictable diffusion kinetics in a protein-rich medium, with the highest levels occurring near the follicular wall and levels decreasing progressively towards the center.

Figure 6.2b is an electron microscopic image of a fully grown human follicle showing the internal location of the oocyte and associated cumulus cells within the follicular fluid (also termed liquor folliculi). As the follicle grows, during which expansion of the perifollicular microvasculature is assumed to occur (Fig. 6.2c) the provision of locally high oxygen levels may primarily benefit the mural granulosa (Fig. 6.2b,c) as noted above. In this respect, the immature oocyte and its surrounding corona and unexpanded cumulus oophorus may also be influenced by a putative higher oxygen milieu because this complex is usually opposed to the follicular wall during follicular growth. Prior to meiotic reactivation, the oocyte and its associated cells may be refractory to or not require an elevated oxygen milieu. In this respect, the activity of this complex may remain unchanged from the situation that prevails in the preantral state, where it has been suggested that the oocyte may exist in a severely hypoxic or virtually anoxic environment (Gosden and Byatt-Smith, 1986; Gaulden, 1992). Figure 6.2a is a representative electron microscopic image of a primary follicle indicating the relative absence of perifollicular vessels detectable by the presence of red blood cells.

A putative static condition within the follicular fluid that could permit the establishment of a dissolved oxygen gradient may change rapidly after the occurrence of the ovulatory stimulus. The preovulatory phase is associated with delamination of the ovarian superficial epithelium at the follicular apex (Van Blerkom and Motta, 1979) and exposure of the underlying connective tissue (Fig. 6.2e). These investigators also showed that leakage of follicular fluid into spaces within the overlying connective tissue and its accumulation between cells of the apical superficial epithelium are early events in the peri-apical region of preovulatory follicles in rodent and rabbit. Fluid leakage from the antrum may be a proximal cause of delamination of the superficial epithelium and focal vascular degeneration within the apical theca. After the LH surge, contractions of perifollicular smooth muscle-like cells (myoid cells; O'Shea, 1970) may have a direct role in changing the geometry of the follicle, perhaps by enabling or causing portions of the follicular wall to invaginate and thereby increasing the relative fluid pressure within the antrum (Owman et al., 1979). After ovulation induction, alterations in follicular structure and architecture, combined with fluid exudation into spaces between peri-apical tissues, may contribute to intrafollicular turbulence and disruption of a putative follicular phase oxygen gradient. During the preovulatory phase, expansion of the cumulus oophorus by hydration of the intercellular hyaluronic acid matrix leads to an attenuation of the contact with the follicular wall and displacement of the oocyte towards the center of the follicle (Fig. 6.2b). The inward movement of this complex may also create turbulence within the follicular antrum. Assuming that intrafollicular levels of dissolved oxygen become uniform, increased oxygen availability within the follicle may be permissive for cumulus granulosa differentiation and expansion during the early luteal phase. If so, the normality of cumulus cell function may directly influence the normality of oocyte maturation and the acquisition of developmental competence. Whether oxygen levels have a direct effect on the oocyte is unknown. However, for most of its life (e.g., Fig. 6.2a), the immature oocyte may exist in an oxygen-limiting environment. Oxygen tension has been suggested to affect the developmental competence of mouse oocytes in vitro (Eppig and Wigglesworth, 1998), and an abrupt rise in oxygen concentration has been proposed to regulate the resumption of meiosis in vivo after the LH surge (Zeilmaker et al., 1972). Collectively, these findings suggest that differences in the average oxygen content of follicular fluid measured at aspiration may accurately reflect preovulatory levels. Additional investigation is required to determine the validity of these notions of intrafollicular oxygen gradients and fluid dynamics for the human ovary. However, the recent introduction of culture systems that can partially support the

growth of individual preantral follicles (Smitz et al., 1996; Abir et al., 1999; Smitz and Cortvrindt, 1999) may be one approach to determine the relationship between the establishment of oocyte competence and microvascular expansion, perifollicular blood flow rates, and intrafollicular oxygenation in vivo, since none of these actions occurs in follicular explants.

The results of Van Blerkom et al. (1997) would tend to discount the possibility that oxygen is a significant trigger of resumed meiosis in women, because comparable frequencies of MII oocytes were observed in fully grown follicles with follicular fluid containing dissolved oxygen at both the low and high ranges. This finding needs to be confirmed with larger numbers of oocytes, especially for those oocytes that failed to progress beyond the germinal vesicle stage after ovulation induction. However, chromosomal analysis of MII oocytes from follicles with different oxygen contents and blood flow characteristics has suggested that a potentially important relationship exists between oocyte competence and Doppler indices. Of the type B follicles examined by Van Blerkom et al. (1997), 74% of MII oocytes showed abnormalities in chromosomal organization and alignment on the metaphase spindle. In contrast, only 8% of oocytes from relatively well-oxygenated type A follicles were classified as abnormal. Some of the abnormalties detected included the occurrence of individual chromosomes detached from the spindle (Fig. 6.1h, color plate) and chromosomes occurring in a single, compact mass (Fig. 6.1i, color plate) or as multiple clusters scattered throughout the cytoplasm (Fig. 6.1j,k, color plate). A portion of the MII spindle in a presumably normal, living human oocyte as observed by conventional laser confocal microscopy after staining with DNA-specific probes is shown in Fig. 6.1g (color plate). Bataggalia et al. (1996) reported that defects in spindle organization and chromosomal alignment occurred in over 80% of normal-appearing MII oocytes obtained during natural menstrual cycles in women of advanced reproductive age (40–45 years). Their results showed spindle malformations that would be expected to be associated with chromosomal malsegregation. These defects were comparable to those observed by Van Blerkom et al. (1997) for normal-appearing MII oocytes obtained from follicles with poor blood flow indices in younger women undergoing superovulation for IVF.

Currently available evidence suggests that preovulatory oocyte maturation in follicles with poor or inadequate perifollicular blood flow correlates with reduced developmental competence after fertilization. With respect to issues of intrinsic and extrinsic influences on competence, whether a certain proportion of immature oocytes are predisposed to incompetence prior to entrance into the follicular growth and ovulatory pathway is a critical question, but one that is difficult to address experimentally in the human. It is not known whether immature oocytes become more susceptible to intrafollicular conditions and influences as women age, a possibility of particular relevance in infertility treatments where exogenous gonadotropin-stimulated follicular recruitment occurs against a background of diminished ovarian reserve that begins around age 33 years (Navot et al., 1991; Dor et al., 1996; Hull et al., 1996; Lass et al., 1997) and which has been correlated with increased frequencies of degenerate (Navot et al., 1991) and incompetent oocytes (Lim and Tsakok, 1997). In a clinical setting, virtually all oocytes available for analysis come from women undergoing IVF procedures. In practice, most of the oocytes routinely available for experimental or analytical purposes represent a highly self-selected class, namely, those that failed to fertilize. To-date, virtually all MII oocytes that have been examined for cytoplasmic and chromosomal defects (for review see Van Blerkom, 1994) have come from infertile women older than 35 years of age. Issues of maternal age and fertility are potentially confounding factors related to the question of whether the immature oocytes of some women may be predisposed to incompetence prior to recruitment or are more susceptible than others to intrafollicular conditions after recruitment.

We have used the mouse model to examine potential effects of repeated superovulation on oocyte competence in young animals (Van Blerkom and Davis, 2001). This study was designed to determine whether repeated superovulations in young mice, spaced one to six weeks apart, influenced oocyte competence at the nuclear level. The organization of the MII spindle and alignment of chromosomes were examined with DNA-specific fluorescence probes and by anti-tubulin immunostaining of newly ovulated oocytes. The study also used MII oocytes that matured in vitro after harvest at the germinal vesicle stage, from preantral follicles in the same stimulated/ovulated ovaries.

The mouse system appears to be an appropriate one experimentally to address questions of intrafollicular influences on oocyte competence, because earlier work indicates that a single cycle of superovulation can have adverse downstream effects on competence that include reduced fertility, elevated frequencies of pre- and postimplantation mortality, and a significant association with fetal growth retardation and certain congenital abnormalties (Vanderhyden et al., 1986; Edgar et al., 1987; Sakai and Endo, 1987; Elmazar et al., 1989; Fossum et al., 1989; Vogel and Spielmann, 1992; Ertzeid et al., 1993; Ma et al., 1997).

As shown in Table 6.1, a progressive increase in the frequency of spindle defects and aberrant chromosomal alignments occurred with each round of superovulation, and similar frequencies were observed for each round when intervals of superovulation were spaced one to six weeks apart. The oocytes examined in this study appeared normal at the light microscope level (e.g., Fig. 6.1*l*, color plate), but when examined by fluorescence microscopy, highly elongated and malformed spindles with malaligned or detached chromosomes were observed at ovulation (i.e., 14 hours after administration of an ovulatory dose of hCG; Fig. 6.1*q,r*, color plate). The color plate Fig. 6.1*m,n* demonstrates spindle organization (anti-tubulin immunofluorescence) and equatorial chromosomal alignment in a normal MII mouse oocyte. The number of ovulated oocytes that contained both defective spindles and numerous cytoplasmic microtubular asters increased significantly after the second round of superovulation. Cytoasters are not a typical constituent of normal

Table 6.1. Frequency of spindle defects in intact metaphase II mouse oocytes matured in vivo or in vitro after each of four rounds of superovulation spaced either one or four weeks apart

| | Frequency of spindle defects after four rounds of superovulation | | | |
| | One week interval | | Four week interval | |
Round	In vivo[a]	In vitro[b]	In vivo[a]	In vitro[b]
1	7/229 (3%)	0/82 (0)	8/167 (5%)	1/101 (1%)
2	26/160 (16%)	1/108 (<1%)	19/132 (14%)	1/60 (2%)
3	49/162 (30%)	0/69 (0)	53/166 (32%)	0/87 (0%)
4	75/128 (59%)	0/101 (0)	119/189 (63%)	0/54 (0%)

Notes:

[a] Intact metaphase II oocytes collected from the oviducts at 14 hours after treatment with human chorionic gonadotrophin.

[b] Metaphase II oocytes matured in vitro for 14 hours after collection at the germinal vesicle stage from the same superovulated ovaries as used in the in vivo maturation.

MII mouse oocytes, and their occurrence suggests that repeated superovulation might have adverse consequences on cytoplasmic stability during meiotic maturation in vivo. In contrast, oocytes retrieved at the germinal vesicle stage from the same ovaries and matured in vitro to MII over a 14-hour period (maturation frequency >90%) were normal (comparable to images shown in Fig. 6.1*m,n*, color plate). The findings reported by Van Blerkom and Davis (2001) indicate that repeated superovulation of young mice is associated with aberrant activity of the microtubular organizing centers, and this adversely affects the normality of spindle organization and the ability of spindle microtubules to capture chromosomes and to align them appropriately. At ovulation, the occurrence of cytoplasmic asters, detached chromosomes, and malformed spindles is very similar to the situation that develops in normal mouse oocytes after approximately 24 hours of culture and is associated with loss of developmental competence (Eichenlaub-Ritter et al., 1986; Eichenlaub-Ritter and Boll, 1989). Aging in the mouse is also associated with an increased frequency of changes in chromosomal alignment that are developmentally lethal in superovulated oocytes (Saito et al., 1993). The normality of oocytes from the same ovaries after maturation in vitro suggests that, with repeated superovulation, an increasing propor-

tion of oocytes that appear normal at ovulation contain nuclear defects. These defects may result from aberrant cytoplasmic activities or physiology that occurred during maturation in vivo.

As noted above, Bataggalia et al. (1996) reported that approximately 80% of MII oocytes aspirated from antral follicles of naturally cycling women between 40 and 45 years of age contained abnormally organized spindles with malaligned or detached chromosomes. Cytoplasmic asters have also been detected in these oocytes but not in the oocytes of younger women (20–25 years of age), which contained normal spindles and normally aligned chromosomes (D. Battagalia, personal communication). Battagalia and Miller (1997) proposed that an increased prevalence of age-related 'intrinsic defects' (oocyte specific) or adverse 'extrinsic factors' (follicle specific) may result from abnormal or asynchronous nuclear and cytoplasmic maturation, the consequence of which for women of advanced reproductive age may be high frequencies of oocyte aneuploidy. For the mouse, Van Blerkom and Davis (2001) suggested that aberrant cytoplasmic maturation during the terminal stages of meiosis is follicle specific. The finding that nuclear progression and cytoplasmic organization are normal for MII oocytes that matured in vitro from the germinal vesicle stage after recovery from preantral follicles in superovulated ovaries raises the intriguing possibility that, for the mouse, aging of the oocyte cytoplasm without evident damage to DNA integrity (Van Blerkom and Davis, 2001) may be accelerated in some proportion of oocytes when preovulatory maturation occurs in vivo. However, these results may also be relevant for other mammals, including the human, if they indicate that the normality of maturation in vivo is susceptible to intrafollicular conditions, the adverse effects of which on the oocyte may be subtle and not evident at the light microscopic level but which become evident during early embryogenesis.

For the mouse, superovulation was associated with significant changes in ovarian structure characterized by nodules of hypertrophied granulosa that become more abundant with repeated cycles of superovulation, even with cycles spaced weeks apart (Van Blerkom and Davis, 2001). As suggested by Szoltys et al. (1994) from histological findings in superovulated rat ovaries, proximity of preantral or early antral follicles to these regions may be an important factor in determining the normality of preovulatory maturation during subsequent natural or stimulated cycles. For example, paracrine and autocrine-acting growth factors, steroids, or other regulatory molecules that target the follicle may occur in these regions at high concentrations. If accumulated in antral fluid at abnormal levels during follicle growth, normal mural and cumulus granulosa cell function and developmentally critical signaling pathways between the oocyte and granulosa may be perturbed. If continued study demonstrates that extrinsic factors differentially influence the normality of meiotic maturation for the corresponding oocyte within cohorts of stimulated follicles, the mouse may offer a clinically relevant system to ask why only some oocytes are affected.

Follicular angiogenesis

During each menstrual cycle, repair of capillaries damaged by follicular rupture and transformation of the residual granulosa into a vascularized endocrine organ (the corpus luteum) involves the rapid proliferation of perifollicular endothelial cells and the formation of a nascent vasculature within the ovulated follicle. It is not surprising, therefore, that analysis of follicular aspirates at ovum retrieval for IVF has demonstrated a complex mixture of growth factors in this fluid, including those known to be involved in angiogenesis (Klein et al., 1996; reviewed by Van Blerkom, 2000). To-date, most biochemical studies of follicular angiogenesis have focused on vascular endothelial growth factor (VEGF), with primary emphasis on its suggested role in corpus luteum development and possible association with ovarian dysfunction and pathologies, such as hyperstimulation syndrome (Kumat et al., 1995; Neulen et al., 1995; Abramov et al., 1997; Doldi et al., 1997; Lee et al., 1997a,b; Rizk et al., 1997; Yamamoto et al., 1997; Agrawal et al., 1998, 1999; Anasti et al., 1998; Artini et al., 1998; Ferrara et al., 1998; Ludwig et al., 1998, 1999). Leptin, which has been recently shown to be a potent promoter of angiogenesis in vitro (Bouloumie et al., 1998; Sierra-Honigmann et al., 1998), is present in preovulatory human follicular fluid (Cioffi et al., 1997; Karlsson et al., 1997; Barroso et al., 1999) and it has been suggested that it may have a similar function in the ovarian follicle (Van Blerkom, 1998, 2000). Both leptin and VEGF are expressed by granulosa cells in vivo and the levels of both proteins appear to be upregulated significantly in granulosa cells when cultured in the presence of hCG (Neulen et al., 1995; Doldi et al., 1997; reviewed by Messinis and Milingos, 1999).

The possibility that oxygenation and angiogenic factors, such as VEGF, may have central roles in preovulatory follicular angiogenesis is suggested by the finding that, as for other systems, VEGF expression is upregulated under hypoxic conditions (Shweiki et al., 1992, 1993), including in cells in the rat corpus luteum that experience severe hypoxia because of deficient vascularization (Ferrara et al., 1998). If the level of VEGF expression by granulosa cells is oxygen sensitive, a hypothetical mechanism of regulation may be one in which an initially low oxygen content is a sufficient stimulus to upregulate VEGF expression by granulosa cells sensitized by FSH to recognize hypoxia during early follicular development and antral expansion. Van Blerkom et al. (1997) measured VEGF concentrations in several hundred follicular fluids after the dissolved oxygen content had been determined at aspiration. The results showed a slight tendency towards higher VEGF levels in relatively well-oxygenated follicles, but differences between follicles with different oxygen contents were not considered to be statistically or biologically significant. For leptin, Cioffi et al. (1997) reported that the concentration of this regulatory protein in follicular aspirates was follicle specific, ranging from a low of 1 ng/ml to a high of 87 ng/ml. Although based on a small number of patients, outcome results described in this study of 26 women undergoing IVF showed no apparent correlation between leptin concentration in follicular fluid and competence for the corresponding oocyte. Barroso et al. (1999) measured leptin and VEGF levels in 55 follicular aspirates from 16 patients undergoing IVF. Their findings indicated that VEGF and leptin concentrations in aspirates were follicle specific and occurred over a wide range (VEGF: 63–3300 pg/ml, leptin: 3–52 ng/ml). Interestingly, the only developmentally significant correlation with competence was reported to be a possible adverse effect of exceptionally high leptin and VEGF concentrations. In these instances, the corresponding oocytes resulted in embryos that on day 3 of culture were presumed to have reduced potential based on morphological criteria. If confirmed, these findings suggest that measurements of the levels of these two factors in periovulatory follicular aspirates may not be clinically useful indicators of competence for embryos that appear to develop normally through the early cleavage stages. However, even these values may not accurately reflect levels of expression during the follicular phase because hCG has been shown to elevate significantly levels VEGF synthesis (Agrawal et al., 1998; Artini et al., 1998).

Further study is required to determine levels of angiogenic factor expression during follicle growth, and in particular, the extent to which, if any, they are stage specific and can be clearly correlated with expansion of the perifollicular microvasculature, changes in perifollicular blood flow indices, and increased intrafollicular oxygenation. Since a low oxygen environment seems to be the state in which oocytes and follicles exist for most of their life, it seems reasonable to suggest that the expression of angiogenic factors may be an early response of granulosa cells to gonadotropin stimulation, perhaps by activation of an intrinsic ability of these cells to respond to hypoxia, as has been described for other systems (Bunn and Poyton, 1996; Van Blerkom, 1998).

Alternatively, the expression of VEGF, leptin, and other growth factors by granulosa cells may have a relatively minor role in perifollicular events and rather may serve to establish intrafollicular conditions that promote vascularization or steroidogenesis in anticipation of corpus luteum development and activity (Ferrara et al., 1998). Kumat et al. (1995) showed the presence of VEGF within the theca during the follicular phase by immunostaining; vessel expansion or blood flow through an existing microvasculature may be significantly influenced by VEGF production in the immediate vicinity of the perifollicular capillary bed. Recently, Antczak and Van Blerkom (2000) demonstrated that subpopulations of human and mouse granulosa cells express receptors and proteins that are specific, in combination, to endothelial cells. These investigators also showed that under certain conditions of culture, mural and cumulus granulosa cells form an expansive complex of interconnecting tube-like structures composed of hundreds of cells surrounding a fluid-filled lumen. The endothelial-like properties of certain granulosa cells and the capillary-like nature of the in vitro network led to the suggestion that some proportion of granulosa cells may have an inherent capacity to behave like endothelial cells; if similar morphogenetic events occur in vivo, these cells may have the ability to establish a primitive vascular-like network. Although this notion is a highly speculative one, the development of a primitive intrafollicular 'vasculature' may occur progressively in both mural and cumulus granulosa during follicular growth and preovulatory development in response to quantitative or qualitative changes in angiogenic factor expression within the follicle. It will be of interest to determine whether the expression of endothelial-like capacities by granulosa cells involves similar regulatory and signaling pathways to those used by true endothelial cells, including those influenced by hypoxia. The existence of a primitive vascular-like network in vivo will require detailed analysis of intact follicles to show both its presence and its capacity to achieve functional communication with endothelial cells derived from perifollicular capillaries. The clear demonstration of such an activity would extend understanding of whether vascularization of a normal corpus luteum involves elements derived from both intrafollicular and extrafollicular compartments. If such a relationship is indicated, the results could begin to explain follicle-specific differences in corpus luteum development and function; this may well be relevant in understanding cellular and molecular etiologies of pathological conditions such as hypervascularization associated with the ovarian hyperstimulation syndrome. Alternatively, the in vitro network observed by Antczak and Van Blerkom (2000) may be a granulosa cell activity that occurs in culture and, as such, is not indicative of a morphogenetic process associated with normal follicular and corpus luteum development. Nevertheless, studies of the differential activities and functions of granulosa cells are likely to result in a more comprehensive understanding of follicular biology in general, and possible origins and causes of follicle-specific vascularity and blood flow in particular.

VEGF and other angiogenic factors such as leptin may have additional roles in follicular and corpus luteum development. Ferrara et al. (1998) showed that experimental disruption of VEGF receptor activity in the rat ovary is associated with vascular degeneration, the creation of ischemic conditions within the corpus luteum, and inhibition of progesterone release by unaffected luteinized granulosa cells. A diminished pregnancy potential has been associated with unusually high VEGF levels in follicular aspirates of women with idiopathic and age-related infertility. In these women, VEGF concentrations have been reported to be severalfold higher (Friedman et al., 1998) than is typical (Van Blerkom et al., 1997). A presumed reduction in embryo competence on day 3 of culture has also been associated with high VEGF and leptin levels detected at ovum retrieval (Barroso et al., 1999). In this regard, elevated leptin levels have been shown to reduce granulosa cell progesterone production significantly by antagonizing the action of insulin (Brannian et al., 1999). After ovulation induction, overexpression of leptin in specific preovulatory follicles may negatively influence progesterone synthesis and could alter the intrafollicular milieu and normal signaling pathways between oocyte and cumulus. This may be especially relevant with respect to granulosa cell function and apoptosis in the preovulatory follicle (Oosterhuis et al., 1998) since both estrogen and progesterone have been shown to have an anti-apoptotic effect on these cells (Billig et al., 1993; Luciano et al., 1994).

Whether overexpression of VEGF (and possibly other angiogenic promoters and growth factors) adversely affects granulosa cell function or is related to abnormalities in perifollicular vascular development and blood flow awaits further study. If confirmed, however, the results could provide fundamentally new insight into the regulation of growth factor expression and granulosa cell activity, which, in turn, may influence oocyte competence. For example, defective signaling within the granulosa or between the granulosa and theca may result from receptor defects that preclude expansion of the capillary bed or increased perifollicular circulation. In this hypothetical circumstance, intrafollicular oxygen levels may remain unchanged. In such instances, factor overexpression in the affected follicle(s) of some women could indicate that the granulosa cells are refractory to downregulation (receptor defect?) or that no downregulation has occurred. For women of advanced reproductive age, Gaulden (1992) suggested that the inability of the perifollicular capillary bed to expand may be a direct result of an existing network that is too distant from the follicular wall to benefit from or be stimulated by factors originated from within the follicle.

Whether the result of receptor inadequacy/defect

or the relative location of the perifollicular vascular bed with respect to the follicular wall, if high levels of VEGF and other angiogenic factors are associated with diminished competence for the corresponding oocyte then the results would tend to suggest the existence of a developmentally significant relationship between the intrafollicular milieu and the ability of the oocyte to progress normally after fertilization. Understanding the nature of this relationship at the molecular and cellular levels presents formidable challenges when it is considered that the biochemistry of follicular fluid is highly complex and stage specific. The following is a short summary of some of the more important questions associated with the biology of the human follicle, answers to which will go a long way in explaining how oocyte competence may be determined by the development of unique follicular characteristics:

- what factors produced within the follicle, if any, are involved in perifollicular angiogenesis
- what regulatory mechanisms determine follicle-specific perifollicular blood flow rates and microvascular expansion
- to what extent is follicular fluid physiology and biochemistry determined by perifollicular blood flow
- do ovarian follicles develop an oxygen-sensing capacity during growth and, if so, do they respond to hypoxia by upregulating angiogenic and other growth factors or receptors to increase intrafollicular oxygenation
- why are blood flow rates increased in only some follicles and is this increase specifically related to follicles characterized as fully grown at ovulation induction; the latter may be an important issue since competent oocytes can originate from follicles that are less than fully grown at aspiration
- what are the consequences for normal granulosa cell proliferation and function when follicles remain undervascularized, have no detectable blood flow, or experience no change in the dissolved oxygen content of follicular fluid
- why are levels of factors such as leptin and VEGF abnormally high in the follicles of certain women, and what are the regulatory mechanisms that

determine factor expression at the transcriptional or translational levels?

Follicular determinants of competence: clinical relevance

For clinical purposes, one of the most relevant questions is: why do preovulatory oocytes that mature in follicles with poor blood flow indices have diminished embryo competence? It is not known whether specific intrafollicular conditions occur in these follicles that perturb developmentally critical signaling between granulosa cells, or between the oocyte and cumulus. Elucidating the role of such conditions/signals will require a more comprehensive understanding than currently exists of the specific paracrine and autocrine interactions that characterize the molecular dialogue between follicular components. In the same respect, continued investigation is required to determine what, if any, aspects of oocyte cytoplasmic physiology are sensitive to or are influenced by intrafollicular conditions or aberrant signaling/communication within the granulosa compartment. Reduced oocyte competence associated with abnormalties in meiotic spindle organization and chromosomal alignment detected in mouse and human oocytes could result from a relatively small reduction in intracellular pH (Van Blerkom, 1996). This, in turn, could have a significant and adverse impact on the dynamics of spindle microtubule formation, stability, or function (Gaulden, 1992). The notion that changes in oocyte physiology may have profound effects on embryo competence needs to be first clearly demonstrated in other systems, such as the mouse or cow, that are amenable to experimental manipulation. For the human, application of these findings in infertility treatment (as described above) would be supported if reduced oocyte competence results from follicle-specific intrafollicular conditions or influences and if the occurrence of these conditions/influences could be indicated by a readily detectable phenotype, such as differential perifollicular blood flow or vascularity. In this respect, the recent findings that cytoplasmic structure and organization at the pronuclear stage may be an early indication of human embryo competence may be particularly relevant. The appearance of a sub-plasmalemmal zone of translucent cytoplasm (initially described by Payne et al. (1997) as a cytoplasmic flare) that often progresses to involve the entire cytocortex (pronuclear halo; Scott and Smith, 1998) has been reported to be a clinically significant indicator of normal developmental potential during the preimplantation stages (Scott et al., 2000) and of competence after transfer (Scott and Smith, 1998; Scott et al., 2000). Garello et al. (1999) correlated pronuclear orientation, with respect to the first and second polar bodies, with the normality of cleavage during three days of culture. Significant deviations from a relatively perpendicular orientation were reported to predispose the affected embryos to common cleavage anomalies such as fragmentation, unequal cell divisions, and early developmental arrest. These investigators suggested that competence may be adversely influenced by certain pronuclear orientations, possibly reflecting aberrant distributions of regulatory proteins or nascent transcripts within the cytoplasm (Edwards and Beard, 1997), or by altering the normal pattern by which the plane of the first cleavage division bisects the single-cell embryo. Van Blerkom et al. (2000) examined the distribution of mitochondria in living human pronuclear and cleavage-stage embryos (followed either by measurements of the net ATP content of individual blastomeres or by anti-tubulin immunofluorescence) to determine the relationship between mitochondrial distribution and microtubular organization. Their results indicated that specific patterns of perinuclear mitochondrial aggregation and microtubular organization are related, and that asymmetrical mitochondrial distributions at the pronuclear stage can result in some proportion of blastomeres with reduced mitochondrial inheritance and diminished ATP-generating capacity during later development. While the inability to divide appears to be a development consequence for an affected blastomere; for the embryo, reduced competence may occur during cleavage if several blastomeres inherit a mitochondrial complement inadequate to support normal cellular functions.

The association between the normality of preimplantation embryogenesis and pronuclear orientation, cortical cytoplasmic organization, and mitochondrial distribution at the single-cell stage suggests that these events may have a common origin related to stage-specific changes in the structure of the cytoplasm, which may primarily involve microtubules (Van Blerkom et al., 1995, 2000). If a common etiology is established, such results could begin to explain how differences in cytoplasmic organization at the single-cell stage are consistent with or permissive of normal preimplantation development in the human. They would also explain, the extent to which they may have already been influenced or determined in the oocyte by virtue of specific intrafollicular influences on ooplasmic physiology.

Application of granulosa cell DNA libraries to the question of competence

While immunologically based assays have demonstrated that follicular fluid has a complex biochemistry containing such macromolecules as regulatory proteins, growth factors, and other bioactive agents, their precise functions, targets, and interactions in the growing and preovulatory follicle are largely unknown, as is their relationship to competence. Another approach to investigate follicular biology as it relates to competence is subtractive analysis of complementary DNA (cDNA) libraries derived from mRNA transcribed by granulosa cells in follicles that have demonstrable characteristics suggestive, on current evidence, of differential competence. With this method, it is possible to detect virtually all transcripts that may be specific for follicle, stage and cell type. It is also possible to detect transcripts that undergo significant up- or downregulation during follicular development. We have used this approach to construct subtractive libraries of mRNA expressed by mural and cumulus granulosa cells obtained from aspirates of fully grown human follicles on the same ovary but with different perifollicular blood flow indices (those occurring in type A but not in type B follicles: J. Van Blerkom and J. Cioffi, unpublished data). Table 6.2 presents a preliminary survey of known genes, identified from public domain human genomic databases, that were expressed in two follicle-specific mural granulosa cell libraries derived from two type A follicles (minus two type B libraries) on the same ovary in two patients. A cursory inspection of the number and types of gene transcripts detected in mural granulosa cells from type A (but not type B) follicles further demonstrates the apparent complexity of gene expression in the fully grown, stimulated human follicle. Whether these transcripts are truly follicle specific or the result of significant over-expression in type A follicles will need to be determined by analysis of additional libraries from similar types of follicle. It should be noted that transcripts for two regulatory factors discussed above, VEGF and leptin, are not included in this list because their expression was common to both types of follicle. The constellation of putative follicle-specific genes shown in Table 6.2 presents a daunting task to select, for a detailed study, specific or interesting genes with expression that may be related to known follicular processes or oocyte competence. While the function or relevance in follicular biology is obscure at present for most of the detected genes, others may provide important insights into differences in molecular expression between follicles. For instance, the levels of angiogenic and steroidogenic activity may be related to the expression of hypoxia-inducible factor 1 (HIF-1) and steroidogenic acute regulatory protein expression (StAR), respectively. The expression of the former is of particular interest because this transcription factor mediates the expression of at least 28 genes involved in cellular responses to hypoxia (Semenza, 1999), including the upregulation of VEGF (Mazure et al., 1997; Agani and Semenza, 1998). If confirmed, the apparent absence or underexpression of HIF-1 mRNA in two libraries from type B follicles examined to date may be related to poor perifollicular blood flow or vascular development in this type of follicle.

The expression of StAR in type A follicles may also be relevant to granulosa cell function and apoptosis. StAR is a protein that stimulates the first step in steroid hormone biosynthesis, namely, the translocation of cholesterol from the outer mitochondrial membrane to the inner mitochondrial membrane, where P450 enzymes cleave the cholesterol side-chain and convert it into pregnenolone. It is not known whether the apparent underexpression of StAR in type B follicles is associated with reduced levels of steroidogenesis and higher frequencies of apoptosis for the corresponding granulosa cells, which could indicate an intrafollicular milieu that is inconsistent with the generation of a competent oocyte. LH and hCG upregulate StAR expression in granulosa cells at both the mRNA and protein levels (Strauss et al., 1999). It is unclear why StAR transcription was not detected or was significantly downregulated in type B follicles, where hCG was presumably present and sufficiently active within the follicle to initiate the meiotic maturation cascade for the oocyte. Further study will be required to determine whether differential gene expression between follicles, as described above, is related to differential follicular characteristics and competence. It is also important to reemphasize that the validity and consistency of genes identified in granulosa cell mRNA expression libraries will need to be confirmed. During this process, the array of genes that are novel or truly follicle specific will undoubtedly change and become more defined. However, the detection of regulatory protein expression by human granulosa cells is an important first step in efforts to provide clinically applicable correlates of follicular phenotypes and competence. In this regard, we are presently examining the possibility that HIF-1 expression is a hypoxia-mediated response by gonadotropin-sensitized granulosa cells that, in a normal follicle, initiates a coordinated expression of angiogenic and other growth factors to increase ambient intrafollicular oxygen levels.

In combination, molecular aspects of follicular biology, noninvasive analyses of follicle-specific characteristics (such as perifollicular blood flow), and outcome for the corresponding oocyte provide a

Table 6.2. Genes unique to or significantly over-expressed in type A human follicles[a]

Acetyl coenzyme A transporter	G-rich sequence factor-1
Acidic calponin (human, kidney, mRNA, 1607 nt)	GC20 protein
ACTB β-actin (β_1-actin)	GDP dissociation inhibitor
Activating transcription factor family member ATF6	Glutamine synthetase (E.C. 6.3.1.2)
ADP/ATP	Gorilla β_2-microglobulin
ADS39	Granulocyte –macrophage 2 activator protein
AH receptor	Heat shock protein 70
Alcohol dehydrogenase chi polypeptide (ADH5)	Heat shock protein 86
Aldolase C gene for fructose 1,6-bisphosphate aldolase	Heat shock protein 90
All-1 gene	Herpesvirus-associated ubiquitin-specific protease
Amyloid precursor protein	*hH3.3B* gene for histone H3.3
Apolipoprotein A1 regulatory protein	Histone deacetylase 3 mRNA
Arginine-rich nuclear protein mRNA	Histone H3.
Arylacetamide deacetylase	Histone H3.3
ATP binding	Histone RNA hairpin-binding protein
B-cell translocation gene-2 polypeptide cDNA	Homeobox protein CDX4 (CDX4) gene
Bcl2/adenovirus E1B 19kDa interacting protein 2	Homolog of Nedd5 (HNedd5)
Beta-2-microglobulin mRNA (GOGOB2M)	Hypoxia-inducible factor 1 α
Bruton's tyrosine kinase	Importin β
Butylcholinesterase	Interferon-responsive transcription factor
Calmodulin	Laminin receptor
calmodulin-1	Lanosterol 14-demethylase
Capping protein α-subunit isoform	Lanosterol 14-demethylase cytochrome P450 (CYP51)
CASK mRNA	Lipocortin II
CD24 signal	Lipoma preferred partner (LPP)
Chaperonin (heat shock protein 60)	Lupus autoantigen (small nuclear ribonucleoprotein)
Cyclin G_1	*memc* mRNA
Cytochrome B561, HCYTO B561	Microsomal aldehyde dehydrogenase
Cytochrome *c*	Mitochondrial 2,4-dienoyl CoA
Cytochrome *c* oxidase gene for subunit VIIc	Mitochrondrial 3-ketoacyl CoA thiolase β-subunit
Cytoplasmic dynein intermediate chain isoform IC-2	Morphogenetic protein receptor type I ALK-6
Cytoplasmic dynein light chain 1 (hdlc1)	mRNA for 80K-L
Cytoplasmic 3-hydroxy-3-methylglutaryl coenzyme A synthase	mRNA for synaptotagmin
Cytovillin 2	mRNA from HIV-associated non-Hodgkin's disease
Decorin	Multispanning membrane
Diabetes-associated peptide 3 (DAP-3)	Myosin regulatory light chain
Dihydropyrimidinase-related protein	*N*-Myristoyltransferase
DNA-binding protein TAXREB107	NADH dehydrogenase subunit
Dynein light chain 1 (hdlc1)	NADH:ubiquinone oxidoreductase subunit B13 mRNA
Dyskeratosis congenita gene (dkc1)	*ncx1* gene (exon 12)
EB1	Nuclear protein 220
EBD3 Cri-du-chat critical region mRNA	Nuclear ribonucleoprotein particle (hnRNP) C protein
Elongation factor 1 α-subunit	oligodendrocyte myelin glycoprotein (OMG)
Estetrol-binding protein 4	p54 *nrb* gene
FMR (Fragile site mental retardation) gene	Plakophilin 2a and b
FRG1	Poly(A)-binding protein II

Table 6.2 (*cont.*)

Proteasome subunit HsN3	Telomeric DNA sequence, clone 16QTEL038, read
Protein kinase, PKX1	Tenascin
Prothymosin α	Tetratricopeptide repeat protein
Putative cytokine 21 (HC21)	Thyroid autoantigen
ras GTPase-activating-like protein	Thyroid autoantigen mRNA
Ras-related (human, genomic/mRNA, 1980)	Thyroid receptor interactor (TRIP7)
Ribosomal protein L37a	Tigger 1 transposable element
Ribosomal protein L9	TPM3R1 DNA sequence
Ribosomal protein S6 mRNA	Transcription factor ETR103 mRNA, complete ods
RY-1 mRNA for putative nucleic acid-binding protein	Transcriptional activator
S signal recognition particle subunit 9 (SRP9)	Translational initiation factor (elF-2), α-subunit mRNA
Scaffold attachment factor A	*tre* oncogene (clone 210)
Secreted protein K39 3′ portion including the poly-A tail	Tryptophanyl tRNA synthetase (WRS)
Serine kinase SRPK2 mRNA	UEV-1 (UBE2V) alternatively spliced incompletely processed
smg GDS-associated protein SMAP	Vacuolar proton ATPase, subunit E
SOD-2 for manganese superoxide dismutase	Zinc finger DNA-binding protein 89 kDa (ZBP-89)
Squalene epoxidase	Zinc finger protein factor ETR103
Steroidogenic acute regulatory protein gene	Zinc finger protein, transcription factor

Notes:

nt, nucleotides.

[a] Genes or gene products given.

truly singular opportunity to understand, in detail, the processes, events, and extent to which the unique developmental competence of each human embryo is established while resident as an oocyte within the follicle. In conjunction with oocyte gene expression libraries, this approach can provide new insights into the basic biology of the human oocyte and the mechanisms by which extrinsic factors and epigenetic forces may influence or regulate this biology. For clinical purposes, these results can lead to a better understanding and characterization of follicular normality and greater confidence in the utility of information obtained from ovarian ultrasonographic evaluations. Ultimately, molecular analysis of follicular gene expression may provide protein markers associated with competence, and new approaches to the causes and treatments of follicular dysfunction and pathology.

REFERENCES

Abir, R., Roizman, P., Fisch, B., et al. (1999). Pilot study of isolated human follicles cultured in collagen gels for 24 hours. *Human Reproduction*, **14**, 1299–301.

Abramov, Y., Barak, V., Nisman, B., and Schenker, J. (1997). Vascular endothelial growth factor plasma concentrations correlate to the clinical picture in severe ovarian hyperstimulation syndrome. *Fertility and Sterility*, **67**, 261–5.

Agrawall, R. Conway, G., Sladkevicius, P., et al. (1998). Serum vascular endothelial growth factor and Doppler blood flow velocities in in vitro fertilization: relevance to ovarian hyperstimulation syndrome and polycystic ovaries. *Fertility and Sterility*, **70**, 651–8.

Agrawall, R., Tan, S.-L., Wild, S., et al. (1999). Serum vascular endothelial growth factor concentrations in in vitro fertilization cycles predict the risk of ovarian hyperstimulation syndrome. *Fertility and Sterility*, **71**, 287–93.

Alikani, M., Cohen, J., Tomkin, G., et al. (1999). Human embryo fragmentation in vitro and its implications for pregnancy and implantation. *Fertility and Sterility*, **71**, 836–42.

Agani, F. and Semenza, G. (1998). Mersalyl is a novel inducer of vascular endothelial growth factor gene expression and hypoxia-inducible factor 1 activity. *Molecular Pharmacology*, **54**, 749–54.

Anasti, J., Kalantaridou, S., Kimzey, L., et al. (1998). Human follicular fluid vascular endothelial growth factor concentrations are correlated with luteinization in spontaneously developing follicles. *Human Reproduction*, **13**, 1144–7.

Antczak, M. and Van Blerkom, J. (1999). Temporal and spatial aspects of fragmentation in early human embryos: possible effects on developmental competence and association with the differential elimination of regulatory proteins from polarized domains. *Human Reproduction*, **14**, 429–47.

Antczak, M. and Van Blerkom, J. (2000). The vascular character of ovarian follicular granulosa cells: phenotypic and functional evidence for an endothelial-like cell population. *Human Reproduction*, **15**, 2306–18.

Artini, P., Fasciani, A., Mori, M., et al. (1998). Changes in vascular endothelial growth factor concentrations and the risk of ovarian hyperstimulation syndrome in women enrolled in an in vitro fertilization program. *Fertility and Sterility*, **70**, 560–4.

Bahl, P., Pugh, N., Chui, D., et al. (1999). The use of transvaginal power Doppler ultrasonography to evaluate the relationship between perifollicular vascularity and outcome in in-vitro fertilization treatment cycles. *Human Reproduction*, **14**, 939–45.

Barroso, G., Barrionuevo, M., Rao, P., et al. (1999). Vascular endothelial growth factor, nitric oxide, and leptin follicular fluid levels correlate negatively with embryo quality in IVF patients. *Fertility and Sterility*, **72**, 1024–6.

Battaglia, D. and Miller, M. (1997). The aging oocyte. *Endocrinologist*, **7**, 1–5.

Battaglia, D., Goodwin, P., Klein, N., and Soules, M. (1996). Influence of maternal age on meiotic spindle assembly in oocytes from naturally cycling women. *Human Reproduction*, **11**, 2217–22.

Billig, H., Furuta, I., and Hsueh, A.(1993). Estrogens inhibit and androgens enhance ovarian granulosa cell apoptosis. *Endocrinology*, **134**, 245–52.

Bouloumie, A., Drexler, H., Lafontan, M., and Busse, R. (1998). Leptin, the product of the *ob* gene, promotes angiogenesis. *Circulation Research*, **83**, 1059–66.

Brannian, J., Zhao, Y., and McElroy, M. (1999). Leptin inhibits gonadotropin-stimulated granulosa cell progesterone production by antagonizing insulin action. *Human Reproduction*, **14**, 1445–8.

Bunn, H. and Poyton. R. (1996). Oxygen sensing and molecular adaptations to hypoxia. *Physiological Reviews*, **76**, 839–85.

Campbell, S., Bourne, T., Waterstone, J., et al. (1993). Transvaginal color flow imaging of the preovulatory follicle. *Fertility and Sterility*, **60**, 433–8.

Cioffi, J., Van Blerkom, J., Antczak, M., et al. (1997). The expression of leptin and its receptors in preovulatory human follicles. *Molecular Human Reproduction*, **3**, 467–72.

Chui, D., Pugh, N., Walker, S., et al. (1997). Follicular vascularity – the predictive value of transvaginal power Doppler ultrasonography in an in vitro fertilization programme. A preliminary study. *Human Reproduction*, **12**, 191–6.

Collins, W., Jurkovic, D., Bourne, T., et al. (1991). Ovarian morphology, endocrine function and follicular blood flow during the peri-ovulatory period. *Human Reproduction*, **6**, 319–24.

Coulam, C., Goodman, C., and Rinehart, J. (1999). Colour Doppler indices of follicular blood flow as predictors of pregnancy after in-vitro fertilization and embryo transfer. *Human Reproduction*, **14**, 1979–82.

Doldi, N., Bassan, M., Messa, A., and Ferrari, A. (1997). Expression of vascular endothelial growth factor in human luteinizing granulosa cells and its correlation with the response to controlled ovarian hyperstimulation. *Gynecologic Endocrinology*, **11**, 263–7.

Dor, J., Seidman, D., and Ben-Shlomo, I. (1996). Cumulative pregnancy rate following in-vitro fertilization: the significance of age and infertility aetiology. *Human Reproduction*, **11**, 425–8.

Edgar, D., Whallet, K., and Mills, J. (1987). Effects of high dose and multiple-dose gonadotropin stimulation on mouse oocyte quality assessed by preimplantation development following in vitro fertilization. *Journal of In Vitro Fertilization and Embryo Transfer*, **4**, 273–6.

Edwards, R. (1986). Causes of early pregnancy loss. *Human Reproduction*, **1**, 185–98.

Edwards, R. and Beard, H. (1997). Oocyte polarity and cell determination in early mammalian embryos. *Molecular Human Reproduction*, **3**, 863–905.

Eichenlaub-Ritter, U. and Boll, I. (1989). Age-related non-disjunction, spindle formation and progression through maturation of mammalian oocytes. *Progress in Clinical Biological Research*, **318**, 259–69.

Eichenlaub-Ritter, U., Chandely, A., and Gosden, R. (1986). Alterations to the microtubular cytoskeleton and increased disorder of chromosome alignment in spontaneously ovulated mouse oocytes aged in vivo: an immunofluorescence study. *Chromosoma*, **94**, 337–45.

Elmazar, M., Vogel, R., and Spielmann, H. (1989). Maternal factors influencing development of embryos from mice superovulated with gonadotropins. *Reproductive Toxicology*, **3**, 135–8.

Eppig, J. and Wigglesworth, K. (1998). Factors affecting the developmental competence of mouse oocytes grown in vitro: oxygen concentrations. *Human Reproduction*, **13**, 664–9.

Ertzeid, G., Storeng, R., and Lyberg, T. (1993). Treatment with gonadotropins impaired implantation and fetal development in mice. *Journal of Assisted Reproduction and Genetics*, **10**, 286–91.

Ferrara, N., Chen, H., Davis-Smith, T., et al. (1998). Vascular endothelial growth factor is essential for corpus luteum angiogenesis. *Nature Medicine*, **4**, 336–40.

Fossum, G., Davidson, A., and Paulson, R. (1989). Ovarian hyperstimulation inhibits embryo implantation in the mouse. *Journal of In Vitro Fertilization and Embryo Transfer*, **6**, 7–10.

Friedman, C., Seifer, D., Kennard, E., et al. (1998). Elevated levels of follicular fluid vascular endothelial growth factor is a marker of diminished pregnancy potential. *Fertility and Sterility*, **70**, 836–9.

Garello, C., Baker, H., Rai, J., et al. (1999). Pronuclear orientation, polar body placement, and embryo quality after intracytoplasmic sperm injection and in-vitro fertilization: further evidence for polarity in human oocytes? *Human Reproduction*, **14**, 2588–95.

Gaulden, M. (1992). The enigma of Down syndrome and other trisomic conditions. *Mutation Research*, **269**, 69–88.

Gerris, J., De Neubourg, D., Mangelschoots, K., et al. (1999). Prevention of twin pregnancy after in vitro fertilization or intracytoplasmic sperm injection based on strict embryo criteria: a prospective randomized clinical trial. *Human Reproduction*, **14**, 2581–7.

Gosden, R. and Byatt-Smith, J. (1986). Oxygen concentration gradient across the ovarian follicular epithelium: model, predictions and implications. *Human Reproduction*, **1**, 65–8.

Gregory, L., Booth, A., Wells, C., and Walker, S. (1994). A study of the cumulus–corona cell complex in in-vitro fertilization and embryo transfer: a prognostic indicator of the failure of implantation. *Human Reproduction*, **9**, 1308–17.

Hoover, L., Baker, A., Check, J., et al. (1995). Evaluation of a new embryo grading system to predict pregnancy rates following in vitro fertilization. *Gynecology and Obstetrics Investigations*, **40**, 151–7.

Huey, S., Abuhamad, A., Barroso, G., Hsu, M., et al. (1999). Perifollicular blood flow Doppler indices, but not follicular pO_2, pO_2, or pH, predict oocyte developmental competence in vitro fertilization. *Fertility and Sterility*, **72**, 707–12.

Hull, M., Fleming, C., Hughes, A., and McDermott, A. (1996). The age-related decline in female fecundity: a quantitative controlled study of implantation capacity and survival of individual embryos after in vitro fertilization. *Fertility and Sterility*, **65**, 783–90.

Karlsson, C., Lindell, K., Svensson, E., et al. (1997). Expression of functional leptin receptors in the human ovary. *Journal of Clinical Endocrinology and Metabolism*, **82**, 4144–8.

Klein, N., Battaglia, D., Miller, P., et al. (1996). Ovarian follicular development and the follicular fluid hormones and growth factors in normal women of advanced reproductive age. *Journal of Clinical Endocrinology and Metabolism*, **81**, 1946–51.

Kumat, B., Brown, L., Manseau, E., et al. (1995). Expression of vascular permeability/vascular endothelial growth factor by human granulosa and theca lutein cells: role in corpus luteum development. *American Journal of Pathology*, **146**, 157–65.

Lass, A., Silye, R., Abrams, D.C., et al. (1997). Follicular density in ovarian biopsy of infertile women: a novel method to assess ovarian reserve. *Human Reproduction*, **12**, 1028–31.

Lee, A., Christenson, L., Patton, P., et al. (1997a). Vascular endothelial growth factor production by human luteinized granulosa cells in vitro. *Human Reproduction*, **12**, 2756–61.

Lee, A., Christenson, L., Stouffer, R., et al. (1997b). Vascular endothelial growth factor concentrations in serum and follicular fluid of patients undergoing in vitro fertilization. *Fertility and Sterility*, **68**, 305–11.

Lim, A. and Tsakok, M. (1997). Age-related decline in fertility: a link to degenerative oocytes? *Fertility and Sterility*, **68**, 265–71.

Luciano, A., Parralardo, A., Ray, C., and Peulso, J. (1994). Epidermal growth factor inhibits granulosa cell apoptosis by stimulating progesterone synthesis and regulating the distribution of intracellular free calcium. *Biology of Reproduction*, **51**, 646–54.

Ludwig, M., Gembruch, U., Bauer, O., and Diedrich, K. (1998). Serum concentrations of vascular endothelial growth factor cannot predict the course of severe ovarian hyperstimulation syndrome. *Human Reproduction*, **13**, 30–2.

Ludwig, M., Jelkmann, W., Bauer, O., and Diedrich, K. (1999). Prediction of severe ovarian hyperstimulation syndrome by free serum vascular endothelial growth factor concentration on the day of human chorionic gonadotropin administration. *Human Reproduction*, **14**, 2437–41.

Ma, S., Kalousek, D., Yuen, B., and Moon, Y. (1997). Investigation of effects of pregnant mare serum gonadotropin (PMSG) on the chromosomal complement of CD-1 mouse embryos. *Journal of Assisted Reproduction and Genetics*, **14**, 162–9.

Mazure, N., Chen, E., Laderoute, K., and Giaccia, A. (1997). Induction of vascular endothelial growth factor by hypoxia is regulated by a phosphatidylinositol 3-kinase/Akt signaling pathway in Ha-*ras* transformed cells through a hypoxia inducible factor-1 transcriptional element. *Blood*, **90**, 3322–31.

Messinis, I. and Milingos, S. (1999). Leptin in human reproduction. *Human Reproduction Update*, **5**, 52–63.

Nargund, G., Bourne, T., Doyle, P., et al. (1996a). Association between ultrasound indices of follicular blood flow, oocyte recovery, and preimplantation embryo quality. *Human Reproduction*, **11**, 109–13.

Nargund, G., Doyle, P., Bourne, T., et al. (1996b). Ultrasound derived indices of follicular blood flow before HCG administration and the prediction of oocyte recovery and preimplantation embryo quality. *Human Reproduction*, **11**, 2515–17.

Navot, D., Bergh, P., Williams, M., et al. (1991). Poor oocyte quality rather than implantation failure as a cause of age-related decline in female fertility. *Lancet*, **337**, 1375–7.

Nayudu, P., Gook, D., Lopata, A., et al. (1987). Follicular characteristics associated with viable pregnancy after in vitro fertilization in humans. *Gamete Research*, **18**, 37–55.

Nayudu, P., Lopata, A., Jones, et al. (1989a). An analysis of human oocytes and follicles from stimulated cycles: oocyte morphology and associated follicular fluid characteristics. *Human Reproduction*, **4**, 558–67.

Nayudu, P., Gook, D., Hepworth, G., et al. (1989b). Prediction of outcome in human in vitro fertilization based on follicular and stimulation response variables. *Fertility and Sterility*, **51**, 117–25.

Neulen, J., Yan, Z., Raczek, S., et al. (1995). Human chorionic gonadotropin-dependent expression of vascular endothelial growth factor/vascular permeability factor in human granulosa cells: importance in ovarian hyperstimulation syndrome. *Journal of Clinical Endocrinology and Metabolism*, **80**, 1967–71.

Oosterhuis, G., Micggelsen, H., Lambalk, C., et al. (1998). Apoptotic cell death in human granulosa-lutein cells: a possible indicator of in vitro fertilization outcome. *Fertility and Sterility*, **70**, 747–9.

O'Shea, J. (1970). An ultrastructural study of smooth muscle-like cells in the theca externa of ovarian follicles in the rat. *Nature Records*, **167**, 127–38.

Owman, C., Sjoberg, N., Wallach, E., et al. (1979). Neuromuscular mechanisms of ovulation. In: *Human Ovulation: Mechanisms, Prediction, Detection and Induction*, Hafez, H.S.E., ed. Elsevier/North-Holland Biomedical Press, Amsterdam, pp. 57–100.

Payne, D., Flaherty, S., Barry, M., and Matthews, C. (1997). Observations on polar body extrusion and pronuclear formation in human oocytes using time-lapse cinematography. *Human Reproduction*, **12**, 532–41.

Rizk, B., Aboulghar, M., Smitz, J., and Ron-El., R. (1997). The role of vascular endothelial growth factor and interleukins in the pathogenesis of severe ovarian hyperstimulation syndrome. *Human Reproduction Update*, **3**, 255–66.

Sakai, N. and Endo, A. (1987). Potential teratogenicity of gonadotropin treatment for ovulation in the mouse offspring. *Teratology*, **36**, 229–33.

Saito, H., Koike, K., Saito, T., et al. (1993). Aging changes the alignment of chromosomes after human chorionic gonadotropin stimulation may be a possible cause of decreased fertility in mice. *Hormone Research*, **39**(Suppl. 1), 28–31.

Scott, L. and Smith, S. (1998). The successful use of pronuclear embryo transfers the day following oocyte retrieval. *Human Reproduction*, **13**, 1003–13.

Scott, L., Alvero, R., Leondires, M., and Miller, B. (2000). The morphology of human pronuclear embryos is positively related to blastocyst development and implantation. *Human Reproduction*, **15**, 2394–403.

Semenza, G. (1999). Regulation of mammalian O_2 homeostasis by hypoxia-inducible factor 1. *Annual Reviews in Cellular and Developmental Biology*, **15**, 551–78.

Shweiki, D., Itin, A., Soffer, D., and Keshet, E. (1992). Vascular endothelial growth factor induced by hypoxia may mediate hypoxia-initiated angiogenesis. *Nature*, **359**, 843–5.

Shweiki, D., Itin, A., and Neufeld, G. (1993). Patterns of expression of vascular endothelial growth factor (VEGF) and VEGF receptors in mice suggest a role in hormonally regulated angiogenesis. *Journal of Clinical Investigation*, **91**, 2235–43.

Sierra-Honigmann, M., Nath, A., Murakami, C., et al. (1998). Biological action of leptin as an angiogenic factor. *Science*, **281**, 1683–6.

Smitz, J. and Cortvrindt, R. (1999). Oocyte in vitro maturation and follicle culture: current clinical achievements and future directions. *Human Reproduction*, **14**(Suppl. 1), 145–61.

Smitz, J., Cortvrindt, R., and Van Steirteghem, A. (1996). Normal oxygen atmosphere is essential for the solitary long-term culture of early pre-antral mouse follicles. *Molecular Reproduction Development*, **45**, 466–75.

Steptoe, P. and Edwards, R. (1978). Birth after the reimplantation of a human embryo. *Lancet*, **ii**, 366.

Stranger, J., Eadle, D., and Morris, D. (1999). Follicle vascularization associated with follicle development. In: *Proceedings of the 11th World Congress on In Vitro Fertilization and Human Reproductive Genetics*, Sydney, Australia, abstract 0–130.

Strauss, J., Kallen, C., Christenseon, L., et al. (1999). The steroidogenic acute regulatory protein (StAR): a window into the complexities of intracellular cholesterol trafficking. *Recent Progress in Hormone Research*, **54**, 369–95.

Suzuki, T., Sasano, H., Takaya, R., et al. (1998). Cyclic changes of vasculature and vascular phenotypes in normal human ovaries. *Human Reproduction*, **13**, 953–9.

Szoltys. M., Galas, J., Jablonka, A., and Tabarowski, Z. (1994).

Some morphological and hormonal aspects of ovulation and superovulation in the rat. *Journal of Endocrinology*, **141**, 91–100.

Van Blerkom, J. (1994). Developmental failure in human reproduction associated with chromosomal abnormalities and cytoplasmic pathologies in meiotically mature oocytes. In: *The Biological Basis of Early Reproductive Failure in the Human: Applications to Medically Assisted Conception*, Van Blerkom, J. ed. Oxford University Press, Oxford, pp. 283–325.

Van Blerkom, J. (1996). The influence of intrinsic and extrinsic factors on the developmental potential and chromosomal normality of the human oocyte. *Journal of the Society for Gynecologic Investigation*, **3**, 3–11.

Van Blerkom, J. (1997). Can the developmental competence of early human embryos be predicted effectively in the clinical IVF laboratory? *Human Reproduction*, **12**, 1610–14.

Van Blerkom, J. (1998). Epigenetic influences on oocyte developmental competence. Follicular oxygenation and perifollicular vascularity. *Journal of Assisted Reproduction and Genetics*, **15**, 226–34.

Van Blerkom, J. (2000). Intrafollicular influences on human oocyte developmental competence: perifollicular vascularity, oocyte metabolism, and mitochondrial function. *Human Reproduction*, **15**(Suppl. 2), 173–88.

Van Blerkom, J. and Davis, P. (2001). Differential effects of repeated superovulation on cytoplasmic and spindle organization in metaphase II mouse oocytes matured in vivo and in vitro. *Human Reproduction*, **16**, 757–64.

Van Blerkom, J. and Motta, P. (1979). *The Cellular Basis of Mammalian Reproduction*. Urban and Schwarzenberg, Baltimore, MD, pp. 5–108.

Van Blerkom, J., Davis, J.P., Merriam, J., and Sinclair, J. (1995). Nuclear and cytoplasmic dynamics of sperm penetration, pronuclear formation, and microtubule organization during fertilization and early preimplantation development in the human. *Human Reproduction Update*, **1**, 429–61.

Van Blerkom, J., Antczak, M., and Schrader, R. (1997). The developmental potential of the human oocyte is related to the dissolved oxygen content of follicular fluid: association with vascular endothelial growth factor levels and perifollicular blood flow characteristics. *Human Reproduction*, **12**, 1047–55.

Van Blerkom, J., Davis, P., and Alexander, S. (2000). Differential mitochondrial between blastomeres in cleavage stage human embryos: determination at the pronuclear stage and relationship to microtubular organization, ATP content and developmental competence. *Human Reproduction*, **15**, 2621–33.

Vanderhyden, B.C., Rouleau, A., Walton, E.A., and Armstrong, D.T. (1986). Increased mortality during early embryonic development after in-vitro fertilization of rat oocytes. *Journal of Reproductive Fertility*, 77, 401–9.

Vogel, R. and Spielmann, H. (1992). Genotoxic and embryotoxic effects of gonadotropin-hyperstimulated ovulation of murine oocytes and preimplantation embryos, and term fetuses. *Reproductive Toxicology*, **6**, 329–33.

Yamamoto, S., Konishi, I., Tsuruta, Y., et al. (1997). Expression of vascular endothelial growth factor (VEGF) during folliculogenesis and corpus luteum formation in the human ovary. *Gynecologic Endocrinology*, **11**, 371–81.

Zaidi, J., Jurovic, D., Campbell, S., et al. (1995). Luteinized unruptured follicle: morphology, endocrine function and blood flow changes during the menstrual cycle. *Human Reproduction*, **10**, 44–9.

Zeilmaker, G., Hulsmann, W., Wensinck, F., and Verhamme, C. (1972). Oxygen-triggered oocyte maturation in vitro and lactate utilization by mouse oocytes and zygotes. *Journal of Reproduction and Fertility*, **9**, 151–2.

Zoller, L. and Weisz, J. (1979). A quantitative cytochemical study of glucose-6-phosphate dehydrogenase and (5–3α-hydroxysteroid dehydrogenase activity in the membrana granulosa of the ovulable type of follicle in the rat. *Histochemistry*, **62**, 125–35.

7

Unresolved and basic problems in assisted reproductive technology

Jim Cummins

Murdoch University, Perth, Western Australia

Introduction

Assisted Reproductive Technology (ART) is now a maturing science. Louise Brown, the first IVF baby, turned 21 in 1999. I well remember the horror that was expressed by many at this "unnatural" procedure, including some distinguished reproductive scientists (many of whom, incidentally, swallowed their qualms and went on to lucrative careers in ART). Today much of this has died down, although the meaningless term "the IVF debate" still raises its head periodically. To set the stage, I thought I would have a quick look at how reproductive technology is perceived today. I want to digress then to evaluate a rather personal vision of how infertility may be a trait deeply entwined with our evolutionary history. I will finish by giving a sketch of current trends in ART and a summary of unanswered questions.

When I first started putting my thoughts together, I took the liberty of putting out a series of open-ended questions to various lists and e-mail groups on the Internet (one of which, SperMail, I have been running since 1994). What came back was fascinating (and given in detail in the Appendix to this chapter). However, it soon became apparent that I was simply generating ever expanding lists of questions, and any scientist worth his or her salt can easily do this. I had to find some way of pulling this morass of technical detail into perspective: after all, with the information explosion doubling roughly every five to seven years, whatever list I came up with would soon be redundant. (Even the term "informa-tion explosion" is itself exploding, with the Alta Vista search engine turning up over 7000 pages containing this phrase.) With the flood of genetic information generated by the Human Genome Project, the need to control and understand the data has even generated a new science in its own right: bioinformatics (Franklin, 1993).

I started to get dizzy. Examining the potential technical developments of ART was starting to turn into a Mandelbrot set: every increase in magnification simply revealed ever more complexity. For example, one could write a whole chapter just on how (and why) sperm–egg recognition occurs; how the in vivo situation may differ from in vitro and the genetic mechanisms underlying it (Hall and Frayne, 1999). Besides, I have only recently co-written a chapter on crystal ball gazing in andrology (Cummins and Jequier, 1999). While I will try to identify some of the key trends, I found it more rewarding to look at ART from the perspective of human biology. In particular, I want to look at the question of human infertility in the light of "Darwinian medicine" (Nesse and Williams, 1995, 1998). To be blunt, why does infertility exist in the first place? Is it a disease or a symptom? How did societies deal with it before ART? How are we dealing with it today? What shifts in attitude can we detect? In a culture that pretends that everyone can do anything, and that all one needs is the right mental attitude, money, or plastic surgeon, how can we deal with the loss of personal control that infertility implies? (I'm not going to attempt that last one, by the way!)

ART in today's society

I thought I would set the stage by looking through the pages of *The Times* (London). As I write these words, the leading story on *The Times*' www page (http://www.the-times.co.uk/news/pages/Times/frontpage.html) is, "Inquiry launched into missing embryos. Women undergoing fertility treatment at two Hampshire clinics are today (Saturday) waiting for news after it was discovered that frozen embryos have gone missing" (*The Times*, 23 September, 2000).

Here are three more stories from *The Times*.

A woman aged 30 who was the youngest in the country when she started having IVF [in vitro fertilization] treatment 13 years ago is expecting her first baby. Susan Young, from Heywood, Greater Manchester, began the fertility treatment at the age of 17 shortly after marrying Paul, now 45. Early expectations turned to disappointment as the years went by with no sign of a child. She had almost given up hope of conceiving when she was told by staff at the IVF unit at St Mary's Hospital, in Manchester, that she was four months pregnant. (*The Times*, 2 October, 1999)

The mother of a 17-year-old girl demanded fertility treatment on the NHS for her daughter because she had apparently been trying unsuccessfully to get pregnant for a year. The mother took her daughter to her doctor to ask for the teenager to be put on an IVF programme. The girl has not been identified but is believed to be living at home with her mother and has a steady boyfriend. (*The Times*, 13 November, 1999)

Gay fathers are doing what comes naturally. So Tony Barlow and Barrie Drewitt are not content with their twins, Aspen and Saffron. They want another girl and mean to get one, whatever people say. As homosexuals, they acquired their twins from the eggs of a selected American donor, Tracie McCune, fertilised by the men in vitro and implanted in a surrogate child-bearer. The process cost £200,000, which they can well afford as they are millionaires. For their third child, the men will use another of Mrs McCune's fertilised embryos, of which 24 are now in a freezer. They will use a new surrogate, relations with the previous woman having broken down over the fee. (*The Times*, 2 June, 2000).

Children as a commodity?

What's going on? Are babies becoming commodities to be bought and sold? It would appear so, at least in the rip-roaring commercial world of United States capitalism. A site called "Ron's Angels (http://www.ronsangels.com/) offers "models" eggs and sperm to the highest bidder over the Internet, under the guise of social Darwinism and "improving our species."

The site uses a second-hand reference (in *Scientific American*) to a paper entitled "Impact of market value on human mate choice decisions" (Pawlowski and Dunbar, 1999). This paper concluded ". . . female market value is determined principally by women's fecundity (and, to a lesser extent, reproductive value), while male market value is determined by men's earning potential and the risk of future pair-bond termination (the conjoint probability that the male will either die or divorce his partner during the next 20 years . . . these selection preferences strongly influence the levels of demands that men and women make of prospective partners (although older males tend to overestimate their market value)."

The site's author takes this one step further, to a very Hollywood-based view of mate choice: "This is Darwin's 'Natural Selection' at its very best." he gloats, "The highest bidder gets youth, beauty and social skills. 'Natural Selection' is choosing genes that are healthy and beautiful. This 'Celebrity Culture' that we have created does better economically than any other civilization in our history. We are excited by beauty."

Conflicts and rivalry in reproduction

It is easy to get sanctimonious about such enterprises (the term "californication" comes to mind). However, I suspect that this entrepreneur has touched a live nerve in American society, and one that may run deep in human culture. Children have probably always been regarded as part gift, part commodity, part burden. The deep divide in all societies over the mother's "right" to abortion versus the "right to life" of the fetus is a measure of this uneasy vision of procreation. Mammalian reproduction at its root carries conflicting interests between males and females and between mothers and the children they may bear (Haig, 1996). These conflicts are not always resolved amicably.

Violence in some form is never far from the surface of human activity. The book, *Demonic Males: Apes and the Origins of Human Violence* (Wrangham and Peterson, 1996) specifically targets male primates as the major source of war, genocide, rape, and inter-group genocide. This emerged from studies on the proclivity of adult male chimpanzees to attack, maim, and kill other adult males that they discover near their territory (Wrangham, 1999). Infanticide of rival males' offspring by invading dominant males is of course known in many animal groups (Daly and Wilson, 1983) (and occurs in human societies, as I will outline below). However, Hrdy's unsettling book on motherhood (Hrdy, 1999) points out that abortion and murder both of one's own and competitors' offspring are female reproductive options that most cultures have resorted to. Moreover, this is not limited to humans (Hrdy, 1977). Among chimpanzees, for example, careful observation shows that actual reproductive success varies widely and is closely related to social dominance. Dominant females achieve their status by a mix of opportunistic coalitions, aggression, and even infanticide against rivals. As a result, they wean young every four to five years compared with nine to ten years for subordinates (Pusey et al., 1997; Wrangham 1997)

It is clear to me that humans are determined to use ART in whatever way they can. They are not in the least interested in the technicalities and are obviously willing to try anything to conceive despite the restrictions politicians (mostly old and male) wish to impose on them. This is because the urge to reproduce – at any cost – lies deep in our evolutionary history.

Assisted reproductive technology and the law

ART is now clearly an integral part of society and increasingly being subjected to the scrutiny of public policy-makers. However, this is extremely variable between and within countries. In Australia, for example, the laws range from being extremely restrictive, as in Western Australia (no embryo research, no diagnostic tests, no access to ART by single women), to non-existent, as in Queensland and New South Wales. However, clinics are generally bound by a code of laboratory practice and subject to regular inspections by the Reproductive Technology Accreditation Committee appointed by the Fertility Society of Australia.

The impact of assisted reproductive technology on demography

We can identify some clear trends by looking at the European experience. According to a report prepared for the European Society for Human Reproduction and Embryology (ESHRE) in 1997 there were 203 411 cycles of treatment initiated (N. Andersen and N. Andersen: personal communication: a preliminary account is at http://ferti.net/med/fertimagazine/congressreport/eshre2000_18.asp). The multiple pregnancy rate varied from 0.8% in Scandinavia, reflecting very tough restrictions on the numbers of embryos permitted to be implanted, to 7.7% in southern and eastern Europe. This is well below the 39% reported from the USA, where the only effective control over clinics appears to be via litigation or the refusal to provide Federal funding for embryo research. There are now strong calls to limit the risks of multiple pregnancies by carrying out only single embryo replacement (Templeton, 2000).

The availability of ART ranged from 330 cycles per million head of population in Portugal to 1538 in Finland. There was an overall "take-home baby rate" of a very respectable 22% (even young, fertile couples only have about a 25% chance of successful conception in any cycle). In Iceland, with only a single clinic, ART produced a staggering 3.5% of all children born. Denmark and the Netherlands were not far behind, and in fact the birth rate from ART in Denmark is now approaching 4% of the total (Skakkebaek et al., 2000). One could predict that if ART reaches high levels of efficiency then the birth rate to infertile couples could equal or even exceed (with multiple pregnancies) their proportion of around 8–10% in the general population (World Health Organization, 1991). Here in Western Australia we are well behind international trends: there were 384 ART births out of a total of 25 677 in 1998, giving a proportion of 1.5% (A. Burmas of the Reproductive Technology Council, personal communication).

What does the public think?

Public perception of ART is also changing. A large survey on the public perception of infertility and its treatment has been reported for European countries, the USA and Australia (Adashi et al., 2000). Infertility was perceived as a disease by less than half of the people surveyed, but general awareness about the definition and incidence of infertility was relatively low. Nevertheless, half the people polled claimed to know someone affected by infertility. Most (approximately 90%) knew about IVF, but less than 25% knew about the chances of success. When informed that the cost of three IVF cycles is roughly equivalent to that of a hip replacement, 70% agreed that IVF should be reimbursable.

Controls and quality assurance

As a sign of the times, ESHRE has now issued strict new guidelines for the operation of clinics (Gianaroli et al., 2000). These identify a number of novel and in some cases questionable techniques that have been proposed recently. These include the freezing of oocytes and ovarian tissue (Rutherford and Gosden, 1999), in vitro maturation of oocytes (Smith et al., 2000), cytoplasmic transfer (Barritt et al., 1999), immature sperm injection (Sousa et al., 1999; Silber et al., 2000), and novel methods of embryo implantation. To these I would personally add the rather poorly justified practices of zona opening to assist hatching (De Vos and Van Steirteghem, 2000) and in vitro sperm maturation (Tesarik and Greco, 1999;

Tesarik et al., 2000a,b). More remote but still advocated by some, are attempts to "cure" male infertility by germ cell transplantation (Cooke and Saunders, 2000; Ogawa et al., 2000). The ESHRE report concludes on a cautionary note: "However, additional studies are necessary before admitting these procedures to the standard technique protocols which are routinely performed in IVF laboratories." Cynically, I have to say this caution is novel to ART as many developments such as spermatid injection have been pushed along by clinics without any appropriate (i.e. infertile) animal models (Cummins, 1998). Similar rigor is being advocated for progress and training in clinical andrology (Cummins, 1998; Cummins and Jequier, 1999; Comhaire, 2000; Rowe et al., 2000).

Reproductive health and personal rights

The right to have a family is, of course, enshrined in the United Nations Declaration of Human Rights. Article 16 contains the following (http://www.unhchr.ch/map.htm):

1 Men and women of full age, without any limitation due to race, nationality or religion, have the right to marry and to found a family. They are entitled to equal rights as to marriage, during marriage and at its dissolution.
2 Marriage shall be entered into only with the free and full consent of the intending spouses.
3 The family is the natural and fundamental group unit of society and is entitled to protection by society and the State.

In the USA, a working draft document from the National Institute of Child Health and Development (NICHD; (http://www.nichd.nih.gov/strategicplan/cells/reproductive.cfm) states "The ability to have children is one of the most basic human values. It encompasses not only the desire to have children but also to have them at a time and in a manner that their future health, both physical and mental, is best assured." The draft identified three main research goals with a view to fulfilling these ideals:

• reducing the incidence of unwanted pregnancy
• progressing towards desired levels of fertility

• reducing morbidity from diseases and disorders of the reproductive system.

This draft was based on the World Health Organization definition of reproductive health. Reproductive health is not merely the absence of disease or disorders of the reproductive process, but rather it is a condition in which the reproductive process is accomplished in a state of complete physical, mental, and social well-being. This implies that people have the ability to reproduce, that women can go through pregnancy and childbirth safely, and that reproduction is carried to a successful outcome, i.e., infants survive and grow up healthy. It implies further that people are able to regulate their fertility without risks to their health and they are safe in having sex.

Aging of the population

One clear trend that is unlikely to change in the twenty-first century (if we survive), is the increasing age and life expectancy of the human population. Many populations are aging more rapidly than their governments admit. For example, it has been forecast that by the year 2050 in the G7 group of industrialized countries (Canada, France, Germany, Italy, Japan, UK, and the USA) the dependency ratio of people over 65 to those in the work-force will be between 6% (UK) and 40% (Japan) higher than official forecasts (Horiuchi, 2000; Tuljapurkar et al., 2000). This inexorable trend is coupled with delays in decisions to commence reproduction: actually a long-term trend in human evolution that I discuss below in more depth.

Age sets a fundamental limit to female reproductive life (Gosden and Finch, 2000; te Velde, 2000). There is a trend for decreased fecundity with age in both men (Ford et al., 2000) and women (Dorland et al., 1998). This, coupled with a general inclination to defer child-bearing, appears to be a major component in the increasing social costs of reproductive medicine (Mosher and Pratt, 1991; van Noorde-Zaadstra et al., 1991; te Velde and Beets, 1992; Stephen, 2000). The overall cost of treatment for women over 38 years of age is 3.6-fold higher than that for younger women (Suchartwatnachai et al., 2000). The Germans even have a word, Torschlüsspanik ("door-closing-panic"),

for the anxiety felt by young women as they pass though their peak of fecundity without a suitable partner (Rheingold, 1988). This is not a new phenomenon, as increased life expectancy and reduced fecundity are a fundamental aspect of the human life cycle and are discussed below.

Age, environment, and life expectancy

One emerging issue that interacts with age at pregnancy is that human life expectancy may be profoundly modified by events around the time of implantation and by maternal age at conception. In mice, for example, very young and older mothers produce offspring with significantly lower body and gonadal weights, presumably because of maternal differences in circulating hormones such as estradiol and testosterone (Wang and Vom Saal, 2000). This effect appears to be associated with reduced embryo growth rates but not with apoptosis. The authors suggest that similarly altered endocrine states may be associated with traits seen in human offspring, such as cryptorchidism and testicular cancer (Bernstein et al., 1986, 1988; Key et al., 1996). In rats, protein deprivation of mothers in the preimplantation stage of embryo development leads to significantly reduced neonatal birthweights, postnatal growth rates, increased hypertension, and altered organ-to-body weight ratios in both male and female offspring (Kwong et al., 2000). Extrapolating from rodent models to the human is always problematic. However, there is good evidence that low birthweights (in particular, altered fetal-to-placental weight ratios) can have profound effects on human life expectancy and on the likelihood of developing serious illness late in life (Robinson et al., 1994; Seamark and Robinson, 1995). Intriguingly, the timing of intercourse within a cycle is thought to influence the primary sex ratio and to affect the likelihood of preterm delivery (James, 2000). The human primary sex ratio is markedly affected by social stress (e.g., war; Lerchl, 1997) and by seasonality and temperature (Lerchl, 1998a,b). Together with the dizygotic twinning rate, it is also proposed to be a sensitive indicator of long-term environmental impacts on human reproduction (James, 1998a,b). These teasing demographic relationships will undoubtedly affect our interpretation of environmental impacts on human and animal reproductive health, in particular the contentious issue of declining sperm counts (Lerchl and Nieschlag, 1996; Swan and Elkin, 1999; Swan et al., 2000).

Evolution of subfecundity in the human life cycle

I want to digress at this point to consider how infertility may fit in with our evolutionary history. Among primates, humans have an unusual reproductive pattern with cryptic estrus (Sillén-Tulberg and Møller, 1993), moderate sexual dimorphism, and great elaboration of the penis and breasts as secondary sexual signals (Lerchl, 1997). Along with only one other mammal – a species of toothed whale (Peccei, 1995) – humans have a genetically programmed period of female infertility at late maturity. The menopause almost certainly evolved to reinforce cultural transmission between generations – the "grandmother hypothesis" (Hawkes et al., 1998, 2000). By contrast, it has also been established that women who are able to give birth late in life also have increased life expectancy (Perls et al., 1997). This complex set of trade-offs between fecundity and life history is discussed further below.

Apoptosis, atresia, and the aging ovary

The vast majority of oocytes undergo atresia in fetal life. From a peak of seven million in mid-gestation, girl babies are born with about two million, and this declines to half a million at puberty (Baker, 1982). Of these, only a few are ever released, In women the recruitment of follicles into the growth phase declines from about 15 per day in young women, to one per day in women aged 40. This steady decline continues into the menopause (Leidy et al., 1998), which is triggered when the mean number of remaining follicles reaches a critical lower threshold

of about 1100 (Gosden and Faddy, 1998). It has been suggested that, besides eliminating excess oocytes, atresia may also serve as a selective mechanism against abnormal mitochondria (Krakauer and Mira, 1999). If this hypothesis is correct, then a key to oocyte atresia may lie in the central role that mitochondria play in the initiation of apoptosis and in regulating calcium metabolism (Cummins, 2000b). Apoptosis is clearly implicated in other aspects of the ovarian cycle (Gosden and Spears, 1997; Kaipia and Hsueh, 1997; Amsterdam et al., 1999), and in atresia (Morita and Tilly, 1999). The relevance here is that many forms of ovulatory disorders appear to be related simply to advancing age rather than to any specific pathology (Gosden and Finch, 2000). It is understandable that both atresia and significant numbers of spontaneous abortions increase with age, as such selection is a powerful mechanism for eliminating potential germline defects. This is in keeping with the "disposable soma" theory of human aging (Kirkwood and Rose, 1991). With the increasing age of women seeking ART, it is essential for clinics to be aware of these unpalatable biological truisms.

Sperm competition and sexual competition

Our relatively small testes suggests that sperm output per se is relatively unimportant in humans, indicating perhaps a low evolutionary intensity of sperm competition (Smith, 1984; Cummins, 1990; Gomendio and Roldán, 1993; Gomendio et al., 1998). This is an enormously complex issue that I can only touch on here. Sperm competition occurs when more than one male mates with a single female during her fertile period (Birkhead and Møller, 1998; Birkhead, 2000). There is increasing evidence that the differing interests and conflicts between genders that are set up by such competitive mating systems may benefit female fitness (Evans and Magurran, 2000) and be a central driving force in evolutionary speciation (Arnqvist et al., 2000). Tensions between the genetic "interests" of males and females in eutherian mammals also leads to the phenomenon of genomic imprinting (Latham, 1999) and to problems in pregnancy such as diabetes and pre-eclampsia (Haig, 1996).

Men are about 10–15% taller than women, and this sexual dimorphism suggests that we evolved a pattern of effective moderate polygyny through "serial monogamy" (Short, 1997). Some form of polygyny – serial or simultaneous – is practiced in over 80% of human cultures (Short, 1994; Shoumatoff, 1995; Lerchl, 1997). Most women in pre-contraceptive gathering–hunting societies appeared to have assured that births were spaced about every four years. This was by a combination of lactational amenorrhea, infanticide, or avoidance of intercourse (Daly and Wilson, 1983). In ecological terms, humans can be classified as "K" selected, with large body size and slow rates of growth and reproductive turnover (Short, 1985). I suspect that an underlying theme of human evolution is that reproductive success was relatively less important than social or cultural success. Widespread subfertility may be, therefore, simply a nonadaptive consequence of evolutionary pressures on factors other than fecundity.

It is known that genes controlling in particular male reproductive traits evolve rapidly (Wyckoff et al., 2000). Moreover, relaxed selection pressure (in *Drosophila*) can lead to the accumulation of mildly deleterious mutations (Lynch et al., 1999). Hominids, in general, suffer a remarkably high deleterious mutation rate (Eyre-Walker and Keightley, 1999), which may help to explain why the human testis is notably inefficient compared with other primates for which data are available (Amann and Howards, 1980). Much of this inefficiency results from high levels of apoptotic wastage, possibly selective against mitotic and meiotic errors (Blanco-Rodriguez, 1998). This "quality control" measure in spermatogenesis, significantly, is mediated by p53, which controls apoptosis by regulating mitochondrial wall permeability (Allemand et al., 1999; Li et al., 1999; Print and Loveland, 2000). There is, therefore, reasonably strong circumstantial evidence that the poor performance of the human testis is a trait that has evolved in concert with our increased lifespan potential and tendency to accumulate deleterious mutations with age (Short, 1997).

Reproductive success and the social ladder

One indirect approach that can be used to study the relationship between individual fertility and long-term reproductive success (they are the same) is that of genealogy. In cultures that practice patrilinearity, surname persistence can be a rough guide to paternity – although anthropologists are careful to distinguish between "biological" and "jural" fatherhood (Shoumatoff, 1995). However, Jones (1996) has pointed out that most genealogies give misleading information about lines of descent. Obviously, everyone alive today must have had fertile ancestors. However, when one traces cohorts of surnames forward in time it is clear that they tend to become extinct surprisingly rapidly. As an example, in the UK, 300 families claim descent from William the Conqueror yet only one can prove unbroken descent through the male line (Shoumatoff, 1995). All of the 5000 feudal knighthoods listed in the *Domesday Book* of 1086–1087 are now extinct, and the average duration of a hereditary title in the Middle Ages was only three generations. In general, male-inherited surnames last only about 200 years (R. Cann, personal communication): the Chinese are down to about 200 common surnames and the Koreans to 80. In the English nobility, the practice of double-barrelling names was used as a device to retain inheritance for a daughter in a family with no sons. This was done provided she could find a partner willing to add her name to his (or to abandon his own) (Shoumatoff, 1995). One spin-off of the low level of fecundity among the aristocracy was a massive increase in the wealth of the Church, through bequests from spinsters and widows. At one point, it owned about a third of England – although this was enhanced by a tradition of younger sons entering the priesthood coupled, of course, with an official insistence on celibacy (Shoumatoff, 1995).

One has to be careful in extrapolating from genealogical data, as patrilines can disappear for reasons other than infertility (death, celibacy, homosexuality, adoption, female infertility). However, one long-term analysis of English genealogical records from 1359 to 1986 shows that 31.7% of families produced no males destined to reproduce (Dewdney, 1986). This may have been even higher in preindustrial societies (Shoumatoff, 1995). One fascinating analysis (Fisher, 1958) concerns the Australian census of 1912. In this, it was found that 50% of all children were parented by only one in nine of the men and one in seven of the women (Heron, 1914). Similar wide variations in long-term reproductive success between women emerges from a longitudinal study of nuclear and mitochondrial DNA in Québec's Saguenay valley (Heyer, 1995).

Turning to pre-industrial societies, among Yanomamo Indians there is highly unbalanced reproductive success, particularly between men. In one cohort of 113 men, 16 (14%) had more than 50% of all the grandchildren that could be traced, while 50 (44%) had three or fewer. Four headmen had 191 grandchildren between them (Chagnon, 1972). This study had its problems in that inbreeding meant that many children were counted twice. Moreover, the Yanomamo at the period of study were (and still are) unusually aggressive, with high levels of polygyny for a few successful men and weaker individuals opting for bachelorhood. An untested report suggests that the men also carried out infanticide when raiding villages to obtain wives (Bloom, 1995): rather like lions taking over a new pride and killing the cubs of their genetic rivals (Daly and Wilson, 1994). However imperfect, this study on the Yanomamo points out the high variation in reproductive success that can exist between individuals in a gathering–hunting society. It also reinforces the point that fecund men tend to have fecund sons: the four most successful men in the study cited above were father–son pairs. The converse is true: there are significant familial associations for male infertility (Lilford et al., 1994).

Paternity assurance

The question of tracing reproductive success is muddied by problems of false paternity and extra-marital intercourse. Human societies have always had doubts about paternity assurance. Since the Middle Ages, for example, Jewishness has been passed on in a matrilineal fashion despite ancient patrilineal traditions (a legacy of mass rapes in Europe) (Shoumatoff, 1995). Estimates of paternal discrepancy based on blood grouping vary from 1.4% to a massive (and notorious) 30% in lower income groups in England (Baker and Bellis, 1995). Jequier (1985) found a 10% pregnancy rate in the consorts of azoospermic men awaiting vasectomy reversal. This situation is not unique to humans. Among chimpanzees, more than half the offspring in one study were fathered by "furtive matings" with extra-troop males (Gagneux et al., 1997). This is an amazing statistic given the levels of violence found between males of rival groups in territorial competition (Wrangham and Peterson, 1996); moreover such "furtive matings" have never been observed (Pusey et al., 1997; Wrangham, 1997). This appears to be a widespread phenomenon. There are surprisingly high levels of false paternity through "sneak" extra-pair copulations in supposedly monogamous birds (Birkhead, 1998, 2000). It is, therefore, entirely possible for a woman in an infertile relationship to resolve her dilemma by an extra-pair copulation while retaining the benefits of consortship with her infertile (but possibly socially successful) partner. This taboo topic goes deep into human culture (Baker and Bellis, 1995). Male fear of cuckoldry and the consequent asymmetry of laws to control female, but not male, reproduction is widespread. It probably reaches its most repellent outcome in female genital mutilation to reduce female sexual desire (Ng, 2000).

Life expectancy and fecundity trade-off: is infertility a disease?

"Hang on, what's all this to do with ART?" I can sense you thinking at this point. My reason for this digression is my suspicion that an underlying theme of human evolution is that reproductive success was relatively less important than social or cultural success. Widespread subfertility may be, therefore, simply a nonadaptive consequence of evolutionary pressures on factors other than fecundity. This may reflect an evolutionary trade-off between investment in fecundity and investment in longevity and cultural development (Kirkwood, 1987, 2000; Kirkwood and Rose, 1991; Westendorp and Kirkwood, 1998). Incidentally, this is not a novel notion. The tendency for fertility to decline as groups ascend the social ladder was first noted by Pliny the Younger in the first century AD. He railed against the failure of the Roman ruling classes to have large families and thus maintain the Empire. Fisher (1930) even traced the idea back to the Greek philosopher Hesiod, in the eighth century BC, who said, "May it befall that an only begotten son maintain the ancestral home, for thus wealth is increased in a house." In fact, the earliest systematic examination of the link between social stratum and fertility was published by Galton (1869). He looked at one situation, the decline in fertility among the English peerage. Of 31 hereditary peerages that he studied, 12 were extinct. Galton found an explanation for peerage extinction that he described with characteristic immodesty as "simple, adequate and novel." A sizeable number of newly created peers and their sons had married heiresses. Galton wrote: "my statistical lists showed, with unmistakable emphasis, that these marriages are peculiarly unprolific. We might have expected that an heiress, who is the sole issue of a marriage, would not be so fertile as a woman who has many brothers and sisters. Comparative infertility must be hereditary in the same way as other physical attributes and I am assured that it is so in the case of domestic animals. Consequently the issue of a peer's marriage with an heiress frequently fails and his title is brought to an end." In a fascinating more recent study, analysis of genealogical data also shows that older women tend to produce less fertile sons (E.R. te Velde, personal communication).

Other aspects of human (and some primates) reproduction, such as cryptic estrus (Sillén-Tulberg and Møller, 1993) and menstruation (Finn, 1998) likewise may be nonadaptive features that have emerged as side-effects of selective pressures on other behavioral and physiological traits. This is not to deny that infertility may be a *symptom* of underlying disease (Dickey et al., 2000). However, many causes of human infertility are either unknown or may result from minor and age-related variations in the genetic control of gametogenesis (Gosden and Faddy, 1998; Eddy, 1999; Gosden and Finch, 2000) or in hormone receptor functions (Gottlieb et al., 1999; Huhtaniemi, 2000). (See http://www.mcgill.ca/androgendb/ for a search list of androgen receptor mutation.)

Current trends

I stated earlier that I do not wish to concentrate on detailed technical lists – there is a risk I might move into another lovely German term, a Korinthenkacker. I'll leave you to find out the scatological meaning of that for yourself, but basically it means one "who couldn't find a forest because he or she is too busy applying a magnifying glass to the bark of one tree" (Rheingold, 1988). (I also run the risk of turning into a Fachidiot, a narrow-minded technological specialist who cannot foresee the consequences of his work. Fachidiots tend, in turn, to lead to a Schlimmbesserung, a technological so-called improvement that is actually an egregiously inappropriate tinkering that makes things worse (Rheingold, 1988). Some religious zealots might argue that ART itself is a good example of the latter!)

However, one does not need a crystal ball to identify clear technical trends in ART. For example, there is a move towards extended (blastocyst) culture and selection of superior embryos for improving implantation rates and reducing the chances of multiple pregnancies (Gardner et al., 2000; Toledo et al., 2000). Against these technical trends must be set the risk of inducing long-term developmental and life-expectancy problems through extended exposure of preimplantation embryos to imperfect or inadequate culture conditions (Kwong et al., 2000; Quinn, 2000). Other rapidly changing factors include improvements in ovulation induction protocols and the introduction of recombinant gonadotropins and gonadotropin-releasing hormone agonists and antagonists (Thornton, 2000). I would not be surprised to see a marked simplification of procedures in IVF, avoiding the risks of ovarian hyperstimulation (Janssens et al., 2000). Moreover, we will probably soon be able to unravel the genetic and cytoskeletal problems associated with failed IVF fertilization (Rawe et al., 2000; Sutovsky and Schatten, 2000). Other developments include the possibility of splitting embryos to improve the chances of pregnancy for couples with poor prospects for successful IVF. Such iatrogenic monozygotic twinning would of course be a form of cloning, but it appears to happen already, particularly in cases where assisted hatching is carried out supposedly to improve implantation (Schieve et al., 2000). There is little doubt that cloning (Wakayama et al., 1998) and stemcell technology, coupled with genetic manipulation, will make it possible to treat some forms of genetically determined infertility (Krawetz et al., 1999; Ogawa et al., 2000; Russell and Griswold, 2000), but whether this will be accepted by society seems doubtful. Recent puzzling observations on the declining efficiency of cloning with successive generations without any alterations to telomeres (Wakayama et al., 2000) suggests that there is still much to be understood before cloning technology leads to immortality.

I am on pretty solid ground in predicting that the major changes in our understanding of human reproduction will emerge from molecular biology. We already have a reasonable grasp on the Y chromosome genes that control spermatogenesis and affect male fertility (Simoni et al., 1999; Saxena et al., 2000), and genetic counseling will undoubtedly play a major role in the ART laboratory (Tuerlings et al., 1997), as will preimplantation genetic diagnosis (Geraedts et al., 1999). The Human Genome Project, coupled with the ability to generate thousands of novel mouse strains with specific genes knocked out or modified, will undoubtedly open the way to a better understanding of the complex gene hierarchies involved in reproduction. These sets of genes control germ cell differentiation (Olaso and Habert, 2000), gametogen-

esis (Kierszenbaum, 1994; Eddy, 1999), germ cell apoptosis (Morita and Tilly, 1999; Print and Loveland, 2000) and the endocrine and paracrine control of gonadal function (Weinbauer and Wessels, 1999). On a cautionary note, current methods for producing genetic knockouts in inbred mouse strains can produce very unpredictable phenotypic results depending on the genetic background (Sigmund, 2000). One promising technique to understand spermatogenesis is by study of the mRNAs carried by sperm as a genetic "history" of their development (Kramer and Krawetz, 1997; Miller, 2000). We have almost no understanding so far of the factors that control the transition from primary to growing follicles in the ovary (Fortune et al., 2000), nor of the interactions between nuclear and cytoplasmic genes in oogenesis and early embryonic development (Cummins, 2000a,b, 2001). (See http://www.thescientist.com/ry200/sep/mccann_p8_00904.htm for developments in the Jackson Laboratory in creating mouse genetic models of disease and DNA microarrays for monitoring complex genetic systems.)

On a final note, the contentious issue of declining sperm counts and reproductive anomalies in relation to the environment (Lerchl and Nieschlag, 1996; Swan et al., 1997, 2000) will probably not disappear. There are now clear links between testicular cancer and poor semen quality in men with infertility (de Kretser, 2000; Jacobsen et al., 2000) and in Vietnam veterans with a history of exposure to toxins (Tarone et al., 1991). The common link is almost certainly via environmentally mediated Sertoli cell and urogenital dysfunction in early childhood (Depue et al., 1983 Forman et al., 1994).

Conclusions

I have to conclude that many aspects of human infertility are inextricably linked with our evolutionary history. When I point this out to my students, invariably someone says "what about the population explosion?" According to the International Programs Center, US Bureau of the Census, the population of the world, projected to the time of writing,

is 6099418836 (http://www.census.gov/cgi-bin/
ipc/popclockw). Every minute today, 249 new
people are born but only 103 die, leaving a natural
increase of 146. Even the horror of the human
immunodeficiency virus and acquired immunodeficiency syndrome (HIV/AIDS) is unlikely to stem this
inexorable advance, although the world population
is likely to plateau sometime in the twenty-first
century. Of course, the population explosion is unrelated to human fecundity; rather it reflects improvements in public health and reductions in perinatal
mortality. Most of the "advanced" countries have
populations that are actually in decline, and at least
18 countries like Russia and Japan are in severe risk
of depopulation (Pearce, 1999). The HIV/AIDS pan-
demic, like all before, will undoubtedly run its
course (Diamond, 1997). The human genome is
replete with genetic fossils of ancient viral invasions
(including HIV-like sequences dating back 30
million years or so) that have become more-or-less
peacefully incorporated (Löwer et al., 1996; Yang et
al., 1999).

The notion that infertility may be natural is hard to
accept, as we are conditioned to view infertility as a
disease requiring medical treatment. Certainly, this
is tacitly accepted by most health authorities,
although the resources actually allocated for treatment pale in comparison to the costs of dealing with,
say, smoking-related premature deaths. Here in
Australia, more is gambled on a single horse race
(the Melbourne Cup) than is allocated to reproductive medicine annually. However, many genetically
based ailments such as sickle-cell anemia, thallase-
mia and cystic fibrosis are maintained by natural
selective forces (Nesse and Williams, 1995). Given
the way society is increasingly turning to technology
to give us control over our lives, I have to conclude
that ART is here to stay.

REFERENCES

Adashi, E.Y., Cohen, J., Hamberger, L., et al. (2000). Public perception on infertility and its treatment: an international
survey. *Human Reproduction*, **15**, 330–4.

Allemand, I., Anglo, A., Jeantet, A.Y., Cerutti, I., and May, E.
(1999). Testicular wild-type p53 expression in transgenic mice
induces spermiogenesis alterations ranging from differentiation defects to apoptosis. *Oncogene*, **18**, 6521–30.

Amann, R.P. and Howards, S.S. (1980). Daily spermatozoal production and epididymal spermatozoal reserves of the human
male. *Journal of Urology*, **124**, 211–15.

Amsterdam, A., Gold, R.S., Hosokawa, K., et al. (1999). Crosstalk
among multiple signaling pathways controlling ovarian cell
death. *Trends in Endocrinology and Metabolism*, **10**, 255–62.

Arnqvist, G., Edvardsson, M., Friberg, U., and Nilsson, T. (2000).
Sexual conflict promotes speciation in insects. *Proceedings of
the National Academy of Sciences USA*, **97**, 10460–4.

Baker, T.G. (1982). Oogenesis and ovulation. In: *Reproduction in
Mammals. Book 1. Germ Cells and Fertilization*, 2nd edn,
Austin, C.R. and Short, R.V., eds. Cambridge University Press,
Cambridge, UK, pp. 17–45.

Baker, R.R. and Bellis, M.A. (1995). *Human Sperm Competition.
Copulation, Masturbation and Infidelity*, Chapman & Hall,
London.

Barritt, J., Cohen, J., Willandsen, S., Scott, R.T., and Brenner, C.A.
(1999). Mitochondrial inheritance and the incidence of
heteroplasmy after ooplasmic transplantation. *Fertility and
Sterility*, **72** (Suppl. 1), S31.

Bernstein, L., Depue, R.H., Ross, R.K., Judd, H.L., Pike, M. C., and
Henderson, B. E. (1986). Higher maternal levels of free estradiol in first compared to second pregnancy: early gestational
differences. *Journal of the National Cancer Institute*, **76**,
1035–9.

Bernstein, L., Pike, M.C., Depue, R.H., Ross, R.K., Moore, J.W.,
and Henderson, B. E. (1988). Maternal hormone levels in early
gestation of cryptorchid males: a case-control study. *British
Journal of Cancer*, **58**, 379–81.

Birkhead, T.R. (2000). *Promiscuity. An Evolutionary History of
Sperm Competition and Sexual Conflict*. Faber and Faber,
London.

Birkhead, T.R. (1998). Sperm competition in birds. *Reviews in
Reproduction*, **3**, 123–9.

Birkhead, T.R. and Møller, A.P. (eds.) (1998). *Sperm Competition
and Sexual Selection*. Academic Press, London.

Blanco-Rodriguez, J. (1998). A matter of death and life – the significance of germ cell death during spermatogenesis.
International Journal of Andrology, **21**, 236–48.

Bloom, H. (1995). *The Lucifer Principle. A Scientific Expedition
into the Forces of History*. Atlantic Monthly Press, New York.

Chagnon, N.A. (1972). Tribal social organization and genetic
microdifferentiation. In: *The Structure of Human
Populations*, Harrison, G.A. and Boyce, A.J., eds. Oxford
University Press, London, pp. 252–82.

Comhaire, F. (2000). Clinical andrology: from evidence-base to ethics. The "E" quintet in clinical andrology. *Human Reproduction*, **15**, 2067–71.

Cooke, H.J. and Saunders, P.T.K. (2000). Germ cell transplantation – a fertile field. *Nature Medicine*, **6**, 16–17.

Cummins, J.M. (1990). Evolution of sperm form: levels of control and competition. In: *Fertilization in Mammals*, Bavister, B.D., Cummins, J.M. and Roldan, E.R.S., eds. Serona Symposia, Norwall, MA, pp. 51–64.

Cummins, J.M. (1998). Potential pitfalls in male reproductive technology. In: *The Male Gamete: from Basic Science to Clinical Applications*, Gagnon, C., ed. Cache River Press, Vienna, IL, pp. 417–27.

Cummins, J.M. (2000a). Fertilization and elimination of the paternal mitochondrial genome. *Human Reproduction*, **15**, (Suppl 2) 92–101.

Cummins, J.M. (2000b). Mitochondrial dysfunction and ovarian aging. In: *Female Reproductive Aging*, te Velde, E.R., Pearson, P.L. and Broekmans, F.J., eds. Parthenon, New York, pp. 207–24.

Cummins, J.M. (2001). Mitochondria: potential roles in embryogenesis and nucleo-cytoplasmic transfer. *Human Reproduction Update*, **7**, 217–28.

Cummins, J.M. and Jequier, A.M. (1999). Gazing into the crystal ball: future diagnosis and management. In: *Disorders of Male Infertility*, Glover, T.D. and Barratt, E.L.R., eds. Cambridge University Press, Cambridge, UK.

Daly, M. and Wilson, M. (1983). *Sex, Evolution and Behavior*, 2nd edn. PWS, Publishers, Boston, MA.

Daly, M. and Wilson, M. (1994). Evolutionary psychology of male violence. In: *Male Violence*, Archer, J., ed. Routledge, London. pp. 253–89.

de Kretser, D.M. (2000). Testicular cancer and infertility. *British Medical Journal*, **321**, 781–2.

Depue, R.H., Pike, M.C., and Henderson, B.E. (1983). Estrogen exposure during gestation and risk of testicular cancer. *Journal of the National Cancer Institute*, **71**, 1151–5.

De Vos, A. and Van Steirteghem, A. (2000). Zona hardening, zona drilling and assisted hatching: new achievements in assisted reproduction. *Cells Tissues Organs*, **166**, 220–7.

Dewdney, A.K. (1986). Computer recreations. Branching phylogenies of the Paleozoic and the fortunes of English family names. *Scientific American*, **254**, 12–16.

Diamond, J. (1997). *Guns, Germs and Steel. A Short History of Everybody for the Last 13 000 Years*. Jonathan Cape, Random House, London.

Dickey, R.P., Taylor, S.N., Rye, P.H., Lu, P.Y., and Sartor, B.M. (2000). Infertility is a symptom, not a disease. *Fertility and Sterility*, **74**, 398.

Dorland, M., van Kooij, R.J., and te Velde, E.R. (1998). General ageing and ovarian ageing. *Maturitas*, **30**, 113–18.

Eddy, E.M. (1999). The effects of gene knockouts on spermatogenesis. In: *The Male Gamete: From Basic Science to Clinical Applications*, Gagnon, C., ed. Cache River Press, Vienna, IL, pp. 23–36.

Evans, J.P. and Magurran, A.E. (2000). Multiple benefits of multiple mating in guppies. *Proceedings of the National Academy of Sciences USA*, **7**, 10074–6.

Eyre-Walker, A. and Keightley, P. D. (1999). High genomic deleterious mutation rates in hominids. *Nature*, **397**, 344–7.

Finn, C.A. (1998). Menstruation – a nonadaptive consequence of uterine evolution. *Quarterly Review of Biology*, **73**, 163–73.

Fisher, R.A. (1930). *The Genetical Theory of Natural Selection*, 2nd edn. Oxford University Press, Oxford.

Fisher, R.A. (1958). *The Genetical Theory of Natural Selection*, 2nd edn. Dover Press, New York.

Ford, W.C.L., North, K., Taylor, H., Farrow, A., Hull, M.G.R., and Golding, J. (2000). Increasing paternal age is associated with delayed conception in a large population of fertile couples: evidence for declining fecundity in older men. *Human Reproduction*, **15**, 1703–8.

Forman, D., Pike, M.C., Davey, G., et al. (1994). Aetiology of testicular cancer: association with congenital abnormalities, age at puberty, infertility, and exercise. *British Medical Journal*, **308**, 1393–9.

Fortune, J.E., Cushman, R.A., Wahl, C.M., and Kito, S. (2000). The primordial to primary follicle transition. *Molecular and Cellular Endocrinology*, **163**, 53–60.

Franklin, J. (1993). Bioinformatics changing the face of information. *Annals of the New York Academy of Sciences*, **700**, 145–52.

Gagneux, P., Woodruff, D. S., and Boesch, C. (1997). Furtive mating in female chimpanzees. *Nature*, **387**, 358–9.

Galton, F. (1869). *Hereditary Genius. An Inquiry into its Laws and Consequences*. Macmillan, London.

Gardner, D.K., Lane, M., Stevens, J., Schlenker, T., and Schoolcraft, W. B. (2000). Blastocyst score affects implantation and pregnancy outcome: towards a single blastocyst transfer. *Fertility and Sterility*, **73**, 1155–8.

Geraedts, J., Handyside, A., Harper, J., et al. (1999). ESHRE Preimplantation Genetic Diagnosis (PGD) Consortium: preliminary assessment of data from January 1997 to September 1998. *Human Reproduction*, **14**, 3138–48.

Gianaroli, L., Plachot, M., van Kooij, R., and Committee of the Special Interest Group on Embryology (2000). ESHRE guidelines for good practice in IVF laboratories. *Human Reproduction*, **15**, 2241–6.

Gomendio, M. and Roldán, E.R. (1993). Coevolution between male ejaculates and female reproductive biology in eutherian mammals. *Proceedings of the Royal Society of London, Series B: Biological Science*, **252**, 7–12.

Gomendio, M., Harcourt, A.H., and Roldán, E.R.S. (1998). Sperm competition in mammals. In: *Sperm Competition and Sexual Selection*, Birkhead, T.R. and Møller, A.P., eds. Academic Press, San Diego, CA, pp. 667–775.

Gosden, R.G. and Faddy, M.J. (1998). Biological bases of premature ovarian failure. *Reproduction, Fertility and Development*, **10**, 73–8.

Gosden, R.G. and Finch, C.E. (2000). Definition and character of reproductive aging and senescence. In: *Female Reproductive Aging*, te Velde, E.R., Pearson, P.L., and Broekmans, F.J., eds. Parthenon Publishing, New York, pp. 11–25.

Gosden, R.G. and Spears, N. (1997). Programmed cell death in the reproductive system. *British Medical Bulletin*, **53**, 644–61.

Gottlieb, B., Beitel, L.K., Lumbroso, R., Pinsky, L., and Trifiro, M. (1999). Update of the androgen receptor gene mutations database. *Human Mutation*, **14**, 103–14.

Haig, D. (1996). Altercation of generations – genetic conflicts of pregnancy. *American Journal of Reproductive Immunology*, **35**, 226–32.

Hall, L. and Frayne, J. (1999). Non-functional fertility genes in humans: contributory factors in reduced male fertility? *Human Fertility*, **2**, 36–41.

Hawkes, K., O'Connell, J.F., Jones, N.G.B., Alvarez, H., and Charnov, E.L. (1998). Grandmothering, menopause, and the evolution of human life histories. *Proceedings of the National Academy of Sciences USA*, **95**, 1336–9.

Hawkes, K., O'Connell, J.F., and Blurton Jones, N.G. (2000). Why do women have a mid-life menopause? Grandmothering and the evolution of human longevity. In: *Female Reproductive Aging*, te Velde, E.R., Pearson, P.L., and Broekmans, F.J., eds. Parthenon, New York, pp. 27–41.

Heron, D. (1914). Note on reproductive selection. *Biometrika*, **X**, 419–20.

Heyer, E. (1995). Mitochondrial and nuclear genetic contribution of female founders to a contemporary population in northeast Quebec. *American Journal of Human Genetics*, **56**, 1450–5.

Horiuchi, S. (2000). Greater lifetime expectations. *Nature*, **405**, 744–5.

Hrdy, S.B. (1977). Infanticide as a primate reproductive strategy. *American Scientist*, **65**, 40–9.

Hrdy, S.B. (1999). *Mother Nature: A History of Mothers, Infants, and Natural Selection*, Pantheon Books, New York.

Huhtaniemi, I. (2000). Mutations of gonadotrophin and gonadotrophin receptor genes: what do they teach us about reproductive physiology? *Journal of Reproduction and Fertility*, **119**, 173–86.

Jacobsen, R., Bostofte, E., Engholm, G., et al. (2000). Risk of testicular cancer in men with abnormal semen characteristics: cohort study. *British Medical Journal*, **321**, 789–92.

James, W.H. (1998a). Dizygotic twinning rates and the possibility that the decline in sperm counts is a cohort phenomenon. *International Journal of Epidemiology*, **27**, 538.

James, W.H. (1998b). Was the widespread decline in sex ratios at birth caused by reproductive hazards? *Human Reproduction*, **13**, 1083–4.

James, W.H. (2000). Why are boys more likely to be preterm than girls? Plus other related conundrums in human reproduction. *Human Reproduction*, **15**, 2108–11.

Janssens, R.M.J., Lambalk, C.B., Vermeiden, J.P.W., Schats, R., and Schoemaker, J. (2000). In-vitro fertilization in a spontaneous cycle: easy, cheap and realistic. *Human Reproduction*, **15**, 314–18.

Jequier, A.M. (1985). Non-therapy related pregnancies in the consorts of a group of men with obstructive azoospermia. *Andrologia*, **17**, 6–8.

Jones, S. (1996). *In the Blood. God, Genes and Destiny*. Flamingo. London.

Kaipia, A. and Hsueh, A.J. (1997). Regulation of ovarian follicle atresia. *Annual Review of Physiology*, **59**, 349–63.

Key, T.J., Bull, D., Ansell, P., et al. (1996). A case-control study of cryptorchidism and maternal hormone concentrations in early pregnancy. *British Journal of Cancer*, **73**, 698–701.

Kierszenbaum, A.L. (1994). Mammalian spermatogenesis in vivo and in vitro – a partnership of spermatogenic and somatic cell lineages. *Endocrinology Reviews*, **15**, 116–34.

Kirkwood, T.B. (1987). Immortality of the germ-line versus disposability of the soma. *Basic Life Science*, **42**, 209–18.

Kirkwood, T.B.L. (2000). Similarities of general and reproductive aging. In *Female Reproductive Aging*, te Velde, E.R., Pearson, P.L., and Broekmans, F.J., eds. Parthenon, New York, pp. 43–7.

Kirkwood, T.B. and Rose, M.R. (1991). Evolution of senescence: late survival sacrificed for reproduction. *Philosophical Transactions of the Royal Society London: Series B Biological Science*, **332**, 15–24.

Krakauer, D.C. and Mira, A. (1999). Mitochondria and germ-cell death. *Nature*, **400**, 125–6.

Kramer, J.A. and Krawetz, S.A. (1997). RNA in spermatozoa – implications for the alternative haploid genome. *Molecular Human Reproduction*, **3**, 473–8.

Krawetz, S.A., Kramer, J.A., and McCarrey, J.R. (1999). Reprogramming the male gamete genome: a window to successful gene therapy. *Gene*, **234**, 1–9.

Kwong, W.Y., Wild, A.E., Roberts, P., Willis, A.C., and Fleming, T.P. (2000). Maternal undernutrition during the preimplantation period of rat development causes blastocyst abnormalities and programming of postnatal hypertension. *Development*, **127**, 4195–202.

Latham, K.E. (1999). Mechanisms and control of embryonic genome activation in mammalian embryos. *International Review of Cytology*, **19**, 71–124.

Leidy, L.E., Godfrey, L.R., and Sutherland, M.R. (1998). Is follicular atresia biphasic? *Fertility and Sterility*, **70**, 851–9.

Lerchl, A. (1997). Comparative biology of reproduction. In: *Andrology. Male Reproductive Health and Dysfunction*, Nieschlag, E. and Behre, H.M., eds. Springer-Verlag, Berlin, pp. 12–22.

Lerchl, A. (1998a). Changes in the seasonality of mortality in Germany from 1946 to 1995: the role of temperature. *International Journal of Biometeorology*, **42**, 84–8.

Lerchl, A. (1998b). Seasonality of sex ratio in Germany. *Human Reproduction*, **13**, 1401–2.

Lerchl, A. and Nieschlag, E. (1996). Decreasing sperm counts? A critical (re)view. *Experimental and Clinical Endocrinology and Diabetes*, **104**, 301–7.

Li, P.-F., Dietz, R., and von Harsdorf, R. (1999). p53 regulates mitochondrial membrane potential through reactive oxygen species and induces cytochrome *c*-independent apoptosis blocked by Bcl-2. *EMBO Journal*, **18**, 6027–36.

Lilford, R., Jones, A.M., Bishop, D.T., Thornton, J., and Mueller, R. (1994). Case-control study of whether subfertility in men is familial. *British Medical Journal*, **309**, 570–3.

Löwer, R., Löwer, J., and Kurth, R. (1996). The viruses in all of us: characteristics and biological significance of human endogenous retrovirus sequences. *Proceedings of the National Academy of Sciences USA*, **93**, 5177–84.

Lynch, M., Blanchard, J., Houle, D., et al. (1999). Perspective: spontaneous deleterious mutation. *Evolution*, **53**, 645–63.

Miller, D. (2000). Analysis and significance of messenger RNA in human ejaculated spermatozoa. *Molecular Reproduction and Development*, **56**, 259–64.

Morita, Y. and Tilly, J.L. (1999). Oocyte apoptosis: like sand through an hourglass. *Developmental Biology*, **213**, 1–17.

Mosher, W.D. and Pratt, W.F. (1991). Fecundity and infertility in the United States: incidence and trends. *Fertility and Sterility*, **56**, 192–3.

Nesse, R.M. and Williams, G.C. (1995). *Why we get Sick. The New Science of Darwinian Medicine*. Times Books, New York.

Nesse, R.M. and Williams, G.C. (1998). Evolution and the origins of disease. *Scientific American*, **279**, 58–65.

Ng, F. (2000). Female genital mutilation; its implications for reproductive health. An overview. *British Journal of Family Planning*, **26**, 47–51.

Ogawa, T., Dobrinski, I., Avarbock, M.R., and Brinster, R.L.

(2000). Transplantation of male germ line stem cells restores fertility in infertile mice. *Nature Medicine*, **6**, 29–34.

Olaso, R. and Habert, R. (2000). Genetic and cellular analysis of male germ cell development. *Journal of Andrology*, **21**, 497–511.

Pawlowski, B. and Dunbar, R.I.M. (1999). Impact of market value on human mate choice decisions. *Proceedings of the Royal Scociety of London, Series B, Biological Science*, **266**, 281–6.

Pearce, F. (1999). Counting down. *New Scientist*, October **2**, 20–21.

Peccei, J.S. (1995). The origin and evolution of menopause: the altriciality-lifespan hypothesis. *Ethology and Sociobiology*, **16**, 425–49.

Perls, T.T., Alpert, L., and Fretts, R.C.C. (1997). Middle-aged mothers live longer. *Nature*, **389**, 133.

Print, C.G. and Loveland, K.L. (2000). Germ cell suicide: new insights into apoptosis during spermatogenesis. *Bioessays*, **22**, 423–30.

Pusey, A., Williams, J., and Goodall, J. (1997). The influence of dominance rank on the reproductive success of female chimpanzees. *Science*, **277**, 828–31.

Quinn, P. (2000). Review of media used in ART laboratories. *Journal of Andrology*, **21**, 610–15.

Rawe, V.Y., Olmedo, S.B., Nodar, F.N., Doncel, G.D., Acosta, A.A., and Vitullo, A. D. (2000). Cytoskeletal organization defects and abortive activation in human oocytes after IVF and ICSI failure. *Molecular Human Reproduction*, **6**, 510–16.

Rheingold, H. (1988). *There's a Word for It*. Severn House. London.

Robinson, J.S., Seamark, R.P., and Owens, J.A. (1994). Placental function. *Australian and New Zealand Journal of Obstetrics and Gynaecology*, **34**, 240–6.

Rowe, P.J., Comhaire, F.H., Hargreave, T.B., and Mahmoud, A.M.A. (2000). *WHO Manual for the Standardized Investigation, Diagnosis and Management of the Infertile Male*. Cambridge University Press, Cambridge, UK.

Russell, L.D. and Griswold, M.D. (2000). Spermatogonial transplantation – an update for the millennium. *Molecular and Cellular Endocrinology*, **161**, 117–20.

Rutherford, A.J. and Gosden, R.G. (1999). Ovarian tissue cryopreservation: a practical option? *Acta Paediatrica*, **88** (Suppl. 433), 13–18.

Saxena, R., de Vries, J.W.A., Repping, S., et al. (2000). Four DAZ genes in two clusters found in the AZFc region on the human Y chromosome. *Genomics*, **67**, 256–67.

Schieve, L.A., Meikle, S.F., Peterson, H.B., Jeng, G., Burnett, N.M., and Wilcox, L.S. (2000). Does assisted hatching pose a risk for monozygotic twinning in pregnancies conceived through in vitro fertilization? *Fertility and Sterility*, **74**, 288–94.

Seamark, R.F. and Robinson, J.S. (1995). Potential health problems stemming from assisted reproduction programmes. *Human Reproduction*, **10**, 1321–2.

Short, R.V. (1985). Species differences in reproductive mechanisms. In: *Reproduction in Mammals, Vol. 4, Reproductive Fitness*, 2nd edn., Austin, C.R., and Short, R.V., eds. Cambridge University Press, Cambridge, UK, pp. 24–61.

Short, R.V. (1994). A man's a man for a' that. In: *The Differences Between the Sexes*, Short, R.V., and Balaban, E., eds. Cambridge University Press, Cambridge, UK, pp. 451–6.

Short, R.V. (1997). The testis – the witness of the mating system, the site of mutation and the engine of desire. *Acta Paediatrica*, **86**(Suppl. 422), 3–7.

Shoumatoff, A. (1995). *The Mountain of Names. A History of the Human Family*, 2nd edn. Kodansha International, New York.

Sigmund, C.D. (2000). Viewpoint: are studies in genetically altered mice out of control? *Arteriosclerosis, Thrombosis and Vascular Biology*, **20**, 1425–9.

Silber, S.J., Johnson, L., Verheyen, G., and Van Steirteghem, A. (2000). Round spermatid injection. *Fertility and Sterility*, **73**, 897–900.

Sillén-Tulberg, B. and Møller, A. P. (1993). The relationship between concealed ovulation and mating system in Anthropoid primates: a phylogenetic analysis. *American Naturalist*, **141**, 1–25.

Simoni, M., Bakker, E., Eurlings, M.C.M., et al. (1999). Laboratory guidelines for molecular diagnosis of Y-chromosomal microdeletions. *International Journal of Andrology*, **22**, 292–9.

Skakkebaek, N.E., Leffers, H., Rajpert-De Meyts, E., Carlsen, E., and Grigor, K.M. (2000). Should we watch what we eat and drink? (Report on the International Workshop on Hormones and Endocrine Disrupters in Food and Water: Possible Impact on Human Health, Copenhagen, Denmark, 27–30 May 2000.) *Trends in Endocrinology and Metabolism*, **11**, 291–3.

Smith, R.L. (1984). Human sperm competition. In: *Sperm Competition and the Evolution of Animal Mating Systems*, Smith, R.L., ed. Academic Press, London, pp. 601–59.

Smith, S.D., Mikkelsen, A.L., and Lindenberg, S. (2000). Development of human oocytes matured in vitro for 28 or 36 hours. *Fertility and Sterility*, **73**, 541–4.

Sousa, M., Barros, A., Takahashi, K., Oliveira, C., Silva, J., and Tesarik, J. (1999). Clinical efficacy of spermatid conception: analysis using a new spermatid classification scheme. *Human Reproduction*, **14**, 1279–86.

Stephen, E.H. (2000). Postponement of childbearing and its effect on the prevalence of subfecundity. In: *Female Reproductive Aging*, te Velde, E.R., Pearson, P.L., and Broekmans, F.J., eds. Parthenon, New York, pp. 59–70.

Suchartwatnachai, C., Wongkularb, A., Srisombut, C., Choktanasiri, W., Chinsomboon, S., and Rojanasakul, A. (2000). Cost-effectiveness of IVF in women 38 years and older. *International Journal of Gynecology and Obstetrics*, **69**, 143–8.

Sutovsky, P. and Schatten, G. (2000). Paternal contributions to the mammalian zygote: fertilization after sperm–egg fusion. *International Review of Cytology*, **195**, 1–65.

Swan, S.H. and Elkin, E.P. (1999). Declining semen quality: can the past inform the present? *Bioessays*, **21**, 614–21.

Swan, S.H., Elkin, E.P., and Fenster, L. (1997). Have sperm densities declined – a reanalysis of global trend data. *Environmental Health Perspectives*, **105**, 1228–32.

Swan, S.H., Elkin, E.P., and Fenster, L. (2000). The question of declining sperm density revisited: an analysis of 101 studies published 1934–1996. *Environmental Health Perspectives*, **108**, 961–6.

Tarone, R.E., Hayes, H.M., Hoover, R.N., et al. (1991). Service in Vietnam and risk of testicular cancer. *Journal of the National Cancer Institute*, **83**, 1497–9.

Templeton, A. (2000). Avoiding multiple pregnancies in ART – Replace as many embryos as you like – one at a time. *Human Reproduction*, **15**, 1662.

Tesarik, J. and Greco, E. (1999). Assisted reproduction for testicular failure: management of germ cell maturation arrest. *Current Opinion in Obstetrics and Gynecology*, **11**, 283–8.

Tesarik, J., Balaban, B., Isiklar, A., et al. (2000a). In-vitro spermatogenesis resumption in men with maturation arrest: relationship with in-vivo blocking stage and serum FSH. *Human Reproduction*, **15**, 1350–4.

Tesarik, J., Mendoza, C., Anniballo, R., and Greco, E. (2000b). In-vitro differentiation of germ cells from frozen testicular biopsy specimens. *Human Reproduction*, **15**, 1713–16.

te Velde, E.R. (2000). Concepts in female reproductive aging. In: *Female Reproductive Aging*, te Velde, E.R., Pearson, P.L., and Broekmans, F.J., eds. Parthenon, New York, pp. 49–57.

te Velde, E. and Beets, G. (1992). Are subfertility and infertility on the increase? *Journal of Fertility Research*, **6**, 5–8.

Thornton, K.L. (2000). Advances in assisted reproductive technologies. *Obstetrics and Gynecology Clinics of North America*, **27**, 517–27.

Toledo, A.A., Wright, G., Jones, A.E., et al. (2000). Blastocyst transfer: a useful tool for reduction of high-order multiple gestations in a human assisted reproduction program. *American Journal of Obstetrics and Gynecology*, **183**, 377–9.

Tuerlings, J.H.A.M., Kremer, J.A.M., and Meuleman, E.J.H. (1997). The practical application of genetics in the male infertility clinic. *Journal of Andrology*, **18**, 576–81.

Tuljapurkar, S., Li, N., and Boe, C. (2000). A universal pattern of mortality decline in the G7 countries. *Nature*, **405**, 789–92.

van Noorde-Zaadstra, B., Looman, C.W.N., Alsbach, H., Habbema, J.D.F., te Velde, E.R., and Karbaat, J. (1991). Delaying childbearing: effect of age on fecundity and outcome of pregnancy. *British Medical Journal*, **302**, 1361–5.

Wakayama, T., Perry, A.C., Zuccotti, M., Johnson, K.R., and Yanagimachi, R. (1998). Full-term development of mice from enucleated oocytes injected with cumulus cell nuclei. *Nature*, **394**, 369–74.

Wakayama, T., Shinkai, Y., Tamashiro, K.L.K., et al. (2000). Aging: cloning of mice to six generations. *Nature*, **407**, 309–10.

Wang, M.-H. and Vom Saal, F. S. (2000). Maternal age and traits in offspring. *Nature*, **407**, 469–470.

Weinbauer, G.F. and Wessels, J. (1999). 'Paracrine' control of spermatogenesis. *Andrologia*, **31**, 249–62.

Westendorp, R.G.J. and Kirkwood, T.B.L. (1998). Human reproductive activity at the price of reproductive success. *Nature*, **396**, 743–6.

World Health Organization (1991). *Infertility: a Tabulation of Available Data on the Prevalence of Primary and Secondary Infertility*, 3rd edn. World Health Organization, Geneva.

Wrangham, R.W. (1997). Subtle, secret female chimpanzees. *Science*, **277**, 774–5.

Wrangham, R.W. (1999). Evolution of coalitionary killing. *American Journal of Physical Anthropology*, **110**, 1–30.

Wrangham, R. and Peterson, D. (1996). *Demonic Males: Apes and the Origins of Human Violence*. Houghton Mifflin, MA, Boston.

Wyckoff, G.J., Wang, W., and Wu, C.I. (2000). Rapid evolution of male reproductive genes in the descent of man. *Nature*, **403**, 304–9.

Yang, Y., Bogerd, H.P., Peng, S., Wiegand, H., Truant, R., and Cullen, B. R. (1999). An ancient family of human endogenous retroviruses encodes a functional homolog of the HIV-1 Rev protein. *Proceedings of the National Academy of Sciences USA*, **96**, 13404–8.

Appendix

Here are some responses to my e-mail list of general questions.

Professor David Handelsman, of the University of Sydney wrote: "Two issues you do not mention but which I see as fundamental and practical problems awaiting potentially feasible solutions are (a) how can we switch on meiosis in tissue culture, and (b) how to develop in vitro culture of spermatogenic cells from stem cells."

Another correspondent, who prefers to remain anonymous, wrote: "What is good egg quality? How do nuclear and cytoplasmic genes interact? How can we switch on meiosis in vitro? What do we do with the information? Does the zona pellucida act as a genetically selective filter for sperm?"

Dean Morbeck, of the Midwest Center for Reproductive Health in Minneapolis wrote: "For what it's worth, here are some areas I feel are potentially rate-limiting for ART. How can we assess cytoplasmic vitality, what aspects of stimulation protocols affect the percentage of good, healthy eggs obtained, and what culture conditions are necessary to nurture less-robust genetically normal eggs/embryos? All of these tie in with the question of how to improve implantation rate of embryos (i.e., viability of embryos – not uterine receptivity – though that actually deserves its own chapter!)."

Greg Buchold from Taylor Hall University of North Carolina came up with the most impressive list.

The Diet of Sperms (with apologies to Martin Luther) A list to delimit the important questions in male germ cell biology:

1 What initiates premeiotic S phase and is it distinct from mitotic S phase initiation? What factors bind to origins and initiate replication?

2 What regulates SPB/centrosome duplication and separation and their ability to produce meiotic I and II spindles?

3 What allows homologous chromosome pairing in meiotic prophase and keeps sister chromatids coherent in the first meiotic division?

4 What is the mechanism to determine sites for, initiation, and resolution of meiotic recombination?

5 Which gene products show alternative splicing in meiotic and haploid cells? Does this involve a germ cell specific alteration in the recognition site for splice site initiation and/or *trans* splicing factors?

6 Does transcription enhancement (overall increase) in pachytene spermatocytes and round spermatids require meiosis (or at least germ cell specific) transcription factors or RNApolII associated factors?

7 What are the positive and negative regulators of entry to the first meiotic division and how do they coordinate each other?

8 How does exit from the first meiotic division differ from that in meiosis II or mitosis?

9 What is the nature of the gap phase of secondary spermato-

cytes and how is S phase suppressed and meiosis II division initiated?

10 How do haploid cells maintain an arrested state and can this be disrupted in mammalian cells?

11 What transcription factors are required for spermiogenesis?

12 How is transcription termination in step 9 spermatids achieved and how are messages stably stored during the remainder of spermiogenesis?

13 How is chromatin progressively modified from pachytene to spermatids to achieve a fully condensed sperm nucleus?

14 How is the tail formed and its functions activated to produce forward and hyperactivated motility?

15 What is the nature of the acrosomal contents and what is their role in fertilization?

16 What is required for migration through the oviduct? Is binding required for sperm survival?

17 What factors allow storage of sperm in epididymis or sperm vesicles in nonmammals?

18. What modifications are produced by epididymal transit to sperm? What is the function of accessory gland products?

19 What are the modifications to sperm mitochondria to allow their function in fertilization/motility and targeting their destruction by ubiquitin-mediated destruction prior to/after fusion?

20 What factors are involved in sperm–egg interaction for zona binding and fusion with the egg?

21 Does the sperm determine the axis of polarity? How is the sperm centrosome kept from interfering with the female meiotic spindle until the completion of oocyte meiosis? Does the sperm contribute to reinitiation of meiosis in oocytes?

22 What is the nature of germ pole plasm/P granules/chromatoid body/nuage and how is it regulated for germline functions and initiation of meiosis?

23 What is the role for PGCs [primordial germ cells] in induction of other tissues in embryogenesis?

24 How do PGCs migrate to the gonadal ridge?

25 What is the nature of germ cell–support cell paracrine signalling and its role in survival/proliferation/differentiation of both lineages?

26 What microenvironment is required for germ cell development? (a) interactions with basement membrane/serum factors, (b) immune privilege, (c) altered nutritional requirements.

27 What is the nature of germ cell syncytia/cytoplasmic bridges? Are they effecting any functions other than synchronization and mRNA/protein sharing between haploid cells? How does this transport occur and is it regulated?

28 Why are there a stereotypical number of spermatogonial divisions and how is this achieved?

29 What is required to be an uncommitted germ cell stem cell (A0) and how is the division to produce two stem cells vs. one stem cell and one A1 (spermatogonium) produced?

30 How is totipotency or pluripotency achieved by the germline and how is senescence avoided?

31 How is telomere lengthening specifically induced in germ cells (including signal transduction to initiate this process)?

32 How is the wave of spermatogenesis (asynchronous yet spatially organized division of A0s) produced and what is the functional advantage of this system over random or synchronous (seasonal?) germ cell production?

33 Does the apoptotic machinery differ in germ cells? If so, how and what function does this fulfil?

34 What role does the endocrine axis play in initiation of pubertal development/maintenance of spermatogenesis?

35 What is the target of 12p amplification in GCTs [germ cell tumors] and the other less frequently altered genes? Which cell type is altered in GCTs? What determines the difference between GCTs appearing as yolk sac tumors, choriocarcinomas, embryonal carcinomas, or seminomas? Why are GCTs so easily eradicated?

36 Why does the germline require reduced temperature with elevated temperatures leading to transformation?

37 What is the nature of sex-determination and what functions/gene products provide male-specific advantages?

The NICHD draft discussion paper on http://www.nichd.nih.gov/strategicplan/cells/ reproductive.cfm lists the following priority research areas:

Differentiate between successful (e.g., full-term deliveries), less favorable (e.g., multiple gestations, pre-term births) and adverse ART outcomes, using large-scale statistical research, standardized criteria and unified assessments. Develop standardized definitions of "success" and "adverse outcomes." Adverse outcomes, in particular, lack standard definition and tend to be underreported because they may become apparent only over time.

Increase scientists' understanding of the development of primordial germ cells to mature oocytes and sperm through differentiation, meiosis, and maturation in an effort to evaluate the "quality" of eggs and sperm.

Enhance detection of abnormalities in preimplantation embryos; advance technology of preimplantation genetic diagnosis.

Understand what constitutes a receptive uterine environment and how receptivity can be enhanced. Understand how a healthy blastocyst–maternal tissue interaction during implantation leads to a healthy pregnancy, and to the well-being of children born as a result of ART.

Elucidate the multifactorial causes that lead to subfertility or infertility in couples and how these factors, both male and female, interact. Develop effective methods with minimal side effects to treat these causes.

Understand the nature of the abnormalities either parent brings into the treatment setting, and identify those that may constitute risks to the offspring. Understand age-related fertility factors. These issues require basic science research to help differentiate normal from abnormal gametes, as well as epidemiological risk-factor assessments.

Understand the effects of gynecologic disorders, such as tubal disease or polycystic ovarian syndrome (PCOS), on fertility rates and the prevention of infertility. Understand how these disorders may affect the choice of infertility treatments.

Understand the long-term effects of ART interventions on parental and child health. For example, in women, this includes the possible connection between ovulation induction and ovarian cancer; in men, the transmission of impaired fertility.

Improve the culturing of immature sperm and ova. Conduct basic research into cryopreservation and subsequent maturation of oocytes.

Utilize knowledge gained from basic stem cell research for understanding reproductive processes and for novel therapeutics.

Part II

Techniques: present and future

8

Influences of culture media on embryo development

Barry Bavister[1] and Jay Baltz[2]

[1]Department of Biological Sciences, University of New Orleans, and the Audubon Institute,
Center for Research of Endangered Species, New Orleans, USA
[2]Ottawa Health Research Institute, Ottawa Hospital, and University of Ottawa, Ottawa, Canada

Introduction

Clinical human in vitro fertilization (IVF) should, more accurately, be called in vitro production (IVP) since this term encompasses embryo development in vitro as well as fertilization. It has been practiced successfully since 1978. However, the average clinical pregnancy success rate (37%; Anon., 2000) is low even though multiple embryos are transferred. Poor viability of most IVP embryos is implicated as a major cause of the low pregnancy rate because, in the majority of transfer procedures, none of the embryos implants, as evidenced by failure to establish a clinical pregnancy as well as by absence of hCG secretion after transfer. Embryo transfer and uterine receptivity problems are also implicated.

Most published clinical studies do not report the proportion of the total IVP embryo cohort that failed to develop in vitro, and embryos used for transfer are selected from among those that do develop. Therefore, the *average* competence/viability as a proportion of all fertilized/cleaving ova is probably substantially lower than is apparent from the Society for Assisted Reproductive Technologies (SART) data, and may be as low as about 5% per IVP embryo (Table 8.1). The analysis in Table 8.1 probably underestimates embryo viability because it assumes that only the transferred embryos are viable; nevertheless, it illustrates that the overall efficiency of human IVP is much lower than is inferred from clinical pregnancy rates. Of those embryos that do implant successfully (fetal heartbeat detected), a considerable proportion (18%; Anon., 2000) is lost before term, lowering the

Table 8.1. Estimated efficiency of human in vitro production[a] by denominator

Denominator	No.[b]	Clinical pregnancy rate (%)	Live baby rate (%)
Transfer procedure	1	37[c]	30[c]
Embryos transferred	3	12	10
Embryos more than 2 cells	10 (5)[d]	4 (7)	3 (6)
Ova fertilized	12 (6)[d]	3 (6)	3 (5)
Mature ova collected and inseminated	15 (12)[d]	2 (3)	2

Notes:
[a] Encompassing embryo development and fertilization.
[b] Estimates for an "average" IVP cycle.
[c] From ASRM/SART registry data, 1997 (Anon., 2000).
[d] "Good" embryos or ova selected in parentheses.

average US livebirth rate resulting from IVP to 30% per embryo transfer. While this rate has increased substantially during the 1990s, there is still need for improvement. Pregnancy rates may be increased by transferring numerous (e.g., more than three) embryos to each patient, but this often results in multiple pregnancies. As shown in Table 8.1, transferring only one embryo under present conditions would likely decrease the livebirth rate to around 10%. More attention needs to be paid to improving the average quality (developmental competence and viability after transfer) of human IVP embryos. Recent use of culture media capable of supporting embryo development up to the blastocyst stage has provided clear evidence that many of these cleavage stage embryos are not developmentally competent (Dawson et al., 1995; Gardner, 1998; Gardner et al., 1998a,b), which appears, in part, to be caused by a high frequency of chromosome anomalies in IVP embryos (Winston, 1996; Munne and Cohen, 1998; Kligman et al., 1996; Winston et al., 1991). In contrast, using singleton transfers with embryos derived from oocytes matured in vitro (IVM), a high pregnancy rate (54%) was achieved in a large series (>4500) of cattle blastocyst transfers (Hasler, 1998). We should aim for similar high success rates with single embryo transfers in the human.

By increasing our understanding of the relationships between embryos and the artificial environment in which they are placed, we should be able to make striking improvements in the average quality of IVP embryos. The nature of this relationship is becoming clearer as genetic and epigenetic mechanisms that regulate normal embryo development are studied.

Regulation of embryo development

Gene expression

It has been recognized for several years that gene expression is modified in IVP embryos, which may help to explain pre- or postimplantation developmental defects (for review see Niemann and Wrenzycki, 2000; Wrenzycki et al., 2001) though many chromosome defects clearly originate before fertilization. In bovine IVP embryos, expression of specific marker genes was particularly affected by the presence of serum in the culture medium, and glucose transporter mRNA was downregulated compared with control embryos produced in vivo (Niemann and Wrenzycki, 2000). Abnormal, biallelic expression of the H19 gene occurred in mouse embryos that were cultured in Whitten's medium, while near-normal expression of only the maternal allele was observed in KSOM-AA medium, which also supported better blastocyst development (Doherty et al., 2000). Using different simple culture media, the presence or absence of serum, or even

altering the concentration of Na^+ changed RNA and protein synthesis patterns (Poueymirou et al., 1989; Ho et al., 1994; Wrenzycki et al., 1999). Mouse embryos developing in vivo had significantly greater insulin-like growth factor (IGF) II expression than either cultured embryos derived from ova fertilized in vivo or IVF embryos (Stojanov et al., 1999).

In view of these examples of the proven ability of culture media to alter gene expression, it is remarkable that the frequency of developmental defects after transfer of IVP embryos is generally quite low. One exception is the "giant fetus" syndrome reported with sheep and cattle IVP embryos. This anomaly appears to be induced by some properties of the culture medium, including serum component(s) (Thompson et al., 1995; Rieger, 1998). At day 70 of gestation, levels of IGF-II mRNA in bovine fetuses derived from IVP blastocysts were altered compared with controls (Blondin et al., 2000). Abnormal fetal development (exencephaly) was reported following transfer of mouse blastocysts that developed in medium containing amino acids that generated NH^{4+} (Lane and Gardner, 1994). Presumably, gene expression is perturbed during embryo culture. However, this defect has not been reported in other species, even though most culture media now contain amino acids. Because the timing of preimplantation development, which is critically important for normal development (discussed below), is regulated by the *ped* gene (Goldbard and Warner, 1982; Brownell and Warner, 1988; Warner et al., 1998; Cao et al., 1999), it would be interesting to know if expression of this gene is affected by culture media.

Epigenetic mechanisms

Regulation of intracellular pH and embryo quality
Until very recently, almost no attention was paid to the role of intracellular pH (pH_i) in supporting normal development of IVP mammalian embryos, nor to the influence of the culture medium on pH_i. This was a remarkable oversight, for several reasons. It is well recognized that pH_i is a critically important epigenetic regulator of somatic cell functions (Roos

and Boron, 1981; Gillies, 1982; Busa and Nuccitelli, 1984; Boron, 1987) controlling enzyme reactions, including metabolism, membrane transport processes, etc. In somatic cells, pH_i plays a pivotal role in controlling metabolism through key enzymes such as phosphofructokinase (PFK), a major regulator of glycolysis the activity of which is highly influenced by pH over a narrow range (Paetkau and Lardy, 1967; Busa and Nuccitelli, 1984). Some potent growth factors such as epidermal growth factor (EGF) appear to act via alterations in pH_i (Pouyssegur et al., 1985; Li et al., 1991; Wakabayshi et al., 1992), usually through an Na^+/H^+ antiporter that becomes operational in very early embryos (see below). With such extensive background on pH_i as a regulator of somatic cell functions, we should expect that cells of preimplantation embryos are not different in this fundamental respect and that alterations in pH_i will have important consequences for embryo development. This prediction is specifically supported for embryos because pH_i changes are functionally linked to increased protein synthesis and/or to intracellular Ca^{2+} levels in toad (*Xenopus*) and sea urchin (*Lytechinus*, *Strongylocentrotus spp.*) eggs and embryos (Grainger et al., 1979; Busa and Nuccitelli, 1984; Schackmann and Chock, 1986; Grandin and Charbonneau, 1989, 1991a,b, 1992). In mammals, there is clear evidence from studies with mice and hamsters (Zhao et al., 1995; Edwards et al., 1998a; Lane et al., 1998) that maintenance of pH_i within a narrow range is essential for embryo development (see below). Similarly, when pH_i was experimentally adjusted to below normal levels in sea urchin cleavage stage embryos, cell division was impaired, with symptoms ranging from complete inhibition of cleavage to production of anucleate fragments and uneven cleavage (Dube and Epel, 1985). This description of defects produced by low pH_i is remarkably similar to the morphological anomalies observed in "poor-quality" human embryos (Wolf et al., 1988; Veeck, 1991). Some of these poor-quality human embryos (i.e., those with low morphological scores and/or developmental competence) could have reduced ability to regulate pH_i when compromised by culture conditions that

challenge these mechanisms (Edwards et al., 1998a,b). Moreover, the "DDK" syndrome in mice (failure to maintain compaction and a lack of cell–cell communication in morulae) was ascribed to abnormally low pH_i (below 6.7) in the blastomeres (Leclerc et al., 1994). Indeed, this failure of normal development could be recreated simply by lowering pH_i to this level for as little as 1 hour using the weak acid butyrate (Leclerc et al., 1994). Most importantly, this DDK defect could be overcome by experimentally raising pH_i with a weak base (methylamine) (Buehr et al., 1987).

In hamsters, blastocyst production from cleavage stage embryos was doubled using the intracellular acidifying agent DMO (5,5-dimethyl-2,4-oxalolidinedione) or by increasing atmospheric carbon dioxide concentration (Carney and Bavister, 1987; McKiernan and Bavister, 1990), strongly supporting the idea that pH_i is abnormally elevated in cultured embryos. Elevation of pH_i could disrupt metabolism, perhaps by stimulating PFK and causing upregulation of glycolysis (Barnett and Bavister, 1996). This might help to explain excessive lactate production in vitro: cultured human, rat, and sheep embryos generate prodigious amounts of lactic acid (Gott et al., 1990; Gardner et al., 1993), implying disproportionately high activity of the glycolytic pathway as well as an inability to metabolize the excess lactic acid via conversion to pyruvate and oxidative phosphorylation. Accumulated lactic acid readily perturbs pH_i since it is a membrane-permeant weak acid (de Hemptinne et al., 1983). Alternatively, increased lactic acid production by the embryo may be a compensatory response to elevated pH_i (Barnett and Bavister, 1996). Whatever the explanation, it is abundantly clear that pH_i needs to be given prominent attention in the search for normal mediators of development that may be disturbed in IVP embryos.

Mechanisms regulating intracellular pH

The major pH_i-regulatory mechanisms are HCO_3^-/Cl^- exchangers, which decrease pH_i, and Na^+/H^+ antiporters and $Na^+,HCO_3^-/Cl^-$ exchangers, which increase pH_i (Roos and Boron, 1981;

Boron, 1987; Boyarsky et al., 1988a,b; Tonnessen et al., 1990). The HCO_3^-/Cl^- exchangers export the weak base HCO_3^- in exchange for Cl^-, thus allowing recovery from alkalosis. They are encoded by the AE (anion exchanger) gene family (Alper, 1994), with three known members (AE1–3). The Na^+/H^+ antiporters export H^+ in exchange for Na^+, thus allowing recovery from acidosis. The Na^+/H^+ antiporters are encoded by members of the NHE (Na^+/H^+ exchanger) gene family, with six known members (NHE1–6) (Orlowski and Grinstein, 1997). Activity of the $Na^+,HCO_3^-/Cl^-$ exchanger has been detected in a wide variety of cells (Roos and Boron, 1981; Boron, 1987; Boyarsky et al., 1988a,b; Tonnessen et al., 1990) and was recently cloned (Wang et al., 2000). It imports Na^+ and HCO_3^- in exchange for Cl^-, increasing pH_i by increasing intracellular HCO_3^-. A key feature of these transporters is that they are activated by changes in pH_i. The Na^+/H^+ antiporter and $Na^+,HCO_3^-/Cl^-$ exchanger are inactive unless pH_i falls below a threshold, or set-point, at which transport is activated (Roos and Boron, 1981; Aronson et al., 1982; Vaughan-Jones, 1988). Conversely, the HCO_3^-/Cl^- exchanger is activated when pH_i rises above the set-point (Olsnes et al., 1986; Vaughan-Jones, 1988). How they sense pH_i is not fully understood, although sensor regions in both AE and NHE proteins have been identified (Wakabayshi et al., 1992; Zhang et al., 1996). A variety of factors, including growth factor activation and metabolic changes as well as cell differentiation, can cause a change in the set-point (Alper, 1994; Orlowski and Grinstein, 1997). Possibly, inappropriate culture media could impair the developmental ability of IVP embryos by compromising their ability to regulate pH_i.

Capacity to regulate intracellular pH

It was reported that amino acids included in the culture medium were able to buffer pH_i in cultured mouse embryos and substantially reduced intracellular acidosis caused by weak acids in the medium (Edwards et al., 1998b). This effect of amino acids was most pronounced at the zygote stage of development, was less noticeable in 2-cell embryos, and was virtually absent by the morula stage. This sug-

gests that the ovum undergoing fertilization is exceptionally sensitive to perturbations of intracellular homeostasis; cellular damage at this stage may manifest itself as development proceeds.

Regulation of intracellular pH in embryos

Regulation against acidosis

Mouse embryos were initially reported to lack the ability to recover from acidosis by specific mechanisms. When acidosis was induced by the NH_4Cl pulse method, 2-cell CF1 strain mouse embryos exhibited a recovery that did not continue above pH_i 7.0 and the recovery was not significantly inhibited by absence of external Na^+ or by amiloride, indicating a lack of Na^+/H^+ antiporter activity (Baltz et al., 1990). More recently, however, a robust pH_i regulation against acidosis in Quackenbush strain (QS) mice has been reported, with initial recoveries about threefold slower than those of hamster 2-cell embryos (Gibb et al., 1997). The apparent conflict in these data, and the discovery of robust Na^+/H^+ antiporter activity in hamster 2-cell embryos (below), led us recently to compare pH_i regulation among several strains of mice (Steeves et al., 2001). A preliminary set of experiments was carried out under the same conditions as for hamster embryos (below). The ability of mouse 2-cell embryos to recover from induced acidosis was found to be low and very variable compared with hamster 2-cell embryos; it also appeared to vary between strains. Based on the preliminary data, 2-cell embryos from CF1, BDF, and BalbC strains were selected for direct comparison (QS strain mice were not available). CF1, BDF, and BalbC 2-cell embryos recovered from acidosis at a rate that was seven- to tenfold slower than hamster 2-cell embryos; however, the recovery required external Na^+ and was inhibited by amiloride, indicating a low but measurable Na^+/H^+ antiporter activity. If, however, the embryos were exposed to a period in Na^+-free medium (which prevents recovery) immediately after acidosis, recovery by BalbC strain embryos was stimulated upon reintroduction of Na^+ to a rate that was almost fivefold higher than without the Na^+-free period, and which was comparable to recovery in the hamster and QS strain mice. In contrast, neither BDF nor CF1 embryos exhibited this stimulation. Consequently, it appears that there are substantial differences between mouse strains in regulation of pH_i by Na^+/H^+ antiporter.

Golden hamster embryos at all early stages (zygote, 2-cell, and 8-cell) regulate pH_i against acidosis by Na^+/H^+ antiporter activity (Lane et al., 1998). This regulation is very robust at each stage, with the fastest recovery at the 2-cell stage of those stages assessed. Recovery from acidosis was found to be appropriately dependent on external Na^+ and inhibited by an amiloride derivative, EIPA. The threshold pH_i (set-point) below which the antiporter is activated in hamster embryos was 7.1–7.2 (Lane et al., 1998), the same as in the mouse (Steeves et al., 2001). Antiporter activity was required for normal development in the face of mild acidosis (Lane et al., 1998). Bovine embryos at the 2-, 4-, and 8- to 16-cell stages exhibited robust recoveries from acidosis that were Na^+-dependent and inhibited by EIPA (5-(N-ethyl-N-isopropyl)amiloride hydrochloride), indicating Na^+/H^+ antiporter activity (Lane and Bavister, 1999). Rates of recovery were comparable to those in hamster embryos.

Humans are the only primates in which pH_i regulation in embryos has been addressed. Human cleavage stage embryos were unable to recover from a mild acidosis (to approximately pH_i 7.0) (Dale et al., 1998), suggesting that these embryos do not possess active pH_i-regulatory mechanisms in the acid range. However, human blastocysts, under the same conditions, did recover from acidosis, indicating that a change in pH_i-regulatory mechanisms may occur after compaction in humans. In contrast, we found that human embryos at the 2- to 8-cell stages could indeed recover from acidosis, and this recovery depended upon external Na^+ (Phillips et al., 2000). In media lacking HCO_3^-/CO_2, recovery was inhibited by amiloride but proceeded only to about pH 6.9 and not above. However, in the presence of HCO_3^-/CO_2, the pH_i of human embryos recovered up to about 7.2, while amiloride had no effect. These data indicate that there are possibly two mechanisms active in human embryos: a Na^+/H^+ antiporter active up to approximately 6.9, and another HCO_3^--dependent mechanism active up to 7.2 (Phillips et al., 2000). We could not resolve the regulatory mechanisms into two separate components in HCO_3^-/CO_2-containing medium. These data also provide a possible explanation for the apparent conflict with the findings of Dale et al. (1998), who used HCO_3^--free media and did not produce an acidosis low enough to reach the apparent active range of the Na^+/H^+ antiporter that we identified.

The above findings in human embryos indicate that the methods developed for elucidating pH_i-regulatory mechanisms in rodent embryos can also be effectively used in primates. They underscore that there are possibly important differences in pH_i regulation between the embryos of rodents and primates. However, it is not clear exactly which pH_i-regulatory mechanisms are active in human preimplantation embryos. Because of the severe restrictions on the quality, quantity, and availability of human embryos for research, it is unlikely that this question can be resolved satisfactorily with human embryos. Therefore, research into regulation of pH_i in primate embryos needs to be conducted with appropriate model species.

Regulation against alkalosis by HCO_3^-/Cl^- exchanger

Mouse embryos from zygotes through blastocysts have robust HCO_3^-/Cl^- exchanger activity that relieves alkalosis (Baltz et al., 1991; Zhao et al., 1995; Zhao and Baltz, 1996). Activity is greatest at the post-pronuclear zygote and 2-cell stages, and it decreases at the morula stage as the embryo passes from the alkaline oviduct into the more neutral uterus (Zhao and Baltz, 1996). Exchanger activity is required for both the maintenance of baseline pH_i and for embryo development when external pH is alkaline (Zhao et al., 1995) such as that in the oviduct (Maas et al., 1977, 1984). The HCO_3^-/Cl^- exchanger isoform responsible for this activity is likely to be encoded by $AE2$, although $AE3$ mRNA appears after the zygote stage and may contribute later (Zhao et al., 1995). The threshold for activating the exchanger is essentially unchanged during preimplantation development, at pH 7.1–7.2 (Zhao and Baltz, 1996). Hamster embryos are similar to mouse embryos, having robust HCO_3^-/Cl^- exchanger activity that regulates pH_i against alkalosis at the zygote and 2-cell stages (Lane et al., 1999a). This activity is necessary for development when mild external alkalosis is present. The threshold for activation is approximately pH 7.2 at the 2-cell stage, similar to the mouse. In contrast, bovine IVM–IVF embryos do not exhibit robust regulation against an induced alkalosis at the 2- or 8- to 16-cell stages, with recovery from NH_4Cl-induced alkalosis being slow and incomplete (with recovery failing to decrease pH_i below approximately 7.8). The Cl^- removal assay showed that there was detectable HCO_3^-/Cl^- exchanger present in bovine embryos, but its ability to regulate against alkalosis was limited, and there was little protection against a small alkalosis induced by external weak base (Lane and Bavister, 1999). Therefore, it appears that bovine embryos, at least those derived from IVM–IVF, are less able to regulate pH_i against alkalosis in vitro than mouse or hamster embryos (that began development in vivo), although there is some detectable HCO_3^-/Cl^- exchanger activity.

Dale et al. (1998) found that human embryos from zygotes through blastocysts could recover from an alkalosis produced by increasing external pH to approximately 8. The mechanism of this recovery was not probed in embryos. However, a similar recovery in fresh human metaphase II (MII) oocytes was sensitive to DIDS (4,4′-diisothiocyanostilbene-2,2-disulfonate), indicating recovery mediated by a Cl^- transport-requiring mechanism such as HCO_3^-/Cl^- exchange. We examined the mechanism of recovery from alkalosis in spare human cleavage stage embryos. Human embryos at the 2- to 8-cell stages recovered from NH_4Cl-induced alkalosis, and the recovery depended on external Cl^-. Furthermore, rapid alkalinization occurred upon external Cl^- removal and this was inhibited by DIDS (Phillips et al., 2000). These findings indicate regulation against alkalosis by HCO_3^-/Cl^- exchanger activity in the human embryo. The threshold for activating the exchanger in human embryos was approximately pH 7.2 (Phillips et al., 2000), comparable to values in mouse and hamster.

Regulation in unfertilized eggs and during fertilization

Given the high HCO_3^-/Cl^- exchanger activity in pronucleate ova and subsequent embryo stages, it is surprising that ovulated, unfertilized mouse and hamster ova have little or no HCO_3^-/Cl^- exchanger activity and no ability to recover from alkalosis (Lane et al., 1999a; Phillips and Baltz, 1999). In both species, activity appears slowly after initial egg activation, with full activity 7–9 hours after sperm–egg fusion. The onset of HCO_3^-/Cl^- exchanger activity appears to depend on activation of existing exchangers, since *AE2* mRNA is present in both ova and zygotes, and upregulation is unaffected by blockage of protein synthesis or by disruption of the cytoskeleton (Phillips and Baltz, 1999). Similarly, in hamsters, Na^+/H^+ antiporter activity and regulation against acidosis appears only several hours after egg activation. The time course is similar to upregulation of the HCO_3^-/Cl^- exchanger in mouse, and upregulation is also independent of protein synthesis or an intact cytoskeleton, indicating activation of preexisting antiporters (Lane et al., 1999b). This study also showed that the mechanism of antiporter activation is dependent on protein kinase C (PKC).

In rodents, then, it appears that there is little or no capacity for pH_i regulation before the middle of the 1-cell stage, approximately the time when the pronuclei are formed and the same period when mitochondria are clustering around the pronuclei (Barnett et al., 1996). Activation of pH_i-regulatory mechanisms and mitochondrial clustering may be functionally related, but how the appearance of this capacity is regulated is not known. In the hamster, activating PKC can partially activate Na^+/H^+ antiporter activity in unfertilized eggs (Lane et al., 1999b). In both hamster and mouse, suppression of the Ca^{2+} transients that follow egg activation and lowering the baseline Ca^{2+} concentration using the chelator BAPTA (1,2-bis(aminophenoxy)ethane-*N,N,N,′N′*-tetraacetic acid) can partially, but not fully, suppress development of pH_i regulatory capacity (Lane et al., 1999b; Phillips and Baltz, 1999). However, preliminary evidence in the mouse (K.P. Phillips and J.M. Baltz, unpublished data) indicated that release from MII arrest alone may be necessary and sufficient for subsequent upregulation of HCO_3^-/Cl^- exchanger activity: cycloheximide-induced egg activation (via cyclin degradation) produces upregulation in the absence of any Ca^{2+} transients. Conversely, Sr^{2+}-induced Ca^{2+} transients, which effectively cause upregulation of exchanger activity, are unable to do so if the metaphase spindle is first disrupted and entry into the cell cycle thus prevented (K.P. Phillips and J.M. Baltz, unpublished data). However, the mechanisms regulating the appearance of pH_i regulatory activity after egg activation are far from clear and need to be elucidated.

The situation in nonrodent species may be different. Dale et al. (1998) reported that the ability to recovery from alkalosis induced by increased external pH existed in human MII oocytes, and that this recovery was blocked by DIDS, indicating HCO_3^-/Cl^- exchanger activity in oocytes. In contrast, they did not find an ability to recover from acidosis in eggs or in any embryonic stage before the blastocyst. However, such an ability *was* evident in more extensive studies of human cleavage stage embryos (Phillips et al., 2000) and, therefore, the question of what regulates pH_i in human or other primate oocytes remains to be determined. In cows, Na^+/H^+ antiporter activity was detectable in IVM-derived unfertilized ova, although the activity was much lower than that seen in embryos (Lane and Bavister, 1999). Consequently, it is not clear whether activation of pH_i-regulatory mechanisms resulting from fertilization is a feature of early development in nonrodent species. With respect to human IVP embryos, it is important to find (i) when the different pH_i-regulatory mechanisms are activated during development, and (ii) if the timing and/or activity of these mechanisms is perturbed by suboptimal culture conditions, which could account for observed developmental anomalies. Such anomalies could include defective activation of the embryonic genome (Schramm and Bavister, 1999).

Regulation of intracellular calcium and embryo quality

Compared with the amount of recent work on pH_i regulation in embryos and effects of altering pH_i on development, there is very little information on intracellular Ca^{2+} regulation. Subcellular organization is regulated by intracellular Ca^{2+} concentration (Wu et al., 1996), so we should expect that Ca^{2+} homeostasis is critically important for embryogenesis. Lowering intracellular Ca^{2+} using calcium channel blockers (nifedipine or verapamil), or a calcium chelator (BAPTA), or even simply changing the extracellular Ca^{2+} and Mg^{2+} concentrations, markedly improved development of hamster ova to blastocysts (Lane and Bavister, 1998). This improvement was noted even when exposure to treatments was for only 6 hours, suggesting that the ovum undergoing fertilization is exceptionally sensitive to perturbations in intracellular Ca^{2+} levels. Because blocking voltage-gated membrane calcium channels during this time enhanced subsequent embryo development, it may be inferred that exposure of 1-cell embryos to culture media alters the cell membrane potential. This is an exciting possibility with implications for both basic and applied embryology that needs further study.

Summary

Maintenance of normal intracellular levels of H^+ and Ca^{2+} is critically important for normal embryo development in vitro. In several animal species, pH_i-regulatory mechanisms become activated during early development. Perturbation of these mechanisms by components of culture media has adverse consequences for normal embryo development, either during the preimplantation period or possibly after embryo transfer.

Composition of culture media

Single-stage versus sequential media

Until recently, most embryo culture was done using a single formulation to support development from

1-cell to blastocyst. This approach met with mixed results. Recently, efforts have been made to devise multistep or sequential media that provide specific components for cleavage stages and for morulae/blastocysts. This approach attempts to mimic the changing environment within the female reproductive tract as the embryo passes from the oviduct to the uterus. The groundwork for developing sequential culture media was laid years ago (Bavister, 1995). Kane and Foote (1970) showed that rabbit zygotes could develop to the morula stage in the absence of free amino acids, but then required amino acids to develop into blastocysts (Kane, 1987). Mouse and human blastocyst development in vitro was improved by withholding addition of glucose to the medium until after the first two cleavage divisions (Chatot et al., 1989; Brown and Whittingham, 1992; Conaghan et al., 1993). Bovine embryo IVP was improved by using a simple medium with particular amino acids and energy substrates for cleavage stages followed by a complex medium containing serum for supporting blastocyst development (Pinyopummintr and Bavister, 1996a,b). Addition of glycine and/or alanine to the culture medium greatly increased bovine blastocyst development, cell numbers, and hatching (Lee and Fukui, 1996). Using nonessential amino acids for cleavage stage development and then adding the essential amino acids enhanced mouse embryo development in vitro (Gardner and Lane, 1993). Based on data such as these, sequential media for human blastocyst IVP have been devised and appear to improve pregnancy rates (Gardner and Lane, 1998). All this information strongly supports the concept that different stages of preimplantation embryos require different medium components, some of which may be harmful if included too early in development. There is still need for improvement in sequential media formulations to optimize IVP of embryos and maximize their viability.

Growth factors and hormones

It has been suggested that growth factors may emanate either from the embryo (autocrine secretion) or from co-cultured somatic cells or other embryos (paracrine secretion). There is little hard evidence for either mode of secretion from studies on embryo development with growth factors in the culture medium. In one study, granulocyte–macrophage colony-stimulating factor increased the proportion of bovine blastocysts when it was added from about the midpoint of fertilization (de Moraes and Hansen, 1997). However, the low proportion of blastocysts produced in all the treatments relative to other studies suggest that the culture conditions used in this study were not adequate. It would be interesting to know if growth factors can influence development when the control culture medium produces 40% or more blastocysts, as in many reports (e.g., Lee and Fukui, 1996; Pinyopummintr and Bavister, 1996a,b). Studies with mice seem to support the idea that growth factors may help under suboptimal conditions. Various growth factors (IGF-I, IGF-II, platelet-activating factor (PAF) (stimulated IVF development) of mouse zygotes when they were cultured at suboptimal ratios of embryos:culture medium volume (O'Neill, 1997). Inclusion of growth factors (platelet-derived growth factor, mouse leukemia-inhibiting factor) in culture media did not improve rabbit blastocyst cell numbers, although addition of fetal bovine serum did (Giles and Foote, 1997). Insulin increased blastocyst cell numbers and hatching in IVP mouse embryos but had no detectable effect on bovine blastocysts (Mihalik et al., 2000). It has been suggested that endogenously produced growth factors such as transforming growth factor α might function as embryo survival factors (Brison and Schultz, 1997). Whether this is a response to the stress imposed by artificial culture conditions or a true physiological mechanism is unknown.

In contrast to the generally weak evidence for a role of specific growth factors on embryo development in vitro, there is quite good evidence that IVM of oocytes in the presence of growth factors, especially EGF, has a pronounced positive effect on the quality of the MII oocytes as judged by blastocyst development following IVF (Lonergan et al., 1996). This effect could well be mediated via the cumulus cells rather than directly on the oocytes.

Evidence for paracrine embryotrophic growth factor effects has been very weak. Much controversy, if not confusion, has been generated by proponents of "co-culture" using somatic cells of various types to assist embryo development. The evidence is strongly in favor of a conditioning effect whereby specific components of the medium are altered by somatic cells towards the optimum for supporting embryo development (Bavister, 1995; Edwards et al., 1997). One study (Edwards et al., 1997) showed that oviduct cells were the most effective: they increased levels of L-lactate and pyruvate in the culture milieu (SOF medium) and reduced the glucose concentration to approximately half. All these changes are known to enhance embryo development; in this study, mimicking them by adjusting the medium formulation significantly increased (almost sixfold) the proportion of bovine zygotes that developed into blastocysts. Therefore, it seems most likely that claims made for "embryotrophic factors" secreted by cultured somatic cells are attributable simply to modification of the chemical environment. Obviously, it is much easier to modify the formulation of the embryo culture medium, avoiding additional work involved in generating somatic cell monolayers, and the variability introduced by an additional cultured cell line, in addition to the danger of introducing pathogenic organisms into the embryo culture environment. A study purporting to show an embryotrophic effect of metalloproteinase inhibitor secreted by oviduct cells was invalidated because there was no statistically significant improvement in embryo development (Satoh et al., 1994). There do not appear to be any reports of somatic cell co-culture, operating via secretion of embryotrophic growth factors, that stand up to rigorous scrutiny. However, this is not to say that paracrine growth factor effects do not exist. A recent study in the cat demonstrated that the age and quality of embryos influenced the development of companion embryos cultured in the same dish (Spindler and Wildt, 2000). The quality of embryos was based on their metabolism of glucose. Although not conclusive, this study provides good indirect evidence for paracrine embryo-

trophic factors. A direct effect of heparin-binding EGF on human embryo development to blastocyst was demonstrated in an exceptional study using serum-free medium (Sargent et al., 1998). Moreover, 80% of the blastocysts hatched, whereas it is typical in serum-free media for most blastocysts to fail to escape from the zona pellucida. Supplementing culture medium with IGF-I increased development of human blastocysts and the number of cells in the inner cell mass, an effect mediated via IGF-I receptors (Lighten et al., 1998). This result suggests that maternal IGF-I may help to support human blastocyst development.

Although embryos developing in vivo are exposed to a variety of hormones at different concentrations during development, there is, surprisingly, very little evidence for a positive effect of hormones on embryo development in vitro. One exception is the preliminary report that development of hamster 1-cell embryos is enhanced by luteinizing hormone, although follicle-stimulating hormone and prolactin were both inhibitory (Ji and Bavister, 1998).

Protein supplementation

It is common practice to add protein to embryo culture media, either in the form of blood serum (a nonphysiological fluid) or serum derivatives such as human serum albumin or Synthetic Serum Substitute, which is misleadingly named because it is another derivative of blood serum. There are several reasons to avoid using serum or serum proteins for this purpose: (i) they may be unnecessary; (ii) they can be dangerous for the health of the embryo or the embryo transfer recipient through contamination with pathogenic organisms such as the prions causing Creutzfeldt–Jakob disease or the new human variant form; (iii) serum is implicated in anomalies of gene expression; and (iv) the high variability of different batches of serum or serum derivatives can affect embryo development and/or viability. Serum proteins can inhibit embryo development. The proportion of bovine zygotes that cleaved was significantly reduced when serum was added to the culture medium just prior to the first cleavage division (Pinyopummintr and Bavister, 1994). Positive effects of PAF on mouse embryo development may be reduced in the presence of serum albumin because this protein can compete with PAF (O'Neill, 1997). In human IVP, pregnancy and/or implantation rates were reduced when embryos were frozen or thawed in medium containing human serum albumin from pooled sera (Warnes et al., 1997). Studies in animals and in humans have shown that embryo development can take place without any protein in the medium (Caro and Trounson, 1986; Keskintepe and Brackett, 1996; Pinyopummintr and Bavister, 1996a,b; Schramm and Bavister, 1996; Rinehart et al., 1998), and babies have been born after transfer of embryos that developed in protein-free media (Caro and Trounson, 1986; McKiernan and Bavister, 1994). Macromolecules used as alternatives to proteins include polyvinylalcohol (PVA) and hyaluronate (McKiernan and Bavister, 1994; Keskintepe and Brackett, 1996; Rinehart et al., 1998; Gardner et al., 1999).

There are also, however, some studies that report a supportive role, if not a need, for serum components to support blastocyst development in vitro. Either blastocysts failed to develop in protein-free media or development was enhanced by serum or serum proteins (Pinyopummintr and Bavister, 1991; Seshagiri and Hearn, 1992; Thompson et al., 1992; Schramm and Bavister, 1996; Biggers et al., 1997).

In summary, there is no absolute need to include serum components in culture media for cleavage stage embryo development. Any beneficial effects of serum such as pH buffering or chelation of metal ion contaminants can be achieved instead with amino acids and/or EDTA (ethylenediaminetetraacetic acid) (Fissore et al., 1989). However, more research is needed to identify and replace the components of serum that stimulate blastocyst development. The ability to use a completely protein-free medium for blastocyst production would not only eliminate concerns about pathogens but also help to standardize media formulations and thereby reduce batch variability problems.

Metabolism of cultured embryos

There is much evidence that the metabolism of IVP embryos is altered by the culture medium (Barnett and Bavister, 1996). For example, different culture media differentially alter glycolysis (Krisher et al., 1999); the activity of this pathway is associated with embryo developmental competence and viability (Leese, 1991; Lane and Gardner, 1996). In general, increased glycolytic activity is inversely proportional to embryo development and may be combined with reduced oxidative metabolism (the Crabtree effect; Seshagiri and Bavister, 1991). The metabolism of mouse and rat blastocysts developed in vivo was perturbed after only a few hours in culture; specifically, glycolysis was increased while pyruvate oxidation was reduced (Lane and Gardner, 1998). This manifestation of the Crabtree effect (Seshagiri and Bavister, 1991) was reduced or eliminated by adding amino acids and vitamins to the culture medium. The converse appears to be true with oocyte maturation, increased glycolytic activity being associated with improved developmental competence, but this may well be because of the needs of the cumulus cells that were nurturing the oocytes (Krisher and Bavister, 1999). A key factor in the success of the "G1/G2" sequential culture media is the inclusion of EDTA in medium G1 to inhibit glycolysis (Gardner and Lane, 1996; Gardner, 1998). A fundamental question that remains to be answered is: why is glycolysis elevated in IVP embryos? A possible answer is that this pathway is upregulated by a rise in pH_i, though why this pH_i increase should occur is unknown. Deletion of glucose from the culture medium for human IVP embryos improved their quality, although pregnancy rates were not different (Coates et al., 1999); perhaps a low level of glucose would be beneficial (Bavister, 1999; Ludwig et al., 2001). The absence of glucose from the culture medium for CF1 mouse embryos was detrimental to their development and viability (Gardner and Lane, 1996). A study with hamster embryos showed that lowering the glucose concentration to 0.5 mmol/l, while having little or no effect on preimplantation embryo development compared with no glucose or

5 mmol/l glucose, greatly increased the proportion of transferred embryos developing into viable fetuses compared with that seen in the absence of glucose (Ludwig et al., 2001). Glutamine, which can be directly metabolized via the tricarboxylic acid cycle, stimulated morula and blastocyst development in human IVP embryos; it also increased pyruvate uptake and lactate production (Devreker et al., 1998). The presence of glutamine was also important for development of "blocking" strains of mouse embryos (Chatot et al., 1989; Gardner and Lane, 1996). In cultured mouse embryos, the concentration of lactate in the medium altered lactate and pyruvate metabolism; this effect was most pronounced at the zygote stage (Lane and Gardner, 2000) and might be partially mediated via the ability of extracellular lactate to lower pH_i (de Hemptinne et al., 1983; Edwards et al., 1998a).

There have been few reports on success in improving embryo development with vitamins. Addition of Eagle's vitamins helped to restore the normal balance between glycolysis and oxidative metabolism in cultured mouse embryos (Lane and Gardner, 1998) and increased glucose uptake and lactate production in sheep embryos (Gardner et al., 1994). Pantothenic acid, an essential component for biosynthesis of coenzyme A, stimulated blastocyst development in cultured hamster embryos and, more importantly, increased the proportions of near-term fetuses derived from these embryos (McKiernan and Bavister, 2000).

Timing of development

The timing of embryo development can be affected by inherent properties of each embryo (Goldbard and Warner, 1982; Brownell and Warner, 1988; Warner et al., 1998; Cao et al., 1999) as well as by characteristics of the culture medium (e.g., Pinyopummintr and Bavister, 1996a,b). Both of these areas need examination, because development timing is critically important for successful embryogenesis, as shown in both animal and human IVP studies. In studies with hamster and cattle embryos, embryo development and viability were directly related to the speed of development (McKiernan and Bavister, 1994; Gonzales et al., 1995; van Soom et al., 1997; Hasler, 1998). High clinical pregnancy rates were achieved when embryos were selected for transfer based on the proportions of 8-cell embryos that had formed by 67 hours after insemination (Racowsky et al., 2000). Using a strictly defined, narrow time window for embryo examination eliminated a problem inherent in several other studies comparing 'day 3' and 'day 5' embryo transfer outcomes. In these reports, embryos transferred on day 3 were at various stages of cleavage and, most likely, were widely different in their viability. Some of these studies reported an improvement in pregnancy rates with blastocyst transfers compared with day 3 embryos, which is not surprising when slow-cleaving embryos that had an increased likelihood of being nonviable were selected for transfer. In the study by Racowsky et al. (2000), when one to three or more acceptable embryos were found by 67 hours after insemination, either embryo transfer was performed on day 3 or transfer was postponed until day 5 when embryos had developed in culture to the blastocyst stage. There was no difference in ongoing pregnancy rates (percentage of transfers) between these two procedures (40–55%). An acceptable pregnancy rate (33%) was still obtained with day 3 embryo transfers even when there were no embryos on day 3 that met the timing and morphological criteria, but there were no ongoing pregnancies after day 5 embryo transfers. The lack of pregnancies in the latter group was correlated with significantly lower values for the numbers and percentages of day 5 blastocysts and expanded blastocysts, compared with the group that had three or more quality 8-cell embryos on day 3. These observations indicate that blastocysts developing from slow-cleaving embryos are nonviable. This is consistent with a study using hamster embryos (McKiernan and Bavister, 1994). The study by Racowsky et al. (2000) also reveals that the in vivo environment is superior to current embryo culture media, because slow-cleaving embryos were "rescued" by the uterine environment when they were transferred on day 3 but did not survive after culture to day 5 before being transferred. The relationship between timing of embryo development and embryo viability was reviewed by Bavister (1995, 2002). Embryo development timing remains the simplest, noninvasive criterion for selection of embryos for transfer, although it should be used in conjunction with other measures such as morphology.

Conclusions

Substantial progress has been made in understanding the regulation of preimplantation development in animals, as well as in assessing their substrate and nutrient needs at different stages of development. With this information, new culture media have been designed that substantially improve embryo development, as evidenced by higher frequencies of blastocyst production with increased cell numbers and greater viability post-transfer. The trend in animal embryo culture is towards completely protein-free, "minimalist" media that are consistent in their composition and free from possible pathogenic agents. This information needs to be examined and applied to human IVP much more widely and rapidly than it has been in order to enhance the quality of human embryos and thereby to increase the efficiency of ART. Two key areas in urgent need of examination are the differential effects of culture media on pH_i and intracellular Ca^{2+}, and the elimination of serum proteins from the entire series of media used for IVP of human embryos.

REFERENCES

Alper, S.L. (1994). The band 3-related anion exchanger gene family. *Cellular Physiology and Biochemistry*, **4**, 265–81.

Anon. (2000). Assisted reproductive technology in the United States: 1997 results generated from the American Society for Reproductive Medicine/Society for Assisted Reproductive Technology Registry. *Fertility and Sterility*, **74**, 641–53.

Aronson, P.S., Nee, J., and Suhm, M. (1982). Modifier role of internal H^+ in activating the Na^+–H^+ exchanger in renal microvillus membrane vesicles. *Nature (London)*, **299**, 161–3.

Baltz, J.M., Biggers, J.D., and Lechene, C. (1990). Apparent absence of Na^+/H^+ antiport activity in the 2-cell mouse embryo. *Developmental Biology*, **138**, 421–9.

Baltz, J.M., Biggers, J.D., and Lechene, C. (1991). Relief from alkaline load in 2-cell stage mouse embryos by bicarbonate–chloride exchange. *Journal of Biological Chemistry*, **266**, 17212–17.

Barnett, D. and Bavister, B.D. (1996). What is the relationship between the metabolism of preimplantation embryos and their development in vitro? *Molecular Reproduction and Development*, **43**, 105–33.

Barnett, D.K., Kimura, J., and Bavister, B.D. (1996). Translocation of active mitochondria during hamster preimplantation embryo development studied by confocal laser scanning microscopy. *Developmental Dynamics*, **205**, 64–72.

Bavister, B.D. (1995). Culture of preimplantation embryos: facts and artifacts. *Human Reproduction Update*, **1**, 91–148.

Bavister, B.D. (1999). Glucose and culture of human embryos. *Fertility and Sterility*, **72**, 233–4.

Bavister, B.D. (2002). Timing of embryo development. In: *Assessment of Mammalian Embryo Quality: Invasive and Non-invasive Techniques*, van Soom, A. and Boerjan, M., Kluwer, eds. Academic, Dordrecht, pp. 139–55.

Biggers, J.D., Summers, M.C., and McGinnis, L.K. (1997). Polyvinyl alcohol and amino acids as substitutes for bovine serum albumin in culture media for mouse preimplantation embryos. *Human Reproduction Update*, **3**, 125–35.

Blondin, P., Farin, P.W., Crosier, A.E., Alexander, J.E., and Farin, C.E. (2000). In vitro production of embryos alters levels of insulin-like growth factor-II messenger ribonucleic acid in bovine fetuses 63 days after transfer. *Biology of Reproduction*, **62**, 384–9.

Boron, W.F. (1987). Intracellular pH regulation. In: *Membrane Transport Processes in Organized Systems*, Andreoli, T.E., Hoffman, J.F., Fanestil, D.D. and Schultz, S.G., eds. Plenum Press, New York, pp. 39–51.

Boyarsky, G., Ganz, M.B., Sterzel, R.B., and Boron, W.F. (1988a). pH regulation in single glomerular messangial cells. I. acid extrusion in the absence and presence of HCO_3^-. *American Journal of Physiology*, **255**, C844–56.

Boyarsky, G., Ganz, M.B., Sterzel, R.B., and Boron, W.F. (1988b). pH regulation in single glomerular messangial cells. II. Na^+-dependent and -independent Cl^-–HCO_3^- exchangers. *American Journal of Physiology*, **255**, C857–69.

Brison, D.R. and Schultz, R.M. (1997). Apoptosis during mouse blastocyst formation: evidence for a role for survival factors including transforming growth factor alpha. *Biology of Reproduction*, **56**, 1088–96.

Brown, J.J.G. and Whittingham, D.G. (1992). The dynamic provision of different energy substrates improves development of one-cell random-bred mouse embryos in vitro. *Journal of Reproduction and Fertility*, **95**, 503–11.

Brownell, M.S. and Warner, C.M. (1988). Ped gene expression by embryos cultured in vitro. *Biology of Reproduction*, **39**, 806–11.

Buehr, M., Lee, S., McLaren, A., and Warner, A. (1987). Reduced gap junctional communication is associated with the lethal condition characteristic of DDK mouse eggs fertilized by foreign sperm. *Development*, **101**, 449–59.

Busa, W.B. and Nuccitelli, R. (1984). Metabolic regulation via intracellular pH. *American Journal of Physiology*, **246**, R409–38.

Cao, W., Brenner, C.A., Alikani, M., Cohen, J., and Warner, C.M. (1999). Search for a human homologue of the mouse Ped gene. *Molecular Human Reproduction*, **5**, 541–7.

Carney, E.W. and Bavister, B.D. (1987). Regulation of hamster embryo development in vitro by carbon dioxide. *Biology of Reproduction*, **36**, 1155–63.

Caro, C.M. and Trounson, A. (1986). Successful fertilization, embryo development, and pregnancy in human in vitro fertilization (IVF) using a chemically defined culture medium containing no protein. *Journal of In Vitro Fertilization and Embryo Transfer*, **3**, 215–17.

Chatot, C.L., Ziomek, C.A., Bavister, B.D., Lewis, J.L., and Torres, I. (1989). An improved culture medium supports development of random-bred 1-cell mouse embryos in vitro. *Journal of Reproduction and Fertility*, **86**, 679–88.

Coates, A., Rutherford, A.J., Hunter, H., and Leese, H.J. (1999). Glucose-free medium in human in vitro fertilization and embryo transfer: a large-scale, prospective, randomized clinical trial. *Fertility and Sterility*, **72**, 229–32.

Conaghan, J., Handyside, A.H., Winston, R.M.L., and Leese, H.J. (1993). Effects of pyruvate and glucose on the development of human preimplantation embryos in vitro. *Journal of Reproduction and Fertility*, **99**, 87–95.

Dale, B., Menezo, Y., Cohen, J., DiMatteo, L., and Wilding, M. (1998). Intracellular pH regulation in the human oocyte. *Human Reproduction*, **13**, 964–70.

Dawson, K.J., Conaghan, J., Ostera, G.R., Winston, R.M.L., and Hardy, K. (1995). Delaying transfer to the third day post-insemination, to select non-arrested embryos, increases development to the fetal heart stage. *Human Reproduction*, **10**, 177–82.

de Hemptinne, A., Marrannes, R., and Vanheel, B. (1983). Influence of organic acids on intracellular pH. *American Journal of Physiology*, **245**, 178–83.

de Moraes, A.A. and Hansen, P.J. (1997). Granulocyte-macrophage colony-stimulating factor promotes development of in vitro produced bovine embryos. *Biology of Reproduction*, **57**, 1060–5.

Devreker, F., Winston, R.M., and Hardy, K. (1998). Glutamine improves human preimplantation development in vitro. *Fertility and Sterility*, **69**, 293–9.

Doherty, A.S., Mann, M.R., Tremblay, K.D., Bartolomei, M.S., and Schultz, R.M. (2000). Differential effects of culture on imprinted H19 expression in the preimplantation mouse embryo. *Biology of Reproduction*, **62**, 1526–35.

Dube, F. and Epel, D. (1985). The hierarchy of requirements for an elevated pH$_i$ during development of sea urchin embryos. *Cell*, **40**, 657–66.

Edwards, L.J., Batt, P.A., Gandolfi, F., and Gardner, D.K. (1997). Modifications made to culture medium by bovine oviduct epithelial cells: changes to carbohydrates stimulate bovine embryo development. *Molecular Reproduction and Development*, **46**, 146–54.

Edwards, L.J., Williams, D.A., and Gardner, D.K. (1998a). Intracellular pH of the preimplantation mouse embryo: effects of extracellular pH and weak acids. *Molecular Reproduction and Development*, **50**, 434–42.

Edwards, L.J., Williams, D.A., and Gardner, D.K. (1998b). Intracellular pH of the mouse preimplantation embryo: amino acids act as buffers of intracellular pH. *Human Reproduction*, **13**, 3441–8.

Fissore, R.A., Jackson, K.V., and Kiessling, A.A. (1989). Mouse zygote development in culture medium without protein in the presence of ethylenediaminetetraacetic acid. *Biology of Reproduction*, **41**, 835–41.

Gardner, D.K. (1998). Development of serum-free media for the culture and transfer of human blastocysts. *Human Reproduction*, **13**(Suppl. 4), 218–25.

Gardner, D.K. and Lane, M. (1993). Amino acids and ammonium regulate mouse embryo development in culture. *Biology of Reproduction*, **48**, 377–85.

Gardner, D.K. and Lane, M. (1996). Alleviation of the '2-cell block' and development to the blastocyst of CF1 mouse embryos: role of amino acids, EDTA and physical parameters. *Human Reproduction*, **11**, 2703–12.

Gardner, D.K. and Lane, M. (1998). Culture of viable human blastocysts in defined sequential serum-free media. *Human Reproduction*, **13**(Suppl. 31), 48–159.

Gardner, D.K., Lane, M., and Batt, P. (1993). Uptake and metabolism of pyruvate and glucose by individual sheep preattachment embryos developed in vivo. *Molecular Reproduction and Development*, **36**, 313–29.

Gardner, D.K., Lane, M., Spitzer, A., and Batt, P.A. (1994). Enhanced rates of cleavage and development for sheep zygotes cultured to the blastocyst stage in vitro in the absence of serum and somatic cells: amino acids, vitamins, and culturing embryos in groups stimulate development. *Biology of Reproduction*, **50**, 390–400.

Gardner, D.K., Schoolcraft, W.B., Wagley, L., Schlenker, T., Stevens, J., and Hesla, J. (1998a). A prospective randomized trial of blastocyst culture and transfer in in-vitro fertilization. *Human Reproduction*, **13**, 3434–40.

Gardner, D.K., Vella, P., Lane, M., Wagley, L., Schlenker, T., and Schoolcraft, W.B. (1998b). Culture and transfer of human blastocysts increases implantation rates and reduces the need for multiple embryo transfers. *Fertility and Sterility*, **69**, 84–8.

Gardner, D.K., Rodrieguez-Martinez, H., and Lane, M. (1999). Fetal development after transfer is increased by replacing protein with the glycosaminoglycan hyaluronan for mouse embryo culture and transfer. *Human Reproduction*, **14**, 2575–80.

Gibb, C.A., Poronnik, P., Day, M.L., and Cook, D.I. (1997). Control of cytosolic pH in two-cell mouse embryos: roles of H^+-lactate cotransport and Na^+/H^+ exchange. *American Journal of Physiology: Cell Physiology*, **273**, C404–19.

Giles, J.R. and Foote, R.H. (1997). Effects of gas atmosphere, platelet-derived growth factor and leukemia inhibitory factor on cell numbers of rabbit embryos cultured in a protein-free medium. *Reproduction, Nutrition and Development*, **37**, 97–104.

Gillies, R.J. (1982). Intracellular pH and proliferation in yeast, tetrahymena, and sea urchin eggs. In: *Intracellular pH: Its Measurement, Regulation and Utilization in Cellular Functions*, Nuccitelli, R. and Deamer, D.W., eds. Alan R. Liss, New York, pp. 314–59.

Goldbard, S.B. and Warner, C.M. (1982). Genes affect the timing of early mouse embryo development. *Biology of Reproduction*, **27**, 419–24.

Gonzales, D.S., Pinheiro, J.C., and Bavister, B.D. (1995). Prediction of the developmental potential of hamster embryos in vitro by precise timing of the third cell cycle. *Journal of Reproduction and Fertility*, **105**, 1–8.

Gott, A.L., Hardy, K., Winston, R.M.L., and Leese, H.J. (1990). Non-invasive measurement of pyruvate and glucose uptake and lactate production by single human preimplantation embryos. *Human Reproduction*, **5**, 104–8.

Grainger, J.L., Winkler, M.M., Shen, S.S., and Steinhardt, R.A. (1979). Intracellular pH controls protein synthesis rate in the sea urchin egg and early embryo. *Developmental Biology*, **68**, 396–406.

Grandin, N. and Charbonneau, M. (1989). Intracellular pH and the increase in protein synthesis accompanying activation of *Xenopus* eggs. *Biology of the Cell*, **67**, 321–30.

Grandin, N. and Charbonneau, M. (1991a). Changes in intracellular free calcium activity in *Xenopus* eggs following imposed intracellular pH changes using weak acids and weak bases. *Biochimica et Biophysica Acta*, **1091**, 242–50.

Grandin, N. and Charbonneau, M. (1991b). Intracellular pH and intracellular free calcium responses to protein kinase C activators and inhibitors in *Xenopus* eggs. *Development*, **112**, 461–70.

Grandin, N. and Charbonneau, M. (1992). The increase in intracellular pH associated with *Xenopus* egg activation is a $Ca(2+)$-dependent wave. *Journal of Cell Science*, **101**, 55–67.

Hasler, J.F. (1998). The current status of oocyte recovery, in vitro embryo production, and embryo transfer in domestic animals, with an emphasis on the bovine. *Journal of Animal Science*, **76**(Suppl. 3), 52–74.

Ho, Y., Doherty, A.S., and Schultz, R.M. (1994). Mouse preimplantation embryo development in vitro: effect of sodium concentration in culture media on RNA synthesis and accumulation and gene expression. *Molecular Reproduction and Development*, **38**, 131–41.

Ji, W.Z. and Bavister, B.D. (1998). Direct effects of gonadotropic hormones on in vitro development of early cleavage stage hamster embryos. *Biology of Reproduction*, **58**(Suppl. 1), 93.

Kane, M.T., (1987). In vitro growth of preimplantation rabbit embryos. In: *The Mammalian Preimplantation Embryo*, Bavister, B.D. ed. Plenum Press, New York, pp. 193–217.

Kane, M.T. and Foote, R.H. (1970). Culture of two- and four-cell rabbit embryos to the expanding blastocyst stage in synthetic media. *Proceedings of the Society for Experimental Biology and Medicine*, **133**, 921–5.

Keskintepe, L. and Brackett, B.G. (1996). In vitro developmental competence of in vitro-matured bovine oocytes fertilized and cultured in completely defined media. *Biology of Reproduction*, **55**, 333–9.

Kligman, I., Benadiva, C., Alikani, M., and Munne, S. (1996). The presence of multinucleated blastomeres in human embryos is correlated with chromosomal abnormalities. *Human Reproduction*, **11**, 1492–8.

Krisher, R.L. and Bavister, B.D. (1999). Enhanced glycolysis after maturation of bovine oocytes in vitro is associated with increased developmental competence. *Molecular Reproduction and Development*, **53**, 19–26.

Krisher, R.L., Lane, M., and Bavister, B.D. (1999). Developmental competence and metabolism of bovine embryos cultured in semi-defined and defined culture media. *Biology of Reproduction*, **60**, 1345–52.

Lane, M. and Bavister, B.D. (1998). Calcium homeostasis in early hamster preimplantation embryos. *Biology of Reproduction*, **59**, 1000–7.

Lane, M. and Bavister, B.D. (1999). Regulation of intracellular pH in bovine oocytes and cleavage stage embryos. *Molecular Reproduction and Development*, **54**, 396–401.

Lane, M. and Gardner, D.K. (1994). Increase in postimplantation development of cultured mouse embryos by amino acids and induction of fetal retardation and exencephaly by ammonium ions. *Journal of Reproduction and Fertility*, **102**, 305–12.

Lane, M. and Gardner, D.K. (1996). Selection of viable mouse blastocysts prior to transfer using a metabolic criterion. *Human Reproduction*, **11**, 1975–8.

Lane, M. and Gardner, D.K. (1998). Amino acids and vitamins prevent culture-induced metabolic perturbations and associated loss of viability of mouse blastocysts. *Human Reproduction*, **13**, 991–7.

Lane, M. and Gardner, D.K. (2000). Lactate regulates pyruvate uptake and metabolism in the preimplantation mouse embryo. *Biology of Reproduction*, **62**, 16–22.

Lane, M., Baltz, J.M., and Bavister, B.D. (1998). Regulation of intracellular pH in hamster preimplantation embryos by the Na^+/H^+ antiporter. *Biology of Reproduction*, **59**, 1483–90.

Lane, M., Baltz, J.M., and Bavister, B.D. (1999a). Bicarbonate/chloride exchange regulates intracellular pH of embryos but not oocytes of the hamster. *Biology of Reproduction*, **61**, 452–7.

Lane, M., Baltz, J.M., and Bavister, B.D. (1999b). Na^+/H^+ antiporter activity in hamster embryos is activated during fertilization. *Developmental Biology*, **208**, 244–52.

Leclerc, C., Becker, D., Buehr, M., and Warner, A. (1994). Low intracellular pH is involved in the early embryonic death of DDK mouse eggs fertilized by alien sperm. *Developmental Dynamics*, **200**, 257–67.

Lee, E.S. and Fukui, Y. (1996). Synergistic effect of alanine and glycine on bovine embryos cultured in a chemically defined medium and amino acid uptake by in vitro-produced bovine morulae and blastocysts. *Biology of Reproduction*, **55**, 1383–9.

Leese, H.J. (1991). Metabolism of the preimplantation mammalian embryo. *Oxford Reviews in Reproductive Biology*, **13**, 35–72.

Li, M., Morley, P., Asem, E.K., and Tsang, B.K. (1991). Epidermal growth factor elevates intracellular pH in chicken granulosa cells. *Endocrinology*, **129**, 656–62.

Lighten, A.D., Moore, G.E., Winston, R.M., and Hardy, K. (1998). Routine addition of human insulin-like growth factor-I ligand could benefit clinical in vitro-fertilization culture. *Human Reproduction*, **13**, 3144–50.

Lonergan, P., Carolan, C., Van Langendonckt, A., Donnay, I., Khatir, H., and Mermillod, P. (1996). Role of epidermal growth factor in bovine oocyte maturation and preimplantation embryo development in vitro. *Biology of Reproduction*, **54**, 1420–9.

Ludwig, T.E., Lane, M., and Bavister, B.D. (2001). Differential effects of hexoses on hamster embryo development in culture. *Biology of Reproduction*, **64**, 1366–74.

Maas, D.H.A., Storey, B.T., and Mastroianni, L. (1977). Hydrogen ion and carbon dioxide content of the oviductal fluid of the rhesus monkey. *Fertility and Sterility*, **28**, 981–5.

Maas, D.H.A., Stein, B., and Metzger, H. (1984). pCO_2 and pH measurements within the rabbit oviduct following tubal microsurgery: reanastomosis of previously dissected tubes. *Advances in Experimental Medicine and Biology*, **169**, 561–70.

McKiernan, S.H. and Bavister, B.D. (1990). Environmental variables influencing in vitro development of hamster 2-cell embryos to the blastocyst stage. *Biology of Reproduction*, **43**, 404–13.

McKiernan, S.H. and Bavister, B.D. (1994). Timing of development is a critical parameter for predicting successful embryogenesis. *Human Reproduction*, **9**, 2123–9.

McKiernan, S.H. and Bavister, B.D. (2000). Culture of one-cell hamster embryos with water soluble vitamins: pantothenate stimulates blastocyst production. *Human Reproduction*, **15**, 157–64.

Mihalik, J., Rehak, P., and Koppel, J. (2000). The influence of insulin on the in vitro development of mouse and bovine embryos. *Physiological Research*, **49**, 347–54.

Munne, S. and Cohen, J. (1998). Chromosome abnormalities in human embryos. *Human Reproduction Update*, **4**, 842–55.

Niemann, H. and Wrenzycki, C. (2000). Alterations of expression of developmentally important genes in preimplantation bovine embryos by in vitro culture conditions: implications for subsequent development. *Theriogenology*, **53**, 21–34.

Olsnes, S., Tonnessen, T.I., and Sandvig, K. (1986). pH-regulated anion antiport in nucleated mammalian cells. *Journal of Cell Biology*, **102**, 967–71.

O'Neill, C. (1997). Evidence for the requirement of autocrine growth factors for development of mouse preimplantation embryos in vitro. *Biology of Reproduction*, **56**, 229–37.

Orlowski, J. and Grinstein, S. (1997). Na^+/H^+ exchangers of mammalian cells. *Journal of Biological Chemistry*, **272**, 22373–6.

Paetkau, V. and Lardy, H.A. (1967). Phosphofructokinase. Correlation of physical and enzymatic properties. *Journal of Biological Chemistry*, **242**, 2035–42.

Phillips, K.P. and Baltz, J.M. (1999). Intracellular pH regulation by HCO_3^-/Cl^- exchange is activated during early mouse zygote development. *Developmental Biology*, **208**, 392–405.

Phillips, K.P., Leveille, M.C., Claman, P., and Baltz, J.M. (2000). Intracellular pH regulation in human preimplantation embryos. *Human Reproduction*, **15**, 896–904.

Pinyopummintr, T. and Bavister, B.D. (1991). In vitro-matured/in vitro-fertilized bovine oocytes can develop into morulae/blastocysts in chemically-defined, protein-free culture media. *Biology of Reproduction*, **45**, 736–42.

Pinyopummintr, T. and Bavister, B.D. (1994). Development of bovine embryos in a cell-free culture medium: effects of type of serum, timing of its inclusion and heat inactivation. *Theriogenology*, **41**, 1241–9.

Pinyopummintr, T. and Bavister, B.D. (1996a). Energy substrate requirements for in vitro development of early cleavage stage bovine embryos. *Molecular Reproduction and Development*, **44**, 193–9.

Pinyopummintr, T. and Bavister, B.D. (1996b). Effects of amino acids on in vitro development of cleavage stage bovine embryos into blastocysts. *Reproduction, Fertility and Development*, **8**, 835–41.

Poueymirou, W.T., Conover, J.C., and Schultz, R.M. (1989). Regulation of mouse preimplantation development: differential effects of CZB medium and Whitten's medium on rates and patterns of protein synthesis in 2-cell embryos. *Biology of Reproduction*, **41**, 317–22.

Pouyssegur, J., Franchi, A., L'Allemain, G., and Paris, S. (1985). Cytoplasmic pH, a key determinant of growth factor-induced DNA synthesis in quiescent fibroblasts. *FEBS Letters*, **190**, 115–19.

Racowsky, C., Jackson, K.V., Cekleniak, N.A., Fox, J.H., Hornstein, M.D., and Ginsburg, E.S. (2000). The number of eight-cell embryos is a key determinant for selecting day 3 or day 5 transfer. *Fertility and Sterility*, **73**, 558–64.

Rieger, D. (1998). Effects of the in vitro chemical environment during early embryogenesis on subsequent development. *Archives of Toxicology*, **Suppl. 20**, 121–9.

Rinehart, J., Chapman, C., McKiernan, S., and Bavister, B. (1998). A protein-free chemically defined embryo culture medium produces pregnancy rates similar to human tubal fluid (HTF) supplemented with 10% synthetic serum substitute (SSS). *Human Reproduction*, **13**(Abstract Book 1), O-116.

Roos, A. and Boron, W.F. (1981). Intracellular pH. *Physiological Reviews*, **61**, 296–434.

Sargent, I.L., Martin, K.L., and Barlow, D.H. (1998). The use of recombinant growth factors to promote human embryo development in serum-free medium. *Human Reproduction*, **13**(Suppl. 4), 239–48.

Satoh, T., Kobayashi, K., Yamashita, S., Kikuchi, M., Sendai, Y., and Hoshi, H. (1994). Tissue inhibitor of metalloproteinases (TIMP-1) produced by granulosa and oviduct cells enhances in vitro development of bovine embryo. *Biology of Reproduction*, **50**, 835–44.

Schackmann, R.W. and Chock, P.B. (1986). Alteration of intracellular [Ca^{2+}] in sea urchin sperm by the egg peptide speract. Evidence that increased intracellular Ca^{2+} is coupled to Na$^+$ entry and increased intracellular pH. *Journal of Biological Chemistry*, **261**, 8719–28.

Schramm, R.D. and Bavister, B.D. (1996). Development of in vitro fertilized primate embryos into blastocysts in chemically defined, protein-free culture medium. *Human Reproduction*, **11**, 1690–7.

Schramm, R.D. and Bavister, B.D. (1999). Onset of nucleolar and extranucleolar transcription and expression of fibrillarin in macaque embryos developing in vitro. *Biology Reproduction*, **60**, 721–8.

Seshagiri, P.B. and Bavister, B.D. (1991). Glucose and phosphate inhibit respiration and oxidative metabolism in cultured hamster eight-cell embryos: evidence for the 'Crabtree effect'. *Molecular Reproduction and Development*, **30**, 105–11.

Seshagiri, P.B. and Hearn, J.P. (1992). Protein-free culture media that support in vitro development of Rhesus monkey blastocysts. *Assisted Reproductive Technology and Andrology*, **3**, 225–32.

Spindler, R.E. and Wildt, D.E. (2000). Influence of companion embryo age and quality on in vitro development of felid embryos. *Biology of Reproduction*, **62**(Suppl. 1), 318–19.

Steeves, C.L., Lane, M., Bavister, B.D., Phillips, K.P., and Baltz, J.M. (2001). Differences in intracellular pH regulation by Na$^+$/H$^+$ antiporter among 2-cell mouse embryos derived from females of different strains. *Biology of Reproduction*, **65**, 14–22.

Stojanov, T., Alechna, S., and O'Neill, C. (1999). In-vitro fertilization and culture of mouse embryos in vitro significantly retards the onset of insulin-like growth factor-II expression from the zygotic genome. *Molecular Human Reproduction*, **5**, 116–24.

Thompson, J.G., Simpson, A.C., Pugh, P.A., and Tervit, H.R. (1992). In vitro development of early sheep embryos is superior in medium supplemented with human serum compared with sheep serum or human serum albumin. *Animal Reproductive Science*, **29**, 61–8.

Thompson, J.G., Gardner, D.K., Pugh, P.A., McMillan, W.H., and Tervit, H.R. (1995). Lamb birth weight is affected by culture system utilized during in vitro pre-elongation development of ovine embryos. *Biology of Reproduction*, **53**, 1385–91.

Tonnessen, T.I., Sandvig, K., and Olsnes, S. (1990). Role of Na$^+$–H$^+$ and Cl$^-$–HCO$_3^-$ antiports in the regulation of cytosolic pH near neutrality. *American Journal of Physiology: Cell Physiology*, **258**, C1117–26.

van Soom, A., Ysebaert, M.T., and de Kruif, A. (1997). Relationship between timing of development, morula morphology, and cell allocation to inner cell mass and trophectoderm in in vitro-produced bovine embryos. *Molecular Reproduction and Development*, **47**, 47–56.

Vaughan-Jones, R.D. (1988). Regulation of intracellular pH in cardiac muscle. In: *Proton Passage Across Cell Membranes*, Bock, G. and Marsh, J., eds. Wiley, Chichester, UK, pp. 23–46.

Veeck, L.L. (1991). Preembryo grading. In: *Atlas of the Human Oocyte and Early Conceptus*, Veeck, L.L., ed. Williams & Wilkins, Baltimore, MD, pp. 121–49.

Wakabayshi, S., Fafournoux, P., Sardet, C., and Pouyssegur, J. (1992). The Na^+/H^+ antiporter cytoplasmic domain mediates growth factor signals and controls H^+-sensing. *Proceedings of the National Academy of Sciences USA*, **89**, 2424–8.

Wang, C.Z., Yano, H., Nagashima, K., and Seino, S. (2000). The Na^+-driven HCO_3^-/Cl^- exchanger: cloning, tissue distribution, and functional characterization. *Journal of Biological Chemistry*, **275**, 35486–90.

Warner, C.M., Cao, W., Exley, G.E., et al. (1998). Genetic regulation of egg and embryo survival. *Human Reproduction*, **13**(Suppl. 3), 178–90.

Warnes, G.M., Payne, D., Jeffrey, R., et al. (1997). Reduced pregnancy rates following the transfer of human embryos frozen or thawed in culture media supplemented with normal serum albumin. *Human Reproduction*, **12**, 1525–30.

Winston, N.J. (1996). Developmental failure in preimplantation human conceptuses. *International Reviews of Cytology*, **164**, 139–88.

Winston, N.J., Braude, P.R., Pickering, S.J., et al. (1991). The incidence of abnormal morphology and nucleocytoplasmic ratios in 2-, 3-, and 5-day human pre-embryos. *Human Reproduction*, **6**, 17–24.

Wolf, D.P., Gerrity, M., and Kopf, G.S. (1988). Morphology of human eggs and embryos. In: *In Vitro Fertilization and Embryo Transfer*, Wolf, D.P., Bavister, B.D., Gerrity, M., and Kopf, G.S., eds. Plenum Press, New York, pp. 147–88.

Wrenzycki, C., Herrmann, D., Carnwath, J.W., and Niemann, H. (1999). Alterations in the relative abundance of gene transcripts in preimplantation bovine embryos cultured in medium supplemented with either serum or PVA. *Molecular Reproduction and Development*, **53**, 8–18.

Wrenzycki, C., Herrmann, D., Keskintepe, L., et al. (2001). Effects of culture system and protein supplementation on mRNA expression in pre-implantation bovine embryos. *Human Reproduction*, **16**, 893–901.

Wu, G.J., Simerly, C., Zoran, S.S., Funte, L.R., and Schatten, G. (1996). Microtubule and chromatin dynamics during fertilization and early development in rhesus monkeys, and regulation by intracellular calcium ions. *Biology of Reproduction*, **55**, 260–70.

Zhang, Y., Chernova, M.N., Stuart-Tilley, A.K., Jiang, L., and Alper, S.L. (1996). The cytoplasmic and transmembrane domains of AE2 both contribute to regulation of anion exchange by pH. *Journal of Biological Chemistry*, **271**, 5741–9.

Zhao, Y. and Baltz, J.M. (1996). Characterization of bicarbonate/chloride exchange during preimplantation mouse embryo development. *American Journal of Physiology: Cell Physiology*, **271**, C1512–20.

Zhao, Y., Chauvet, P.J.-P., Alper, S.L., and Baltz, J.M. (1995). Expression and function of bicarbonate/chloride exchangers in the preimplantation mouse embryo. *Journal of Biological Chemistry*, **270**, 24428–34.

9

Cryopreservation of immature and mature gametes

John K. Critser[1], Yuksel Agca[2], and Erik J. Woods[2]

[1]College of Veterinary Medicine, University of Missouri, Columbia, USA
[2]Cryobiology Research Institute, Indiana University School of Medicine, Indianapolis, USA

Introduction

The development of preimplantation mammalian embryos is a well-orchestrated series of events that naturally occurs following female and male gamete interaction in the female reproductive tract. A better understanding of spermatogenesis, oogenesis, and fertilization/embryo development could enable endless opportunities to manipulate and/or interfere with these events, allowing: (i) the development of better animal production programs, (ii) conservation of endangered species, and (iii) advances in biomedical research and human reproductive medicine. During the last half of the twentieth century, there have been considerable advancements in mammalian reproductive technologies, including in vitro production of preimplantation embryos, spermatozoa and embryo sexing, and even cloning in some species. However, in most cases, management of noncryopreserved reproductive cells (i.e., oocytes, spermatozoa) and tissues (i.e., ovarian tissue, testicular tissue) is very problematic because of difficulties in donor–recipient synchronization and the potential for transmission of infectious pathogens, which cumulatively limit widespread application of these techniques. Therefore, there is an urgent need for the development of optimum gamete cryopreservation methods.

Today frozen–thawed spermatozoa and embryos have become an integral component of animal agriculture, laboratory animal genome banking, human sperm banking and infertility programs. However, although widely implemented, the protocols currently used to cryopreserve bull sperm, for example, are still suboptimal and cannot be extrapolated to other species, including human, mouse, pig, and ram (Watson, 2000). Similarly, embryo-freezing protocols successfully used for mice and cattle have yielded little success when applied to embryos from some other species or to a related cell type, oocytes. To-date, with the exception of mouse oocytes, oocytes from almost all mammalian species studied have proven very difficult to cryopreserve successfully (Bernard and Fuller, 1996; Shaw et al., 2000). Recently, there is a growing interest to understand the underlying biological fundamentals responsible for these low survival rates in an effort to develop better cryopreservation methods for oocytes (Critser et al., 1997; Parks, 1997).

Additionally, there is growing interest in developing technologies for the optimal isolation and cryopreservation of the earliest stage of male (i.e. spermatogonia, spermatids) and female (i.e. primordial follicles) germlines, with subsequent maturation to the desired stage in vitro. Recently, there have been increasing efforts directed toward improvements in follicular recruitment and in vitro maturation in some mammalian species (Leibfried-Rutledge et al., 1997). Female gamete maturation, fertilization, and embryo development entirely under in vitro conditions from primordial follicles has been achieved in mice (Eppig and O'Brien, 1996); however, techniques for most other species are still early in their development. Furthermore, with the recent advances made in intracytoplasmic sperm injection (ICSI), and gamete isolation

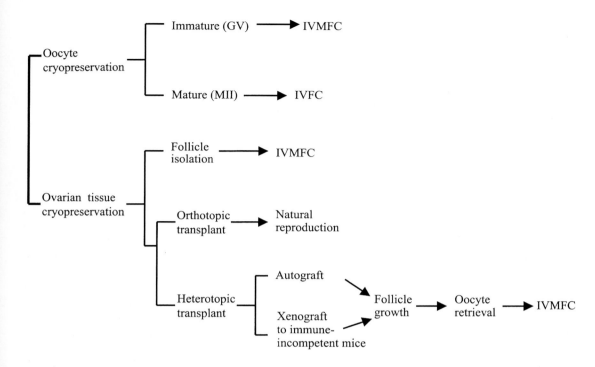

Fig. 9.1. Possible options for restoring fertility using cryopreserved immature and mature female germlines. AI, artificial insemination; IVMFC, in vitro maturation, fertilization, and culture; IVFC, in vitro fertilization and culture; GV, germinal vesicle; MII, metaphase II.

and maturation (Palermo et al., 1992; Roy and Greenwald, 1996), close attention has been given to cryopreservation of gametes in the form of gonadal tissue (i.e., ovarian tissue and testicular tissue) containing various developmental stages of male (spermatogonia, spermatids, spermatozoa) and female (primordial, secondary, tertiary follicles) germlines (Oktay et al., 1998, Hovatta, 2000a,b) (Figs. 9.1 and 9.2). Testing the developmental competence of cryopreserved reproductive cells and tissues requires availability of optimal in vitro assay methods. However, limited success has been achieved using in vitro culture of spermatogonia. Live fetuses have been obtained following transplantation of both fresh and frozen–thawed spermatogonia; however, full-term development from in vitro matured sper-

matogonia has not been demonstrated (Ogawa et al., 2000).

This chapter is intended to provide a brief overview of our current understanding of mammalian gamete cryobiology and how cryopreserved immature and mature male and female gametes can be used in assisted reproductive technology (ART).

Fundamental cryobiology

The relationship between the frozen state and living systems has fascinated mankind for years. As early as 1683, Robert Boyle observed that some fish and frogs could survive subzero (degrees centigrade) temperatures for short periods of time if a fraction of their body water remained unfrozen (Boyle, 1683). Successful application of cryopreservation was first demonstrated in 1948 by Polge, Smith, and Parkes (Polge et al., 1949) by serendipitous discovery of the cryoprotective properties of glycerol for bull sperm and, subsequently, for red cells (Smith, 1950). More

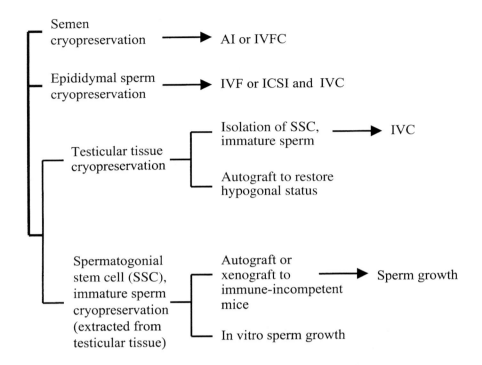

Fig. 9.2. Possible options for restoring fertility using cryopreserved immature and mature male germ lines. AI, artificial insemination; IVF, in vitro fertilization; IVFC, in vitro fertilization and culture; IVC, in vitro culture; ICSI, intracytoplasmic sperm injection.

recently, scientists interested in the natural phenomena and biomedical applications associated with freezing biological systems have begun to investigate the fundamental processes governing the relationship. It is well known that decreased temperature results in the suppression of metabolic activity and, thus, in a reduction of the rate at which deterioration of an unnourished biological system would occur. The freezing process, however, is not benign; it generally induces extreme variations in chemical, thermal, and electrical properties that could be expected to alter intracellular organelles, cellular membranes, and the delicate cell–cell interaction systems inherent in tissues and organs. Indeed, given the extreme complexity of even the simplest biological cells, it is remarkable that a

reversible state of suspended animation by freezing is possible at all.

The relative damage to biological cells in suspension caused by freezing was first described by Peter Mazur in the 1960s, in an elegant model that defined the relationship between cell membrane permeability, cell volume, cooling rate, and the phase transition from liquid to solid aqueous solutions (Mazur, 1963, 1970). As the suspension temperature falls below its melting point, there will usually be some supercooling before the first ice nucleus develops (around −5°C). Between −5 and −15°C, ice forms in the external medium, but the cell cytoplasm remains unfrozen and supercooled, presumably because the plasma membrane blocks the growth of ice crystals into the cytoplasm. The supercooled water inside the cells has a higher chemical potential than that of water outside and, therefore, it flows out of the cells osmotically and freezes externally. The subsequent physical events in the cell depend on cooling velocity. If cooling is sufficiently slow, the cell is able to lose water rapidly enough by exosmosis to concentrate intracellular solutes sufficiently to eliminate supercooling and maintain the chemical potential of intracellular water in equilibrium with that of extracellular water. The result is that the cell dehydrates and does not freeze intracellularly. But, if the cell is cooled too rapidly, it is not able to lose water fast enough to maintain equilibrium. As a result, the cell will become increasingly supercooled and eventually will attain equilibrium by freezing intracellularly (Mazur, 1970).

In cells that survive freezing, the usual finding is that plots of percent survival versus cooling rate form inverted U-shapes (Mazur, 1970). There is a critical cooling rate for which survival is at a maximum, but the numerical value of that critical rate can vary a thousandfold depending upon the cell type. The drop in survival at supraoptimal rates results from intracellular freezing, and with few exceptions, high survival demands that the cooling rate be sufficiently low to avoid such internal freezing. Although rates low enough to prevent internal freezing injury are necessary for high survival, freezing at very slow rates can also cause injury and lower survival through the high solute concentrations that form during freezing.

A cell that has survived cooling to low subzero temperatures still faces the challenge of warming and thawing. The rate of warming can exert effects on survival comparable to those associated with the rate of cooling. The effects depend on whether the prior rate of cooling had been high enough to induce intracellular freezing or low enough to produce cell dehydration. In the former case, if the cells are not killed outright by lysis owing to large ice crystal formation, they will end up with an accumulation of smaller ice crystals from the residual intracellular water. These thermodynamically unstable smaller crystals may undergo a process called recrystalization, in which they fuse to form larger crystals during warming if the warming rate is low enough. This process can be just as damaging as cooling-induced intracellular ice formation and can also lead to cell death. If cells are cooled slowly enough to preclude intracellular freezing, the response to warming rate is highly variable among cell types. In some cells,

warming rate makes little or no difference, but in others, rapid or slow warming appears mandatory (Mazur, 1984).

As a general rule, artificially induced freeze tolerance is correlated inversely with the complexity of the biological system. Single cells can be considered two compartment systems, with water moving from the inside of the cell to the medium outside upon the precipitation of extracellular water as ice. The structure of tissues and organs is much more complex. In multicellular tissues, water might have to traverse several layers of cells before it reaches the outside medium. However, the "outside" of the structure is not necessarily the "outside" relevant to the principles previously outlined. This is fortunate because, as one can imagine, it could take a very long time for water to diffuse through dozens if not hundreds of layers of cells before reaching the "outside." It is appropriate in this context to define the outside of a tissue in the process of freezing as the lumen of the nearest capillary. This definition would imply that there are at least four compartments in series: (i) cells separated from capillaries by other cells, (ii) cells adjacent to the capillary lumens, (iii) the solution in the capillary lumens, and (iv) the true equilibrated external solution (Mazur, 1984). This compartmentalization (as well as the sheer size of most organs and tissues) can result in damaging chemical and thermodynamic gradients.

Since the introduction of glycerol as a cryoprotective agent (CPA) by Polge et al. (1949) and the discovery of the widely applicable permeating CPA dimethyl sulfoxide (DMSO) by Lovelock and Bishop (1959), many investigators have attempted the preservation of cells or tissues, mostly through empirical methods. Most cell suspension cryopreservation protocols have been built around the use of molar concentrations of permeating CPAs to enable freezing survival. By using these artificial CPAs, much flexibility has been added to the cryopreservation process. For example, human red cells need to be cooled at a rate of around 1000°C/min for optimal survival without CPA addition. In the presence of 3.3 mol/l (30%) glycerol, however, survival of this cell type remains around 90% over a several hundredfold range in cooling rates. As can be expected, the higher the CPA concentration, the greater the likelihood of osmotic damage during the addition/removal of the substance; consequently, more care is necessary in these processes. With these considerations in mind, it is interesting to note that the same general procedure can be used to yield 70–90% survival of human red cells, mouse embryos, and fetal rat pancreases: suspension of cells in 2M glycerol or DMSO, seeding with an ice crystal to avoid supercooling, cooling at about 0.5°C/min, thawing at 1–4°C/min, and slowly removing the CPA from the thawed cells (Brown et al., 1976; Leibo et al., 1978).

These solutes, however, can have dramatic osmotic effects upon cells. Cells exposed to such high concentrations of permeating solutes undergo extensive initial dehydration followed by rehydration and potential gross swelling when the solutes are removed. This shrinkage and or swelling is capable of causing damage or even cell death. (Mazur and Schneider, 1986). Since most cell membranes are permeable to water and such additives, a coupled flow of both occurs. The dynamics of the coupled flow dictates cell volume and intracellular concentrations during cryopreservation processing (McGrath, 1997). In general, we may expect coupled flow when CPAs are added, during freezing, during thawing, and when CPAs are removed from cells. The resultant dynamics of cell volume change are important in relation to possible membrane damage by mechanical means such as plasma membrane stretching (Mazur and Schneider, 1986). Thus, impermeable solutes such as sucrose are often added to dilution media to prevent excessive osmotic swelling during the post-thaw CPA wash-out procedures. The dynamics of the coupled flow also determine the intracellular concentration of CPA prior to cooling and/or freezing (Diller and Lynch, 1984). Investigators often seek particular states (fully equilibrated, maximally shrunken, etc.) prior to cooling or freezing. Solidification of water, which naturally occurs in aqueous physiological solutions during slow or rapid freezing, provides the driving force for the flow of water and permeable solutes during this process (Mazur, 1963). The amount and state of intracellular water is related to

the likelihood of intracellular ice formation, which, in turn, is linked to lethal cell damage in many cases (Mazur, 1963).

Overview of female reproductive biology

Oogenesis

The mammalian ovary contains thousands of resting primordial follicles arrested at prophase of meiosis I at the time of birth. However, by puberty these numbers drop to approximately 3000 in the mouse and approximately 500 000 in the human. In contrast to spermatogonia in the testes, oocytes in the ovaries do not have the ability to replicate and are progressively depleted throughout the reproductive history of the female. The life cycle of the female gamete is schematically shown in Figure 9.3. Primordial follicles are recruited and begin to grow in size while becoming surrounded by multiple layers of granulosa cells as they develop (Fig. 9.4). Fully grown immature oocytes are characterized by the large prophase nucleus, called the germinal vesicle (GV). Under the influence of the gonadotropins follicle-stimulating hormone (FSH) and luteinizing hormone (LH), in the last phase of oocyte growth, fully grown GV oocytes experience nuclear membrane breakdown and a series of subsequent nuclear and cytoplasmic maturational changes. They then arrest at metaphase of the second meiotic division (MII) until sperm activation (Eppig, 1996). Mature oocytes are recognized by the presence of the first polar body and freely existing meiotic spindle fibers in the cytoplasm. Folliculogenesis involves significant structural and biochemical changes at the level of the nucleus, oolemma, granulose–oocyte complexes, and cytoskeletal elements, eventually forming one of the largest cells (80–120 μm diameter) of the mammalian body (Wassarman, 1988). The duration of this process from primordial follicle to fully mature oocytes varies among species (Eppig, 1996).

Since oocyte growth is a dynamic process during which tremendous changes take place, each developmental stage has different cryobiological properties.

DEVELOPMENTAL EVENTS

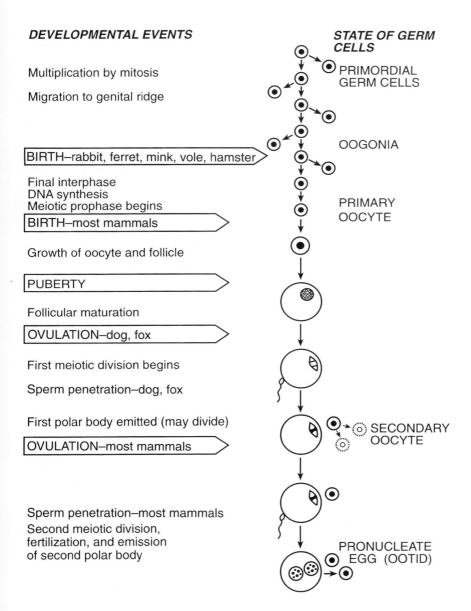

STATE OF GERM CELLS

Multiplication by mitosis

Migration to genital ridge

PRIMORDIAL GERM CELLS

OOGONIA

BIRTH–rabbit, ferret, mink, vole, hamster

Final interphase
DNA synthesis
Meiotic prophase begins

BIRTH–most mammals

PRIMARY OOCYTE

Growth of oocyte and follicle

PUBERTY

Follicular maturation

OVULATION–dog, fox

First meiotic division begins

Sperm penetration–dog, fox

First polar body emitted (may divide)

OVULATION–most mammals

SECONDARY OOCYTE

Sperm penetration–most mammals
Second meiotic division,
fertilization, and emission
of second polar body

PRONUCLEATE EGG (OOTID)

Fig. 9.3. Generalized diagram of oogenesis in mammals. The life cycle of female gametes from embryonic stages through reproductive maturity is represented. (Reproduced with permission from Baker, 1972.)

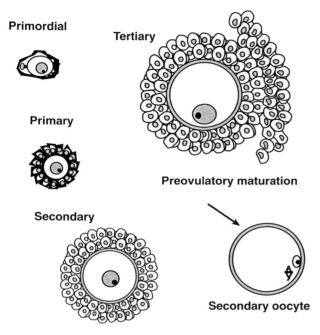

Fig. 9.4. Generalized diagram of folliculogenesis in mammals. Growth and differentiation of the follicle unit starting from a non-growing pool of primordial follicles, entering growth phase and ending with the oocyte–cumulus complex undergoing meiosis I in the tertiary follicle prior to ovulation. (Reproduced with permission from Leibfried-Rutledge et al., 1997.)

Therefore, cytoskeletal elements, cell cycle progression, organelle movement, spindle morphogenesis, and somatic cell interaction with the oolemma are important determining factors for the development of stage-specific cryopreservation protocols (Albertini, 1995). For example, GV oocytes have a nuclear content that is protected by an envelope and they do not possess meiotic spindle fibers. Following maturation, the GV breaks down and meiotic spindles form in the cytoplasm, which makes them more vulnerable to the detrimental effects of cryopreservation processing (Eroglu et al., 1998).

The ability to cryopreserve earlier stages of oocytes (i.e, primordial follicle, GV stage) has many advantages, since they are more abundant. In some

species, it is now possible to mature GV oocytes in vitro, fertilize them in vitro and then develop them into a live fetus following embryos transfer (Candy et al., 1994). Further attempts have been made to isolate intact primordial follicles from various mammalian species. To-date, very limited success has been achieved in the development of entirely in vitro systems. A promising report by Eppig and O'Brien (1996), however, did demonstrate two-step growth including primordial follicle development into primary follicles and subsequent culture to MII stage.

To-date, typical cryopreservation efforts for female gametes have been directed towards primordial follicles, GV, and MII oocytes. Currently, there are major efforts to develop cryopreservation methods for oocytes isolated from tertiary follicles at the GV or MII stage for many mammalian species. These efforts have generally met with very limited success (Shaw et al., 2000). There are advantages and disadvantages to cryopreserving oocytes at the GV or the MII stage (Critser et al., 1997). The isolation of GV oocytes avoids the need for exogenous gonadotropin stimulation and could generate a readily available source of oocytes. The major limiting factor making this technology usable, however, remains the inefficiency of in vitro maturation systems. To-date, significant progress has been made with the in vitro culture of follicles and in vitro maturation of GV oocytes isolated from tertiary follicles in mice, cows, sheep, and pigs. However, with the exception of mice, full development resulting in livebirths from primordial follicles has not been reported. Livebirths have been achieved in orthotopic transplantation of cryopreserved ovarian tissue from mice, rats, and, most importantly, sheep (Gosden et al., 1994; Gunasena et al., 1997; Aubard et al., 1998;). Cryopreservation of ovarian tissue slices containing predominantly primordial follicles and transplantation into immunodeficient mice has been proposed as an alternative approach to obtain MII oocytes; however, livebirths have been limited to mice using this technique (Carroll and Gosden, 1993).

Cryopreservation of immature and mature female gametes

The establishment of long-term preservation methods for mammalian oocytes at the desired developmental stage has significant importance in improving ART for human and various animal species. However, the determination of reliable methods for oocyte cryopreservation has been challenging. The first livebirth obtained from cryopreserved MII mouse oocytes, using a slow cooling protocol in the presence of DMSO, was reported nearly a quarter of a century ago (Whittingham, 1977). Subsequent studies in other mammalian species utilizing 1.5 mol/l CPA (DMSO or 1,2-propanediol (PROH)) and cooling rates of 0.3–0.5°C/min (seeding the samples at -7°C) to -40 or -80°C have been disappointing (Parks and Ruffing, 1992; Bernard and Fuller, 1996; Critser et al., 1997). These attempts have shown that it is possible to obtain livebirths from cryopreserved human (Al-Hasani et al., 1986; Chen, 1986; Porcu et al., 1997), and bovine (Fuku et al., 1992; Lim et al., 1992) oocytes, but with extremely low rates of success.

The application of exogenous gonadotropins in ART produces supernumerary oocytes, and often embryos. Oocyte cryopreservation could contribute to human ART by: (i) providing an alternative to embryo cryopreservation, (ii) allowing donated eggs to be screened for potential infectious diseases (e.g., hepatitis virus B and C and human immunodeficiency virus), and (iii) allowing restoration of fertility of female patients after successful cancer therapy. Currently used human oocyte cryopreservation protocols are those used for mouse embryos or slight modifications of these methods. The mouse protocols were primarily developed by trial and error adjustments of cooling and warming rates, and choice of CPA and CPA concentration. However, in general, success rates with mammalian oocyte cryopreservation have been extremely low and do not satisfy the current need. Research efforts have made cryosurvival of mouse oocytes superior over other mammalian oocytes. Although successful cryopreservation of oocytes has been a goal of many

scientists since the early 1980s, the actual importance of this technology has been highlighted by advancements in ART, such as ovum pick-up, in vitro oocyte maturation, fertilization and embryo culture, and ICSI (Leibfried-Rutledge et al., 1997). These improvements have resulted, in part, in an increased efficiency of producing pregnancies from fewer and fewer transferred embryos. Therefore, more embryos are now cryopreserved than ever before. Efficient cryopreservation protocols for oocytes would allow ART laboratories to create fewer embryos and avoid the problems associated with long-term embryo storage.

Recently, it has been realized that it is crucial to achieve a fundamental understanding of the nature of damage to oocytes during the multiple steps involved in the cryopreservation procedure, such as CPA addition/removal, cooling, and warming. The ability for successful cryopreservation of mammalian oocytes is highly dependent upon an understanding of the fundamental cryobiological factors that determine viability or death post-thaw. A better understanding of the mechanisms responsible for poor post-thaw survival could also lead to answers for the prevention of such damage. The major sites of damage during oocyte cryopreservation are at the organelle/subcellular level and, therefore, are generally more complex than the issues related to successful embryo freezing (Albertini, 1995). The adverse effects of cryopreservation on subcellular structures has been well documented in terms of loss of one or more requisite structural and/or functional component, such as microtubules, microfilaments, cytoplasmic organelles, zona pellucida glycoproteins, and plasma membrane integrity (Glenister et al., 1987; Kola et al., 1988; Van Blerkom, 1989; Pickering et al., 1990; Van Blerkom and Davis, 1994). Results from these studies indicate that oocytes are an extremely sensitive cell type compared with developing embryos, and there may be no simple, universal protocol that can be used for cryopreserving oocytes across species and among developmental stages. Investigations of human oocyte cryopreservation have been very limited because of the limited availability of fresh oocytes and the legal/ethical restrictions in experimentally testing developmental competence. In addition, many studies of human oocyte cryopreservation have also been more empirical, using embryo cryopreservation strategies (Bernard and Fuller, 1996). Integration of the information gained regarding the effects on subcellular structures has indicated several distinct sites of cryoinjury, including microfilament and microtubule depolymerization, zona hardening owing to premature cortical granule release, and sodium ion toxicity (Stachecki et al., 1998a,b). It has been determined that, in general, the type of injury caused during cryopreservation is consistent among species. However, the severity of the injury has been found to vary among species and between stages (GV or MII). These fundamental characteristics are often species and cell type specific and, therefore, need to be investigated on this basis (Hunter et al., 1992; Ruffing et al., 1993; Le Gal et al., 1994; Ben-Yosef et al., 1995; Agca et al., 1998).

Fundamental cryobiological studies that have been initiated to address these problems include studies focused on oolemma permeability and temperature-dependent osmotic characteristics, and studies that determined the effects of cryopreservation procedures on the integrity of the oolemma and ultrastructural units, including microtubules, microfilaments, and cortical granule vesicles of oocytes. Future studies will likely focus on the integration of these interrelated fields to develop enhanced cryopreservation protocols for oocytes.

Plasma membrane permeability characteristics

Estimation of several membrane transport parameters such as the hydraulic conductivity (L_p), CPA permeability, and the reflection coefficient are important in predicting the likelihood of cell injury during cryopreservation (Mazur et al., 1984; Gilmore et al., 2000). By measuring the temperature dependence of L_p and CPA permeability, one can obtain estimates of the activation energy for these parameters and can use this information to calculate optimal cooling rates to minimize cell injury and

subsequently enhance cell survival (Karlsson et al., 1996). It has been demonstrated that oocytes from various species and developmental stages (i.e., GV and MII) responded differently when they were exposed to CPAs at different temperatures. Agca et al. (1999) estimated that the activation energy for L_p for bovine GV oocytes (23.84 kcal/mol (5.7 kJ/mol)) was threefold higher than that for MII oocytes (8.46 kcal/mol (2.0 kJ/mol)). Similarly, Le Gal et al. (1995) estimated an activation energy of L_p for MII oocytes from goat (16.10 kcal/mol (3.8 kJ/mol)) as twofold higher than those for human and bovine MII oocytes. Interestingly, another study estimated 8.61 kcal/mol (2.0 kJ/mol) as the activation energy for L_p for MII human oocytes (Hunter et al., 1992), which is very similar to the bovine value. Considering the scarcity of human oocytes for research, the bovine oocyte would seem to be a good model for the development of human MII oocyte cryopreservation strategies.

It has also been demonstrated that the osmotically inactive cell volume fraction of oocytes increases after maturation (Le Gal et al., 1994). This difference was determined to be caused by involvement of the actin filaments located in the cortical region of the cytoplasm, which suggests a role for cytoskeletal organization in the permeation kinetics of oolemma. Ford et al. (2000) have demonstrated that expression of a water channel protein (aquaporin-9) in rat oocytes decreases from the GV to the MII stage. Aquaporins can drastically change the rate of water transport across the plasma membrane during CPA addition and removal, as well as during cooling and warming. This information is further evidence that oocyte cryopreservation protocols for different stages need to be optimized independently.

Cryoprotective agents

Although CPAs are required in essentially all current cryopreservation methods, they can also cause detrimental effects in oocytes (Vincent et al., 1990; Vincent and Johnson, 1992; George et al., 1996). The developmental stage of the oocyte affects the cell's membrane permeability properties and, consequently, the optimal procedures needed to add and remove CPAs effectively (Critser et al., 1997; Parks, 1997). Previous studies indicate that the extent of damage (reduced microfilament density, cortical granule exocytosis) increases if CPAs are added at a higher temperature (37 °C). However, addition and removal of CPAs at a lower temperature (4 °C) appears to reduce the detrimental effects as assessed by post-thaw fertilization (Schroeder et al., 1990; Karlsson et al., 1996). It is known that cumulus cells and tranzonal processes have a metabolic role and also play a crucial role in the maturation process of GV oocytes (Brower and Schultz, 1982; Albertini and Rider, 1994). Younis et al. (1996) demonstrated the harmful effects of high glycerol concentrations on F-actin organization around the cortex and in the transzonal processes of GV oocytes from the rhesus monkey. Bouquet et al. (1993) obtained aneuploid embryos from MII mouse oocytes exposed to 1.5 mol/l DMSO, suggesting that CPAs induced spindle damage.

Alterations of zona pellucida glycoproteins, especially ZP2, are reported to be responsible for zona hardening in mouse oocytes (Moller and Wassarman, 1989). As with oocytes from other species, low in vitro fertilization (IVF) rates for frozen–thawed human oocytes are partly caused by zona hardening. Exposing mouse and human oocytes to DMSO and PROH before freezing results in significant premature exocytosis of cortical granules (Schalkoff et al., 1989). ICSI has been employed after human oocyte freezing and thawing to overcome this problem and resulted in a livebirth (Porcu et al., 1997).

Chilling injury

Oocytes exposed to low temperatures also experience a substantial degree of disruption of their cytoskeletal elements (e.g., spindle fiber integrity) (Pickering et al., 1990; Aman and Parks, 1994), cortical granules (Vincent and Johnson, 1992), and plasma membrane (Arav et al., 1996). Disruption of the cytoskeletal elements is likely to lead to aneuploidy in murine embryos (Kola et al., 1988; Bouquet et al., 1995); disruptions of the cortical granules and plasma membrane are likely to lead to poor fertiliza-

tion and cell death, respectively (Vincent and Johnson, 1992; George and Johnson, 1993). It has been reported that chilling of GV and MII bovine as well as human oocytes to 0 °C causes depolymerization of the cytoskeletal elements, resulting in reduced developmental rates following fertilization (Pickering et al., 1990; Martino et al., 1996a). The nature of the cell plasma membrane with regard to its low-temperature behavior and its role in cell survival is being progressively understood (Muench et al., 1996). A study by Arav et al. (1996) indicated that irreversible oolemma lipid phase changes occur during cooling. According to this study, the membrane lipid phase transition of bovine GV oocytes occurred between 13 and 20°C, while a very broad phase transition, which centered around 10°C, was observed for MII oocytes. It is also well known that intracellular calcium plays an important role in mammalian fertilization (Miyazaki et al., 1993). Ben-Yosef et al. (1995) demonstrated that chilling is associated with calcium oscillations in MII oocytes, which may potentially hamper normal post-thaw fertilization. These studies indicate that cryopreservation of either GV or MII oocytes using current slow-cooling protocols will result in low survival for different reasons.

Rall and Fahy (1985) introduced an ultra-rapid, nonequilibrium cooling approach as an alternative to conventional slow freezing. Since the effects of chilling on the developmental potential of oocytes from many species are widely recognized, ultra-rapid cooling methods have been used to cryopreserve mouse (Nakagata, 1989; Wood et al., 1993; Rayos et al., 1994), human (Yoon et al., 2000), and bovine (Martino et al. 1996b; Vajta et al., 1998) oocytes with varying levels of success. Martino et al. (1996b) reported a protocol in which in vitro matured oocytes were exposed to 5.5 mol/l ethylene glycol plus 1M sucrose for <30 seconds before plunging the oocytes into liquid nitrogen in order to minimize duration of exposure to low temperatures. Similarly, Vajta et al. (1998) have proposed a new technique that involved achieving vitrification at the tip of the pulled plastic straw (open pulled straw), which has less surface area and a very small CPA volume, allowing vitrification during plunging into liquid nitrogen. However, the osmotic stress and chemical toxicity from the relatively high solute concentrations in vitrification solutions are of great concern and impart procedural challenges that must be carefully controlled (Fahy, 1986; Hotamisligil et al., 1996; Agca et al., 2000).

Osmotic and ionic stress

Cells generally demonstrate an ideal osmotic response (i.e. they follow a linear relationship between cell volume and the reciprocal of the surrounding medium osmolality; the Boyle–van't Hoff relationship). How oocytes tolerate changes in osmotic pressure and the associated volume changes plays an important role in the outcome of cell survival during cryopreservation. Therefore, in order to develop optimal cryopreservation methods, there is a need to determine the membrane permeability parameters discussed above, the osmotically inactive volume, and the osmotic tolerance limits in order to avoid excessive shrinkage and swelling during the addition and removal of CPAs. Additionally, the relatively large size of oocytes can lead to difficult technical challenges when considering the need for addition and removal of permeating CPAs while maintaining the cells within tolerated osmotic conditions. These changes in cell volume affect several parameters that play a role in the cryosurvival of oocytes, including integrity of the plasma membrane (McWilliams et al., 1995; Hotamisligil et al., 1996) and subcellular organelles. Furthermore, those parameters have to be determined for each species and for each developmental stage (McWilliams et al., 1995; Hotamisligil et al., 1996; Pedro et al., 1997; Agca et al., 2000).

Bovine and human oocytes behave as ideal osmometers over the ranges 265–800 mOsm and 230–1400 mOsm, respectively (Ruffing et al., 1993; Newton et al., 1999). Pedro et al. (1997) demonstrated that a 30 minute exposure of MII mouse oocytes to a 72.5 mOsm sucrose solution significantly lowered their morphological integrity. By comparison, GV bovine oocytes appeared to be more sensitive to osmotic stress than MII oocytes,

supporting the need for development of stage-specific cryopreservation protocols. Particularly, nonequilibrium cryopreservation protocols (e.g., vitrification) require the use of relatively high concentrations of CPAs (approximately 6 mol/l). Cortical granule kinetics is one of the most important elements affecting fertilizability of oocytes. Ultrastructural observation on vitrified bovine GV and MII oocytes revealed that GV oocytes are more vulnerable to CPA addition than the MII stage (Fuku et al., 1995).

Sodium chloride is the major component of holding and cryopreservation solutions, and during slow cooling it is often the primary electrolyte solute responsible for the high osmolalities associated with solute damage (Lovelock, 1954; Mazur, 1984; Stachecki et al., 1998a). Biggers et al. (1993) have shown that high sodium chloride concentrations are detrimental to embryo development. Stachecki et al. (1998b) simply replaced sodium chloride with choline chloride, resulting in improved mouse oocyte survival after slow cooling.

Cryopreservation of the male gamete

Spermatogenesis

The adult male gonads are highly organized organs, with two structurally distinct compartments that are separated by a cellular layer (the blood–testis barrier). Male gametes (spermatozoa) and hormones (androgens) are produced in these compartments under the control of the gonadotrophins FSH and LH. While the formation of mature spermatozoa (spermatogenesis) is taking place within the seminiferous tubules in close association with Sertoli cells, production of androgens occurs in the Leydig cells between the tubules. Spermatogenesis is a highly complex process that is completed through a series of mitotic and meiotic cell divisions and morphological differentiation (Griffin, 2000). Differentiation occurs over a period of weeks to months in order to generate mature spermatozoa; however, this time does vary

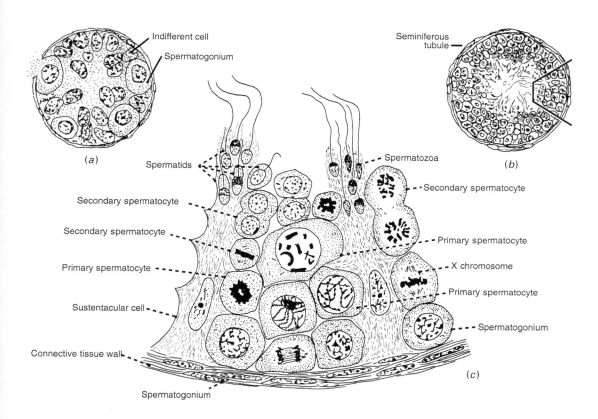

Indifferent cell
Spermatogonium

(a)

Seminiferous tubule

(b)

Spermatids
Secondary spermatocyte
Secondary spermatocyte
Primary spermatocyte
Sustentacular cell
Connective tissue wall
Spermatogonium

Spermatozoa
Secondary spermatocyte
Primary spermatocyte
X chromosome
Primary spermatocyte
Spermatogonium

(c)

Fig. 9.5. Generalized diagram of spermatogenesis as it occurs in the seminiferous tubules of the mammalian testes. Cross-sections of a seminiferous tubule prior to (a) and after (b) puberty are shown. A section of the tubule illustrating the stages of spermatogenesis is also depicted (c). (Reproduced with permission from Arey, 1974.)

among species (Clermont, 1972; Gao et al., 1997). The evolution of the male gamete is schematically represented in Fig. 9.5. The process can be divided into four major steps: (i) mitotic proliferation in which large numbers of cells are produced; (ii) meiotic division, in which diploid chromosome becomes haploid and the formation of the first and second spermatocytes and round spermatids occurs; (iii) spermiogenesis, where essential parts of the spermatozoa such as the tail, mid-piece, and acrosome region develop; and (iv) spermiation, or the release of spermatozoa into the lumen of the

seminiferous tubule for further maturation and storage in the epididymis. Although epididymal sperm are capable of moving forward, they cannot participate in normal fertilization until they undergo the capacitation process, which is essentially a series of physiological changes and substantial modifications in the plasma membrane lipid configuration (Wassarman, 1988). Unlike oogenesis, the process of spermatogenesis continues throughout the male lifespan. Spermatagonial stem cells are capable of self-replication and continuously produce progeny cells. Although the morphology of mammalian sperm significantly varies in regard to tail length and acrosomal head shape (Fig. 9.6), mature mammalian spermatozoa typically have a plasma membrane surrounding three distinct regions: (i) the head, containing the condensed haploid nucleus; (ii) the anterior region, consisting of the acrosome and the

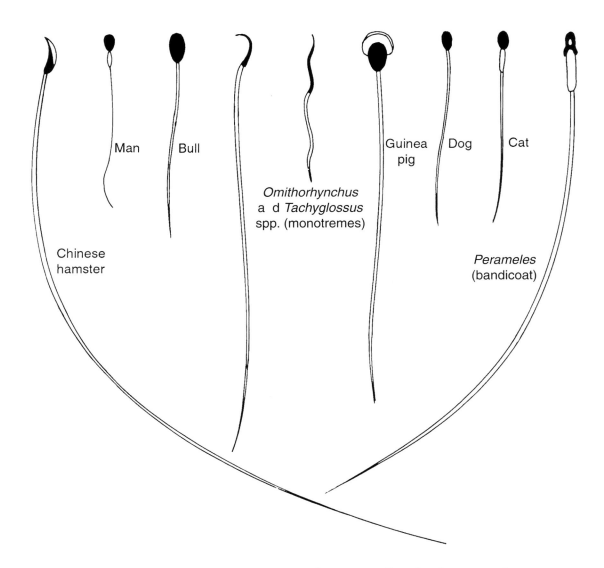

Fig. 9.6. Morphology of mammalian spermatozoa. Morphology varies dramatically from species to species. (Redrawn with permission from Austin, 1965.)

mid-piece containing the mitochondria; and (iii) the tail, which generates forward propulsion. Functional integrity of each of these sperm structures has to be well preserved in order for normal fertilization via artificial insemination (AI) or IVF.

Cryopreservation of mature spermatozoa

Cryopreservation of ejaculated sperm

Following the first known report of cryopreservation of mammalian spermatozoa (canine spermatozoa; Spallanzani, 1776), no significant advancements were made until the discovery of the cryoprotective properties of glycerol for bull sperm (Polge et al., 1949) and the advancement of semen extenders (e.g., egg yolk and skim milk; Watson, 1995). With the availability of these compounds, cryopreserved semen has since become extensively used in AI and IVF programs, with few significant changes to the original protocols (Parrish et al., 1986). Successful semen cryopreservation has allowed significant advancements in agriculture, by making available an international exchange of germplasm of genetically superior animals; in biotechnology, by allowing scientifically important murine lines to be efficiently stored; in conservation of endangered species through genome resource banking; and in human reproductive medicine.

Successful cryopreservation of human and bovine spermatozoa has evolved empirically, typically using 100–200°C/min cooling rates in the presence of glycerol buffered with egg yolk-citrate medium. The success rates have been, for the most part, satisfactory following either AI or IVF in these species. Consequently, the fundamental cryobiological properties that determine survival following cryopreservation processing have, for the most part, been ignored. However, if one looks critically at the percentage of post-thaw, fully functional spermatozoa, the success is still relatively low (Holt, 2000). Loss of viability may not be an issue where sperm counts are normal, but for oligozoospermic samples, these losses may be very significant. With the development of ICSI procedures, and the availability of techniques for surgical sperm retrieval, there is an increased need to be able to cryopreserve low numbers of sperm successfully and to improve freezing techniques in order to maximize survival. The wide use of cryopreserved spermatozoa for ART using surgically collected spermatozoa creates the need for further studies to improve post-thaw survival of this material.

The "standard" mammalian sperm cryopreservation protocol has limitations, and success rates vary among species (Hammerstedt et al., 1990; Watson, 2000). Indeed, in some species appropriate methods are yet to be determined; when the standard protocol has been tried in species such as pigs, mice, and sheep, for instance, it failed in most reported cases (Curry et al., 1994). These imperfections suggest that the empirically obtained cryopreservation protocols must be re-examined, with close attention given to the exact nature of sperm cryoinjury in order to determine species-specific cryopreservation protocols (Holt, 2000). Recently, along with sperm motility, more sensitive criteria have been proposed to assess sperm "viability" objectively, including energy status, plasma membrane integrity, membrane lipid phase transition temperature, integrity of subcellular elements, and acrosome/chromosome morphology (Drobnis et al., 1993; Willoughby et al., 1996).

Biochemical changes have been assessed following exposure to various combinations of extenders with different permeating CPAs to minimize osmotic pressure and achieve membrane stabilization (De Leeuw et al., 1993). Spermatozoa cryopreservation consists of a series of nonphysiological steps that involve hypertonic CPA addition, cooling, warming, and CPA removal. Several studies have focused on the biophysical conditions that determine optimal CPA addition and removal, and the cooling and warming rates (Gao et al., 1995; Morris et al., 1999). With this type of approach, it becomes theoretically possible to calculate the minimal number of CPA addition steps required prior to cooling to avoid osmotic stress, as well as optimal cooling rates to avoid intracellular ice formation. Various aspects of sperm cryopreservation, such as chemical composition of extenders and their effects on the sperm plasma membrane, osmotic tolerance limits, hydraulic conductivity, and CPA permeability have been studied (Gilmore et al., 1999). These studies suggest that the spermatozoa of each species have different cryobiological properties as well as varying degrees of sensitivity to manipulation (pipetting, centrifugation), osmotic tolerance, and cold-shock sensitivity (membrane lipid phase transition temperatures) (Katkov and Mazur, 1999; Phelps et al., 1999). There is evidence that cryopreservation processing affects all aspects of sperm structure. Cytological evaluation following cryopreservation has revealed extensive damage to the plasma membrane, acrosomal region, and sperm tail configuration (Henry et al., 1993; Willoughby et al., 1996;

Garner et al., 1997). In order to develop improved methods of sperm cryopreservation, it seems to be most appropriate to consider the physical changes sperm undergo during this process; advances made to manage these changes could no doubt significantly increase survival rates (Gao et al., 1995).

Improvements in cryopreservation of human spermatozoa have been attempted by incorporating different CPAs and semen extenders, in particular by altering the cooling rates (Ragni et al., 1990; Henry et al., 1993; Gilmore et al., 1997). With human spermatozoa, a very broad response curve exists with little difference in survival observed following cooling at 1°C/min up to 100°C/min (Henry et al., 1993). Cooling rates for optimum sperm recovery may be predicted using theoretical models based on measured osmotic behavior of the cells combined with physical/chemical knowledge of the freeze media (Gilmore et al., 2000).

Cryopreservation of epididymal sperm

In some cases, recovery of ejaculate is not possible, and collection of mature spermatozoa from the epididymis is required. This technique has been a common practice for the collection of sperm from captive wildlife species because of unexpected death, as well as collection and routine cryopreservation of sperm from specific mouse strains. Currently, mature, viable spermatozoa retrieved from the epididymis are routinely used (either as fresh or cryopreserved material) for IVF and ICSI procedures in human reproductive medicine (Devroey et al., 1995). The development of surgical techniques, such as percutaneus epididymal sperm aspiration and microsurgical epididymal sperm aspiration, in combination with ICSI, provide options for treatment for azoospermia (Craft et al., 1995; Tournaye et al., 1999). Such surgical approaches underscore the importance of developing optimal methods to cryopreserve epididymal sperm. More studies need to be done to improve the functional integrity of epididymal spermatozoa after cryopreservation in order to minimize the need for repeated surgical intervention.

ICSI has been widely used in ART for sperm of low motility and poor quality and has offered effective ways to achieve fertilization with such sperm. For example, in human males with obstructed or non-obstructed testes conditions, sperm counts are typically low with poor motility. These sperm samples generally do not survive well following cryopreservation, but by combining cryopreservation with ICSI procedures, it is now possible to circumvent this problem. Indeed, several studies clearly suggest that in human reproductive medicine the use of cryopreserved epididymal spermatozoa with the aid of ICSI results in fertilization and pregnancy success rates comparable to those obtained with non-cryopreserved spermatozoa, or spermatozoa aspirated from the epididymis (Oates et al., 1996; Holden et al., 1997; Hutchon et al., 1998). Sperm cryopreservation combined with ICSI is also a valuable tool since it reduces the number of procedures required for pregnancy success (Oates et al., 1996; Nudell et al., 1998). Despite some sporadic positive reports in species other than humans (including cattle and mice) success, for the most part, has not been forthcoming (Goto et al., 1990; Wakayama et al., 1998).

Perhaps one of the most important achievements in male germ cell preservation in recent years was the demonstration of full-term development from immotile freeze-dried mouse spermatozoa that were injected into mouse oocytes following storage at room temperature over a 3-month period in a dried state (Wakayama and Yanagimachi, 1998). Although the technique is not highly efficient, improvement would allow the storage of male genomes at ambient temperatures and furthermore allow transportation without cryostorage.

Cryopreservation of immature male germ cells

Cryopreservation of spermatogonia

The successful demonstration of spermatogonial stem cell transplantation and subsequent recolonization and differentiation in seminiferous tubules of busulphan-treated immunodeficient mice was a major milestone in reproductive science (Brinster and Avarbock, 1994; Brinster and Zimmermann,

1994). To-date, this technique has been used for transplantation of spermatogonial stem cells from various mammalian species, including mouse, rat, hamster, monkey, bull, dog, and rabbit (Clouthier et al., 1996; Ogawa et al., 1999; Schlatt et al., 1999). However, while mature spermatozoa have been recovered in mice, rats and hamsters, the stem cells did not differentiate beyond the stage of spermatogonial expansion in the other species. Despite the limited success achieved in these higher species, there is no doubt that this technique would serve as a novel approach to manipulate the male germline in some species since current methods of in vitro growth are still inefficient.

Spermatogonial stem cell lines have the ability to undergo replication and meiotic recombination during spermatogenesis. Therefore, the ability to establish cryopreserved spermatogonial stem cell lines that are capable of differentiation under in vitro conditions could significantly improve our understanding of spermatogenesis. Spermatogonial stem cells from laboratory animals, farm animals, wild animals, and from humans could be stored until appropriate recipients were available or until optimal in vitro culture conditions were developed. This could also facilitate genetic modification by transfection of spermatogonial stem cells with desired genes (Dobrinski et al., 1999; Nagano et al., 2000). With this technology, it would be possible to create laboratory animals to study specific gene regulation, as well as to create farm animals capable of producing important pharmaceutical compounds (Chan, 1999). Alternatively, recent studies have shown that rat and hamster testicular cells transplanted to the seminiferous tubules of immunodeficient mice will generate rat or hamster spermatogenesis and produce normal appearing rat or hamster spermatozoa, opening the possibility of xenogeneic testicular cell transplantation for other species. It is, therefore, theoretically possible to cryopreserve germ cell lines of endangered animals in the case of unexpected death and produce mature spermatozoa following transplantation into closely related species (Johnston et al., 2000). In the future, cryopreservation of germ cells from young cancer patients who are not able to produce mature spermatozoa would also benefit from this technology (Avarbock et al., 1996). Successful fetal development following injection of round spermatids in both mouse and human oocytes (Kimura and Yanagimachi, 1995; Gianaroli et al., 1999) provides hope for the future application of this technology.

Recently, it has been reported that mature mouse and hamster spermatozoa have been produced from cryopreserved spermatogonial stem cells (Brinster and Nagano, 1998; Ogawa et al., 1999) using a cryopreservation protocol typically used for somatic cell cryopreservation. Using this technique, it was possible to achieve over 70% engraftment in the recipients. These results may suggest that male germ cells from other species can also be cryopreserved with the same efficiency as they resemble stem cells. In the context of cryobiology, there is growing evidence that male and female germ cell lines can be readily cryopreserved because the subcellular structures have little cryosensitivity. Mature spermatozoa show a greater degree of variation in their morphology among species (Fig. 9.6); this is reflected in their survival after cryopreservation (Gao et al., 1997). Similarly, while cryopreservation of isolated and ovarian primordial follicles from many mammalian species has been successful, corresponding survival rates using mature oocytes are still extremely low for most species (Shaw et al., 2000).

It is generally accepted that germ cells have a very limited lifespan in vitro. Recently, a few attempts have been made for long-term culture of spermatogonial stem cells and encouraging results have been obtained. Nagano et al. (1998) have demonstrated that mouse spermatogonial stem cells can be maintained in culture for as long as four months in serum-containing medium, and further recolonize and generate mature spermatozoa following transplantation. Studies on long-term in vitro culture of porcine spermatogonial stem cells are also encouraging. For example, Dirami et al. (1999) were able to culture porcine type A spermatogonial cells for up to 120 hours in Dulbecco's modified Eagle's medium/ Ham's F-12 medium and achieved 50% recovery.

Overall, these studies demonstrate feasibility and the first steps towards establishing a system that will allow spermatogonial stem cells from some animals to be harvested and cryopreserved, while still retaining their ability to proliferate, either following transplantation in vivo or in an in vitro expansion system. However, several areas must be improved for widespread use of this technology, including cryopreservation procedures, transfer technology, enrichment of stem cell populations, and long-term in vitro culture techniques.

Cryopreservation of testicular sperm and testicular tissue

The first known study of testicular tissue cryopreservation was the autologous transplantation of cryopreserved immature rat testis, which resulted in formation of mature spermatozoa (Deanesly, 1954; Parkes and Smith, 1954). Since then there have been advances made in ART, particularly with the successful application of ICSI procedures and in vitro gamete maturation, which have allowed utilization of male germ cells of virtually any quality or developmental stage in order to restore fertility. It was the development of the ICSI procedure (Palermo et al., 1992) that allowed utilization of immotile mature sperm or even round spermatids extracted from testicular tissue (Romero et al., 1996). This procedure can bypass sperm concentration and motility problems to allow successful fertilization. Compared with sperm cryopreservation, tissue cryopreservation presents different considerations, such as cell-to-cell interactions and sufficient CPA permeation to provide optimal cryoprotection (Paynter et al., 1997). There are several occasions in which testicular tissue cryopreservation would be beneficial as a source for germ cell recovery in humans. It could allow prepubertal boys who are undergoing cancer therapy to become fertile postpuberty. Currently, for the prepubertal male there are no clinically applicable options in-so-far as extraction and cryopreservation of mature spermatozoa or round spermatids. Additionally, infertile adult men who are having testicular biopsy could also benefit from improved methods for cryopreservation of testicular tissue. Particularly

in nonobstructive azoospermia, the only way to obtain spermatozoa is from testicular tissue. To-date, these approaches have been successfully used to restore fertility in humans, and livebirths have been reported using testicular spermatozoa extracted from cryopreserved testis biopsies (Fischer et al., 1996; Salzbrunn et al., 1996; Khalifeh et al., 1997; Borini et al., 2000). Furthermore, some studies achieved comparable success with cryopreserved and noncryopreserved testicular spermatozoa (Oates et al., 1996, 1997; Friedler et al., 1997; Marmar, 1998).

There is a growing interest in utilizing cryopreserved testicular tissue containing germ cells of various developmental stages in conjunction with ICSI procedure for young cancer patients. While advanced stage (spermatids) germ cells can be extracted from cryopreserved testicular tissue, there is also the possibility for harvesting earliest stage (spermatogonia) germ cells for further maturation. However, there are potential drawbacks associated with the use of this technique. For instance, it presents the risk of reintroduction of malignant cells into the patient, particularly patients suffering from leukemia or gonadal tumors. Additionally, in vitro sperm maturation techniques will need to be more fully developed and refined in order for these procedures to be commonly applied.

Summary

Successful long-term storage of male and female gametes at any developmental stage or form has significant importance in the advancement of ART. Consequently, there is an urgent need for the development of methodologies for optimal gamete isolation and maturation. A more complete understanding of gamete formation and cellular/molecular properties is essential for the development of more reliable cryopreservation procedures. This synergism between reproductive science and cryobiology will eventually provide better management of livestock and laboratory animal species, enable better conservation of biodiversity, and give hope for infertile people. It can be concluded that cryobanking of germplasm in any form is important to ART for both humans and animals. Considering the rapid advancements currently being witnessed in the field of reproductive biology, any form of long-term storage (cryopreservation, freeze-drying) may have great merit and could potentially add great flexibility to these emerging technologies.

REFERENCES

Agca, Y., Liu, J., Peter, A.T., Critser, E.S., and Critser J.K. (1998). Effect of developmental stage on bovine oocyte plasma membrane water and cryoprotectant permeability characteristics. *Molecular Reproduction and Development*, **49**, 408–15.

Agca, Y., Liu, J., Critser, E.S., McGrath, J.J., and Critser, J.K. (1999). Temperature-dependent osmotic behavior of germinal vesicle and metaphase II stage bovine oocytes in the presence of Me$_2$SO in relationship to cryobiology. *Molecular Reproduction and Development*, **53**, 59–67.

Agca, Y., Liu, J., Rutledge, J.J., Critser, E.S., and Critser, JK. (2000). Effect of osmotic stress on the developmental competence of germinal vesicle and metaphase II stage bovine cumulus oocyte complexes and its relevance to cryopreservation. *Molecular Reproduction and Development*, **55**, 212–19.

Albertini, D.F. (1995). The cytoskeleton as a target for chill injury in mammalian cumulus oocyte complexes. *Cryobiology*, **32**, 551.

Albertini, D.F. and Rider, V. (1994). Patterns of intercellular connectivity in the mammalian cumulus–oocyte complex. *Microscopy Research Technology*, **27**, 125–33.

Al-Hasani, S., van der Ven, H., Diedrich, K., and Krebs, D. (1986). Successful in vitro fertilization of frozen/thawed human oocytes. In: *Reports of a Workshop on Embryos and Oocytes Freezing*, Collection Foundation Marcel Merieux, Annenc, pp. 25–39.

Aman, R.R. and Parks, J.E. (1994). Effects of cooling and warming on the meiotic spindle and chromosomes of in vitro-matured bovine oocytes. *Biology of Reproduction*, **50**, 103–10.

Arav, A., Zeron, Y., Leslie, S.B., Behboodi, E., Anderson, G.B., and Crowe, J.H. (1996). Phase transition temperature and chilling sensitivity of bovine oocytes. *Cryobiology*, **33**, 589–99.

Arey, L.B. (1974). *Developmental Anatomy, A Textbook and Laboratory Manual of Embryology*. Saunders, Philadelphia, PA, pp. 28–61.

Aubard, Y., Newton, H., Scheffer, G., and Gosden, R. (1998). Conservation of the follicular population in irradiated rats by the cryopreservation and orthotopic autografting of ovarian tissue. *European Journal of Obstetrics, Gynecology and Reproductive Biology*, **79**, 83–7.

Austin, C.R (1965). *Fertilization*. Prentice-Hall, Englewood Cliffs, NJ.

Avarbock, M.R., Brinster, C.J., and Brinster, R.L. (1996). Reconstitution of spermatogenesis from frozen spermatogonial stem cells. *Nature Medicine*, **2**, 693–6.

Baker, T. (1972). Oogenesis and ovulation. In: *Reproduction in Animals*, Austin, C.R. and Short, R.V., eds. Cambridge University Press, Cambridge, pp. 14–45.

Ben-Yosef, D., Oron, Y., and Shalgi, R. (1995). Low temperature and fertilization-induced Ca^{+2} changes in rat eggs. *Molecular Reproduction and Development*, **42**, 122–9.

Bernard, A., and Fuller, B.J. (1996). Cryopreservation of human oocytes: a review of current problems and perspectives. *Human Reproduction Update*, **2**, 193–207.

Biggers, J.D., Lawitts, J.A., and Lechene, C.P. (1993). The protective action of betaine on the deleterious effects of NaCl on preimplantation mouse embryos in vitro. *Molecular Reproduction and Development*, **34**, 380–90.

Borini, A., Sereni, E., Bonu, and Flamigni, C. (2000). Freezing a few testicular spermatozoa retrieved by TESA. *Molecular and Cellular Endocrinology*, **169**, 27–32.

Bouquet, M., Selva, J., and Aureoux, M. (1993). Cryopreservation of mouse oocytes: mutagenic effects in the embryo. *Biology of Reproduction*, **49**, 764–9.

Bouquet, M., Selva, J., and Auroux, M. (1995). Effects of cooling and equilibration in DMSO, and cryopreservation of mouse oocytes, on the rates of in vitro fertilization, development and chromosomal abnormalities. *Molecular Reproduction and Development*, **40**, 110–15.

Boyle, R. (1683). *New Experiments and Observations Touching Cold*. London.

Brinster, R.L., and Avarbock, M.R. (1994). Germline transmission of donor haplotype following spermatogonial transplantation. *Proceedings of the National Academy of Sciences USA* **91**, 11303–37.

Brinster, R.L., and Nagano, M. (1998). Spermatogonial stem cell transplantation, cryopreservation and culture. *Seminars in Cell Developmental Biology*, **9**, 401–9.

Brinster, R.L., and Zimmermann, J.W. (1994). Spermatogenesis following male germ-cell transplantation. *Proceedings of the National Academy of Sciences USA*, **91**, 11298–302.

Brower, P.T. and Schultz, R.M. (1982). Intracellular communication between granulosa cells and mouse oocytes: existence and possible nutritional role during oocyte growth. *Developmental Biology*, **90**, 144.

Brown, J., Clark, W.R., Molnar, I.G., and Mullen, Y.S., (1976). Fetal pancreas transplantation for the reversal of streptozotocin induced diabetes in rats. *Diabetes*, **25**, 56–64.

Candy, C.J., Wood, M.J., Whittingham, D.G., Merriman, J.A., and Choudhury, N. (1994). Cryopreservation of immature mouse oocytes. *Human Reproduction*, **9**, 1738–42.

Carroll, J. and Gosden, R.G. (1993). Transplantation of frozen-thawed mouse primordial follicles. *Human Reproduction*, **8**, 1163–7.

Chan, A.W.S. (1999). Transgenic animals: current and alternative strategies. *Cloning*, **1**, 25–46.

Chen, C. (1986). Pregnancy after human oocyte cryopreservation. *Lancet*, **i**, 884–6.

Clermont, Y. (1972). Kinetics of spermatogenesis in mammals: seminiferous epithelium cycle and spermatogonium renewal. *Physiological Review*, **52**, 198–236.

Clouthier, D.E., Avarbock, M.R., Maika, S.D., Hammer, R.E., and Brinster, R.L. (1996). Rat spermatogenesis in mouse testis. *Nature*, **381**, 418–21.

Craft, I., Tsirigotis, M., Bennett, V., et al. (1995). Percutaneous epididymal sperm aspiration and intracytoplasmic sperm injection in the management of infertility due to obstructive azoospermia. *Fertility and Sterility*, **63**, 1038–42.

Critser, J.K., Agca, Y., and Gunasena K.T. (1997). The cryobiology of mammalian oocytes. In: *Reproductive Tissue Banking: Scientific Principles*, Karow, A. and Critser, J.K., eds. Academic Press, New York, pp. 329–57.

Curry, M.R., Millar, J.D., and Watson, P.F. (1994). Calculated optimal cooling rates for ram and human sperm cryopreservation fail to conform with empirical observations. *Biology of Reproduction*, **51**, 1014–21.

Deanesly, R. (1954). Spermatogenesis and endocrine activity in grafts of frozen thaw rat testis. *Journal of Endocrinology*, **11**, 201–6.

De Leeuw, F.E., De Leeuw, A.M., Den Daas, J.H., Colenbrander, B., and Verkleij, A.J. (1993). Effects of various cryoprotective agents and membrane-stabilizing compounds on bull sperm membrane integrity after cooling and freezing. *Cryobiology*, **30**, 32–44.

Devroey, P., Silber, S., Nagy, Z., et al. (1995). Ongoing pregnancies and birth after intracytoplasmic sperm injection with frozen-thawed epididymal spermatozoa. *Human Reproduction*, **10**, 903–6.

Diller, K. and Lynch, M.E. (1984). An irreversible thermodynamic analysis of cell freezing in the presence of membrane permeable additives. II. Transient electrolyte and additive concentrations. *Cryobiology*, **4**, 131–44.

Dirami, G., Ravindranath, N., Pursel, V., and Dym, M. (1999). Effects of stem cell factor and granulocyte macrophage-colony stimulating factor on survival of porcine type A spermatogonia cultured in KSOM. *Biology of Reproduction*, **61**, 225–30.

Dobrinski, I., Avarbock, M.R., and Brinster, R.L. (1999). Transplantation of germ cells from rabbits and dogs into mouse testes. *Biology of Reproduction*, **61**, 1331–9.

Drobnis, E.Z., Crowe, L.M., Berger, T., Anchordoguy, T.J., Overstreet, J.W., and Crowe, J.H. (1993). Cold shock damage is due to lipid phase transitions in cell membranes: a demonstration using sperm as a model. *Journal of Experimental Zoology*, **265**, 432–7.

Eppig, J.J. (1996). The ovary: oogenesis. In: *Scientific Essentials of Reproductive Medicine*, Hillier, S.G., Kitchner, H.C., and Nielson, J.P., eds. Saunders, New York, pp. 147–59.

Eppig, J.J. and O'Brien, M.J. (1996). Development in vitro of mouse oocytes from primordial follicles. *Biology of Reproduction*, **54**, 197–207.

Eroglu, A., Toth, T.L., and Toner, M. (1998). Alterations of the cytoskeleton and polyploidy induced by cryopreservation of metaphase II mouse oocytes. *Fertility and Sterility*, **69**, 944–57.

Fahy, G.M. (1986). The relevance of cryoprotectant toxicity to cryobiology. *Cryobiology* **23**, 1–13.

Fischer, R., Baukloh, V., Naether, O.G., Schulze, W., Salzbrunn, A., and Benson, D.M. (1996). Pregnancy after intracytoplasmic sperm injection of spermatozoa extracted from frozen-thawed testicular biopsy. *Human Reproduction*, **11**, 2197–9.

Ford, P., Merot, J., Jawerbaum, A., Gimeno, M.A., Capurro, C., and Parisi, M. (2000). Water permeability in rat oocytes at different maturity stages: aquaporin-9 expression. *Journal of Membrane Biology*, **176**, 151–8.

Friedler, S., Raziel, A., Soffer, Y., Strassburger, D., Komarovsky, D., and Ron-el, R. (1997). Intracytoplasmic injection of fresh and cryopreserved testicular spermatozoa in patients with non-obstructive azoospermia – a comparative study. *Fertility and Sterility*, **68**, 892–7.

Fuku, E., Kojima, T., Shioya, T., Marcus, G.L., and Downey, B.R. (1992). In vitro fertilization and development of frozen-thawed bovine oocytes. *Cryobiology*, **29**, 485–92.

Fuku, E., Liu, J., and Downey, B.R. (1995). In vitro viability and ultrastructural changes in bovine oocytes treated with a vitrification solution. *Molecular Reproduction and Development*, **40**, 177–85.

Gao, D.Y., Liu, J., Liu, C., et al. (1995). Prevention of osmotic injury to human spermatozoa during addition and removal of glycerol. *Human Reproduction*, **10**, 1109–22.

Gao, D.Y., Mazur, P., and Critser, J.K. (1997). Fundamental cryobiology of mammalian spermatozoa. In: *Reproductive Tissue Banking: Scientific Principles*, Karow, A. and Critser, J.K., eds. Academic Press, New York, pp. 263–313.

Garner, D.L., Thomas, C.A., Joerg, H.W., DeJarnette, J.M., and Marshall, C.E. (1997). Fluorometric assessments of mitochondrial function and viability in cryopreserved bovine spermatozoa. *Biology of Reproduction*, **57**, 1401–6.

George, M.A. and Johnson, M.H. (1993). Cytoskeletal organization and zona sensitivity to digestion by chymotrypsin of frozen-thawed mouse oocytes. *Human Reproduction*, **8**, 612–20.

George, M.A., Pickering, S.J., Braude, P.R., and Johnson, M.H. (1996). The distribution of α- and γ-tubulin in fresh and aged human and mouse oocytes exposed to cryoprotectant. *Molecular Human Reproduction*, **2**, 445–56.

Gianaroli, L., Selman, H.A., Magli, M.C., Colpi, G., Fortini, D., and Ferraretti, A.P. (1999). Birth of a healthy infant after conception with round spermatids isolated from cryopreserved testicular tissue. *Fertility and Sterility*, **72**, 539–41.

Gilmore, J.A., Liu, J., Gao, D.Y., and Critser, J.K. (1997). Determination of optimal cryoprotectants and procedures for their addition and removal from human spermatozoa. *Human Reproduction*, **12**, 112–18.

Gilmore, J.A., Liu, J., and Critser, J.K. (1999). Osmotic tolerance limits of murine spermatozoa in the presence of extender media. *Cryobiology*, **39**, 353–4.

Gilmore, J.A., Liu, J., Woods, E.J., Peter, A.T., and Critser, J.K. (2000). Cryoprotective agent and temperature effects on human sperm membrane permeabilities: convergence of theoretical and empirical approaches for optimal cryopreservation methods. *Human Reproduction*, **15**, 335–43.

Glenister, P.H., Wood, M.J., Kirby, C., and Whittingham, D.G. (1987). Incidence of chromosome anomalies in first-cleavage mouse embryos obtained from frozen-thawed oocytes fertilized in vitro. *Gamete Research*, **16**, 205–16.

Gosden, R.G., Baird, D.T., Wade, J.C., and Webb, R. (1994). Restoration of fertility to oophorectomized sheep by ovarian autografts stored at -196 degrees C. *Human Reproduction*, **9**, 597–603.

Goto, K., Kinoshita, A., Takuma, Y., and Ogawa, K. (1990). Fertilisation of bovine oocytes by the injection of immobilised, killed spermatozoa. *Veterinary Record*, **127**, 517–20.

Griffin, J.E. (2000). Male reproductive function. In: *Textbook of Endocrine Physiology*, Griffin, J.E. and Ojeda, S.R., eds. Oxford University Press, New York, pp. 243–64.

Gunasena, K.T., Lakey, J.R., Villines, P.M., Critser, E.S., and Critser, J.K. (1997). Allogeneic and xenogeneic transplantation of cryopreserved ovarian tissue to athymic mice. *Biology of Reproduction*, **57**, 226–31.

Hammerstedt, R.H., Graham, J.K., and Nolan, J.P. (1990). Cryopreservation of mammalian sperm: what we ask them to survive. *Journal of Andrology*, **11**, 73–88.

Henry, M.A., Noiles, E.E., Gao, D., Mazur, P., and Critser, J.K. (1993). Cryopreservation of human spermatozoa. IV. The effects of cooling rate and warming rate on the maintenance of motility, plasma membrane integrity, and mitochondrial function. *Fertility and Sterility*, **60**, 911–18.

Holden, C.A., Fuscaldo, G.F., Jackson, P., et al. (1997). Frozen-thawed epididymal spermatozoa for intracytoplasmic sperm injection. *Fertility and Sterility*, **67**, 81–7.

Holt, W.V. (2000). Fundamental aspects of sperm cryobiology: the importance of species and individual differences *Theriogenology*, **53**, 47–58.

Hotamisligil, S., Toner, M., and Powers, R.D. (1996). Changes in membrane integrity, cytoskeletal structure, and developmental potential of murine oocytes after vitrification in ethylene glycol. *Biology of Reproduction*, **55**, 161–8.

Hovatta, O. (2000a). Cryopreservation and culture of human primordial and primary ovarian follicles. *Molecular and Cellular Endocrinology*, **169**, 95–7.

Hovatta, O. (2000b). Cryopreservation of testicular tissue. *Molecular and Cellular Endocrinology*, **169**, 113–15.

Hunter, J.E., Bernard, A., Fuller, B.J., McGrath, J.J., and Shaw, R.W. (1992). Measurements of the membrane water permeability (L_p) and its temperature dependence (activation energy) in human fresh and failed-to-fertilize oocytes and mouse oocyte. *Cryobiology*, **29**, 240–9.

Hutchon, S., Thornton, S., Hall, J., and Bishop, M. (1998). Frozen-thawed epididymal sperm is effective for intracytoplasmic sperm injection: implications for the urologist. *British Journal of Urology*, **81**, 607–11.

Johnston, D.S., Russell, L.D., and Griswold, M.D. (2000). Advances in spermatogonial stem cell transplantation. *Reviews in Reproduction*, **5**, 183–8.

Karlsson, J.O.M., Eroglu, A., Toth, T.L., Cravalho, E.G., and Toner, M. (1996). Fertilization and development of mouse oocytes cryopreserved using a theoretically optimized protocol. *Human Reproduction*, **11**, 1296–1305.

Katkov, I.I. and Mazur, P. (1999). Factors affecting yield and survival of cells when suspensions are subjected to centrifugation. Influence of centrifugal acceleration, time of centrifugation, and length of the suspension column in quasi-homogeneous centrifugal fields. *Cell Biochemistry and Biophysics*, **31**, 231–45.

Khalifeh, F.A., Sarraf, M., and Dabit, S.T. (1997). Full-term delivery following intracytoplasmic sperm injection with spermatozoa extracted from frozen-thawed testicular tissue. *Human Reproduction*, **12**, 87–8.

Kimura, Y. and Yanagimachi, R. (1995). Development of normal mice from oocytes injected with secondary spermatocyte nuclei. *Biology of Reproduction*, **53**, 855–62.

Kola, I., Kirby, C., Shaw, J., Davey, A., and Trounson, A. (1988). Vitrification of mouse oocytes results in aneuploid zygotes and malformed fetuses. *Teratology*, **38**, 467–74.

Le Gal, F., Gasqui, P., and Renard, J.P. (1994). Differential osmotic behavior of mammalian oocytes before and after maturation: a quantitative analysis using goat oocytes as a model. *Cryobiology*, **31**, 154–70.

Le Gal, F., Gasqui, P., and Renard, J.P. (1995). Evaluation of intracellular cryoprotectant concentration before freezing of goat oocyte. *Cryo-Letters*, **16**, 3–12.

Leibfried-Rutledge, M.L., Dominko, T., Critser, E.S., and Critser, J.K. (1997). Tissue maturation in vivo and in vitro, gamete and early embryo ontogeny. In: *Reproductive Tissue Banking Scientific Principles*, Karow, A. and Critser, J.K., eds. Academic Press, New York, pp. 23–111.

Leibo, S.P., McGrath, J.J., and Cravalho, E.G. (1978). Microscopic observation of intracellular ice formation in unfertilized mouse ova as a function of cooling rate. *Cryobiology*, **15**, 257–71.

Lim, J.M., Fukui, Y., and Ono, H. (1992). The post-thaw developmental competence of bovine oocytes frozen at various maturation stages followed by in vitro maturation and fertilization. *Theriogenology*, **37**, 351–61.

Lovelock, J.E. (1954). The protective action of neutral solutes against haemolysis by freezing and thawing. *Biochemical Journal*, **56**, 265.

Lovelock, J.E. and Bishop, M. (1959). Prevention of freezing damage to cells by dimethyl sulphoxide. *Nature*, **183**, 1394–5.

Marmar, J.L. (1998). The emergence of specialized procedures for the acquisition, processing, and cryopreservation of epididymal and testicular sperm in connection with intracytoplasmic sperm injection. *Journal of Andrology*, **19**, 517–26.

Martino, A., Pollard, J.W., and Leibo, S.P. (1996a). Effect of chilling bovine oocytes on their developmental competence. *Molecular Reproduction and Development*, **45**, 503–12.

Martino, A., Songsasen, N., and Leibo, S.P. (1996b). Development into blastocysts of bovine oocytes cryopreserved by ultra-rapid cooling. *Biology of Reproduction*, **54**, 1059–69.

Mazur, P. (1963). Kinetics of water loss from cells at subzero temperatures and the likelihood of intracellular freezing. *Journal of General Physiology* **47**, 347–69.

Mazur, P. (1970). Cryobiology: the freezing of biological systems. *Science*, **168**, 939–49.

Mazur, P. (1984). Freezing of living cells: mechanisms and implications. *Cell Physiology* **16**, C125–42.

Mazur, P. and Schneider, U. (1986). Osmotic responses of preimplantation mouse and bovine embryos and their cryobiological implications. *Cell Biophysics*, **8**, 259–85.

Mazur, P., Rall, W.F., and Leibo, S.P. (1984). Kinetics of water loss and the likelihood of intracellular freezing in mouse ova: influence of the method of calculating the temperature dependence of water permeability. *Cell Biophysics*, **6**, 197–214.

McGrath, J. (1997). Quantitative measurement of cell membrane transport: technology and applications. *Cryobiology*, **34**, 315–34.

McWilliams, R.B., Gibbons, W.E., and Leibo, S.P. (1995). Osmotic and physiological responses of mouse zygotes and human oocytes to mono- and disaccharides. *Human Reproduction*, **10**, 1163–71.

Miyazaki, S., Shirakawa, H., Nakada, K., and Honda, Y. (1993). Essential role of the inositol 1,4,5-trisphosphate receptor/Ca^{2+} release channel in Ca^{2+} waves and Ca^{2+} oscillations at fertilization of mammalian eggs. *Developmental Biology*, **158**, 62–78.

Moller, C. and Wassarman, P.M. (1989). Characterization of a proteinase that cleaves zona pellucida glycoprotein ZP2 following activation of mouse eggs. *Developmental Biology*, **132**, 103–12.

Morris, G.J., Acton, E., and Avery, S. (1999). A novel approach to sperm cryopreservation. *Human Reproduction*, **14**, 1013–21.

Muench, J.L., Kruuv, J., and Lepock, J.R. (1996). A two-step reversible-irreversible model can account for a negative activation energy in an Arrhenius plot. *Cryobiology*, **33**, 253–9.

Nagano, M., Avarbock, M.R., Leonida, E.B., Brinster, C.J., and Brinster, R.L. (1998). Culture of mouse spermatogonial stem cells. *Tissue Cell*, **30**, 389–97.

Nagano, M., Shinohara, T., Avarbock, M.R., and Brinster, R.L. (2000). Retrovirus-mediated gene delivery into male germ line stem cells. *FEBS Letters* **475**, 7–10.

Nakagata, N. (1989). High survival rate of unfertilized mouse oocytes after vitrification. *Journal of Reproduction and Fertility*, **87**, 479–83.

Newton, H., Pegg, D.E., Barrass, R., and Gosden, R.G. (1999). Osmotically inactive volume, hydraulic conductivity, and permeability to dimethyl sulphoxide of human mature oocytes. *Journal of Reproduction and Fertility*, **117**, 27–33.

Nudell, D.M., Conaghan, J., Pedersen, R.A., Givens, C.R., Schriock, E.D., and Turek, P.J. (1998). The mini-micro-epididymal sperm aspiration for sperm retrieval: a study of urological outcomes. *Human Reproduction*, **13**, 1260–5.

Oates, R.D., Lobel, S.M., Harris, D.H., Pang, S., Burgess, C.M., and Carson, R.S. (1996). Efficacy of intracytoplasmic sperm injection using intentionally cryopreserved epididymal spermatozoa. *Human Reproduction*, **11**, 133–8.

Oates, R.D., Mulhall, J., Burgess, C., Cunningham, D., and Carson, R. (1997). Fertilization and pregnancy using intentionally cryopreserved testicular tissue as the sperm source for intracytoplasmic sperm injection in 10 men with non-obstructive azoospermia. *Human Reproduction* 12, 734–9.

Ogawa, T., Dobrinski, I., and Brinster, R.L. (1999). Recipient preparation is critical for spermatogonial transplantation in the rat. *Tissue Cell*, 31, 461–72.

Ogawa, T., Dobrinski, I., Avarbock, M.R., and Brinster, R.L. (2000). Transplantation of male germ line stem cells restores fertility in infertile mice. *Nature Medicine*, 6, 29–34.

Oktay, K., Newton, H., Aubard, Y., Salha, O., and Gosden, R.G., (1998). Cryopreservation of immature human oocytes and ovarian tissue: an emerging technology? *Fertility and Sterility*, 69, 1–7.

Palermo, G., Joris, H., Devroey, P., and Van Steirteghem, A.C. (1992). Pregnancies after intracytoplasmic injection of single spermatozoon into an oocyte. *Lancet*, 340, 17–18.

Parkes, A.S. and Smith, A.U. (1954). Storage of testicular tissue at very low temperatures. *British Medical Journal*, 1, 315–16.

Parks, J.E. (1997). Hypothermia and mammalian gametes. In: *Reproductive Tissue Banking: Scientific Principles*, Karow, A.M. and Critser, J.K., eds. Academic Press, New York, pp. 229–61.

Parks, J.E. and Ruffing, N.A. (1992). Factors affecting low temperature survival of mammalian oocytes. *Theriogenology*, 37, 59–73.

Parrish, J.J., Susko-Parrish, J., Leibfried-Rutledge, M.L., Critser, E.S., Eyestone, W.H., and First, N.L. (1986). Bovine in vitro fertilization with frozen-thawed semen. *Theriogenology*, 25, 591–600.

Paynter, S., Cooper, A., Thomas, N., and Fuller, B. (1997). Cryopreservation of multicellular embryos and reproductive tissues. In: *Reproductive Tissue Banking: Scientific Principles*, Karow, A.M. and Crister, J.K., eds. Academic Press, New York, pp. 359–91.

Pedro, P.B., Zhu, S.E., Makino, N., Sakurai, T., Edashige, K., and Kasai, M. (1997). Effects of hypotonic stress on the survival of mouse oocytes and embryos at various stages. *Cryobiology*, 35, 150–8.

Phelps, M.J., Liu, J., Benson, J.D., Willoughby, C.E., Gilmore, J.A., and Critser, J.K. (1999). Effects of Percoll separation, cryoprotective agents, and temperature on plasma membrane permeability characteristics of murine spermatozoa and their relevance to cryopreservation. *Biology of Reproduction*, 61, 1031–41.

Pickering, S.J., Braude, P.R., Johnson, M.H., Cant, A., and Currie, J. (1990). Transient cooling to room temperature can cause irreversible disruption of the meiotic spindle in the human oocyte. *Fertility and Sterility*, 54, 102–8.

Polge, C., Smith, A., and Parkes, A. (1949). Revival of spermato-zoa after vitrification and dehydration at low temperatures. *Nature*, 164, 666.

Porcu, E., Fabbri, R., Seracchioli, R., Ciotti, P.M., Magrini, O., and Flamigni, C. (1997). Birth of a healthy female after intracyto-plasmic sperm injection of cryopreserved human oocytes. *Fertility and Sterility*, 68, 724–6.

Ragni, G., Caccamo, A.M., Dalla-Serra, A., and Guercilena, S. (1990). Computerized slow-staged freezing of semen from men with testicular tumors or Hodgkin's disease preserves sperm better than standard vapor freezing. *Fertility and Sterility*, 53, 1072–5.

Rall, W.F. and Fahy, G.M. (1985). Ice-free cryopreservation of mouse embryos at −196°C by vitrification. *Nature*, 313, 573–5.

Rayos, A.A., Takashashi, Y., Hishinuma, M., and Kanagawa, M. (1994). Quick freezing of unfertilized mouse oocytes using ethylene glycol with sucrose or trehalose. *Journal of Reproduction and Fertility*, 100, 123–9.

Romero, J., Remohi, J., Minguez, Y., Rubio, C., Pellicer, A., and Gil-Salom, M. (1996). Fertilization after intracytoplasmic sperm injection with cryopreserved testicular spermatozoa. *Fertility and Sterility*, 65, 877–9.

Roy, S.K. and Greenwald, G.S. (1996). Methods of separation and in-vitro culture of pre-antral follicles from mammalian ovaries. *Human Reproduction Update*, 2, 236–45.

Ruffing, N.A., Steponkus, P.L., Pitt, R.E., and Parks, J.E. (1993). Osmometric behavior, hydraulic conductivity, and incidence of intracellular ice formation in bovine oocyte at different developmental stages. *Cryobiology*, 30, 562–80.

Salzbrunn, A., Benson, D.M., Holstein, A.F., and Schulze, W. (1996). A new concept for the extraction of testicular sper-matozoa as a tool for assisted fertilization (ICSI). *Human Reproduction*, 11, 752–5.

Schalkoff, E.M., Oskowitz, P.S., and Powers, R.D. (1989). Ultrastructural observations of human and mouse oocytes treated with cryoprotectives. *Biology of Reproduction*, 40, 379–93.

Schlatt, S., Rosiepen, G., Weinbauer, G.F., Rolf, C., Brook, P.F., and Nieschlag, E. (1999). Germ cell transfer into rat, bovine, monkey and human testes. *Human Reproduction*, 14, 144–50.

Schroeder, A.C., Champlin, A.K., Mobraaten, L.E., and Eppig, J.J. (1990). Developmental capacity of mouse oocytes cryopre-served before and after maturation in vitro. *Journal of Reproduction and Fertility*, 89, 43–50.

Shaw, J.M., Oranratnachai, A., and Trounson, A.O. (2000). Fundamental cryobiology of mammalian oocytes and ovarian tissue. *Theriogenology*, 53, 59–72.

Smith, U. (1950). Prevention of heamolysis during freezing and thawing of red blood cells. *Lancet*, 11, 910–11.

Spallanzani, L. (1776). Osservazioni e spezienze interno ai vermicelli spermatici dell'uomo e degli animali. *Opuscoli di Fisica Animale e Vegitabile*, Modena, Italy.

Stachecki, J.J., Cohen, J., and Willadsen, S. (1998a). Detrimental effects of sodium during mouse oocyte cryopreservation. *Biology of Reproduction*, **59**, 395–400.

Stachecki, J.J., Cohen, J., and Willadsen, S.M. (1998b). Cryopreservation of unfertilized mouse oocytes: the effect of replacing sodium with choline in the freezing medium *Cryobiology*, **37**, 346–54.

Tournaye, H., Merdad, T., Silber, S., et al. (1999). No differences in outcome after intracytoplasmic sperm injection with fresh or with frozen-thawed epididymal spermatozoa. *Human Reproduction*, **14**, 90–5.

Vajta, G., Holm, P., Kuwayama, M., et al. (1998) Open pulled straw (OPS) vitrification: a new way to reduce cryoinjuries of bovine ova and embryos. *Molecular Reproduction and Development*, **51**, 53–8.

Van Blerkom, J. (1989). Maturation at high frequency of germinal-vesicle-stage mouse oocytes after cryopreservation: alterations in cytoplasmic, nuclear, nucleolar and chromosomal structure and organization associated with vitrification. *Human Reproduction*, **4**, 883–98.

Van Blerkom, J. and Davis, P.W. (1994). Cytogenic, cellular, and developmental consequences of cryopreservation of immature and mature mouse and human oocytes. *Microscopy Research and Technique*, **27**, 165–93.

Vincent, C. and Johnson, M.H. (1992). Cooling, cryoprotectants, and the cytoskeleton of the mammalian oocyte. *Oxford Review Reproductive Biology*, **14**, 73–100.

Vincent, C., Pickering, S.J., Johnson, M.H., and Quick, S.J. (1990). Dimethyl sulfoxide affects the organisation of microfilaments in the mouse oocyte. *Molecular Reproduction and Development*, **26**, 227–35.

Wakayama, T. and Yanagimachi, R. (1998). Development of normal mice from oocytes injected with freeze-dried spermatozoa. *Nature Biotechnology*, **16**, 639–41.

Wakayama, T., Whittingham, D.G., and Yanagimachi, R. (1998). Production of normal offspring from mouse oocytes injected with spermatozoa cryopreserved with or without cryoprotection. *Journal of Reproduction and Fertility*, **112**, 11–17.

Wassarman, P.M. (1988). Fertilization in mammals. *Scientific American*, **259**, 78–84.

Watson, P.F. (1995). Recent developments and concepts in the cryopreservation of spermatozoa and the assessment of their post-thawing function. *Reproduction, Fertility and Development*, **7**, 871–91.

Watson, P.F. (2000). The causes of reduced fertility with cryopreserved semen. *Animal Reproduction Science*, **60–61**, 481–92.

Whittingham, D.G. (1977). Fertilization in vitro and development to term of unfertilized mouse oocytes previously stored at −196°C. *Journal of Reproduction and Fertility*, **49**, 89–94.

Willoughby, C.E., Mazur, P., Peter, A.T., and Critser, J.K. (1996). Osmotic tolerance limits and properties of murine spermatozoa. *Biology of Reproduction*, **55**, 715–27.

Wood, M.J., Barros, C., Candy, C.J., Carroll, J., Melendez, J., and Whittingham, D.G. (1993). High rates of survival and fertilization of mouse and hamster oocytes after vitrification in dimethyl sulfoxide. *Biology of Reproduction*, **49**, 489–95.

Yoon, T.K, Chung, H.M., Lim, J.M., Han, S.Y., Ko, J.J., and Cha, K.Y. (2000). Pregnancy and delivery of healthy infants developed from vitrified oocytes in a stimulated in vitro fertilization-embryo transfer program. *Fertility and Sterility*, **74**, 180–1.

Younis, A.I., Toner, M., Albertini, D.F., and Biggers, J.D. (1996). Cryobiology of non-human primate oocytes. *Human Reproduction*, **11**, 156–65.

10

Embryonic stem cells

Ann M. Lawler and John D. Gearhart

Johns Hopkins University, Baltimore, USA

Introduction

The possibility that a single source of cells could be used to treat diseases as diverse as Parkinson's disease, diabetes mellitus, multiple sclerosis, cardiomyopathies, liver disease, and muscular dystrophies plus acute conditions such as severe burns, spinal cord injuries, strokes and heart attacks seems as preposterous as the thought 30 years ago that a single compound, a so-called "magic bullet," could be found that would cure all forms of cancer. However, the report of the derivation of human embryonic stem (ES) cells in 1998 (Shamblott et al., 1998; Thomson et al., 1998) and subsequent reports on a variety of other stem cells have brought us to the point of turning the preposterous into a reality at the beginning of the twenty-first century. In fact, clinical trails have already started employing a neuronal stem cell line to treat stroke victims (Kondziolka et al., 2000). However, this rapidly moving field is enmeshed in controversy because of the source of the cells, either fetal tissue or preimplantation embryos. The concurrent discoveries regarding the potential of stem cells derived from a variety of adult tissues has led to the proposal that adult stem cells could be used as an alternative to embryonic stem cells.

Our understanding of the mechanisms that maintain stem cells in an undifferentiated state and the mechanisms that drive differentiation of stem cells to a particular fate, or even of the malleability of differentiated cells, is currently in an embryonic state characterized by rapid growth. In this chapter, we will review the concept of stem cells and the historical development of our knowledge of ES cells, describe the use of stem cells in research and clinical therapy, and describe some of the legal issues surrounding derivation of and research on embryonic stem cells.

Stem cells

Stem cells are defined by two essential features. First is the ability to generate additional stem cells through cell division and second is the ability to generate differentiated cell types with specific functions. The combination of these two features necessitates that stem cells can undergo asymmetric cell divisions resulting in additional stem cells and also differentiated cells. Stem cells are most easily understood in the context of tissues that normally display continuous cell death and replenishment during adult life, such as the hematopoietic system, the epithelial cells lining the digestive tract, and the basal cells of the epidermis. In each of these, a significant fraction of functional cells is replaced on a daily basis with cells derived from a stable population of stem cells. Recently, stem cells have been identified in other organs that do not undergo such an obvious replenishment of functional tissue, including the nervous system and muscle (Gussoni et al., 1999; Gage, 2000). The terms precursor or progenitor cell have, on occasion, been used interchangeably for stem cell. However, both terms can also be applied to cells that do not form a stable population of regenerating cells.

When using the term stem cell, a regenerative capacity is implied in the definition.

Each stem cell population is further defined by a limited spectrum of progeny cell functions. For example, hematopoietic stem cells give rise to both lymphoid stem cells and cells of the myeloid lineage. Lymphoid stem cells, in turn, give rise to thymocytes and B cells, while the stem cells of the myeloid lineage give rise to eosinophils, red blood cells, megakaryocytes, basophils, neutrophils, and macrophages. The epithelial stem cells of the gut are located near the base of the crypts and give rise to four functional cell types: the absorptive cells, goblet cells, enteroendocrine cells, and Paneth cells. Although each stem cell population was previously thought to be restricted in its developmental potential, recent experiments have challenged this notion and suggest that a substantial amount of reprogramming between cell fates is possible under appropriate environmental conditions (Eglitis and Mezey, 1997; Bjornson et al., 1999; Brazelton et al., 2000; Mezey et al., 2000).

Embryonic stem cells

In addition to the features of stem cell replenishment and production of differentiated cell types, ES cells have the exceptional capacity to generate all of the cell types in an adult organism. During mammalian development, a small population of cells fitting this description exists for only a brief period of time in two structures termed the inner cell mass and the epiblast. Just prior to implantation, mammalian embryos develop into blastocysts, cystic structures comprising an outer epithelial layer of trophoblast cells surrounding a fluid-filled cavity. Within the cavity, and attached to the trophoblasts, are a compact clump of cells called the inner cell mass.

The cells of the inner cell mass (ICM) will eventually give rise to all of the cells and tissues of the embryo proper (fetus). Shortly after implantation, the ICM forms a layer of rapidly dividing cells called the epiblast. Within several days of its appearance, the epiblast undergoes gastrulation, a dramatic transformation in which cells detach from the epiblast layer, migrate ventrally and differentiate to form three separate germ layers, the ectoderm, mesoderm, and endoderm. Establishment of ES cell lines requires that the population of ICM or epiblast cells be prevented from undergoing the differentiation events associated with gastrulation and be maintained in an environment that promotes indefinite cell division and inhibits cell differentiation. Since the cells of the ICM or epiblast exist as pluripotent stem cells for only a brief period of time and do not form a stable population of undifferentiated stem cells, they do not fulfill the strict criteria defining stem cells (van der Kooy and Weiss, 2000). In fact, the establishment of continuous cultures of embryonic stem cells can be conceived as an artificial manipulation of cellular phenotype elicited by defined culturing conditions.

Mouse embryonic stem and embryonic germ cells

In 1981, efforts to establish long-term cultures of undifferentiated cells from mouse preimplantation embryos succeeded and the first ES cell lines were described (Evans and Kaufman, 1981; Martin, 1981). ES cells were derived by culturing blastocysts on a layer of fibroblast feeder cells that supplied soluble growth factors and extracellular support. Once the blastocysts attached to the feeder layer, the cells of the ICM proliferated into small clumps. The growing clumps were physically removed from the differentiative influence of the trophoblasts and expanded on fresh feeder layers. Leukemia-inhibiting factor (LIF) was identified as one essential soluble growth factor required for inhibiting the differentiation of ES cells. Subsequently, ES cell lines were derived using LIF alone, without the requirement for fibroblast feeder cells (Nichols et al., 1990). Nonetheless, fibroblast feeder cells are believed to supply additional factors that aid in maintaining undifferentiated ES cells. The first ES cells were derived from the 129/Sv strain of mice, a strain known to have a propensity for developing germ cell tumors (teratomas or teratocarcinomas).

Other stem cell lines, termed embryonal carcinoma (EC) cell lines, had previously been derived from teratocarcinomas. In fact, the term stem cell was originally defined in the 1900s in the context of tumor biology as the proliferating cell giving rise to the tumor. Teratocarcinomas retain a population of stem cells and are malignant tumors, whereas, teratomas do not have a population of stem cells and are benign. Like ES cells, EC cells have the capacity to proliferate indefinitely and can form most of the cells within an embryo but are limited in the ability to form germ cells. EC cells tend to become heteroploid during extended culture, leading to the occasional formation of tumors when placed into a normal mouse embryo. Subsequent attempts to derive ES cells from other strains of mice proved to be more difficult, and this indicated that several genes may influence the derivation of ES cells. A method has been devised to isolate stem cells away from differentiating cells in the initial cultures and has led to improvements in derivation of lines from several strains (Mountford et al., 1998). There is currently no further understanding of the mechanism contributing to genetic differences in stem cell derivation but similar mechanisms may underlay the difficulties faced in attempts to derive ES cells from other species.

Murine ES cells display several defining morphological features in the undifferentiated state and also demonstrate essential functional characteristics when induced to differentiate. Undifferentiated ES cells grow as tight clumps of small cells with a very high ratio of nuclear to cytoplasmic volume. Cell cycle times of 12–16 hours lead to high-density cultures, requiring passaging every second or third day. Despite this high proliferative rate, ES cells remain euploid over extended periods of culture. However, some recurrent karyotypical anomalies have been observed (Liu et al., 1997).

If mouse ES cells are grown in media lacking LIF and removed from the support of a feeder layer, small multicellular aggregates form and grow in suspension. These cellular aggregates are called embryoid bodies, a term originally applied to structures identified in human testicular tumors (Peyron, 1939). Initial differentiation of embryoid bodies leads to the formation of multiple layers, analogous but not equivalent to embryonic germ layers. Extensive cellular differentiation continues, leading to the formation of complex cystic structures. A variety of cell types can be observed in these structures including hematopoietic, endothelial, chondrocytic, and neural cells. Under appropriate culture conditions, embryoid bodies can be induced to form cardiomyocytes that spontaneously initiate rhythmic contractions (Doetschman et al., 1985, 1993). Although some complex processes occur in embryoid bodies, such as multilayering or vascular formation, these processes are uncontrolled and highly variable and display no degree of regularity or patterning that is essential to normal embryogenesis. As such, embryoid bodies must not be confused with embryos.

Another indication of the differentiative capacity of ES cells is determined by transplanting cells back into mice of the same strain or into immunodeficient animals or an immunoprivileged site such as the kidney capsule. The transferred ES cells proliferate and differentiate into teratocarcinomas, tumors resembling germ cell tumors and containing a variety of cell types. ES cells can also be injected into the cavity of blastocysts, where the cells will quickly adhere to and intermingle with the ICM cells. The resulting embryos are termed chimerae, with ES cells contributing to all of the tissues of the animal. The percentage of ES cells relative to host cells within each tissue can vary dramatically between individual chimeric animals. An important measurement of the developmental potential of ES cells is determined by the contribution of ES cells to the germ cells of the chimeric progeny. The ability of ES cells to contribute to the germ cells allows genetic manipulations made in the ES cells to be easily transferred into animals, thereby providing the basis for extremely powerful tests of genetic function (Rossant and Nagy, 1995) and the potential to model human genetic diseases in the mouse.

In the early 1990s, cultures of undifferentiated cells from the primordial germ cells (PGCs) of post-gastrulation mouse embryos were reported (Matsui et al., 1992; Resnick et al., 1992). Following implantation of mammalian embryos, PGCs migrate from the epiblast to an extra-embryonic position near the allantois, presumably avoiding the differentiative signals of the gastrulating embryo. Upon completion of gastrulation, the PGCs begin to proliferate rapidly and migrate back into the embryo and into the genital ridges, structures that will eventually become the gonads, either testes or ovaries. Once PGCs enter the gonads, proliferation declines and the cells begin to differentiate into oogonia or spermatogonia. PGCs are diploid until undergoing meiosis to form either secondary spermatocytes or mature oocytes. PGCs that are isolated during the period of rapid proliferation and cultured with LIF, basic fibroblast growth factor (bFGF), the membrane form of stem cell factor, and an activator of adenylyl cyclase will grow in a manner similar to ES cells. These cell lines were termed embryonic germ (EG) cells to describe the original tissue source. As with ES cells, EG cells are strictly a product of unique in vitro culture conditions and no equivalent cell type exists during normal embryogenesis.

Once established, EG cells lose the requirement for bFGF and stem cell factor (SCF) and resemble ES cells in most aspects including the formation of dense colonies of rapidly proliferating cells, the requirement for LIF and/or feeder cells to remain undifferentiated, the ability to differentiate into embryoid bodies, the ability to form teratocarcinomas when injected into immunoprivileged sites, and the ability to form germ cells within chimerae when injected into blastocysts. Derivation of EG lines was accomplished from mice of several different genetic backgrounds. Besides morphological similarities, ES and EG cells have common expression patterns for several molecular markers including alkaline phosphatase, stage-specific embryonic antigen (SSEA-1), regulator x (Rex) 1 and Oct-4. However, ES and EG cells differ in the state of methylation of specific genes (Solter and Gearhart, 1999), a finding that may be related to loss of parental imprinting in PGCs.

Embryonic stem and germ cells from other species

As the tremendous value of murine ES and EG cells was realized, efforts to establish similar lines from a variety of species began. ES-like cell lines have been reported from Medaka fish, rabbit, hamster, and mink (Prelle et al., 1999). The potential for using ES or EG cell lines for the production of transgenic livestock species led to work on chicken, sheep, cattle, and pig. The chicken cells have a high differentiative capacity, express alkaline phosphatase and SSEA-1, can contribute to chimerae, but have a very low capacity to form germ cells. For sheep and cattle, the potential for using nuclear transfer procedures has diminished the need for establishing long-term ES cell lines. Transgenesis can be accomplished in fetal fibroblast cells, and these cells can be used as donors for nuclear transfer experiments to derive transgenic animals. Establishment of ES-like cells from porcine embryos, either from ICM or PGCs, has been reported by a number of groups (e.g., Prelle et al., 1999). The porcine cell lines tend to have an epithelial morphology but express alkaline phosphatase and produce chimerae through blastocyst injection (Chen et al., 1999).

ES cell lines have also been derived from nonhuman primates. In 1995, Thomson reported the establishment of ES cells from rhesus monkeys (Thomson et al., 1995). The cells were derived from blastocysts in which the trophectoderm cells had been immunosurgically removed and the ICM cells were cultured on mouse embryonic fibroblasts with supplemental LIF. Under these culture conditions, the cells were maintained for over a year in an undifferentiated state. The cell lines expressed alkaline phosphatase, SSEA-3, and SSEA-4, and thus resembled human EC cell lines. Following removal from the feeder layer, the cells differentiated into a variety of cell types and also formed teratocarcinomas in immunodeficient mice. Similar cell lines were also derived from marmosets by the same laboratory (Thomson et al., 1996). No report has been made regarding the ability of these cell lines to produce chimerae following injection into blastocysts.

Human embryonic stem and germ cells

The establishment of ES cell lines from nonhuman primates set the stage for experiments to derive ES or EG cells from humans. In addition to substantial technical challenges, procedures for the procurement of human tissue had to be established. In the case of ES cells, preimplantation embryos were obtained from in vitro fertilization (IVF) procedures. Since federal funds cannot be used for research involving human embryos in the USA, private funding sources were used. In the case of EG cultures, PGCs were obtained from gonadal tissue dissected from fetuses following therapeutic terminations of pregnancy. Research involving fetal tissue is eligible for federal funding under current US National Institutes of Health (NIH) guidelines.

Thomson's group from the University of Wisconsin followed up their success with rhesus monkey and marmoset ES cells by culturing ICM from human blastocysts (Thomson et al., 1998). Both fresh and frozen, cleavage stage human embryos from clinical IVF procedures were used. The embryos were cultured to the blastocyst stage using a two-stage culture media system and the ICMs were immunosurgically isolated and grown on a mouse fibroblast feeder layer following the protocol used for rhesus monkey and marmoset. Both male and female lines were established, maintained for months in an undifferentiated and karyotypically normal state, and analyzed for molecular markers and differentiative capacity. The ES cell lines expressed alkaline phosphatase, the surface markers SSEA-3 and SSEA-4, and had a high level of telomerase. When injected into immunodeficient mice, the ES cells differentiated into teratomas containing cells that are attributed to all three germ layers during normal embryogenesis. In vitro differentiation of the cells occurred when grown without the fibroblast feeder layer or when grown to high density and allowed to form three-dimensional clumps. LIF was not sufficient to prevent differentiation under these circumstances. Differentiation into both endoderm and trophoblast-type cells was evident. In striking contrast to murine ES cells, the human ES cells have a relatively low proliferative rate, with an estimated cell cycle time of three to four days. Since then, another group reported the derivation of cell lines from human blastocysts (Reubinoff et al., 2000). Although, the morphology of the cells is more epithelial than other lines, the cells have the potential to form teratomas containing a variety of cell types.

Report of human EG derivation occurred in the same month as the report from Wisconsin (Shamblott et al., 1998). John Gearhart's group at the Johns Hopkins School of Medicine obtained genital ridges from fetuses and established cultures under the conditions used for establishing murine EG lines, namely using murine STO fibroblast feeder cells expressing a membrane form of SCF and adding human recombinant bFGF, human recombinant LIF and forskolin to the media. Over 90% of the cultures initiated demonstrated characteristics of stem cell lines although the conversion of the cultures into lines that could be passaged over 20 times was variable. The cultures showed alkaline phosphatase staining and also demonstrated the cell surface markers SSEA-1, SSEA-3, SSEA-4, tumor resistant antigen (TRA) 1–60 and 1–81, although the staining with SSEA-3 was weak. There was also variability of staining for the various markers within individual colonies. As with the human ES cell lines, LIF was not sufficient to prevent differentiation in some cases, resulting in the formation of embryoid bodies containing a variety of cell types and tissues. A peculiar feature of the cultures was the extreme difficulty of disaggregating the colonies with trypsin/EDTA (ethylenediaminetetraacetic acid) preparations, leading to low plating efficiencies, inability to grow to high cell densities or derive clonal lines. As with human ES cells, the EG cultures had a relatively long cell cycle time and were passaged approximately once a week.

The development of human ES and EG cell lines has stimulated a barrage of media attention, ranging from excitement over the potential for therapeutic applications to consternation over the use of human embryos or fetal tissue. We will first discuss the research applications of human ES or EG cells (using the term ES cells for simplicity) and then discuss the legal issues surrounding research with these cells.

Research applications

The ability of human ES cells to differentiate in vitro to form embryoid bodies serves as a useful experimental model to explore aspects of embryogenesis, particularly the formation and differentiation of various cell lineages. Although the variability observed in embryoid bodies does not replicate the highly regulated process of normal embryogenesis, the timing of appearance of many structures and cells mimics the time course of some developmental events (Hole, 1999; Doevendans et al., 2000). Numerous processes, such as angiogenesis, hematopoiesis, and cardiomyocyte formation, all occur within a time frame similar to that seen in the embryo. Culture of human ES cells allows these processes to be observed and dissected on a molecular level within the defined conditions of in vitro culture. Recently, experiments with human ES cells demonstrated that various growth factors could skew the differentiation of ES cell aggregates towards cell populations that express markers representative of each of the three embryonic germ layers, although in all cases, the resulting differentiated cells contained a mixture of cell phenotypes. This work confirms the notion that soluble growth factors can influence the fate of ES cell differentiation (Schuldiner et al., 2000).

Ironically, the foundation of comparable work in the mouse system is relatively weak since most efforts have been directed to studying normal embryogenesis. However, there has been progress in establishing culture conditions to derive neuronal precursors (Strubing et al., 1995; Okabe et al., 1996; Brustle et al., 1997; Lee et al., 2000), cardiomyocytes (Maltsev et al., 1993; Wobus et al., 1994, 1997; Klug et al., 1996) and hematopoietic cells (Schmitt et al., 1991; Snodgrass et al., 1992; Keller et al., 1993). The extensive experience with genetic engineering in mouse ES cells could prove to be extremely valuable to test genetic function in human ES cells within the context of the in vitro differentiation system. As in

the situation of using murine ES cells to create mouse models of human genetic diseases, it should be possible to replicate known genetic abnormalities in human ES cells and subsequently test the effects on cellular differentiation. In this way, research on human ES cells could lead to better understanding of the mechanisms underlying common birth defects. Many processes that normally occur during embryogenesis, such as rapid cell proliferation, cell migration, epithelial–mesenchymal transitions, and apoptosis can go awry later in life, leading to cancer. An understanding of these processes within the context of ES cell differentiation could lead to approaches to control various aspects of tumorigenesis.

As our understanding of cellular differentiation grows, it should be possible to generate populations of defined cell types from ES cultures. This may require careful administration of growth factors or inhibitory molecules and provision of appropriate substrates, as well as physical selection based on cell surface molecules. Once defined populations have been obtained, they will be valuable for a variety of drug and toxicity testing. Currently, the pharmaceutical industry is investing heavily in high-throughput assays for therapeutic compounds. The specificity of the assay is critical for selecting the best potential drug candidates. Human ES cells could provide phenotypically or functionally defined cell types that would enhance the efficacy of the tests. Functionally defined cell types could also be used in toxicity tests of environmental compounds. For example, murine ES cell differentiation into cardiomyocytes has been used to measure the embryotoxicity of teratogenic compounds (Scholz et al., 1999).

Therapeutic applications of human embryonic stem cells

The tremendous potential for ES cells to improve the treatment of a variety of diseases relies on the ability of ES cells to form any cell in the body. Differentiated cell types could be produced to replace damaged or diseased cells and tissues. The experimental paradigms that have been described involve transplantation of murine ES cell derivatives into various animal models of disease or injury. Neuronal precursors derived from embryoid bodies have been transplanted into the ventricles of fetal rats during a time of extensive neurogenesis (Brustle et al., 1997). Within two weeks of birth, both neuronal and astrocytic derivatives were identified in multiple locations in the brain. Neuronal derivatives were primarily found in gray matter, while astrocyte derivatives were located in white matter. In a model of paralysis, neuronal derivatives were transplanted into rat spinal cords nine days after traumatic injury (McDonald et al., 1999). After two to five weeks, derivatives of the cells were found up to 8 mm away from the transplantation site and some of the rats demonstrated improvement in hind limb function. Glial precursors have also been generated from ES cells and transplanted into the spinal cords of neonatal myelin-deficient rats, and into the ventricles of fetal rats (Brustle et al., 1999). In both cases, the ES derivatives migrated from the transplantation site and formed myelin sheaths. An enriched population of cardiomyocytes was obtained by genetic selection based on the cardiac myosin heavy chain promoter and was grafted into the hearts of dystrophic mice (Klug et al., 1996). The ES-derived cells integrated into the heart muscle and remained viable for the length of the seven-week experiment. A selection approach has also been used to derive insulin-secreting cells from embryoid bodies. The cells were able to correct hypoglycemia in a mouse model of diabetes (Soria et al., 2000). Hematopoietic cells, including lymphoid cells, have also been derived from ES cells and shown to have long-term repopulating capability following transplantation (Hole, 1999). The function of a number of genes in hematopoiesis has been elegantly tested using this system.

Untested paradigms for ES cell transplantation include derivation of liver cells for hepatitis, muscle cells for muscular dystrophies, skin cells to treat burns, and bone or cartilage to treat osteoarthritis. In addition to restoring function of diseased or damaged tissue, ES cell derivatives could be used as delivery agents for genetic therapies. Derivatives of ES cells could possibly be used to modulate the immune system in order to treat such autoimmune diseases as rheumatoid arthritis, multiple sclerosis, or juvenile onset diabetes. The impact on medical treatment and, hopefully, on quality of life could be enormous.

Legal issues surrounding human embryonic stem cell derivation

Controversies regarding the derivation of human ES cells center primarily on the source of tissue, either human preimplantation embryos from IVF procedures or fetal tissues from therapeutic terminations of pregnancy. US federal regulations concerning the use of fetal tissue for research purposes have existed since 1975 (National Bioethics Advisory Council) (NBAC, 1999). An essential aspect of the process is to protect the patient and insulate the decision to proceed with a pregnancy termination from the decision to use the tissue for research. There must not be any possibility of coercion based on payment or other compensation for proceeding with a termination, including a protocol to ensure that the counselors and physicians involved in the termination procedure do not receive any financial or other benefit derived from the research project. Institutional Review Board oversight of the research plan and the consenting process is required. In 1993, separate legislation was enacted regarding the use of fetal tissue for transplantation purposes (NBAC, 1999). Currently, work with human EG cells has not progressed to the point of use in transplantations and it is not clear whether the fetal tissue transplantation regulations would apply to the use of cells derived from embryonic germ cell lines. The distinction between the use of fetal tissue and the use of preimplantation embryos is evident in the fact that, in the USA, there is currently a ban on the use federal funds to support research involving human embryos, whereas, fetal tissue research is eligible for federal funding. Current NIH guidelines also recommend that research using previously derived human ES cell lines from either source should also be eligible for federal funding.

The legal issues surrounding the use of human preimplantation embryos are substantially more complicated because of the greater number of potential sources. Currently, the most readily available source of human preimplantation embryos is from IVF procedures performed for the treatment of infertile couples. A closely related source are embryos derived from donated oocytes and donated sperm. A final source would be embryos derived by transfer of an adult cell nucleus to a donated oocyte in which the genetic material has been removed.

With recent increases in the effectiveness of IVF procedures, more and more couples have unused, frozen embryos as a result of discontinuation of additional treatment because of successful pregnancy. It is estimated that tens of thousands of frozen embryos are stored in the USA alone. Given the current limited use of embryo donation, only a very small fraction of the frozen embryos will ever be used to establish a pregnancy. The others will be stored indefinitely, discarded, or used in research. All decisions to use preimplantation embryos for research must proceed in a manner that preserves the unique moral status of the embryos. In the UK, the Human Fertilization and Embryology Authority (HFEA, www.hfea.gov.uk) establishes guidelines and monitors IVF clinics, including their research activities. The HFEA Code of Practice of 1998 requires that each research project be licensed by the HFEA and that application for a license should be preceded by ethics committee review as well as peer review to determine scientific merit. Research that is acceptable is restricted to investigation into the causes of congenital abnormalities or miscarriages, techniques to improve contraception, the treatment of infertility, or the detection of genetic abnormalities in preimplantation embryos. Under these guidelines, the derivation of human ES cell lines could be licensed by the HFEA. In late January 2001, the House of Commons voted to permit stem cell research using embryos up to 14 days of age and also to permit the use of somatic cells to generate embryos for the derivation of ES cells (therapeutic cloning, see below). Final approval for ES cell derivation and research in the UK was reached early in 2002.

Very few countries have established national governing bodies with authority similar to the HFEA. In the USA there is no federal agency empowered to license human embryo research. Some individual state laws specifically prohibit human embryo research. US federal law denies the use of federal funds to support research on human embryos, although recently the NBAC and the NIH recommended that federal funds be made available for research with existing human ES cells. Despite the recommendation and the support of numerous scientists and patient advocacy groups (Perry, 2000), allocation of funds to support such research is expected to remain a hotly contested political issue in the USA. In Europe, human embryo research falls under the Council of Europe Treaty Number 164 from the 1997 Convention for the Protection of Human Rights and Dignity of the Human Being with Regard to the Application of Biology and Medicine. Article 18 of Chapter V states that research should ensure adequate protection for the embryo but does not explicitly exclude the use of embryos for derivation of ES cells.

In contrast, the use of donated gametes to generate embryos for research purposes is categorically prohibited by the European treaty. The recommendations of NBAC and existing US regulations also oppose the use of federal funds for research on embryos created solely for research purposes. However, such research could proceed with funding from private sources. In contrast, the guidelines of HFEA do not specifically prohibit the creation of embryos for research purposes.

The final potential source of embryos for the derivation of ES cell lines has the potential benefit of tailoring the ES cells to an individual patient. By using donated oocytes to reprogram the genome from a patient's own cells and form an embryo, it would be possible to derive ES cells with a genetic component identical to the patient. Such cells would eliminate any problems with immune rejection. This approach to the generation of ES lines involves nuclear transfer, which has been used to clone sheep and other animals (Wilmut et al., 1997). The term therapeutic cloning, is used in order to distinguish the process from reproductive cloning, in which the reprogrammed embryo is allowed to develop into a fetus. Although reproductive cloning has garnered considerable opposition and is discussed in Chapter 13, therapeutic cloning has received some favorable support. In the UK, both the HFEA and the Human Genetics Advisory Commission have recommended that research involving therapeutic cloning proceed; however, a final decision has not been made (Dickson and Smaglik, 2000).

Conclusions

As the potential for the tremendous therapeutic value of ES cells grows, controversy over this field of research also grows. Increasing pressure from patient advocacy groups intent on rapidly developing treatments is balanced by groups opposed to the use of human fetal tissue and embryos and also by individuals urging restraint in the face of the uncertain ethical status of therapeutic cloning and the unknown potential ethical dilemmas raised by this technology (Young, 2000). Advocates for the use of ES cells also compete with surprising developments in the field of adult stem cells, which have revealed an amazing level of plasticity in hematopoietic, mesenchymal, and neuronal stem cell populations. Should it prove possible to isolate sufficient numbers of stem cells from adult organs and also to reprogram the cells into fates appropriate for treatment, the need for continued derivation of ES cells might be diminished. At this time, however, concurrent research in the areas of ES and adult stem cells is most likely to yield complementary information of the processes directing differentiation into various cell fates.

The future role of reproductive technologists in this field remains unclear. Certainly, the derivation of human ES cells depended on advances made in embryo culture that permitted the growth of healthy blastocysts. Continued derivation of ES lines will require the procurement of embryos from IVF clinics. If therapeutic cloning is ever employed in the derivation of ES cells, reproductive technologists

have the technical expertise and equipment to perform enucleation of donor oocytes and nuclear fusions. These procedures will, undoubtedly, be permitted in some countries and prohibited in others. It will be up to individuals within the field to determine their level of involvement in this rapidly changing area of research.

Numerous hurdles remain before the full potential of ES cell therapeutics can be tapped. Methods to grow large numbers of undifferentiated cells will need to be optimized. A means to control the initial differentiation process in order to generate precursors of a particular lineage would greatly facilitate differentiation of specific cell types. Elucidation of defined culture conditions, including growth factors and extracellular substrates, to specify differentiation into specific cell types may reduce the need for methods to select for a particular type of cell. Methods to track the cells following transplantation will need to be employed in order to determine the extent to which transplanted cells move throughout the body, and the risk of transplanted cells forming abnormal structures or even tumors. Procedures to manage the potential immune reaction to transplanted cells will also need to be developed unless procedures to establish ES lines from individual patients are used. Based on the number of surprises and controversies arising in stem cell biology at the turn of the twentieth century, the path to ES transplantation therapies will be an exciting one.

REFERENCES

Bjornson, C.R., Rietze, R.L., Reynolds, B.A., Magli, M.C., and Vescovi, A.L. (1999). Turning brain into blood: a hematopoietic fate adopted by adult neural stem cells in vivo. *Science*, **283**, 534–7.

Brazelton, T.R., Rossi, F.M.V., Keshet, G.I., and Blau, H.M. (2000). From marrow to brain: expression of neuronal phenotypes in adult mice. *Science*, **290**, 1775–9.

Brustle, O., Spiro, A.C., Karram, K., et al. (1997). In vitro-generated neural precursors participate in mammalian brain development. *Proceedings of the National Academy of Sciences USA*, **94**, 14809–14.

Brustle, O., Jones, K.N., Learish, R.D., et al. (1999). Embryonic stem cell-derived glial precursors: a source of myelinating transplants. *Science*, **285**, 754–6.

Chen, L.R., Shuie, Y.L., Bertolini, L., Medrano, J.F., BonDurant, R.H., and Anderson, G.B. (1999). Establishment of pluripotent cell lines from porcine preimplantation embryos. *Theriogenology*, **52**, 195–212.

Dickson, D. and Smaglik, P. (2000). UK government backs change in law over stem-cell research. *Nature*, **406**, 815.

Doetschman, T.C., Eistetter, H., Katz, M., Schmidt, W., and Kemler, R. (1985). The in vitro development of blastocyst-derived embryonic stem cell lines: formation of visceral yolk sac, blood islands and myocardium. *Journal of Embryology and Experimental Morphology*, **87**, 27–45.

Doetschman, T., Shull, M., Kier, A., and Coffin, J.D. (1993). Embryonic stem cell model systems for vascular morphogenesis and cardiac disorders. *Hypertension*, **22**, 618–29.

Doevendans, P.A., Kubalak, S.W., An, R.H., et al. (2000). Differentiation of cardiomyocytes in floating embryoid bodies is comparable to fetal cardiomyocytes. *Journal of Molecular and Cellular Cardiology*, **32**, 839–51.

Eglitis, M.A. and Mezey, E. (1997). Hematopoietic cells differentiate into both microglia and macroglia in the brains of adult mice. *Proceedings of the National Academy of Sciences USA*, **94**, 4080–5.

Evans, M.J. and Kaufman, M.H. (1981). Establishment in culture of pluripotential cells from mouse embryos. *Nature*, **292**, 154–6.

Gage, F.H. (2000). Mammalian neural stem cells. *Science*, **287**, 1433–8.

Gussoni, E., Soneoka, Y., Strickland, C.D., et al. (1999). Dystrophin expression in the *mdx* mouse restored by stem cell transplantation. *Nature*, **401**, 390–4.

Hole, N. (1999). Embryonic stem cell-derived haematopoiesis. *Cells, Tissues and Organs*, **165**, 181–9.

Keller, G., Kennedy, M., Papayannopoulou, T., and Wiles, M.V. (1993). Hematopoietic commitment during embryonic stem cell differentiation in culture. *Molecular and Cellular Biology*, **13**, 473–86.

Klug, M.G., Soonpaa, M.H., Koh, G.Y., and Field, L.J. (1996). Genetically selected cardiomyocytes from differentiating embronic stem cells form stable intracardiac grafts. *Journal of Clinical Investigation*, **98**, 216–24.

Kondziolka, D., Wechsler, L., Goldstein, S., et al. (2000). Transplantation of cultured human neuronal cells for patients with stroke. *Neurology*, **55**, 565–9.

Lee, S.H., Lumelsky, N., Studer, L., Auerbach, J.M., and McKay, R.D. (2000). Efficient generation of midbrain and hindbrain neurons from mouse embryonic stem cells. *Nature Biotechnology*, **18**, 675–9.

Liu, X., Wu, H., Loring, J., et al. (1997). Trisomy eight in ES cells is a common potential problem in gene targeting and interferes with germ line transmission. *Developmental Dynamics*, **209**, 85–91.

Maltsev, V.A., Rohwedel, J., Hescheler, J., and Wobus, A.M. (1993). Embryonic stem cells differentiate in vitro into cardiomyocytes representing sinusnodal, atrial and ventricular cell types. *Mechanisms of Development*, **44**, 41–50.

Martin, G.R. (1981). Isolation of a pluripotent cell line from early mouse embryos cultured in medium conditioned by teratocarcinoma stem cells. *Proceedings of the National Academy of Sciences USA*, **78**, 7634–8.

Matsui, Y., Zsebo, K., and Hogan, B.L. (1992). Derivation of pluripotential embryonic stem cells from murine primordial germ cells in culture. *Cell*, **70**, 841–7.

McDonald, J.W., Liu, X.Z., Qu, Y., et al. (1999). Transplanted embryonic stem cells survive, differentiate and promote recovery in injured rat spinal cord [see comments]. *Nature Medicine*, **5**, 1410–12.

Mezey, E., Chandross, K.J., Harta, G., Maki, R.A., and McKercher, S.R. (2000). Turning blood into brain: cells bearing neuronal antigens generated in vivo from bone marrow. *Science*, **290**, 1779–82.

Mountford, P., Nichols, J., Zevnik, B., O'Brien, C., and Smith, A. (1998). Maintenance of pluripotential embryonic stem cells by stem cell selection. *Reproduction, Fertility and Development*, **10**, 527–33.

NBAC (1999). Ethical issues in human stem cell research. www.bioethics.gov

Nichols, J., Evans, E.P., and Smith, A.G. (1990). Establishment of germ-line-competent embryonic stem (ES) cells using differentiation inhibiting activity. *Development*, **110**, 1341–8.

Okabe, S., Forsberg-Nilsson, K., Spiro, A.C., Segal, M., and McKay, R.D. (1996). Development of neuronal precursor cells and functional postmitotic neurons from embryonic stem cells in vitro. *Mechanisms of Development*, **59**, 89–102.

Perry, D. (2000). Patients' voices: the powerful sound in the stem cell debate. *Science*, **287**, 1423.

Peyron, A. (1939). Faits nouveaux relatifs a l'origine et a l'histogenese des embyomes. *Bulletin Association Française Etude Cancer*, **28**, 658–81.

Prelle, K., Vassiliev, I.M., Vassilieva, S.G., Wolf, E., and Wobus, A.M. (1999). Establishment of pluripotent cell lines from vertebrate species – present status and future prospects. *Cells, Tissues and Organs*, **165**, 220–36.

Resnick, J.L., Bixler, L.S., Cheng, L., and Donovan, P.J. (1992). Long-term proliferation of mouse primordial germ cells in culture. *Nature*, **359**, 550–1.

Reubinoff, B.E., Pera, M.F., Fong, C., Trounson, A., and Bongso,

A. (2000). Embryonic stem cell lines from human blastocysts: somatic differentiation in vitro. *Nature Biotechnology*, **18**, 399–404.

Rossant, J. and Nagy, A. (1995). Genome engineering: the new mouse genetics. *Nature Medicine*, **1**, 592–4.

Schmitt, R.M., Bruyns, E., and Snodgrass, H.R. (1991). Hematopoietic development of embryonic stem cells in vitro: cytokine and receptor gene expression. *Genes and Development*, **5**, 728–40.

Scholz, G., Pohl, I., Genschow, E., Klemm, M., and Spielmann, H. (1999). Embryotoxicity screening using embryonic stem cells in vitro: correlation to in vivo teratogenicity. *Cells, Tissues and Organs*, **165**, 203–11.

Schuldiner, M., Yanuka, O., Itskovitz-Eldor, J., Melton, D.A., and Benvenisty, N. (2000). Effects of eight growth factors on the differentiation of cells derived from human embryonic stem cells. *Proceedings of the National Academy of Sciences USA*, **97**, 11307–12.

Shamblott, M.J., Axelman, J., Wang, S., et al. (1998). Derivation of pluripotent stem cells from cultured human primordial germ cells. *Proceedings of the National Academy of Sciences USA*, **95**, 13726–31.

Snodgrass, H.R., Schmitt, R.M., and Bruyns, E. (1992). Embryonic stem cells and in vitro hematopoiesis. *Journal of Cellular Biochemistry*, **49**, 225–30.

Solter, D. and Gearhart, J. (1999). Putting stem cells to work. *Science*, **283**, 1468–70.

Soria, B., Roche, E., Berna, G., et al. (2000). Insulin-secreting cells derived from embryonic stem cells normalize glycemia in streptozotocin-induced diabetic mice. *Diabetes*, **49**, 157–62.

Strubing, C.G., Anhert-Hilger, G., Shan, J., Wiedenmann, B., Hescheler, J., and Wobus, A.M. (1995). Differentiation of pluripotent embryonic stem cells into the neuronal lineage in vitro gives rise to mature inhibitory and excitatory neurons. *Mechanisms of Development*, **53**, 275–87.

Thomson, J.A., Kalishman, J., Golos, T.G., et al. (1995). Isolation of a primate embryonic stem cell line. *Proceedings of the National Academy of Sciences USA*, **92**, 7844–8.

Thomson, J.A., Kalishman, J., Golos, T.G., et al. (1996). Pluripotent cell lines derived from common marmoset (*Callithrix jacchus*) blastocysts. *Biology of Reproduction*, **55**, 254–9.

Thomson, J.A., Itskovitz-Eldor, J., Shapiro, S.S., et al. (1998). Embryonic stem cell lines derived from human blastocysts. *Science*, **282**, 1145–7.

van der Kooy, D. and Weiss, S. (2000). Why stem cells? *Science*, **287**, 1439–41.

Wilmut, I., Schnieke, A.E., McWhir, J., Kind, A.J., and Campbell, K.H. (1997). Viable offspring derived from fetal and adult mammalian cells. *Nature*, **385**, 810–13.

Wobus, A.M., Kleppisch, T., Maltsev, V., and Hescheler, J. (1994). Cardiomyocyte-like cells differentiated in vitro from embryonic carcinoma cells P19 are characterized by functional expression of adrenoceptors and Ca^{2+} channels. *In Vitro Cell and Developmental Biology of Animals*, **30A**, 425–34.

Wobus, A.M., Kaomei, G., Shan, J., et al. (1997). Retinoic acid accelerates embryonic stem cell-derived cardiac differentiation and enhances development of ventricular cardiomyocytes. *Journal of Cellular and Molecular Cardiology*, **29**, 1525–39.

Young, F.E. (2000). A time for restraint. *Science*, **287**, 1424.

11

Modification of the male genome by gene and spermatogonial transplantation

Peter J. Donovan[1], Michael D. Griswold[2], and the late Lonnie D. Russell[3]

[1]Kimmel Cancer Center, Thomas Jefferson University, Philadelphia, USA
[2]Washington State University, Pullman
[3]Formerly of Southern Illinois University School of Medicine, Carbondale,USA

Introduction

Virtually all offspring are chosen by parents or relatives that find certain genetic traits in their mates desirable. We have come to believe that this type of natural selection is the acceptable way that reproduction transpires. Whether it is deemed ethically acceptable or not, assisted reproduction techniques (ART) influence the genetic selection process. In some instances ART rescues defective reproductive systems, perhaps those that are genetically defective. ART techniques provide donor gametes with entirely different or unexpected genetic make-up. ART may be allowing genetically defective gametes to fertilize eggs: gametes that would have not otherwise been successful under natural conditions. We have allowed women to reproduce at ages beyond those considered normal, ages in which time-related mutations may have accumulated. Thus, there has been a general acceptance of ART to fulfill the need of couples to have offspring. Although not intentional, we have come to accept purposeful genetic alteration to overcome barriers to natural reproduction.

Purposeful genetic modification extends beyond the couple's need to have children. There are numerous current efforts to utilize gene therapy to reverse or cure disease processes or even to prevent transmission of undesirable genes to future generations. Gene therapy may have as its purpose the induction of somatic cell mutations that are beneficial only to the individual being treated without the need for the genetic alteration to be passed on to the offspring.

Purposeful genetic modification is a double-edged sword, having a negative side. During gene therapy, there is the possibility that germ cells will incur stable transfection through accidental introduction of the vector to the germ cell line. Genetic alteration in the germ cell line is a consequence of many chemotherapeutic regimens and is monitored in safety testing of pharmaceuticals and food products.

The male and female mammalian reproductive systems are not equally susceptible to stable transfection. In the female, gametes are arrested in development, specifically in prophase of meiosis, prior to birth. They do not resume meiosis until ovulation, and then only one or a few gametes at a time. The male produces sperm continually from the time of puberty. Cell division is constantly occurring in the testis. In fact, it has been said that the human male produces 1000 sperm each time his heart beats. Consequently, the male appears to be more susceptible to purposeful modification of the genome.

This review focuses on the status of purposeful genetic modification of the male germ cell line. It should be noted that this rapidly growing field is in its infancy.

Spermatogonial stem cell transplantation

Spermatogonial transplantation involves removing spermatogonia from a donor and replacing them back into a recipient testis, where they will initiate spermatogenesis. The donor spermatogonia can be harvested from the same animal, the same species,

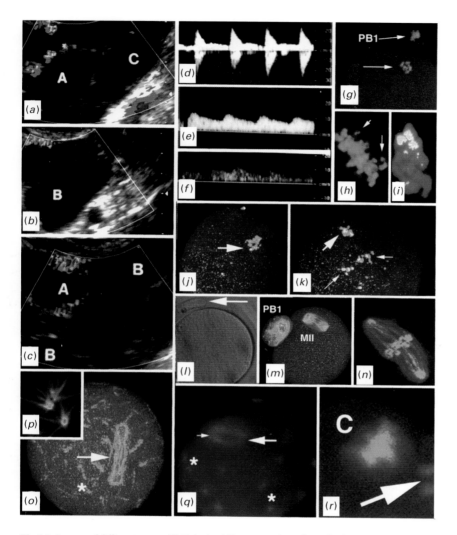

Fig. 6.1. Images of different types of follicle. (*a–c*) Representative color pulsed Doppler ultrasonographic images of three types of follicle (A, B, and C) on the same ovary that have different intrafollicular oxygen contents and perifollicular blood flow characteristics. (*d–f*) A characteristic waveform pattern obtained by pulsed Doppler ultrasonography for types A (*f*), B (*d*), and C (*e*) follicles. (*g–k*) Chromosomal configurations (arrows) in living metaphase II (MII) stage human oocytes from follicles with different dissolved oxygen contents and perifollicular blood flow characteristics after staining with DNA-specific probes and examined by conventional (*g*) and scanning laser confocal microscopy (*h–k*). In comparison with the normal MII configurations observed in oocytes from follicles with relatively high perifollicular blood flow (*g*), chromosomal organization in oocytes with poor or undetectable flow were often displaced from (*j,k*) or abnormally arranged on the metaphase spindle (*h,i*). (*l–r*) DNA fluorescence (*n,r*), anti-γ-tubulin immunofluorescence (*m–q*) in normal appearing MII mouse oocytes (*l*) ovulated after repeated cycles of superovulation. A normal spindle with normal equatorial chromosomal alignment (*m, n*) are shown. The asterisks indicate regions of disorganized microtubular staining (*o*) and cytoplasmic asters (*q*) in conventional epifluorescent images. Two of these cytoplasmic asters are shown as scanning laser confocal image (*p*). The spindle at metaphase II is noted by an arrow (in *o* and *q*) and two displaced chromosomes are shown with an arrow in *r*. PB1, first polar body. (Parts *a–k* are from Van Blerkom et al., 1997; parts *l–r* are from Van Blerkom and Davis, 2001.)

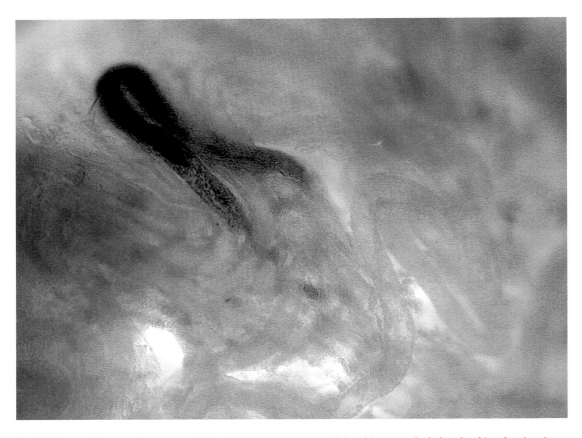

Fig. 11.1. Successfully transplanted spermatogenesis using a LacZ donor will show blue-stained tubules when histochemistry is performed for β-galactosidase.

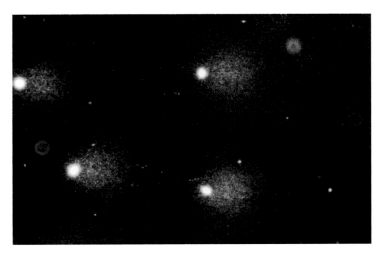

Fig. 16.3. The single-cell electrophoretic COMET assay for assessing the integrity of sperm DNA. Computation of the percentage of the fluorochrome signal that lies in the tail of the Comet provides an indication of the degree of DNA fragmentation.

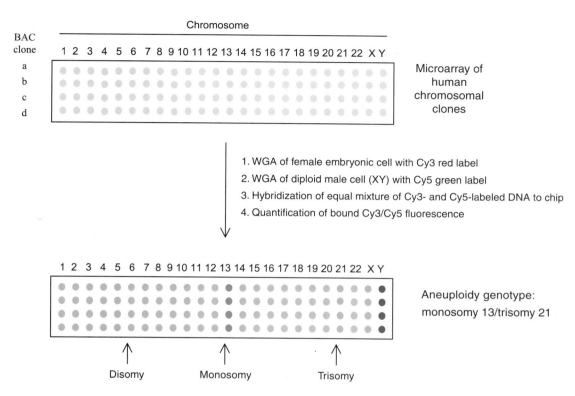

Fig. 12.6. Single-cell analysis of chromosomal aneuploidy using a microarray of human BAC clones. The sets of four BAC clones represent different target loci on each of the 24 chromosomes. The ratio of the bound dyes Cy3 (red) and Cy5 (green) to the microarray is diagnostic for chromosome number. A 1:1 ratio (orange) indicates disomy, a 1:2 ratio (green) indicates monosomy and a 3:2 ratio (red) indicates a trisomy. The ratio of Cy3/Cy5 bound to the X and Y clones varies according to the sex of the test cell. For a female (X,X) test cell, the expected Cy3/Cy5 ratio would be 2:1 for X clones and 2:0 for Y clones. For a male (X,Y) cell, the expected Cy3/Cy5 ratio would be 1:1 for X and Y clones. For example, a cell from a patient with Klinefelter's syndrome should produce ratios of 1:1 for the 22 autosomal clones, 2:1 for X clones and 1:1 for Y clones. In the case of a female cell with a monosomy 13/trisomy 21 genotype as shown here, the expected Cy3/Cy5 ratios would be 1:1 for chromosomes 1–12, 14–20 and 22 (disomy), 1:2 for chromosome 13 (monosomy), 3:2 for chromosome 21 (trisomy), 2:1 for chromosome X (two copies of X), and 2:0 for chromosome Y (absence of Y).

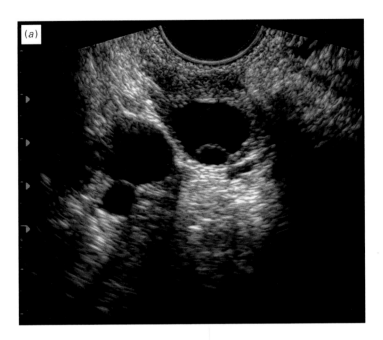

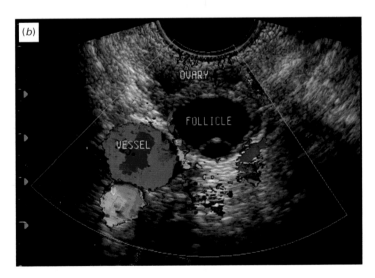

Fig. 18.7. Preovulatory follicles immediately before oocyte retrieval.
(*a*) Gray-scale image. (*b*) Doppler image.

or a different species than the recipient. The word "spermatogonia" in the phrase "spermatogonial transplantation" is a slight misnomer and some confusion might result. Although spermatogonia are the cell type giving rise to other adult cell types of the male germ cell lineage, not all spermatogonia are suitable for spermatogonial transplantation. Numerous types of spermatogonium are found in the testis of mammals, but only a small fraction are *stem cell* spermatogonia. Stem cells are the only germ cells of the testis that have both the division characteristic of self-renewal and differentiation in that they give rise to cells that are committed to the spermatogenic process (de Roiij and Russell, 2000). Therefore, because cell divisions occur in the male, the stem cells are the functional cells employed in spermatogonial stem cell transplantation (SSCT).

A change in the genome of testicular germ cells, other than stem cells, is usually of less impact to the organism than is a change in the stem cell. Stem cells actively produce sperm throughout the lifespan of the individual. If a cell other than a stem cell is genetically altered, the consequences are minor. Genomic changes in cells other than stem cells are limited to the progeny of the subsequent division of that spermatogonium and are only present in the period that it takes the progeny of that one cell to form sperm and for these sperm to go through the epididymis and out of the excurrent duct system.

The spermatogonial stem cell is positioned within the seminiferous tubule in the basal compartment of the testis. Here it is exposed to the elements of the circulatory and lymphatic systems. On the one hand, circulating vectors or mutagenic agents have theoretical access to all spermatogonia (Russell, 1989). On the other hand, virtually all spermatocytes and spermatids are sequestered by junctions formed by Sertoli cells into an adluminal compartment that is far less accessible to circulating molecules in the physiological situation.

The technique

The literature relating to the technique of spermatogonial transplantation is manageable; most is refer-enced herein. SSCT, as pioneered in the laboratory of Dr. Ralph Brinster in 1994 (Brinster and Avarbock, 1994; Brinster and Zimmerman, 1994), is now successfully performed in several laboratories. The technique involves microinjection of a donor cell suspension containing spermatogonial stem cells among many other cell types into one of three sites of a recipient testis: cells can be microinjected into the lumen of seminiferous tubules using a micromanipulator; they can be injected by hand or by micromanipulator into the rete through the testis capsule; they can be injected into the rete through the bundle of efferent ducts (Ogawa et al., 1997). A successful injection, no matter the site of introduction of cells, is dependent on retrograde flow of the donor cell suspension from the rete into other seminiferous tubules.

Prior to microinjection, testis cells are first treated with enzymes to produce a cell suspension. Approximately 5×10^7 cells/ml (Dobrinski et al., 1999a) are used to fill 30–100% of seminiferous tubules. A dye such as trypan blue is generally used to identify the extent of filling of seminiferous tubules. Hopefully, the suspension of cells from prepubertal and adult animals contains the stem cell spermatogonia. It is important to obtain single-cell preparations for the injection, as clumping will clog the injection micropipette.

The recipient testis must be virtually devoid of spermatogenesis. There are two ways to insure that there is a germ cell-depleted recipient. The recipient may be a genetically sterile male whose somatic cells are capable of supporting spermatogenesis (Brinster and Avarbock, 1994). The most common recipient model is the white spotted (W) locus mouse, the germ cells of which lack a functional c-Kit receptor (Brinster and Zimmerman, 1994). Depletion of spermatogenesis may be accomplished by using agents such as busulfan that are cytotoxic to germ cells (Brinster and Avarbock, 1994; Brinster and Zimmerman, 1994). Although busulfan is useful, it is also cytotoxic to bone marrow cells and the dose must be tested in rodents to determine if a particular strain will tolerate the ensuing white cell loss. It is likely that busulfan will not destroy all stem cell spermatogonia and that, with time, there will be both transplanted and reinitiated endogenous spermatogenesis. In this event, a donor marker is needed to distinguish between the two types of spermatogenesis. The marker most commonly used is from a transgenic donor with cells expressing the *LacZ* gene encoding for β-galactosidase. Enzyme activity is seen as a blue reaction product with the substrate 5-bromo-4-chloro-3-indolyl-β-D-galactoside (X-gal) (Fig. 11.1). If a W-locus recipient is used, then any active spermatogeneis is likely to be from the donor (Parreira et al., 1998).

After transplantation, the donor cells are allowed to colonize the recipient testis for periods of several months. The recipient testis can be histologically examined or histochemically analyzed for β-galactosidase activity. The recipient epididymis can be examined for the presence of sperm or the recipient animal can be bred to determine if there are donor-derived offspring. The fine details of the technique are numerous and we suggest the more comprehensive reviews be consulted (Ogawa et al., 1997; Nagano and Brinster, 1998).

Basic results of spermatogonial stem cell transplantation

The most obvious result of SSCT is that cells transplanted into the lumen of recipient seminiferous tubules are capable of dividing and forming sperm. Although stem cells are injected into the tubular lumen, it is apparent that there is some translocation and reorganization of cells within the tubule that results in a normal seminiferous tubule architecture, with stem cell division from the basal compartment leading to more mature cells near the lumen (Russell and Brinster, 1996; Russell et al., 1996). The implication is that the stem cells injected into the tubular lumen must first move to the base of the tubule through Sertoli–Sertoli tight junctions to reside in their normal position along the tunica propria. The successful reorganization of seminiferous tubules after transplantation suggests that spermatogonial translocation is capable of taking place (Parreira et

al., 1999), although the mechanism has not been demonstrated.

Studies have shown that all injected donor somatic cells and most germ cell types are lost shortly after transplantation and that these are engulfed by the recipient's endogenous Sertoli cells (Parreira et al., 1999). Only a very few donor spermatocytes seem to live and complete meiosis. About a month after mouse-to-mouse or rat-to-mouse transplantation, the stem cells have developed into clones of spermatogonia and young spermatocytes and these terminated development as sperm after two months (Parreira et al., 1998). About 30% of the testis is colonized three months post-transplantation. Spermatogenesis is initially confined to small regions within each seminiferous tubule and spermatogenesis then proceeds to expand in both directions along the tubule, advancing at a rate of over 50 μm/day (Nagano et al., 1999).

At least some sperm formed by mouse-to-mouse transplantation are capable of fertilizing eggs and producing offspring (Brinster and Avarbock, 1994). Thus, the transplantation technique has been shown to be a novel transgenic method whereby the entire genome can be substituted utilizing congeneic, allogeneic, and xenogenic protocols.

It appears that the purer the population of donor spermatogonia from which one transplants the greater the transplant success. Markers can be used to assist purification of spermatogonia; animals can be used with testes richer in spermatogonia by virtue of a condition, such as cryptorchidism, that depletes more advanced germ cell types; or one can use cell surface antigens that allow affinity purification of spermatogonia (Shinohara et al., 1999).

Can fertility be restored in infertile animals using SSCT? Testes that possess no germ cells more advanced than spermatogonia and possess few or no spermatogonia have been made fertile using stem cell transplants (Brinster and Avarbock, 1994). In this situation, sterile donors are used with defective somatic cell products (stem cell factor, the ligand for c-Kit), and normal germ cells (Sl mutants). The sterile recipients have c-Kit receptor-deficient germ cells (W-locus mutants) but normal somatic cells. When sterile donors and sterile recipients are used to place both fully functional germ cells and fully functional somatic cells together as the Sl-locus into W-locus mutants, respectively, then fertility ensues (Ogawa et al., 2000).

Transplants other than from donor to congeneic recipient are the most successful since immuno-compatibility is not a factor. However, to transplant across species, it is necessary to use recipients with compromised or virtually deficient immune systems, e.g., nude or SCID mice (Clouthier et al., 1996; Russell and Brinster, 1996). The extent to which strain differences can be tolerated is not known.

Xenogenic transplants have been used to show that the timing of spermatogenesis is programmed by the genome of the germ cell and is apparently not under the influence of the Sertoli cell. When germ cells were transplanted from a rat to a busulfan-treated mouse, the recipient could carry on both transplanted rat spermatogenesis and endogenous mouse spermatogenesis, each occurring at two different rates and each occurring at the characteristic rate of its donor-derived species (França et al., 1998).

The SSCT technique was recently used to solve an old controversy regarding how spermatogenesis was regulated by androgen. There is considerable literature suggesting that germ cells have androgen receptors and an equally large body of literature suggesting that they do not. If germ cells have functional androgen receptors, they may respond directly to stimulation by Leydig cell testosterone. If not, they would most likely be stimulated in their developmental progress by nearby somatic cells. By transplanting androgen-insensitive germ cells from one mouse, having testicular feminization syndrome, into a normal recipient, it was demonstrated that spermatogenesis leading to sperm formation would result (Johnston et al., 2000). Thus, testosterone action appears to be mediated, not by germ cells, but by somatic cells.

The SSCT technique allows one to discriminate between the effects of germ cell and Sertoli cell in animals with defective spermatogenesis. Since mouse knockout models show testicular phenotypes, there is a need to determine if the defect is in the somatic cells or the germ cells. To-date, two such experiments have been performed. In both experiments, germ cells were transplanted from a knockout animal into a normal animal. Since full transplanted spermatogenesis ensued, these results show that the germ cells are not primarily responsible for the phenotype of the null mutant. This then, implicates somatic cells as the primary cause of the defect (Boettger-Tong et al., 2000; Mahato et al., 2000).

Species limitations in transplantation

Only a few species have been tested for their ability to support stem cell transplantation. It is not yet clear that the commonly used mouse model is the best recipient model. Even if all the conditions of successful transplantation can be optimized for other species, it is not clear if SSCT will be successful. To-date, there are some methodological successes in recipient species other than the mouse (Ogawa et al., 1999a,b), but no clear evidence of transplantation success leading to complete spermatogenesis in recipients (Dobrinski et al., 1999a; Hausler and Russell, 1999; Schlatt et al., 1999).

Brinster's laboratory has methodically examined transplant success with increasing donor–recipient phylogenetic disparity. Successful rat-to-rat transplants are technically much more difficult (Jiang and Short, 1998; Ogawa et al., 1999a) than rat-to-mouse transplants (Clouthier et al., 1996; Russell and Brinster, 1996). Even less successful is hamster transplants into mouse (Ogawa et al., 1999b). When even less-closely related species such as dog, rabbit, pig, horse and bull are used as donors into a mouse recipient, there is some seeding of spermatogonia but with little to no development beyond the spermatogonial phase of spermatogenesis (Dobrinski et al., 1999b, 2000). Human transplants into mice have so far proved unsuccessful (Reis et al., 2000).

Phylogenetic diversity appears to be a limiting factor in SSCT success. However, it is of interest to note that the somatic cells of a mouse recipient, for example, can not only tolerate but apparently facilitate the development of germ cells of a rat or a hamster (Clouthier et al., 1996; Russell and Brinster, 1996; Ogawa et al., 1999b) and vice versa (Ogawa et al., 1999a). The timing of germ cell development is different in donor and recipient. It had previously been thought that the cycle exhibited by the Sertoli cell of one species would not match that of another species with a markedly different cycle length. However, as a result of transplants across species, we now believe the somatic cells, especially the Sertoli cells, are more flexible in the phylogenetic-related diversity of cells they can support.

Conditions that enhance transplantation

There is increasing evidence that early spermatogenesis (spermatogonial divisions) can be enhanced in conditions where low levels of intratesticular testosterone exist (Shetty et al., 2000). The degree to which SSCT succeeds can be enhanced by compounds that suppress the stimulation of luteinizing hormone (Ogawa et al., 1998). Testosterone levels are normally low during the early initiation of spermatogenesis, which leads to puberty when spermatogonial development is initiated. Thus, pituitary suppression can enhance transplantation success (Ogawa et al., 1998).

Purification of stem cells by a variety of methods to enhance transplant have been successful (immunoaffinity: Shinohara et al., 1999; cryptorchidism: Shinohara et al., 1999; heat treatment: M.D. Griswold, unpublished observations). There appears to be a direct correlation between the number of stem cells injected and the number of successful transplant sites.

Genetic manipulation of male germ cells

The ability to transplant spermatogonial stem cells immediately created the possibility of a new route for manipulation of the genome. For this to become reality, two hurdles had to be overcome. First, tech-

niques had to be developed for culturing spermatogonia without compromising their viability or stem cell characteristics. Second, techniques had to be developed for gene transfer into spermatogonia. Both conditions have now been successfully accomplished. Brinster and colleagues have shown that stem spermatogonia are preserved during long-term culture (Brinster and Nagano, 1998; Nagano et al., 1998). Introduction of new genetic information into spermatogonia in vitro has relied on the use of murine or avian retroviruses (de Miguel et al., 2000; Nagano et al., 2000) or on transfection techniques (Feng et al., 2000). Retroviruses need to integrate into the host genome for their gene products to be produced by the host cell. Retroviral integration, in turn, requires the host cell to transition through the cell cycle. Therefore, the efficiency of retroviral-mediated gene expression is dependent on the proliferative activity of the host cell. Since stem cells such as stem spermatogonia are thought to be slow cycling cells the efficiency of gene transduction in these types of cell is likely to be low.

To-date, two types of retroviral vector have been used to infect spermatogonia in culture, based on Moloney murine leukemia virus (Mo-MuLV) and avian leukosis virus (ALV) (de Miguel et al., 2000; Nagano et al., 2000). The use of ALV-based vectors requires the use of strains of transgenic mice expressing the ALV receptor tvA. In in vitro studies, ALV-based vectors are more efficient at infecting spermatogonial stem cells than Mo-MuLV-based vectors, but this may simply reflect the availability of retroviral receptors on the stem cell (de Miguel et al., 2000). Mo-MuLV-based vectors bearing an ecotropic envelope infect spermatogonia and it has been estimated that 1 in 280 stem cells becomes infected (Nagano et. al. 2000). Introduction of genes into spermatogonia in vitro and in vivo has also been carried out by lipofection and electroporation, although quantitative data on transduction efficiencies and long-term transfection were not reported (e.g., Muramatsu et al., 1997; Yamazaki et al., 1998; Feng et al., 2000; Nagano et al., 2001). Although the transduction efficiencies are low, collectively these data demonstrate the ability to introduce genetic information into the mammalian germline using a variety of techniques. The ability to introduce foreign DNA into the male germline of mammals should allow techniques to be developed both for animal transgenesis and for the treatment of a variety of types of human infertility. While the above studies also suggest that the germline should be susceptible to viral infection in human somatic gene therapy treatments, previous data suggest that this is not the case. A number of studies in mice suggest that stem spermatogonia are difficult, if not impossible, to infect with viruses even in mice that are viremic (e.g., Jenkins and Copeland, 1985; Ye et al., 1998).

Potential clinical use of spermatogonial stem cell transplantation

There are no guarantees that the SSCT technique can be used clinically or that the technique will attain its full potential. There are potential uses of the SSCT technique for fertility control. It is theoretically possible that men could achieve fertility by employing donor spermatogonia. It should be realized that there are potential histocompatibility problems to overcome in such transfers since the spermatogonial cells end up outside the Sertoli cell barrier. Moreover, there are many ethical considerations prior to undertaking SSCT.

It is well known that irradiation, used to treat cancer, and chemotherapy have deleterious effects on dividing cell populations. A male expecting to undergo chemotherapy in his prepubertal years could freeze spermatogonia cells, which would then be transferred back to his testis after the chemotherapeutic regimen was complete, assuming unwanted cancer cells are not harvested and retransplanted.

It should be borne in mind that the testis of most mammals, such as humans, is more complex than the testis of the rodents in which SSCT has taken place. The number of seminiferous tubules in large mammals often numbers in the hundreds. Techniques to inject these seminiferous tubules with donor germ cells have not yet been fully developed (see below). In spite of the apparent anatomical problems, it is not always necessary to establish

full transplant spermatogenesis throughout the testis, since regional aspiration of sperm could be undertaken in conjunction with intracytoplasmic sperm injection.

SSCT offers the long-term promise of modification of the human genome. This could eliminate or reduce the possibility that certain disease processes would be passed on by transplanted gametes. Modifications in the germ cell genome would, of course, not affect somatic cells in the transplanted individual. The limits to modifications of the genome would no doubt be delineated by a lively debate on the ethical issues involved (Dym, 1994).

At the time of writing this review, it is apparent that great strides have been made towards a reliable ability to incorporate vectors stably into germ cells and have the cells express such vectors. Dr. Ralph Brinster and collaborators, studying primarily rodent models, have been instrumental in developing spermatogonial transplants to the point that the major steps in transgenesis of the germline are now feasible (Russell and Brinster, 1998; Russell et al., 1998). The following breakthroughs are important for germ cell therapy via stem cell transplantation; we note via references beside each step the breakthrough that has been an initial step leading to future practical applications.

1 Isolation of stem cell spermatogonia (albeit, in some instances, with other cell types) (Brinster and Avarbock, 1994; Brinster and Zimmerman, 1994; Shinohara et al., 1999)
2 Culture of spermatogonia (Brinster and Nagano, 1998; Nagano et al., 1998)
3 Establishment of culture conditions to stimulate efficient spermatogonial stem cell proliferation
4 Transfection of dividing spermatogonia in culture (de Miguel et al., 2000; Feng et al., 2000; Nagano et al., 2000)
5 Freezing of stem cell spermatogonia (Avarbock et al., 1996; Brinster and Nagano, 1998)
6 SSCT (Brinster and Avarbock, 1994; Brinster and Zimmerman, 1994 and many of the references listed)
7 Development of transplanted spermatogenesis (many of references listed at the end of this chapter).

All of the above have been accomplished apart from (3), the culture conditions. Developments in this field and practical improvements towards achieving germ cells containing and expressing stable vectors are eagerly awaited.

Potential use of spermatogonia stem cell transplantation in livestock production

Improvements in livestock genetics and production efficiency could be gained through use of SSCT. Breakthroughs in our ability to introduce germ cells into the testes of large mammals, such as pigs (Hausler and Russell, 1999), indicates that transplanted spermatogenesis could be obtained on a large scale. Russell has had success in destroying endogenous spermatogenesis in the recipient animals. The reader is referred to Hausler and Russell (1999) for the rationales for performing transplantation in livestock. Perfection of SSCT in endangered species, has obvious benefits in species preservation.

Conclusions

Recently, there has been greater consideration towards developing methodologies for genetic modifications of the male germ cell line. Substantial progress has been achieved since the development of the spermatogonial transplantation technique in Dr. Ralph Brinster's laboratory. The feasibility of isolation of cells, culture, freezing, genetic modification, and successful transplantation has been demonstrated in a series of reports in the late 1990s. Improving the efficiency of the process must now be a research priority to bring the basic science into practical use.

REFERENCES

Avarbock, M.R., Brinster, C.J., and Brinster, R.L. (1996). Reconstitution of spermatogenesis from frozen spermatogonial stem cells. *Nature Medicine*, **2**, 693–6.

Boettger-Tong, H.L., Johnson, D.S., Russell, L.D., Griswold M.D., and Bishop C.E. (2000). *jsd* (juvenile spermatogonial depletion) mutant seminiferous tubules are capable of supporting transplanted spermatogenesis. *Biology of Reproduction*, **63**, 1185–91.

Brinster, R.L. and Avarbock, M.R. (1994). Germline transmission of donor haplotype following spermatogonial transplantation. *Proceedings of the National Academy of Sciences USA*, **91**, 11303–7.

Brinster, R.L. and Nagano, M. (1998). Spermatogonial transplantation, cryopreservation and culture. *Seminars in Cell and Developmental Biology*, **9**, 401–9.

Brinster, R.L. and Zimmerman, J.W. (1994). Spermatogenesis following male germ-cell transplantation. *Proceedings of the National Academy of Sciences USA*, **91**, 11298–302.

Clouthier, D.E., Avarbock, M.R., Maika, S.D., Hammer R.E., and Brinster,R.L. (1996). Rat spermatogenesis in mouse testes following spermatogonial stem cell transplantation. *Nature*, **381**, 418–21.

de Miguel, M.P., Federspiel, M.J., and Donovan, P.J. (2000). Regulation of growth and survival in the mammalian germline. In: *The Testis: From Stem Cell to Sperm Function*, Goldberg, E., ed. Serona Symposium, Springer Verlag, New York, pp. 55–70.

de Rooij, D. and Russell, L.D. (2000). All you wanted to know about spermatogonia but were afraid to ask. *Journal of Andrology*, **21**, 776–98.

Dobrinski, I., Ogawa, T., Avarbock, M., and Brinster, R.L. (1999a). Computer assisted image analysis to assess colonization of recipient seminiferous tubules by spermatogonial stem cells from transgenic donor mice. *Molecular Reproduction and Development*, **53**, 142–8.

Dobrinski, I., Avarbock, M., and Brinster, R.L. (1999b). Transplantation of germ cells from rabbits and dogs into mouse testes. *Biology of Reproduction*, **61**, 1331–9.

Dobrinski, I., Avarbock, M., and Brinster, R.L. (2000). Germ cell transplantation from large domestic animals into mouse testes. *Molecular Reproduction and Development*, **57**, 270–9.

Dym, M. (1994). Spermatogonial stem cells of the testis. *Proceedings of the National Academy of Sciences USA*, **91**, 11287–9.

Feng, L.X., Ravindranath, N., and Dym, M. (2000). Stem cell factor/c-kit up-regulates cyclin D3 and promotes cell cycle progression via the phosphoinositide 3-kinase/p70 S6 kinase pathway in spermatogonia. *Journal of Biological Chemistry*, **275**, 25572–6.

França, L., Ogawa, T., Avarbock, M., Brinster, R.L., and Russell, L.D. (1998). Germ cell genotype controls cell cycle during spermatogenesis. *Biology of Reproduction*, **59**, 1371–7.

Hausler, C. and Russell, L.D. (1999). Prospects for developing spermatogonial transplantation in domestic animals. In: *The Male Gamete*, Gagnon, C., ed. Cache River Press, Vienna, IL, pp. 37–45.

Jenkins, N.A. and Copeland, N.G. (1985). High frequency germline acquisition of ecotropic MuLV proviruses in SWR/J-RF/J hybrid mice. *Cell*, **43**, 811–19.

Jiang, F.-X. and Short, R.V. (1998). Different fate of primordial germ cells and gonocytes following transplantation. *APMIS*, **106**, 53–63.

Johnston, D., Russell, L., and Griswold, M. D. (2000). Advances in spermatogonial stem cell transplantation. *Reviews in Reproduction*, **5**, 183–8.

Mahato, D., Goulding, E.H., Korach, K.S., and Eddy, E.M. (2000). Spermatogenic cells do not require estrogen receptor-alpha for development or function. *Endocrinology*, **141**, 1273–6.

Muramatsu, T., Shibata, O., Ryoki, S., Ohmori, Y., and Okumura, J. (1997). Foreign gene expression in the mouse testis by localized in vivo gene transfer. *Biochemical and Biophysical Research Communications*, **233**, 45–9.

Nagano, M. and Brinster, R.L. (1998). Spermatogonial transplantation and reconstitution of donor cell spermatogenesis in recipient males. *APMIS*, **106**, 47–57.

Nagano, M., Avarbock, M., Leonida, E., Brinster C., and Brinster, R.L. (1998). Culture of mouse spermatogonial stem cells. *Tissue Cell*, **30**, 389–97.

Nagano, M., Avarbock, M., and Brinster, R.L. (1999). Pattern and kinetics of mouse donor spermatogonial stem cell colonization in recipient testes. *Biology of Reproduction*, **60**, 1429–36.

Nagano, M., Shinohara, T., Avarbock, M.R., and Brinster, R.L. (2000). Retrovirus-mediated gene delivery into male germ line stem cells. *FEBS*, **475**, 7–10.

Nagano, M., Brinster, C.J., Orwig, K.E., Ryu, B.-Y., Avarbock, M.R., and Brinster, R.L. (2001). Transgenic mice produced by retroviral transduction of male germ-line stem cells. *Proceedings of the National Academy of Sciences USA*, **98**, 13090–5.

Ogawa, T., Arechaga, J., Avarbock M., and Brinster, R.L. (1997). Transplantation of testis germinal cells into mouse seminiferous tubules. *International Journal of Developmental Biology*, **41**, 111–21.

Ogawa, T., Dobrinski, I., Avarbock, M.R., and Brinster, R.L. (1998). Leuprolide, a gonadotropin-releasing hormone agonist, enhances colonization after spermatogonial transplantation into mouse testes. *Tissue Cell*, **30**, 583–8.

Ogawa, T., Dobrinski, I., and Brinster, R.L. (1999a). Recipient preparation is critical for spermatogonial transplantation in the rat. *Tissue Cell*, **31**, 461–72.

Ogawa, T., Dobrinski, M., and Brinster, R.L. (1999b). Xenogeneic spermatogenesis following transplantation of hamster germ cells to mouse testes. *Biology of Reproduction*, **60**, 515–21.

Ogawa, T., Dobrinski, I., Avarbock, M.R., and Brinster, R.L. (2000). Transplantation of male germ line stem cells restores fertility in infertile mice. *Nature Medicine*, **6**, 16–33.

Parreira, G., Ogawa, T., Avarbock, M., Brinster, R., and Russell, L.

(1998). Development of testis cell transplants. *Biology of Reproduction*, **59**, 1360–70.

Parreira, G.G., Ogawa, T., Avarbock, M.R., França, L.R., Brinster, R.L., and Russell, L.D. (1999). Development of germ cell transplants: morphometric and ultrastructural studies. *Tissue Cell*, **31**, 241–54.

Reis, M.A., Tsai, M.C., Schlegel, P.N., et al. (2000). Xenogeneic transplantation of human spermatogonia. *Zygote*, **8**, 97–105.

Russell, L.D. (1989) Barriers to entry of substances into seminiferous tubules: compatibility of morphologic and physiologic evidence. In: *Banbury Report 3: Biology of Mammalian Germ Cell Mutagenesis*, Cold Spring Harbor Laboratory Press, Cold Spring Harbor, New York, pp. 3–17.

Russell, L.D. and Brinster, R.L. (1996). Ultrastructural observations of spermatogenesis following transplantation of rat testis cells into mouse seminiferous tubules. *Journal of Andrology*, **17**, 615–27.

Russell, L.D. and Brinster, R.L. (1998). Spermatogonial transplantation. In: *Germ Cell Development, Disruption and Death*, Zirkin, B.R., ed. Serono Symposium, Springer-Verlag, New York, pp. 19–27.

Russell, L.D., França, L.R., and Brinster, R.L. (1996). Ultrastructural observations of spermatogenesis in mice resulting from transplantation of mouse spermatogonia. *Journal of Andrology*, **117**, 603–14.

Russell, L.D., Nagano, M., and Brinster, R.L. (1998). Spermatogonial transplantation. In: *Testicular Function: From Gene Expression to Genetic Manipulation*, Stefanini et al., Springer-Verlag, Berlin, pp. 41–57.

Schlatt, S., Rosiepen, G., Weinbauer, G., Rolf, C., Brook, P., and Nieschlag, E. (1999). Germ cell transfer into rat, bovine, monkey, and human testes. *Human Reproduction*, **14**, 144–50.

Shetty, G., Wilson, G., Huhtaniemi, I., Shuttlesworth, G.A., Reissmann, T., and Meistrich, M.L. (2000). Gonadotropin-releasing hormone analogs stimulate and testosterone inhibits the recovery of spermatogenesis in irradiated rats. *Endocrinology*, **141**, 1735–45.

Shinohara, T., Avarbock, M.R., and Brinster, R.L. (1999). B1- and A6-integrin are surface markers on mouse spermatogonial stem cells. *Proceedings of the National Academy of Sciences USA*, **96**, 5504–9.

Yamazaki, Y., Fujimoto, H., Ando, H., Ohyama, T., Hirota, Y., and Noce, T. (1998). In vivo gene transfer to mouse spermatogenic cells by deoxyribonucleic acid injection into seminiferous tubules and subsequent electroporation. *Biology of Reproduction*, **59**, 1439–44.

Ye, X., Gao, G.P., Pabin, C., Raper, S.E., and Wilson, J.M. (1998). Evaluating the potential of germ line transmission after intravenous administration of recombinant adenovirus in the C3H mouse. *Human Gene Therapy*, **9**, 2135–42.

12

Genetic diagnosis: the future

David Cram[1,2] and David de Kretser[2]

[1]Monash IVF, Melbourne, Australia
[2]Monash Institute of Reproduction and Development, Melbourne, Australia

Male infertility

For many couples who are unable to conceive naturally, the causative or contributory factors underlying their infertility are commonly associated with the male partner (de Kretser et al., 1997). Despite some recent advances in our understanding of reproductive genetics and the availability of new molecular biological techniques to interrogate the genome, the genetic causes of idiopathic male infertility remain elusive. In some infertile men, abnormalities in their semen have been related to specific chromosomal aneuploidies, translocations, and microdeletions of the Y chromosome (de Kretser et al., 1997; Meschede and Horst, 1997). From gene targeting studies in animals, it is clear that many genes encoded on both the sex chromosomes and the autosomes are essential for the expression of male fertility. Current estimates in the human suggest that the interplay of some 2000 different genes are involved in testicular development, germ cell differentiation, meiosis, and the successive stages of spermiogenesis (Bhasin et al., 1998). More specifically, evidence is accumulating that genes associated with chromosome dynamics (the synaptosomal complex, meiosis), DNA repair, the ubiquitin pathway, sperm structure and function, and mRNA localization, stability, and translation are some of the main players that are important for the expression of a normal male fertility phenotype.

Known genetic causes

Yq microdeletions involving spermatogenic genes represent the most significant type of pathogenetic defect identified to date, with a prevalence of ~5% in men with severe primary testicular failure and a sperm density of less than five million per milliliter in their semen (McLachlan et al., 1998). De novo deletions of Yq, the most frequently occurring chromosomal abnormalities in humans, are believed to arise by recombination events between long stretches of highly repetitive sequences (Edwards and Bishop, 1997). Polymerase chain reaction (PCR) analysis of mapped sequence-tagged sites (STSs) has shown that Yq genes important for spermatogenesis are heavily concentrated within three azoospermia factor (AZF) regions known as AZFa, AZFb, and AZFc (Vogt et al., 1996). In humans, deletions within any of the three AZF regions disrupts normal spermatogenesis, causing infertility in otherwise fertile men. Over 90% of all reported Yq deletions are associated with the loss of the AZFc region extending from distal sequences of AZFb through to sequences in close proximity to the junction of the euchromatic and heterochromatic regions (Vogt, 1998). The absence of DAZ (deleted in azoospermia) is tightly linked with this common AZFc deletion and is usually associated with severe oligozoospermia or azoospermia (Reijo et al., 1996; Pryor et al., 1997; Simoni et al., 1997; Vogt, 1998). More recently, an infertile man with a deletion specifically within the DAZ cluster has been identified who has severe hypospermatogenesis (Moro et al., 2000). This demonstrated unequivocally that DAZ is indeed a key gene central to the process of normal sperm production. Of the remaining Yq deletions reported (<10%), most extended in a centromeric direction beyond AZFc through to AZFb and AZFa sequences and were characterized by the loss of both *DAZ* (*AZFc*) and the gene for a member of the RBM (RNA-binding motif) family, *RBM1*, which is located in the distal region of *AZFb*. Men with these more extensive Yq deletions are invariably azoospermic and frequently exhibit testicular pathologies such as germ cell arrest and/or Sertoli cell-only syndrome (Vogt et al., 1996).

Twelve novel genes have recently been identified, cloned, and mapped to Yq (Lahn and Page, 1997). Northern blotting studies have shown that *TTY1*, *PRY*, *TTY2*, *BPY1*, *CDY*, *XKRY*, and *BPY2* are exclusively expressed in the testis whereas *DBY*, *DFFRY*, *TB4Y*, *EIF1AY*, and *UTY* are ubiquitously expressed. Sequencing across the entire *AZFa* region has mapped *DFFRY* and *DBY* to an 800 kb segment (Sun et al., 2000). Mutation screening of 576 infertile and 96 fertile men revealed several natural *DFFRY* polymorphisms and one functionally significant *DFFRY* mutation in a man with nonobstructive azoospermia. Further, several men with a deletion of *DFFRY* were also found to be azoospermic (Sargent et al., 1999; Sun et al., 2000), suggesting that *DFFRY* defects cause spermatogenic failure. Apart from *DFFRY*, no other cases of defective spermatogenesis have been traced to a point mutation in any of the other 11 remaining novel Yq genes or in *DAZ* or *RBM1*. Mutations in any of these Yq genes could account for the genetic basis of infertility in a significant portion of men with idiopathic infertility. Because the Yq region does not undergo any significant homologous recombination with the X chromosome, it is believed to have a higher propensity to acquire new mutations that are passed on in each successive generation. On this basis, it is conceivable that the Yq region has accumulated mutations along its length and, potentially, in functional genes important for normal spermatogenesis. Any of the genes mapped to Yq could, therefore, harbor mutations that would account for unexplained defects in the semen analysis of infertile men. Potential Yq deletions or point mutations in infertile men treated by intracytoplasmic sperm injection (ICSI) would be expected to be vertically transmitted to sons and cause a similar infertility phenotype (Cram et al., 2000).

Another well-established genetic defect causing infertility is the occurrence of mutations in the cystic gene for the fibrosis transmembrane conductance regulator (*CFTR*), which results in bilateral congenital absence of the vas deferens (Chillon et al., 1995). Over 800 mutations in this gene have been identified but screening for all, by current technology, is not cost effective. Consequently, since this is a recessive disorder, screening of the man and his partner for the common mutations can reduce the risk of cystic fibrosis and bilateral congenital absence of the vas deferens to acceptable levels. Where the partner of the affected male is heterozygous for a CFTR mutation, the use of in vitro fertilization (IVF) with testicular sperm retrieval and preimplantation genetic diagnosis (PGD) can avoid having an affected child.

It is well known that the mutations in the gene for the androgen receptor can cause androgen insensitivity syndrome and lead to problems of gender identification (Quigley et al., 1995). More recent studies have shown that point mutations in this gene can result in spermatogenic disruption, although the frequency of finding such patients is low (Wang et al., 1998). Unfortunately, no specific phenotype can be identified that would assist the clinician in ordering an androgen receptor gene analysis. Further studies have linked trinucleotide repeat (TNR) expansions of a CAG (polyglutamine) tract in exon 1 of the androgen receptor with spermatogenic defects (Tut et al., 1997; Dowsing et al., 1999; Mifsud et al., 2001). This observation would be in keeping with the known cause of Kennedy's disease, a late-onset neuromuscular disorder associated with infertility, where the number of CAG repeats is usually in excess of 40. Other studies have failed to show this association between CAG repeat length and spermatogenic failure.

Other genetic defects associated with infertility include those involving gonadotropin-releasing hormone physiology (*Kal 1*), genes for follicle-stimulating hormone (FSH) and luteinizing hormone β-subunits, and genes encoding their receptors (Taipanainen et al., 1997; Latronico et al., 1998; Seminara et al., 1998). In some instances, failure to complete puberty successfully leads the clinician to the diagnosis and appropriate genetic assessment. Finally, there are infertility disorders that have a genetic basis but the precise mechanism is unknown. For instance, the absence of dynein arms, nexin linkages, or radial spokes, all part of the axoneme, are the cause of the immotile cilia syndrome but the specific mechanism remains unclear (Eliasson et al., 1977). Another well-known cause is the presence of the second X chromosome in Klinefelter's syndrome, but we do not know which extra copy of the gene(s) on the X chromosome interacts in the failure of germ cell survival.

Identification of new genetic causes of male infertility

It is anticipated that other major causes of male infertility will be mutations of both X chromosomal and autosomal genes that are expressed in a testis-specific manner (Hoog, 1995). Phenotypic analysis of mutations in male *Drosophila* and gene-targeting experiments in mice have revealed numerous autosomal and X-linked genes that are important for the expression of normal male fertility without associated systemic effects (Bhasin et al., 1998). The functional analysis of sterile male *Drosophila* has identified mutations in genes that cause abnormal testicular development, reduced numbers of germ cells, meiotic arrest, defects in postmeiotic differentiation, abnormal spermatids, and infertility owing to problems in mating behavior. Likewise, studies of mice nullizygous for a myriad of genes has revealed mutations associated with deficient gonadotropin secretion (e.g., colony-stimulating factor 1), impaired Leydig cell function and reduced testosterone levels (e.g., insulin-like growth factor 1), abnormal germ cell development and/or deficiency of germ cells (e.g., bone morphogenetic protein 8), meiotic defects (e.g., heat shock protein 70.2), postmeiotic defects in spermiogenesis (e.g., Bcl-w), and post-testicular defects in sperm maturation. The power of gene knockout technology in revealing candidate fertility genes is elegantly demonstrated for Bcl-w, which is a death-protecting member of the Bcl-2 family of apoptosis-regulating proteins that is expressed in the testis and several other tissues. Expression of Bcl-w in the testis is largely restricted to spermatogonia, spermatocytes, spermatids, and Sertoli cells. Bcl-w-deficient male mice exhibit sterility associated with progressive testicular degeneration in early postnatal life (Print et al., 1998), whereas female Bcl-w-deficient mice display no fertility phenotype. In the adult Bcl-w-deficient male mouse, there is total loss of all germ cells, resulting in a Sertoli cell-only phenotype. Based on the phenotype of Bcl-w-deficient mice, it is possible that some men with nonobstructive azoospermia with Sertoli cell-only syndrome could have mutations in *Bcl-w*.

The functional analysis of new knockout mice will continue to play an important role in the identification of candidate human fertility genes. However, because point mutations are likely to be the major genetic defect associated with infertility in the human, gene knockouts may not reveal phenotypes associated with autosomal recessive infertility where there is partial or no loss of function. Large-scale generation of mouse mutants using whole genome mutagenesis with *N*-ethyl-*N*-nitrosourea (ENU) is becoming an attractive method for identifying genes associated with disease and specific complex traits (Hrabe de Angelis et al., 2000; Nolan et al., 2000). This powerful mutagen induces random DNA point mutations at high frequencies that are sufficient to cover the genome. Following mutagenesis, treated male mice are mated with untreated female mice to produce F1 founders. F1 can then be analyzed for dominant or semidominant phenotypes or bred further to reveal recessive phenotypes. Localization of the causative point mutations on the mouse chromosomes requires linkage evaluation of the heterozygous parental DNA using sequence length polymorphism markers spaced at ~10 cM followed by analysis with more closely linked markers and eventually DNA sequencing. The application of ENU mutagenesis to spermatogenesis should reveal new batteries of candidate male infertility genes in the mouse and define the genetic pathways essential for each developmental stage of this complex process.

With increasing knowledge of the nature of candidate male infertility genes, the next stages of research will involve the identification of human homologs using the DNA sequence data from the human genome project (Venter et al., 2001) and a switch from gene mining to functional genomics. Central to this research will be the identification of human mutations in the candidate genes and estimates of their frequency in infertile men. To facilitate these studies, the availability of large databases containing genomic DNA from infertile men together with detailed clinical information on semen parameters and testicular pathologies will be paramount. Moreover, with the development of automated denaturing high-pressure liquid chromatography (DHPLC), it is now possible to achieve high throughput and rapid mutation detection (Liu et al., 1998) where the nature and location of the mutations are unknown. To detect the presence of the mutation in heterozygous DNA, exonic and intronic sequences encompassing potential mutations can simply be amplified by PCR, denatured to separate the four different strands, and renatured to allow the different combinations of homo- and heteroduplexes to form. Homo- and heteroduplex structures can be differentiated by DHPLC analysis at a specific temperature and acetonitrile gradient that are calculated from the known DNA sequence of the PCR product and its theoretical melting curve. Less-stable heteroduplexes can be distinguished from homoduplexes by their altered migration profiles. DHPLC has already been applied to track gene evolution and successfully to identify elusive mutations in families with a history of genetic disease (Jones et al., 2000). Characterization of the precise nature of newly identified mutations will delineate for the first time clinically relevant genetic–phenotypic correlations and pave the way for the development of new clinical genetic tests for the infertile male. A strategy for the identification of mutations associated with male infertility and the subsequent development of new genetic tests is outlined in Fig. 12.1.

Genetic testing for infertile men prior to in vitro fertilization

In approximately 1 in 25 men, there is some form of subfertility. Male partners in couples with a history of infertility commonly present to a male infertility specialist in an attempt to gain an understanding of the basis of their infertility. With the current available technology, it is essential to make a thorough andrological assessment with a view to characterizing the phenotype of the patient. This must include semen analysis, hormonal analysis, and, where necessary, testicular biopsy. In this way, the phenotype can direct the clinician to the most appropriate genetic test. A schematic approach is illustrated in Fig. 12.2. For instance, the finding of azoospermia, normal-sized testes, a distended epididymal head, the absence of the vas on palpation and a low semen volume with a pH less than 7.2 indicates the diagnosis of bilateral congenital absence of the vas deferens. These findings call for mutation screening of *CFTR* as discussed earlier. Invariably, in 40% of men examined, there will be no known basis for his infertility, indicating that a genetic cause is likely. With the identification of new clinically relevant mutations and more precise phenotype–genetic correlations, the clinician will be able to determine the best treatment options for the couple that preferably, where possible, avoids assisted reproduction.

Identification of a genetic defect in the patient's genome is the first step in developing an approach to therapy. In many instances, this will require functional studies to identify how the particular gene is involved in sperm production. For example, for patients who have expanded CAG repeat tracts in their androgen receptor gene, studies suggest that this can diminish *trans*-activation. Consequently, a therapeutic possibility emerges: namely to stimulate Leydig cell testosterone production with a view to increasing *trans*-activation and thus sperm output. Alternatively, in vitro maturation of gametes may be a possibility to overcome a critical step in spermatogenesis, but such systems are unavailable at present. Some investigations have suggested using spermatogonial transplantation with other species to

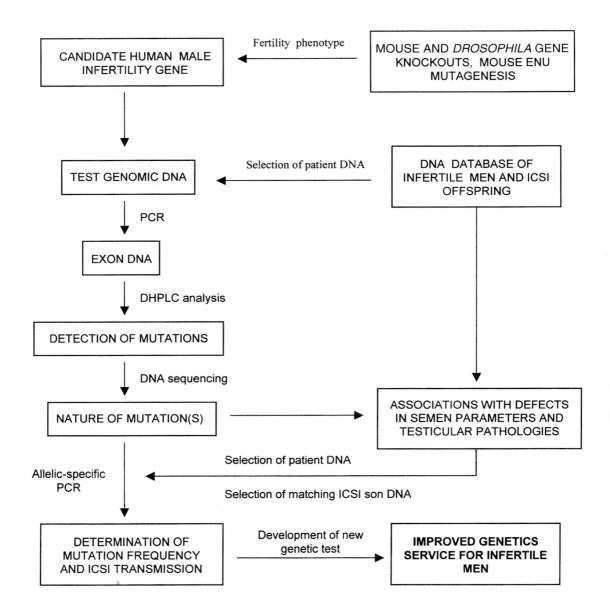

Fig. 12.1. Strategy to identify new genetic causes of male infertility. PCR, polymerase chain reaction; DHPLC, denaturing high-pressure liquid chromatography; ICSI, intracytoplasmic sperm injection; ENU, *N*-ethylnitrosourea.

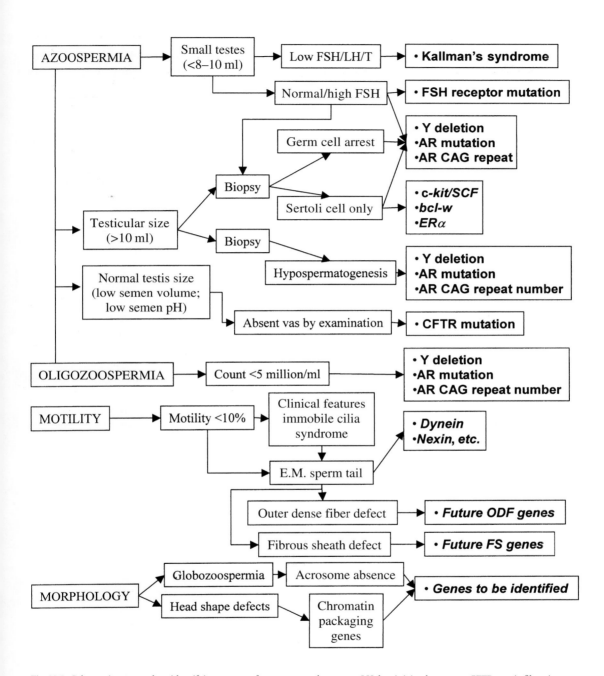

Fig. 12.2. Schematic approach to identifying groups of patients with a potential genetic basis for infertility. Tests indicated in bold are currently available whereas those in bold italics point to future directions. FSH, follicle-stimulating hormone; LH, luteinizing hormone; CFTR, cystic fibrosis transmembrane conductance regulator; T, testosterone; SCF, stem cell factor; ODF, outer denser fibers; FS, fibrous sheath.

allow spermatogenesis to proceed to completion. Whether such approaches are feasible will depend on interspecies regulatory mechanisms and even potential safety issues such as virus transmission. For the majority of men with severe hypospermatogenesis, with or without knowledge of a genetic defect, assisted reproduction will unfortunately be their only option.

Given that a variety of mutations in different genes may cause similar infertility phenotypes, genetic testing will require the fine analysis of multiple loci within the genome. Multiplex PCR and the analysis of PCR products by restriction fragment length polymorphism (RFLP) or allelic sizing will become too labor intensive and costly as more and more causative mutations are revealed. The application of microarray technology will undoubtedly dominate in the new era. An array is essentially an orderly arrangement of known DNA sequences coupled to a solid surface such as glass. Up to 100 000 oligonucleotide sequences can now be accommodated on a single chip (Lipshutz et al., 1999). The arrayed DNA is interrogated by fluorescently labeled genomic DNA from the patient. Hybridization patterns, interpreted by laser scanning, reflect the presence or absence of defined sequences or specific mutations. For targeted genome screens, oligonucleotide arrays (20–25 nucleotides per oligonucleotide) will be the preferred format because larger DNA sequences can sometimes hybridize nonspecifically to related sequences with >80% homology. To ensure high sensitivity and specificity of the hybridization, probe preparation will be paramount. One approach may involve isolation of the patient's DNA from a blood sample and digestion of the DNA with a restriction enzyme to simplify the genome into pieces of ~200 bp in size. Using linker adapter ligation coupled to PCR (Hamilton et al., 1999), it will be possible to amplify and label each fragment with a fluorescent dye such as Cy3 or Cy5.

What would a male infertility chip look like and how will it detect specific DNA variants in patients, DNA? The oligonucleotide array could be designed into four sections containing Yq markers, Y gene mutations, X gene mutations, and autosomal gene mutations (Fig. 12.3). Design of mutant oligonucleotides would require that the mutation be placed centrally to produce maximum disruption of hybridization of normal DNA. The choice of Yq markers will be dictated by our knowledge of Yq sequences from the human genome project, so that Y-specific markers represent functional genes along the length of Yq to cover all reported deletion intervals and surrounding sequences. Consequently, this approach will not only detect deletions by loss of hybridization to sequential markers but also provide detailed information on the deletion endpoints. Eventually, as the precise deletion breakpoints are identified through fine mapping studies using the complete Y sequence as a basis, simple PCR across the joined segments will confirm a deletion by the presence of a productive PCR product. In this case, breakpoint PCR products could be incorporated on the DNA chip. For point mutations in sex chromosomal and autosomal genes, it will be necessary to array four oligonucleotides for each specific mutation: two representing the sense and antisense normal allele and two representing the sense and antisense mutant allele. With the use of replicates of the four oligonucleotide set, this sense and antisense strategy will provide a confirmatory diagnosis for each mutation. To normalize results, DNA from a fertile man can be hybridized in parallel to an identical chip.

Genetic testing of children conceived through intracytoplasmic sperm injection

Once a genetic cause has been identified in the male partner, it would be expected that couples undergoing ICSI treatment will request genetic testing of their offspring to determine unequivocally whether the causative mutation has been inherited or not. For Y chromosomal defects in sperm, it is expected that first-generation sons would inherit their father's mutation and experience a similar fertility phenotype as they reach sexual maturity. Indeed, in limited follow-up studies of male offspring born to fathers with Yq deletions (Kent-First et al., 1996; Page et al., 1999; Cram et al., 2000), all deletions have been

MALE INFERTILITY CHIP WITH (8 x 16) OLIGONUCLEOTIDE ARRAY

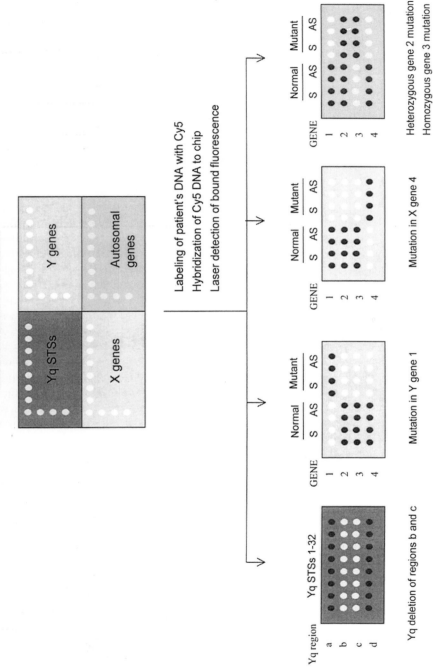

Fig. 12.3. Gene chip microarray technology for the identification of genetic causes of male infertility. Shaded and white circles on the array represent positive and negative hybridization signals, respectively. Oligonucleotides representing normal and mutant alleles are arrayed in quadruplicate. Sense (S) and antisense (AS) oligonucleotides for confirmatory diagnosis are duplicated. Each quadrant of the chip depicts hypothetical examples of microarray results for four infertile men. In quadrant 1, absence of hybridization to STSs 9–24 indicates a man with a deletion of Yq regions b and c. In quadrant 2, hybridization to only mutant oligonucleotides representing a gene 1 mutation indicates a man who has a mutation in this single copy Y gene. The reverse hybridization pattern for genes 2–4 indicates the absence of the test mutation in these genes. In quadrant 3, hybridization to only mutant oligonucleotides representing gene 4 indicates a man who has a mutation in this single copy X gene. The reverse hybridization pattern for genes 1–3 indicates the absence of the test mutation in these genes. In quadrant 4, hybridization to normal and mutant oligonucleotides representing autosomal gene 2 indicates a man heterozygous for the test mutation. Hybridization to only normal oligonucleotides representing genes 1 and 4 confirms the presence of two normal copies of these autosomal genes. However, hybridization to only mutant oligonucleotides representing autosomal gene 3 confirms the presence of two mutant copies of gene 3. STSs, sequence-tagged sites; Cy5, a fluorescent marker molecule.

vertically transmitted to male offspring, although in one case a widening of the father's *AZFc* deletion was reported in his son (Stuppia et al., 1996), indicating that some Yq deletions may be inherently unstable. In situations where Yq mosaicism in the father has been suspected and confirmed by single-sperm Yq PCR, then the chances of transmission will depend on the ratio of sperm carrying deleted and nondeleted Yq. However, for X chromosomal defects, it is likely that the defect would not affect the fertility of first-generation daughters, but would, presumably, cause an infertility phenotype in half of her sons in the next generation.

The number of ICSI cycles that have been used to treat severe male infertility is rapidly increasing worldwide (Tarlatzis and Bili, 2000). For the vast majority of children born by ICSI, no genetic follow up has been conducted for Yq deletions. Furthermore, IVF clinics in general have not been proactive in banking father and sibling DNA samples for retrospective analysis. Therefore, as our knowledge of genetic causes of male infertility increases with time, many couples that have previously undertaken assisted reproduction will become concerned about the fertility of their offspring and request testing for all known mutations. Given that venepuncture is not the ideal method for collecting blood as a source of genomic DNA, it is likely that retrospective samples for testing will be collected by less-invasive procedures such as cheek buccal cell sampling (Rudbeck and Dissing, 1998). This procedure is also simple, rapid, and cost-effective and would provide sufficient DNA from father and son samples to synthesize labeled probes to interrogate a male infertility chip. Through these types of analyzes, the causative mutation in the father will be identified and information regarding transmission of the genetic defect ascertained. In some instances, the family may additionally request DNA fingerprinting to confirm that their own gametes were used in IVF. The use of five microsatellite markers of high heterozygosity (>0.9) is sufficient to confirm parental origins of children born by ICSI (M. Katz and D. Cram, unpublished data).

Female infertility

The genetic causes of female infertility are also largely unknown. A few candidate genes involved in the expression of female fertility have been revealed by gene knockout experiments in mice, including *DAZLA*, an autosomal homolog of Y-specific *DAZ* (Ruggiu et al., 1997), and the gene for growth differentiation factor 9/bone morphogenetic protein 15, which is essential for normal follicular development (Dong et al., 1996; Galloway et al., 2000). In some Swedish women, mutations in genes for FSH have been associated with their infertility. Women with premature ovarian failure may form one of the more interesting groups to screen for potential mutations, particularly for CGG expansions in *FMR1*, which causes fragile X syndrome. Further clues to the identity of other relevant genes will undoubtedly stem from reproduction-failure phenotypes in female mice revealed by gene disruptions and ENU mutagenesis studies. Mutations related to female infertility in the human homologs of the candidate genes could be identified by screening databases of genomic DNA from infertile women by combined DHPLC and DNA sequencing. Once a set of relevant mutations are identified and their frequency in specific groups of infertile women ascertained, routine genetic screening of infertile women prior to assisted reproduction could also be facilitated by a gene chip microarray approach, similar to that proposed for infertile men.

Preimplantation genetic diagnosis

IVF with PGD is an alternative to traditional prenatal diagnosis and provides the opportunity for couples at risk of having a child with a serious genetic condition to start a pregnancy with the knowledge that their embryos will not be affected with the indicated disease. Currently, the two main clinical indications for PGD are risk of aneuploid embryos for infertile couples of advanced maternal age, repeat IVF cycles, or altered karyotype, and the risk of chromosomal translocations and inheritable genetic disease in offspring of fertile couples (Verlinsky and Kuliev, 1999). PGD involves embryo biopsy and analysis of either oocyte polar bodies or one to two blastomeres from cleavage stage embryos. From a technical point of view, PGD is arguably the most advanced form of genetic testing developed because of the limited target DNA in a single cell: ~6pg or two molecules per target allele. With current fluorescent PCR (FL-PCR)-based diagnostic methods, the accuracy of PGD is now >97% which is a level that is rapidly approaching that of prenatal diagnosis (>99.9%).

Since the inception of PGD in 1989, over 2000 clinical cycles have been performed worldwide, resulting in 531 pregnancies and 395 healthy children born (data from European Society of Human Reproduction and Embryology, 2001). Of these children, 289 were tested for chromosomal abnormalities and 106 for single gene disorders. PGD has been successfully applied to a range of single gene disorders including cystic fibrosis, beta thalassemia, Huntington's disease, and myotonic dystrophy as well as X-linked conditions such as fragile X (Verlinsky and Kuliev, 1999, 2000; Vandervors et al., 2000). Overall, there have only been four misdiagnoses worldwide. Regardless of this success, the procedure has not been widely embraced by patients. There are probably a number of factors contributing to this, including the paucity of centers offering PGD; the lack of education of patients, genetic counsellors and clinicians; low IVF pregnancy rates per cycle (~25%); and high cost. Once these issues have been addressed and further incremental improvements are made in the reliability and accuracy of the molecular diagnostic tests, it is likely that PGD will become a more acceptable pathway for couples at genetic risk. In the first decade of the twenty-first century, as the genetic basis of more complex traits are understood from family pedigree studies, PGD requests may extend beyond screening for serious genetic conditions and sex selection towards the identification of embryos with reduced risk of genetic predisposition to adult-onset disease and, possibly, with the potential for desirable physical and social traits.

Preimplantation diagnosis of monogenic disorders

Over 8000 inheritable genetic disorders have been described and the molecular basis for most are now defined at the gene and nucleotide level. In many cases, the DNA variants that cause disease are remarkably heterogeneous. For example, since the association of *CFTR* with cystic fibrosis (Riordan et al., 1989), over 800 different *CFTR* variants have been discovered with the ΔF508 3bp deletion in exon 10 being the most common variant. A complete understanding of all functional genes expressed by the human genome in various tissues together with focused DHPLC studies on DNA samples from families with a history of genetic disease will ultimately identify the full spectrum of gene variants that cause each heritable syndrome. With this knowledge as a basis, we could see population testing at birth for transmission of disease alleles and for predisposition to disease, using oligonucleotide microarrays containing all possible identified gene variants. In the context of PGD, there will be a gradual shift to a microarray-based diagnosis, particularly for genetic predisposition to disease where multiple loci are likely to be involved.

Allelic dropout, defined as the failure of the maternal or paternal gene to amplify by PCR, still represents the main impediment to higher PGD accuracy (Rechitsky et al., 1998). This phenomenon is believed to occur in the first few cycles of PCR and is related to primer performance and the state of the chromosomal DNA. The presence of allelic dropout can cause either a complete misdiagnosis of embryo genotype or a "no diagnosis" scenario that leads to unnecessary embryonic wastage. If the mutation loci of the couple presenting for PGD can be captured together in one amplicon (<1kb in length), then the mutations themselves serve as means of identifying allelic dropout. This approach may be possible for PGD of beta thalassemia because the vast majority of disease-causing mutations are localized to a 1.5kb segment of the β-globin gene. Recent studies in our laboratory have demonstrated that such a PCR fragment can be amplified from single cells with an allelic dropout rate of 10–15%. With further primer design and testing, it may be possible to decrease the effect of allelic dropout further. However, if two mutation loci are physically separated by more than 1 kb, requiring each loci to be captured in two separate amplicons, then allelic dropout in both amplicons can cause a misdiagnosis. One strategy to identify allelic dropout is the co-analysis of either a polymorphic marker (Kuliev et al., 1998) or a single nucleotide polymorphism linked in 100% dysequilibrium with the mutation of interest, which would track the parental allelic contribution to the embryo.

A reduction in allelic dropout rates would lead to improved efficiency and accuracy in PGD genetic testing. Replacement of conventional PCR with FL-PCR, which is approximately 1000 times more sensitive, has significantly reduced the incidence of allelic dropout (Sermon et al., 1998a). New strategies involving more target PCR templates should eventually eliminate this problem. One possible approach would be to amplify the more abundant mRNA in the biopsied blastomeres by reverse transcriptive PCR. This approach would require comprehensive gene expression studies in human preimplantation embryos to determine if maternally and paternally derived disease alleles are expressed at this early embryonic development stage. A second approach would be to amplify the genomic DNA from blastocyst trophectoderm biopsies. Up to 20 trophectoderm cells can be taken without compromising the ability of the blastocyst to develop further in vitro and hatch (Dokras et al., 1990). Whilst no unusual pre- or postnatal abnormalities have been reported following the transfer of biopsied bovine (Shea, 1999) or marmoset monkey (Summers et al., 1988) blastocysts, the outcome of human blastocyst biopsy remains uncertain.

The most common DNA variant encountered in PGD of autosomal recessive disorders like cystic fibrosis and beta thalassemia are nucleotide substitutions or point mutations. Methods for PGD of point mutations such as RFLP (Kuliev et al., 1998), amplification refractory mutation system PCR (ARMS-PCR) (Sherlock et al., 1998), single-strand

conformational polymorphism (El-Hashemite et al., 1997), and denaturing gradient gel electrophoresis (Vrettou et al., 1999) have stemmed from traditional technologies established for prenatal diagnosis where large numbers of fetal cells are available for isolation of genomic DNA. However, while the effectiveness of each of these methods has been amply demonstrated, all suffer from inherent technical difficulties and are both time consuming and labor intensive. For example, RFLP relies on whether the mutation creates or destroys a restriction enzyme site. In many cases, an amenable site is not always available. In ARMS-PCR, where both a conserved primer and two allele-specific primers encompassing the mutation site are used for second round nested PCR, the specificity of the test is solely dependent on the 3′ nucleotide of the allele-specific primers for exact allele discrimination. Further, in many instances, the sequence surrounding the mutation site is unfavorable for design of a robust PCR primer, thus reducing the sensitivity of the assay. Consequently, neither RFLP nor ARMS-PCR is applicable to a wide range of disease-causing point mutations. In the next few years, we will see the introduction of universal point mutation detection systems such as standard DNA sequencing and fluorescent single nucleotide primer extension (FL-SNuPE) which involves extension of a primer that abuts the mutation site by one base with the complementary fluorescently labeled dideoxynucleotide (Piggee et al., 1997). With both of these methods, the mutation can be directly assayed from the sense and antisense DNA strands of the PCR amplicon for confirmatory diagnosis and linked polymorphisms (to identify allelic dropout) analyzed in parallel. We have recently developed FL-SNuPE using DNA sequencing gels to assay reaction products and have successfully applied the method clinically for PGD in two patients with beta thalassemia.

There will eventually be a shift from gel-based detection systems towards more sophisticated solution detection systems that do not require post-PCR processing and analysis. The most promising solution-based technique uses capillary PCR and dual color fluorescence detection on the Lightcycler with internal hybridization probes that can diagnose point mutations (Mangasser-Stephan et al., 1999; Pals et al., 2001) and small deletions (Aoshima et al., 2000). These probes comprise an anchor primer labeled at the 3′ end with fluorescence 1 (e.g., fluorescein) and two allele-specific primers labeled at the 5′ end, one with fluorescence 2 (e.g., LC RED 640) and one with fluorescence 3 (e.g., LC RED 705). The allele-specific primers anneal between the two non-labeled primers (Fig. 12.4). Essentially, a single cell can be amplified by PCR with non-labeled primers and during each PCR cycle the hybridization probes anneal head to tail. If there is a productive annealing of the allele-specific primer, fluorescence energy transfer occurs, producing fluorescence 2 and/or fluorescence 3 emission from the allele-specific primer(s). The amount of fluorescence emission is directly proportional to the product yield and can be measured in real time. For autosomal recessive disorders such as cystic fibrosis, the sense and antisense strand of each allele can also be analyzed simultaneously to give complementary readouts of homozygous normal, heterozygous normal, or homozygous affected at the mutation loci of interest.

TNR expansions are commonly associated with autosomal dominant disorders such as myotonic dystrophy and Huntington's disease as well as X-linked disorders such as fragile X. In human IVF embryos, TNRs can be analyzed by allelic sizing of FL-PCR products on DNA sequencing gels to determine the exact number of repeat units in the normal and expanded alleles (Sermon et al., 1998a,b). This approach is straightforward for couples where the normal alleles of each partner are completely informative. When this is not the case, the use of linked markers is the only method to track normal and expanded alleles. The composition and length of the TNR tract greatly affects its ability to be amplified by PCR. In Huntington's disease, both the normal and expanded CAG tract can be readily amplified and sized (Sermon et al., 1998b). More recently, PCR conditions have been reported that enable amplification of the refractile CGG repeat in normal (6–54 repeats) and premutation (52–200 repeats) *FMR*

alleles associated with fragile X (Sermon et al., 1999). Microarray technology will eventually supersede allelic sizing on gels as a readout of TNR number. In this scenario, oligonucleotides containing a series of TNR repeats differing by one repeat and surrounding conserved gene sequences will be available. Labeled allelic products generated by FL-PCR would simply be hybridized to the array with specificity controlled by the length of the TNR tract sandwiched between the conserved sequence. This approach would rapidly identify normal and affected embryos as well as any additional expansion or contraction of the disease allele that can occur following meiosis mistakes in gametes (Sermon et al., 1998a).

Single-cell genetic analysis of large TNR expansions remains a technical challenge. For example in myotonic dystrophy, CTG expansions can vary between 100 and 4000 repeats, making them refractory to PCR analysis. One promising method called triplet repeat PCR (TP-PCR) could be readily adapted to identify reliably the expanded TNR tract in disease alleles (Warner et al., 1996). In TP-PCR, a conserved primer upstream of the TNR together with a triplet-specific primer containing a non-specific tagged sequence is used in first round PCR to bind randomly along the length of the TNR tract. In a second PCR round, the first-round products are re-amplified using the conserved primer and a primer designed to the nonspecific tag sequence. This produces a ladder of fluorescent products varying by one repeat that represents increasing distance along the TNR expansion. Once PCR conditions are further optimized for a range of long TNR expansions, TP-PCR could be used to provide readouts of products by hybridization to microarrays containing oligonucleotide sequences representing a full ladder of sequences containing increasing TNR length. TP-PCR analysis of both strands of the expanded allele and hybridization to sense and antisense targets on the array would verify the presence of an expanded allele. The identification of expanded TNRs would improve PGD of autosomal dominant disorders by providing a more reliable and accurate diagnosis of patient's embryos. In the future, microarrays with the capacity to diagnose all

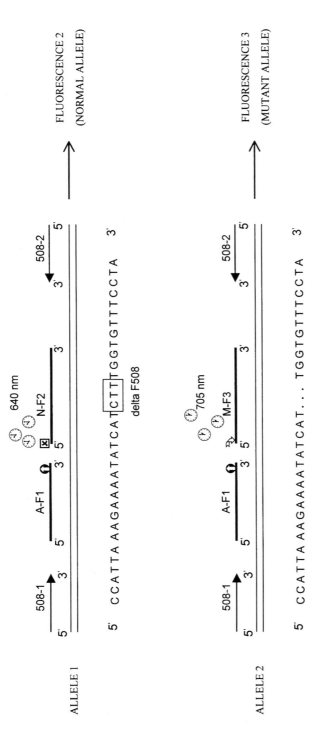

Fig. 12.4. Duel fluorescence detection of the common cystic fibrosis mutation ΔF508 in a single cell. F508-1 and F508-2 are nonlabeled primer pairs for the amplification of *CFTR* (for the cystic fibrosis transmembrane conductance regulator) exon 10 sequences containing the ΔF508 locus. A-F1 denotes the anchor fluorescence 1 primer whereas N-F2 and M-F3 represent allele-specific fluorescence 2 and fluorescence 3 primers that specifically bind to the normal and mutant alleles, respectively. Fluorescence 2 emits at 640 nm and fluorescence 3 emits at 705 nm. The dotted line in the DNA sequence of the mutant allele denotes the loss of CTT (ΔF508 mutation). Detection of F2 and F3 would indicate a cell heterozygous for ΔF508; detection of F2 only would indicate a normal cell and detection of F3 only would indicate a cell homozygous for ΔF508.

types of DNA variant will be developed and used routinely in laboratories performing PGD for single gene disorders.

Preimplantation diagnosis for chromosomal disorders

Chromosomal numerical changes known as aneuploidies are associated with reproduction failure and early embryo loss in the human. Aneuploidy results predominantly from nondysjunction of the chromatids in the first meiotic division of the oocyte and increases with age (Verlinsky and Kuliev, 1999). Trisomy 13, 16, 18, 21, and 22 and monosomy X are commonly found in cleavage stage embryos and also at the blastocyst stage (Magli et al., 2000). These aneuploidies usually cause implantation failure of the blastocyst or spontaneous abortion of the fetus in the first trimester, although a small proportion of trisomy 13, 18 and 21 fetuses can develop to term. The remaining possible trisomies and monosomies almost always result in embryo death. In clinical PGD, transfer of euploid embryos identified by fluorescent in situ hybridization (FISH) significantly increases implantation and pregnancy rates in couples where the female partner is of advanced maternal age (>37 years). Other chromosomal abnormalities such as Robertsonian translocations and reciprocal translocations are another significant cause of repeated miscarriages early in pregnancy. Robertsonian translocations involve the fusion of the centromeres of two acrocentric chromosomes, whereas reciprocal translocations, result from the balanced exchange of genetic material from one chromosome to another. Carriers of these types of translocations are at a high risk of having offspring with an unbalanced chromosomal constitution involving trisomy and monosomy of the two involved chromosomes (Gardner and Sutherland, 1996). PGD of Robertsonian and reciprocal translocations has been successfully performed by FISH using a combination of centromeric and telomeric probes (Munne et al., 2000).

Currently, interphase FISH is the gold standard for the diagnosis of chromosomal abnormalities in IVF embryos (Verlinsky and Kuliev, 2000). Whilst this technique has been developed to a high level of reliability and accuracy, a comprehensive diagnosis is not always possible because of problems with cell fixation, hybridization failure, overlapping and split signals, and subjective visual assessment. Presently, up to 9 of the 23 chromosomes can be assessed by FISH on a single cell. Spectral karyotyping using different combinations of five fluorochromes to paint each chromosome is now possible but requires metaphase chromosome spreads for generating a complete karyogram (Marquez et al., 1998). Although metaphase conversion has been achieved by fusion of mouse (Verlinsky and Evsikov, 1999) or bovine (Willadsen et al., 1999) metaphase oocytes to human blastomeres and polar bodies, spectral karyotyping remains technically difficult and very expensive.

A relatively new method called comparative genomic hybridization (CGH) has the capacity to analyze all 23 chromosomes simultaneously and is currently being explored as a viable alternative to FISH for PGD of chromosomal abnormalities (Voullaire et al., 2000; Wells and Delhanty, 2000). CGH requires whole genome amplification (WGA) technology (Wells et al., 1999) to produce multiple copies of all DNA sequences of the entire genome from a single cell. Test cell DNA is labeled with a red fluorochrome and a diploid control cell is labeled with a green fluorochrome; an equal mixture of each is competitively hybridized to a metaphase spread of a known diploid cell. Fluorescence patterns can then be analyzed by laser detection and results displayed as karyograms. An equal 1:1 weighting of red and green fluorescence along the length of a given chromosome indicates disomy (diploid status), a 3:2 weighting a trisomy and a 1:2 weighting a monosomy. At present, the long hybridization period of 72 hours associated with CGH is not compatible with clinical PGD unless the tested embryos are frozen for a later transfer. In addition, the interpretation of the aneuploid status of some chromosomes remains difficult probably because WGA cannot reliably replicate regions containing a high content of repetitive DNA sequences. Once these problems have been

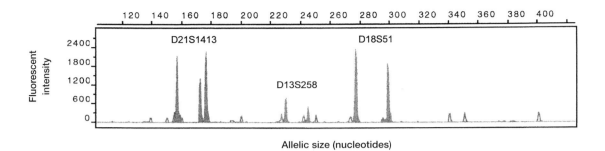

Fig. 12.5. DNA fingerprint of a single buccal cell taken from a child with Down's syndrome. Markers D21S1413, D13S258 and D18S51 were amplified by single cell multiplex fluorescence polymerase chain reaction using primers labeled with either TETRA (green) or 6-FAM (blue), both fluorescent dyes. The fingerprint derived by Genescan analysis shows three green peaks for D21S1413 (tri-allelic pattern) indicative of trisomy 21 and two blue peaks for D13S258 and D18S51 (bi-allelic pattern) indicative of disomy 13 and 18. The open peaks represent internal standards to size the marker alleles.

overcome, CGH has the potential to analyze both chromosomal aneuploidy and translocations in pre-implantation embryos (Wells and Delhanty, 2000).

More rapid PCR-based methods that also operate independently of the status of the genomic DNA will undoubtedly be explored for diagnosis of chromosomal abnormalities in single cells. Multiplex FL-PCR using chromosome-specific polymorphic microsatellite markers with a high degree of heterozygosity (>0.9), also known as DNA fingerprinting, can detect numerical changes in chromosomes from their allelic fingerprints (Adinolfi et al., 1997; Findlay et al. 1998; Sherlock et al., 1998). For example, a bi-allelic pattern for a specific chromosome 21 marker would indicate disomy whereas a tri-allelic pattern would be diagnostic of trisomy 21 or Down's syndrome. As an example, a single buccal cell DNA fingerprint that we obtained from a child with Down's syndrome using markers for chromosomes 13, 18, and 21 is shown in Fig. 12.5. The use of additional primers that amplify other markers on a particular chromosome would provide internal confirmation of the diagnosis and serve as a backup for markers that exhibited allelic dropout or were non-informative because of the presence of two homozygous parental alleles. Access to the complete sequence of the human genome will enable the identification of suitable markers for specific chromosomes and the design of robust primer pairs for single-cell multiplex FL-PCR. Further, the fingerprints derived will also confirm parental origin of the embryonic alleles and identify any potential extraneous DNA contamination in the PCR reaction that could lead to a misdiagnosis of embryonic genotype.

A DNA fingerprinting system to diagnose the common Robertsonian translocation 13q14q could simply comprise a six-plex PCR reaction that targeted polymorphic markers located on the long arm of chromosomes 13 and 14 (three markers per chromosme). The selection of markers with a broad allelic size range will be critical to ensure that one or more diagnose trisomy as a tri-allelic pattern. Tetranucleotide markers are generally preferred to dinucleotide markers because they produce less stutter PCR artifact, which can confound the interpretation of the fingerprints. There are essentially four possible embryonic outcomes with approximate equal probability of occurrence for a couple where one partner carries a balanced 13q14q *trans*-locations. One half of the embryos would either have a normal or a balanced 13,14 chromosome complement, which would both produce bi-allelic patterns for each marker and be indicative of diploidy. In the remaining half of the embryos, chromosomes 13 and 14 would be unbalanced and display tri-allelic and mono-allelic patterns indicative of either trisomy 13/monosomy 14 or trisomy 14/monosomy 13.

More comprehensive analyses of chromosomal aneuploidy in embryos will require the use of more complex DNA fingerprinting systems. This may be limited by the number of primers that can be reliably multiplexed without compromising the performance of individual primer pairs specific for each chromosomal marker. Although recent data from our laboratory have shown that nine primer pairs can work reproducibly in multiplex single cell FL-PCR, it is unlikely that other primers could be added without compromising amplification efficiency. Consequently, for total aneuploidy analysis by DNA fingerprinting, improved WGA methods that more efficiently replicate microsatellite sequences (Dietmaier et al., 1999) will be necessary to generate sufficient DNA template for reliable PCR. In addition, automated robotic platforms and high-throughput capillary electrophoresis will be required to set up and read different combinations of multiplex FL-PCR reactions. Further research is still required to identify a set of specific chromosomal markers that are amenable to WGA. Once verified and tested, these markers will serve as a basis to design a range of DNA fingerprinting systems for the diagnosis of chromosomal aneuploidy.

In the future, a comprehensive analysis of chromosomal aneuploidy will be possible using a gene chip microarray format containing a series of bacterial artificial chromosome clones that represent multiple regions along the length of each of the 23 chromosomes (Fig. 12.6, color plate). Using WGA methods, the test cell from the biopsy could be labeled with red fluorescence (Cy3) and the control cell with a normal karyotype with green fluorescence (Cy5). An equal mixture of the two would then be hybridized to the array and bound fluorescence estimated. A balance of red and green fluorescence for each clone representing a particular chromosome would indicate disomy. However, a predominance of red over green fluorescence by a ratio of 3 : 2 would indicate a trisomy whereas a 1 : 2 ratio would indicate a monosomy. The presence of a consistent pattern of deviation from diploidy for all representative clones of a particular chromosome would confirm the diagnosis and increase the overall accu-

racy and reliability. With the assembly of more detailed chromosomal maps that will stem from the human genome project, it will be possible in the near future also to pinpoint rapidly the precise chromosome breakpoints for individuals with common or unique chromosome translocations that have elected to have PGD. The availability of this information will allow specific PCR primers to be designed that transverse the breakpoint and unequivocally determine the presence or absence of the translocation in IVF embryos.

Preimplantation diagnosis for other genetic disorders and for favorable genotypes

Apart from inherited genetic diseases, the predisposition to adult late-onset disorders primarily relates to environmental and genetic factors and the ability of the body to maintain homeostasis with age. Consequently, the lifetime risk for genetic predisposition to disease is considerably lower than that for a severe inheritable disorder, which is 1 in 4 for an autosomal recessive condition and 1 in 2 for an autosomal dominant condition. For example, a person who carries a p53 suppressor gene mutation has a 50% chance of passing the affected gene on to offspring, with implications for both male and female children. Children who inherit the mutation have a high risk of autosomal dominant familial predisposition to breast cancer, bone and soft tissue sarcomas, leukemia and brain tumors. Their chance of developing a tumor by 30 years is 30% compared with 1% in the general population, and by the age of 70 years the probability increases to 90% (Offit, 1998). Already PGD has been successfully applied to a couple where one partner carried p53 suppressor gene mutations, resulting in the birth of a healthy child without the mutation (Verlinsky et al., 2001). We are also likely to see requests for embryo screening of *BRCA1* and *BRCA2* mutations, which have a 50% chance of being transmitted to offspring. Women who inherit either a *BRCA1* or a *BRCA2* mutation have a 60–80% lifetime risk of developing breast cancer and a 20–40% risk of developing ovarian cancer (Offit, 1998). Familial history of genetic predisposition to inherited cancers will ultimately have a significant bearing on whether a couple at genetic risk would contemplate assisted reproduction and PGD to ensure that their child does not have the genetic potential for the indicated cancer.

The human genome project has already initiated active research to discover susceptibility and resistance genes associated with other major diseases that afflict the human race, such as noninheritable cancers, heart disease, diabetes, arthritis, and autoimmune disease. Further, research will eventually focus on identifying genes and specific polymorphisms that are also associated with favorable phenotypes such as eye color and athletic prowess. With this knowledge, PGD could be seen as a convenient means of having children without predisposition to particular diseases or of having children with desirable traits. At the level of PGD, this would entail genetic testing of multiple loci throughout the genome of either a single cell from cleavage stage embryos or several cells from a blastocyst biopsy. These new applications will depend upon improvements to the reproducibility and accuracy of WGA methods and the availability of gene chips arrayed with oligonucleotides representing disease susceptibility gene variants as well as trait loci. This alternative pathway for PGD may be pursued by some couples and will undoubtedly raise ethical concerns that could override the original purpose of the technology, which was developed for couples with specific fertility and genetic problems. These are issues that need to be widely debated in our society before a clear way forward becomes apparent. There are likely to be a diversity of views and achieving some sort of consensus will be difficult.

Concluding remarks

In this new century, the stage is set for a revolution in functional genomics and human genetics that will give us a much deeper understanding of health and disease and open up new possibilities for assisted reproduction. Central to this revolution will be the gene chip, with the potential to identify genetic variation accurately and quantitate deviation in normal gene expression in specific tissues. Continual development and improvement of existing gene chip technology will enable cost-effective, rapid and high throughput analyses of the patient's genome. In the first decade of the twenty-first century, it is likely that gene chips will be specifically designed to identify the genetic basis of male and female infertility and for PGD of single gene and chromosomal abnormalities. Eventually, total genome screening using gene chips containing all known disease alleles and trait polymorphisms will become a reality. The identification of an individual's genetic blueprint at birth will provide the clinician with powerful tools to assess disease risk and implement appropriate programs and treatments to manage the patient's health and well-being effectively over a lifetime.

With the availability of new genetic tests, there will be many hurdles to overcome, particularly in the areas of assisted reproduction and predisposition to age-specific disease. The dissemination of accurate scientific information for the education of the community, patients, genetic counsellors and clinicians will be an important process so that the implications of new genetic tests are clearly understood at all levels. If this can be achieved, the new revolution in genetics will have profound benefits for human health and the infertile couple.

REFERENCES

Adinolfi, M., Pertl, B., and Sherlock, J. (1997). Rapid detection of aneuploidies by microsatellite and the quantitative fluorescent polymerase chain reaction. *Prenatal Diagnosis*, **17**, 1299–311.

Aoshima, T., Sekido, Y., Miyazaki, T., et al. (2000). Rapid detection of deletion mutations in inherited metabolic diseases by melting curve analysis with LightCycler. *Clinical Chemistry*, **46**, 119–22.

Bhasin, S., Ma, K., Sinha, I., Limbo, M., Taylor, W.E., and Salehian, B. (1998). The genetic basis of male infertility. *Endocrinology and Metabolism Clinics of North America*, **27**, 783–805.

Chillon, M., Casals, T., Mercier, B., et al. (1995). Mutations in the cystic fibrosis gene in patients with congenital absence of the vas deferens. *New England Journal of Medicine*, **332**, 1475–80.

Cram, D.S., Ma, K., Bhasin, S., et al. (2000). Y chromosome analysis of infertile men and their sons conceived through intracytoplasmic sperm injection: vertical transmission of deletions and rarity of de novo deletions. *Fertility and Sterility*, **74**, 909–15.

de Kretser, D.M., Mallidis, C., Ma, K., and Bhasin, S. (1997). Y chromosome deletions and male infertility. *Reproductive Medicine Reviews*, **6**, 37–53.

Dietmaier, W., Hartmann, A., Wallinger, S., et al. (1999). Multiple mutation analyses in single tumor cells with improved whole genome amplification. *American Journal of Pathology*, **154**, 83–95.

Dokras, A., Sargent, I.L., Ross, C., Gardner, R.L., and Barlow, D.H. (1990). Trophectoderm biopsy in human blastocysts. *Human Reproduction*, **5**, 821–5.

Dong, J., Albertini, D.F., Nishimori, K., Kumar, T.R., Lu, N., and Matzuk, M.M. (1996). Growth differentiation factor-9 is required during early ovarian folliculogenesis. *Nature*, **383**, 531–5.

Dowsing, A.T., Yong, E.L., Clark, M., McLachlan, R.I., de Kretser, D.M., and Trounson, A.O. (1999). Linkage between male infertility and trinucleotide repeat expansion in the androgen-receptor gene. *Lancet*, **354**, 640–3.

Edwards, R.G. and Bishop, C.E. (1997). On the origin and frequency of Y chromosome deletions responsible for male infertility. *Molecular Human Reproduction*, **3**, 549–54.

El-Hashemite, N., Wells, D., and Delhanty, J.D. (1997). Single cell detection of beta-thalassaemia mutations using silver stained SSCP analysis: an application for preimplantation diagnosis. *Molecular Human Reproduction*, **3**, 693–8.

Eliasson, R., Mossberg, B., Camner, P., and Afzelius, B.A. (1977). The immotile-cilia syndrome. A congenital ciliary abnormality as an etiologic factor in chronic airway infections and male sterility. *New England Journal of Medicine*, **297**, 1–6.

European Society of Human Reproduction and Embryology (2001). Tenth anniversary of preimplantation genetic diagnosis. (*The 10th Annual Meeting and International Workshop on Preimplantation Genetics* in association with the *3rd International Symposium on Preimplantation Genetics*, Bologne, June 2000.) *Journal of Assisted Reproduction and Genetics*, **18**, 66–72.

Findlay, I., Toth, T., Matthews, P., Marton, T., Quirke, P., and Papp, Z. (1998). Rapid trisomy diagnosis (21,18, and 13) using fluorescent PCR and short tandem repeats: applications for prenatal diagnosis and preimplantation genetic diagnosis. *Journal of Assisted Reproduction and Genetics*, **15**, 266–75.

Galloway, S.M., McNatty, K.P., Cambridge, L.M., et al. (2000).

Mutations in an oocyte-derived growth factor gene (BMP15) cause increased ovulation rate and infertility in a dosage-sensitive manner. *Nature Genetics*, **25**, 279–83.

Gardner, R.J.M. and Sutherland, G.R. (1996). *Oxford Monographs on Medical Genetics*, No. 29: *Chromosome Abnormalities and Genetic Counselling*. Oxford University Press, Oxford.

Hamilton, M.B., Pincus, E.L., Di Fiore, A., and Fleischer, R.C. (1999). Universal linker and ligation procedures for construction of genomic DNA libraries enriched for microsatellites. *Biotechniques*, **27**, 500–2.

Hoog, C. (1995). Expression of a large number of novel testis-specific genes during spermatogenesis coincides with the functional reorganization of the male germ cell. *International Journal of Developmental Biology*, **39**, 719–26.

Hrabe de Angelis, M.H., Flaswinkel, H., Fuchs, H., et al. (2000). Genome-wide, large-scale production of mutant mice by ENU mutagenesis. *Nature Genetics*, **254**, 444–7.

Jones, A.C., Sampson, J.R., Hoogendoorn, B., Cohen, D., and Cheadle, J.P. (2000). Application and evaluation of denaturing HPLC for molecular genetic analysis in tuberous sclerosis. *Human Genetics*, **106**, 663–8.

Kent-First, M.G., Kol, S., Muallem, A., et al. (1996). The incidence and possible relevance of Y-linked microdeletions in babies born after intracytoplasmic sperm injection and their infertile fathers. *Molecular Human Reproduction*, **2**, 943–50.

Kuliev, A., Rechitsky, S., Verlinsky, O., et al. (1998). Preimplantation diagnosis of thalassemias. *Journal of Assisted Reproduction and Genetics*, **15**, 219–25.

Lahn, B.T. and Page, D.C. (1997). Functional coherence of the human Y chromosome. *Science*, **278**, 675–80.

Latronico, A.C., Chai, Y., Arnhold, I.J., Liu, X., Mendonca, B.B., and Segaloff, D.L. (1998). A homozygous microdeletion in helix 7 of the luteinizing hormone receptor associated with familial testicular and ovarian resistance is due to both decreased cell surface expression and impaired effector activation by the cell surface receptor. *Molecular Endocrinology*, **12**, 442–50.

Lipshutz, R.J., Fodor, S.P., Gingeras, T.R., and Lockhart, D.J. (1999). High density synthetic oligonucleotide arrays. *Nature Genetics*, **21**, 20–4.

Liu, W., Smith, D.I., Rechtzigel, K.J., Thibodeau, S.N., and James, C.D. (1998). Denaturing high performance liquid chromatography (DHPLC) used in the detection of germline and somatic mutations. *Nucleic Acids Research*, **26**, 1396–400.

Magli, M.C., Jones, G.M., Gras, L., Gianaroli, L., Korman, I., and Trounson, A.O. (2000). Chromosome mosaicism in day 3 aneuploid embryos that develop to morphologically normal blastocysts in vitro. *Human Reproduction*, **15**, 1781–6.

Mangasser-Stephan, K., Tag, C., Reiser, A., and Gressner, A.M. (1999). Rapid genotyping of hemochromatosis gene mutations on the LightCycler with fluorescent hybridization probes. *Clinical Chemistry*, **45**, 1875–8.

Marquez, C., Cohen, J., and Munne, S. (1998). Chromosome identification in human oocytes and polar bodies by spectral karyotyping. *Cytogenetics and Cell Genetics*, **81**, 254–8.

McLachlan, R.I., Mallidis, C., Ma, K., Bhasin, S., and de Kretser, D.M. (1998). Genetic disorders and spermatogenesis. *Reproduction, Fertility and Development*, **10**, 97–104.

Meschede, D. and Horst, J. (1997). The molecular genetics of male infertility. *Molecular Human Reproduction*, **3**, 419–30.

Mifsud, A., Sim, C.K., Boettger-Tong, H., et al. (2001). Trinucleotide (CAG) repeat polymorphisms in the androgen receptor gene: molecular markers of risk for male infertility. *Fertility and Sterility*, **75**, 275–81.

Moro, E., Ferlin, A., Yen, P.H., Franchi, P.G., Palka, G., and Foresta, C. (2000). Male infertility caused by a de novo partial deletion of the DAZ cluster on the Y chromosome. *Journal of Clinical Endocrinology and Metabolism*, **85**, 4069–73.

Munne, S., Sandalinas, M., Escudero, T., Fung, J., Gianaroli, L., and Cohen, J. (2000). Outcome of preimplantation genetic diagnosis of translocations. *Fertility and Sterility*, **73**, 1209–18.

Nolan, P.M., Peters, J., Strivens, M., et al. (2000). A systematic, genome-wide, phenotype-driven mutagenesis programme for gene function studies in the mouse. *Nature Genetics*, **25**, 440–3.

Offit, K. (1998). *Clinical Cancer Genetics: Risk Counseling and Management.* Wiley-Liss, New York.

Page, D.C., Silber, S., and Brown, L.G. (1999). Men with infertility caused by AZFc deletion can produce sons by intracytoplasmic sperm injection, but are likely to transmit the deletion and infertility. *Human Reproduction*, **14**, 1722–6.

Pals, G., Young, C., Mao, H.S., and Worsham, M.J. (2001). Detection of a single base substitution in a single cell using the LightCycler. *Journal of Biochemical and Biophysical Methods*, **47**, 121–9.

Piggee, C.A., Muth, J., Carrilho, E., and Karger, B.L. (1997). Capillary electrophoresis for the detection of known point mutations by single-nucleotide primer extension and laser-induced fluorescence detection. *Journal of Chromatography A*, **781**, 367–75.

Print, C.G., Loveland, K.L., Gibson, L., et al. (1998). Apoptosis regulator *bcl-w* is essential for spermatogenesis but appears otherwise redundant. *Proceedings of the National Academy of Sciences USA*, **95**, 12424–31.

Pryor, J.L., Kent-First, M., Muallem, A., et al. (1997). Microdeletions in the Y chromosome of infertile men. *New England Journal of Medicine*, **336**, 534–9.

Quigley, C.A., De Bellis, A., Marschke, K.B., el-Awady, M.K., Wilson, E.M., and French, F.S. (1995). Androgen receptor defects: historical, clinical, and molecular perspectives. *Endocrine Reviews*, **16**, 271–321.

Rechitsky, S., Strom, C., Verlinsky, O., et al. (1998). Allele dropout in polar bodies and blastomeres. *Journal of Assisted Reproduction and Genetics*, **15**, 253–7.

Reijo, R., Alagappan, R.K., Patrizio, P., and Page, D.C. (1996). Severe oligospermia resulting from deletions of the azoospermia factor gene on Y chromosome. *Lancet*, **347**, 1290–3.

Riordan, J.R., Rommens, J.M., Kerem, B., et al. (1989). Identification of the cystic fibrosis gene: cloning and characterization of complementary DNA. *Science*, **245**, 1066–73.

Rudbeck, L. and Dissing, L. (1998). Rapid, simple alkaline extraction of human genomic DNA from whole blood, buccal epithelial cells, semen and forensic stains for PCR. *Biotechniques*, **25**, 588–90.

Ruggiu, M., Speed, R., Taggart, M., et al. (1997). The mouse *dazla* gene encodes a cytoplasmic protein essential for gametogenesis. *Nature*, **389**, 73–7.

Sargent, C.A., Boucher, C.A., Kirsch, S., et al. (1999). The critical region of overlap defining the AZFa male infertility interval of proximal Yq contains three transcribed sequences. *Journal of Medical Genetics*, **36**, 670–7.

Seminara, S.B., Hayes, F.J., and Crowley, W.F. (1998). Gonadotropin-releasing hormone deficiency in the human (idiopathic hypogonadotropic hypogonadism and Kallmann's syndrome): pathophysiological and genetic considerations. *Endocrine Reviews*, **19**, 521–39.

Sermon, K., De Vos, A., Van de Velde, H., et al. (1998a). Fluorescent PCR and automated fragment analysis for the clinical application of preimplantation genetic diagnosis of myotonic dystrophy (Steinert's disease). *Molecular Human Reproduction*, **4**, 791–6.

Sermon, K., Goossens, V., Seneca, S., et al. (1998b). Preimplantation diagnosis for Huntington's disease (HD): clinical application and analysis of the HD expansion in affected embryos. *Prenatal Diagnosis*, **18**, 1427–36.

Sermon, K., Seneca, S., Vanderfaeillie, A., et al. (1999). Preimplantation diagnosis for fragile X syndrome based on the detection of the non-expanded paternal and maternal CGG. *Prenatal Diagnosis*, **19**, 1223–30.

Shea, B.F. (1999). Determining the sex of bovine embryos using polymerase chain reaction results: a six-year retrospective study. *Theriogenology*, **51**, 841–54.

Sherlock, J., Cirigliano, V., Petrou, M., Tutschek, B., and Adinolfi, M. (1998). Assessment of diagnostic quantitative fluorescent multiplex polymerase chain reaction assays performed on single cells. *Annals of Human Genetics*, **62**, 9–23.

Simoni, M., Gromoll, J., Dworniczak, B., et al. (1997). Screening for deletions of the Y chromosome involving the DAZ (deleted in azoospermia) gene in azoospermia and severe oligozoospermia. *Fertility and Sterility*, **67**, 542–7.

Stuppia, L., Calabrese, G., Franchi, P.G., et al. (1996). Widening of a Y-chromosome interval-6 deletion transmitted from a father to his infertile son accounts for an oligozoospermia critical region distal to the RBM1 and DAZ genes. *American Journal of Human Genetics*, **6**, 1393–5.

Summers, P.M., Campbell, J.M., and Miller, M.W. (1988). Normal in-vivo development of marmoset monkey embryos after trophectoderm biopsy. *Human Reproduction*, **3**, 389–93.

Sun, C., Skaletsky, H., Rozen, S., et al. (2000). Deletion of azoospermia factor a (AZFa) region of human Y chromosome caused by recombination between HERV15 proviruses. *Human Molecular Genetics*, **9**, 2291–6.

Tapanainen, J.S., Aittomaki, K., Min, J., Vaskivuo, T., and Huhtaniemi, I.T. (1997). Men homozygous for an inactivating mutation of the follicle-stimulating hormone (FSH) receptor gene present variable suppression of spermatogenesis and fertility. *Nature Genetics*, **15**, 205–6.

Tarlatzis, B.C. and Bili, H. (2000). Intracytoplasmic sperm injection. Survey of world results. *Annals of the New York Academy of Sciences*, **900**, 336–44.

Tut, T.G., Ghadessy, F.J., Trifiro, M.A., Pinsky, L., and Yong, E.L. (1997). Long polyglutamine tracts in the androgen receptor are associated with reduced trans-activation, impaired sperm production, and male infertility. *Journal of Clinical Endocrinology and Metabolism*, **82**, 3777–82.

Vandervors, M., Staessen, C., Sermon, K., et al. (2000). The Brussels' experience of more than 5 years of clinical preimplantation genetic diagnosis. *Human Reproduction Update*, **6**, 364–73.

Venter, J.C., Adams, M.D., Myers, E.W., et al. (2001). The sequence of the human genome. *Science*, **291**, 1304–51.

Verlinsky, Y. and Evsikov, S. (1999). A simplified and efficient method for obtaining metaphase chromosomes from individual human blastomeres. *Fertility and Sterility*, **72**, 1127–33.

Verlinsky, Y. and Kuliev, A. (1999). Preimplantation genetic diagnosis. *Reproductive Medicine Reviews*, **7**, 1–10.

Verlinsky, Y. and Kuliev, A. (2000). *An Atlas of Preimplantation Genetic Diagnosis*. Parthenon, New York.

Verlinsky, Y., Rechitsky, S., Verlinsky, O. et al. (2001). Preimplantation diagnosis for p53 tumour suppressor gene mutations. *Reproductive Biomedicine Online*, **2**, 102–105.

Vogt, P.H. (1998). Human chromosome deletions in Yq11, AZF candidate genes and male infertility: history and update. *Molecular Human Reproduction*, **4**, 739–44.

Vogt, P.H., Edelmann, A., Kirsch, S., et al. (1996) Human Y chromosome azoospermia factors (AZF) mapped to different subregions in Yq11. *Human Molecular Genetics*, **5**, 933–43.

Voullaire, L., Slater, H., Williamson, R., and Wilton, L. (2000). Chromosome analysis of blastomeres from human embryos by using comparative genomic hybridization. *Human Genetics*, **106**, 210–17.

Vrettou, C., Palmer, G., Kanavakis, E., et al. (1999). A widely applicable strategy for single cell genotyping of beta-thalassaemia mutations using DGGE analysis: application to preimplantation genetic diagnosis. *Prenatal Diagnosis*, **19**, 1209–16.

Wang, Q., Ghadessy, F.J., Trounson, A., et al. (1998). Azoospermia associated with a mutation in the ligand-binding domain of an androgen receptor displaying normal ligand binding, but defective trans-activation. *Journal of Clinical Endocrinology and Metabolism*, **83**, 4303–9.

Warner, J.P., Barron, L.H., Goudie, D., et al. (1996). A general method for the detection of large CAG repeat expansions by fluorescent PCR. *Journal of Medical Genetics*, **33**, 1022–6.

Wells, D. and Delhanty, J.D. (2000). Comprehensive chromosomal analysis of human preimplantation embryos using whole genome amplification and single cell comparative genomic hybridization. *Molecular Human Reproduction*, **6**, 1055–62.

Wells, D., Sherlock, J.K., Handyside, A.H., and Delhanty, J.D. (1999). Detailed chromosomal and molecular genetic analysis of single cells by whole genome amplification and comparative genomic hybridisation. *Nucleic Acids Research*, **27**, 1214–8.

Willadsen, S., Levron, J., Munne, S., et al. (1999). Rapid visualization of metaphase chromosomes in single human blastomeres after fusion with in-vitro matured bovine eggs. *Human Reproduction*, **14**, 470–5.

13

Cloning mammals

Don P. Wolf and Shoukhrat Mitalipov

Division of Reproductive Sciences, Oregon Regional Primate Research Center, Beaverton, USA

Introduction

Cloning, defined simply as making a copy by asexual reproduction, does not normally occur in mammals, except in the relatively rare cases of identical twinning that results from early embryo separation or splitting. As proven by the existence of identical twins, individual cells or blastomeres in the early preimplantation mammalian embryo are totipotent (able to develop into any cell lineage in the fetus or placenta) as demonstrated decades ago by experiments involving blastomere separation and culture, selective destruction of blastomeres, or embryo bisection (Nicholas and Hall, 1942; Tarkowski, 1959; Willadsen, 1979; Seidel, 1983). A modern, medical definition of cloning would specify a process involving nuclear transfer (NT): to reproduce asexually by transferring a somatic cell or its nucleus (karyoplast) into an enucleated oocyte (cytoplast). Unlike twinning technologies such as blastomere separation and culture or embryo splitting, which produce exact copies or true clones, NT clones may have multiple sources of mitochondrial DNA. Twinning, used in domestic species since the early 1980s, has now been largely abandoned because of poor efficiency except in unique biomedical applications, for example, in the rhesus monkey where sets of identical twins would be extremely useful for vaccine development or other studies involving immune system response (Wolf, 2000).

In the past several years there has been a resurgence of interest and remarkable progress in cloning by somatic cell NT. This option became a possibility in mammals only recently despite the fact that successful NT with embryonic blastomeres as donor nuclei dates back to the pioneering studies of Steen Willadsen (Willadsen, 1986). Then, in the mid 1990s, live offspring were produced in cattle and sheep by NT from embryo-derived, cultured cells (Sims and First, 1994; Campbell et al., 1996) and finally experimentation at the Roslyn Institute in Scotland culminated in the announcement in 1997 of the production of offspring by NT of nuclear donor cells derived from fetal or adult tissue (Wilmut et al., 1997). This latter event forced a revolution in our working assumptions of somatic cell cloning and opened the field to worldwide activity.

Why clone nonhuman mammals?

A major objective of cloning related research at an applied level is to improve the efficiency of the process and to develop or define universal protocols. In a basic research context, understanding the nuclear reprogramming that must occur following NT could impact not only the establishment of routine cloning protocols but also lead to improved insights into early mammalian development and cell cycle regulation, with potential implications for oncogenesis and human health. Parenthetically, defining the relative roles of the nucleus and cytoplasm in mammalian development harkens back to the "fantastical" experiment of Hans Spemann in 1938 (Spemann, 1938) in which he first proposed experimentation involving nuclear transfer.

For agricultural applications, improving the quality

or characteristics of a herd quickly and efficiently is possible with NT, since the ability to replicate large numbers of genetically elite animals, say based on milk production or wool quality, is possible. Indeed one of the strengths of NT from a primary culture or cell line is that the nuclear donor cell is not limiting, thereby allowing the possibility of a very large if not infinite clone size. In an agricultural context, the ability to clone from adult cells carries an important advantage over embryonic or fetal cell cloning as expression of the desired trait can be prescreened in cloning candidates.

Another advantage to NT with cultured cells is an increased efficiency in generating germline-positive, transgenic animals (Cibelli et al., 1998). Conventional methods of transgenesis involve introduction of exogenous DNA into embryos by direct microinjection of multiple copies of a gene construct into pronuclei or by using membrane-disrupted sperm as a carrier along with microinjection. In these cases, germline transmission occurs infrequently, a major disadvantage in efforts to produce a heritable transgenic line (Perry, 2000). With the use of NT, transfection of nuclear donor cells is accomplished in culture, and it is only after selection of cells carrying the desired genes that NT embryos are produced and transferred in efforts to establish pregnancy. The use of NT makes germline transmission a non-issue since all progeny cells are transgenic.

Of course, somatic cell cloning could be used in the preservation or propagation of endangered animals, of founder animals, as described above, in a biomedical context, or for pets. Lazaron BioTechnologies (www.lazaron.com) states that pet cloning (dogs, cats, and horses) is very likely to be affordable to most animal owners by 2005–2010. To prepare for this eventuality, they recommend proper preservation of your pet's living cells now, by cryopreservation of a skin sample.

Cloning protocols

While the fundamentals of cloning by NT are similar among species, the process will likely require a

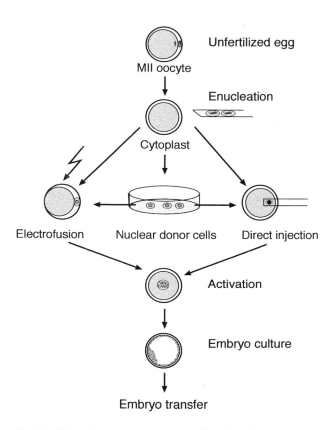

Fig. 13.1. Schematic representation of somatic cell cloning by nuclear transfer.

unique recipe in each (Fig. 13.1; Mitalipov and Wolf, 2000). The prerequisites for cloning start with an extensive knowledge of the endocrinology and gamete/reproductive biology of the species under study. The first requirement is a reliable source of high-quality oocytes, satisfied by harvesting immature oocytes from slaughterhouse ovaries with subsequent in vitro maturation (IVM) or by recovering in vivo matured oocytes following ovarian stimulation. Mature oocytes are then enucleated. This is usually physically by micromanipulation with microscopic confirmation of DNA removal, although early success with chemical enucleation has been reported (Baguisi and Overstrom, 2000). The donor DNA is added either as an isolated nucleus (direct injection) or an intact cell (electro-fused), and the cytoplast is subjected to an activation stimulus, either in conjunction with electrofusion or after a delay, that is designed to initiate development. Modulations of intracellular calcium concentrations are required for this, which can be accomplished by electroporation in the presence of high extracellular calcium, by exposure to ionophores or, in the mouse, by the use of strontium (Wakayama et al., 1998). The second step in activation involves maturation promoting factor (MPF), a complex of two proteins, cyclin B and $p34^{cdc2}$. The latter is a protein kinase with activity regulated by changes in phosphorylation state and by association with cyclins (Nurse, 1990). High levels of MPF preclude those nuclear events downstream from oocyte activation that prestage mitosis. MPF levels, which normally fall following sperm penetration, can be reduced in the cytoplast by exposure to general protein synthesis or specific protein kinase inhibitors. Once produced, developing NT embryos must be stored at low temperature (conventional cryopreservation or vitrification) or grown to a stage suitable for transfer to a synchronized surrogate. Embryo culture may be one of the most challenging aspects to the cloning process since the embryo's nutritional requirements change with development and at present culture conditions do not mimic the in vivo environment very well. In the past, the spectrum of approaches to embryo culture has included everything from in vivo culture in ligated oviducts, to co-culture, and to the use of chemically defined or sequential media.

Embryo transfer in an attempt to establish pregnancy carries its own set of challenges and again the unique characteristics of each species is paramount, for instance, in deciding how many embryos to transfer. In the pig, a large number must be transferred to establish a pregnancy while in a nonhuman primate the consequences of a high-order multiple pregnancy might be unacceptable. The route (oviductal or transcervical) and method (surgical or nonsurgical) of transfer are additional variables. With regards to pregnancy detection and maintenance, the industry as a whole will undoubtedly become more proactive at the very least to document problems and abnormalities as they occur. In the monkey, a monitoring program patterned after the high-risk obstetrical care offered women would be desirable. The high incidence of fetal and neonatal wastage associated with somatic cell cloning in domestic species (see below) also mandates additional, and perhaps exceptional, efforts to improve term birth and neonatal outcomes.

The biology of cloning

Synchrony in cell cycle events between the host cytoplast and the transferred nucleus is important for the creation of a viable NT embryo and for the timing of subsequent developmental events and the maintenance of proper ploidy in NT embryos. The cytoplast must direct the reprogramming of the donor nucleus, a process that involves the activities of MPF and other cell cycle regulatory proteins along with the replacement, by maternal stores, of proteins associated with the donor nucleus (Kikyo and Wolffe, 2000). This long-standing realization of the importance of cell cycle synchrony has led to donor cell manipulation strategies such as serum starvation to force cells into a desirable cell cycle stage (G_0; Wilmut et al., 1997), use of cells naturally in a prolonged G_1 stage (Wakayama et al., 1998), or selection of cells based on size, appearance, or other physical characteristics that may reflect cycle stage and DNA content. Empirically defined variables also include the source and age of the donor animal, the passage number of cultured cells, and even the specific cell line (Rideout et al., 2000). Despite the fundamental importance of genetic reprogramming in NT, the precise molecular events that constitute the process are poorly understood. Clearly, since the DNA sequence information does not usually change as a cell differentiates, reprogramming of a differentiated cell nucleus reflects the reversal of epigenetic changes (heritable changes in gene expression that occur without a change in DNA sequence) that transpire during normal development (Wolffe and Matzke, 1999). In other words, in order for the transferred nucleus to recapitulate the events of early development, it must first be transcriptionally silenced (like a mature gamete?) and then re-establish the temporal, spatial, and quantitative patterns of gene expression associated with normal development. (Campbell, 1999). These patterns might be established at different times depending on the species and the timing of the maternal to embryonic transition in the regulation of development. Differential gene expression is a normal component of development, an example of which is imprinting. In this case, one of the two alleles is uniquely modified (methylated) during gametogenesis and this modification, which is stable, heritable, and erasable, can mark parental alleles and also can be used to inhibit gene activity, since hypermethylated DNA is typically transcriptionally repressed (Bartolomei et al., 2000). Histone acetylation and chromatin structure are also players in this game of selective gene expression (Wolffe and Matzke, 1999). It follows that, if postzygotic loss of methylation imprints is irreversible or developmentally associated epigenetic modifications are not reset appropriately during reprogramming, the inappropriate expression of imprinted alleles may limit the efficiency of cloning. In fact, some of the characteristics of cloned pregnancies – large placenta, oversize embryo, fetal death – are consistent with problems of genomic imprinting (Wolffe and Matzke, 1999). Variable expression of imprinted genes has been associated with manipulations as simple as culturing control embryos under suboptimal conditions (Doherty et al., 2000).

As noted at the outset, cloning by NT produces "genetic replicates" rather than true clones, and this fact carries potential implications for the health and well-being of cloned animals. Mammalian cells contain two distinct genomes: nuclear DNA inherited in a Mendelian fashion and mitochondrial DNA, which is maternally transmitted. In order to achieve maternal transmission, paternal mitochondria originating with the sperm are rapidly and selectively eliminated during fertilization (Sutovsky et al., 1999). With somatic cell NT, accomplished by electrofusion of the entire donor cell with the cyto-

plast, heteroplasmy may result, with mitochondria originating from both the cytoplast and the donor cell. However, recent findings in 10 cloned sheep are consistent with the maintenance of cytoplast-origin mitochondria only and the selective loss of mitochondria from the nuclear donor cells (Evans et al., 1999). Therefore, while heteroplasmy remains a theoretical contributing factor in cloning by the NT process, compatibility between the donor nuclear DNA and the recipient mitochondrial DNA may be the major concern.

What about aging and telomere length? Will newborn animals cloned from adult cells assume the age of their nuclear donors, i.e., will they age prematurely? Telomeres are unique protein–DNA structures that form the termini of eukaryotic linear chromosomes and play a role in the regulation of cell division (Hodes, 1999). Normal cells have a finite replicative lifespan, and a correlation exists between telomere length and senescence because telomeres shorten with each cell division. Measurements of telomere length in one-year-old Dolly and in two other NT-derived sheep (Shiels et al., 1999) indicated shortened telomere length relative to age-matched controls, consistent with the age of the progenitor mammary tissue and with the time that the nuclear donor cells spent in culture before NT. However, a similar analysis of telomere length in calves cloned from fetal fibroblasts indicated significantly longer telomeres than those of newborn or age-matched controls (Lanza et al., 2000). In the mouse, no evidence of premature aging has been reported although careful comparisons have only been made up to one year of age. In these studies, the nuclear donor cells were from – animals of eight to ten weeks of age. This would require that any assessment of premature aging would have to be sensitive to a difference of eight to ten weeks between cloned and control animals (Tamashiro et al., 2000). Cumulina, the first cloned mouse, recently passed away at 3 years of age, the normal lifespan for a laboratory-reared mouse. Obviously, a final answer must await additional results but there is no compelling reason to be overly concerned about premature aging in somatic cell clones at this time.

Table 13.1. Success rates of assisted reproduction and nuclear transfer in cattle

Procedure	Embryos to live calves (%)	Pregnancy rate at 35 days (%)	Abortion rate (%)	Neonatal losses[a] (%)
Artificial insemination/natural mating	—	75	6–8	2–3
Embryos recovered from one animal and transferred to another	50	75	6–8	2–3
Embryos produced by in vitro maturation and in vitro fertilization	20	45–50	8–15	10
Embryos produced by nuclear transfer				
Embryonic donor nucleus	20	25–35	20–25	—
Fetal or adult donor nucleus	15	35	50	30

Notes:
[a] Neonatal losses include those within a few days of birth.

Cloning success

Most experience of NT with embryonic cells as donor nuclei involves ruminants, reflecting extensive commercial interests. However, studies have involved sheep (Willadsen, 1986; Wells et al., 1997), cattle (Bondioli et al., 1990; Stice et al., 1996), rabbit (Stice and Robl, 1988; Collas and Robl, 1990; Yang et al., 1992), mice (Cheong et al., 1993; Kwon and Kono, 1996), goat (Yong and Yuqiang, 1998), pig (Prather et al., 1989), and monkey (Meng et al., 1997). In the period 1995–2000, somatic cell cloning has been accomplished from fetal or adult cells in sheep, cattle, mice, goats, and now pigs (Betthauser et al., 2000; Onishi et al., 2000; Polejaeva et al., 2000); for review see Colman, 2000). As a perspective for evaluating cloning success, pregnancy rates and neonatal outcomes for natural mating (NM)/artificial insemination (AI), for transfers of in vitro-produced (IVP) embryos, as well as for NT embryos produced from embryonic cells are useful and have been summarized for cattle (Table 13.1). In addition, successes have been updated for several other species.

Cattle

The use of NM or AI in cattle is characterized by a pregnancy (non-return) rate of ~75%, a low abor-

tion rate (6–8%) and low neonatal losses (Table 13.1). When embryos produced by NM/AI are flushed nonsurgically and transferred to a synchronized recipient, comparable pregnancy and loss rates are observed, with 50% of embryos transferred resulting in live calves. In contrast, for embryos produced by IVM or in vitro fertilization (IVF), only about 20% of embryos transferred result in live calves and both the abortion and neonatal loss rates are increased. Pregnancy rates (expressed per recipient undergoing ET) at day 35 are in the range of 75%, 75%, and 50% for AI/NM, ET, and IVP, respectively. Note that day 35 pregnancy rates less spontaneous abortion rates expressed in Table 13.1 do not equal term pregnancy rates because losses also occur between days 35 and 90. The average birthweight of ET calves is elevated by 8% compared with calves produced by AI/NM (Wilson et al., 1995). IVP embryos cultured in ligated sheep oviducts give calves of similar birthweight to AI controls, while embryos subjected to in vitro co-culture result in calves that are significantly heavier (Behboodi et al., 1995). These increased birthweights form the basis for the large calf syndrome but by no means represent the complete spectrum of problems in such animals. Elevated weights tend to normalize over time, while severe medical problems are often present that contribute to neonatal losses (Wilson et al., 1995).

Approximately 1000 calves were produced in the 1990s, prior to the Dolly success, by NT with embryonic blastomeres as donor cells (Bondioli et al., 1990; Stice et al., 1996). The efficiency of producing term births from NT embryos approaches that for IVP; for instance, 294 transferred NT embryos resulted in 62 term births (21%). The pregnancy rates of 25–32% for embryonic cell cloning with 20–32% of pregnancies resulting in live calves is in the range established for IVP (Table 13.1). However, in a study of 219 cloned calves, accelerated growth and heavier birthweights (20% larger) were reported compared with full-term siblings produced by ET or AI/NM. This extraordinary in utero growth was transient as yearling calves in all groupings showed comparable percent body weights (Wilson et al., 1995).

The use of cultured inner cell mass cells as the source of donor nuclei is limited to a single report (Sims and First, 1994) wherein 34 blastocysts were transferred into 27 cows with 13 (49%) becoming pregnant and four livebirths (12%).

Efforts to clone from fetal or adult somatic cells are summarized in Table 13.1. While livebirths at 15% of transferred embryos is comparable with other NT or IVP procedures, fetal and neonatal losses have been extraordinary, at 50% and 30%, respectively! Therefore, it can be concluded that embryos cloned by NT, even from embryonic blastomeres or undifferentiated cells, result, upon transfer, in increased fetal wastage throughout pregnancy, high birthweight, perinatal and postnatal death, and poor adaptation to the after birth environment. These negative outcomes appear more severe with fetal or adult somatic cell NT. Also worth noting is that the results in Table 13.1 do not consider the efficiency of development of embryos to a stage suitable for nonsurgical ET nor the number and quality of embryos transferred.

Sheep

With cultured (differentiated) sheep embryonic cells, 23% (235/1015) of the NT embryos produced developed to the blastocyst stage and 196 embryos when transferred resulted in 12 livebirths, for a success rate per embryo transferred of 6.1% (Colman, 2000). A 25% neonatal loss rate is obtained by combining the results of two groups (Campbell, et al., 1996; Wells et al., 1997). The corresponding experience for NT with fetal or adult cells was 16% (145/906) development to blastocyst and a 7.6% livebirth rate (10/131). Neonatal loss rates are not always reported but appear to be high; for instance, in the studies that included the Dolly success, 62% of fetuses were lost, a significantly greater proportion than the estimate of 6% after natural mating.

Goat

Although experience with somatic cell cloning in goats is limited, fetal and neonatal wastage has been low, unlike in sheep and cattle. Both Baguisi and coworkers (1999) and Keefer and coworkers (2000) reported that all pregnancies that reached 60 days were carried to term, birthweights were within normal ranges and, except for one member of a twin set that died at birth, all kids survived and were healthy.

Mouse

The experience in mice is robust for in vitro manipulated embryos and for somatic cell cloning (Wakayama et al., 1998, 1999; Wakayama and Yanagimachi, 1999). If in vitro manipulated embryos were transferred to pseudopregnant hosts, they developed to surviving pups at 50–75% efficiency. This value was calculated, with an assumption or two, from Tamashiro et al. (2000), who conducted comparative studies on normal and cloned pups. Under comparable conditions, NT embryos have high implantation rates (57–71%) but low fetal (5–16%) and full-term (2–3%) developmental rates (Tamashiro et al., 2000). A much higher full-term development rate (21%) was reported recently following NT from an embryonic stem cell line (Rideout et al., 2000) under conditions where a significant dependence upon the cell line used as the source of nuclear donor cells was demonstrated. While pups with elevated birthweight are not obtained for in vitro manipulated or NT embryos, obesity in cloned mice has been observed; body-weights are the same until 9 weeks of age, after which clones are heavier (Tamashiro et al., 2000). Additionally, no physical abnormalities were observed in either a control or cloned group; behavior and motor tests showed that, although there were some developmental delays in clones, there was no evidence of serious adverse effects.

Can we clone all mammalian species?

While it is a little early to bet the farm, there no longer seems to be a compelling case for maintaining that you can not clone a species, provided the prerequisites can be fulfilled for infrastructural support, a detailed knowledge of the reproductive and endocrine biology of the species in question, and a critical mass of competent scientists focused on the challenge. Relevant to this conclusion are the recent successes announced in the pig, a heretofore unclonable species (Betthauser et al., 2000; Onishi et al., 2000; Polejaeva et al., 2000). Commercial interests have funded extensive cloning efforts in this species based on potential applications in organ xenotransplantation. The concept is to clone from porcine cell lines that carry a loss of function mutation in the gene for α-1,3-galactosyl transferase, since α-1,3-galactose, found on pig but not human cells, triggers immune rejection. Other laboratory species receiving attention in somatic cell cloning circles include the rat, the rabbit, and the monkey.

Can we clone humans?

The possibility of cloning humans represents a unique challenge because of ethical issues. Technically, we have the infrastructure well in place, as good as or better than that for any other species, including protocols for oocyte recovery, embryo production, growth, and transfer. With the advent of intracytoplasmic sperm injection (ICSI) and embryo biopsy for preimplantation genetic diagnosis, many laboratories are already experienced in the micro-manipulative techniques required to support NT. In fact, NT is used extensively in the treatment of human infertility by ICSI, and clinical trials are ongoing or envisioned using NT to alleviate infertility secondary to advanced maternal age, where an increase in aneuploidy is an undesirable consequence (Wolf, 2000). If this increase is caused by cytoplasmic incompetence in spindle formation, resulting in errors in chromosome segregation, it could be overcome by allowing maturation of the nucleus from an older oocyte to occur in the presence of the cytoplasmic machinery of a younger oocyte. So NT would be employed to move the germinal vesicle/nucleus from the older patient's immature oocyte to a young donor cytoplast. Other potentials envisioned for NT in assisted reproduction in humans include a treatment for mitochondrial disease, where moving the affected patient's nucleus into the cytoplast of a healthy donor might circumvent the disease, or in creating an egg by NT of a somatic cell into a cytoplast with subsequent polar body abstriction to achieve the haploid state (Takeuchi et al., 2000). Since these NT activities are ongoing or under development, it takes little fortitude to speculate that, from a technical perspective, somatic cell cloning in humans is a realistic possibility. Perhaps it is this possibility that makes the promises of Richard Seed, to be the first to clone a human, so threatening (Wolf, 2000).

The more pressing question is *should* we clone humans. Arguments for somatic cell cloning, to reproduce an existing person, as a source of organs or to circumvent mortality are, when serious, ludicrous and uniformly rejected. However, cogent arguments for reproductive cloning have been made, based on the expression of an individual's reproductive rights. For example, reproductive cloning could be used to propagate the genetic contribution of gays or lesbians, adults with genetic defects (lethal recessive genes), or infertile patients with no germ cells. An argument can also be made for somatic cell NT in support of therapeutic cloning (see Ch. 10), made possible by the discovery in 1998 that human embryonic stem (ES) cells could be isolated and immortalized from the inner cell mass of IVF-pro-duced blastocysts (Thomson et al., 1998). The most useful and important property of these cells is their pluripotency: ability to differentiate in vitro and in vivo into the three major layers of the body. Since diseases like Parkinson's disease or juvenile-onset diabetes mellitus arise from the death or dysfunc-tion of just one or a few cell types, cell-replacement strategies could offer an effective and permanent solution to the abnormal condition barring autoim-mune concerns. Therefore, if you or I wanted to create our own ES cells, nuclear transfer from a skin fibroblast into a cytoplast would be followed by embryo growth and ES cell isolation. Alternatively stocks of "typed" ES cells might be derived from donated embryos from IVF–ET patients. In any case, the idea is that, when needed, ES cells would be propagated in vitro and coaxed to differentiate into specific genotypes for use to replace lost or dysfunc-tional cell populations, to treat immune disorders, or in gene therapy.

Although human cloning, either reproductive or therapeutic, might be technically feasible, legally it can not be supported with federal research dollars in the USA and most other countries, and ethically it is still circumspect. Before the advent of therapeutic cloning, the US National Bioethics Advisory Commission, in a report to President Clinton in June of 1997, concluded that efforts to clone a person would be unsafe, at least now and in the near future, because of the likelihood of creating malformed fetuses. With the advent of human stem cell isolation and the possibility of therapeutic cloning, a different debate has arisen nationally centered on the use of ES cells, generated from IVF-produced embryos, in research. Because of the potential value of these cells in the treatment of human disease, many of the world's scientific societies have registered support for the experimental use of existing human ES cells, but not necessarily for the isolation of additional ES lines, which would require human embryo sacrifice. The current position of the US National Institute of Health is in favor of funding research on human stem cells derived from the destruction of embryos in privately funded clinics (Annas, 2000) and it

would appear that ES cell research will be supported in both the USA and the UK.

The future of cloning

At the practical level, improvements in cloning effi-ciency are desirable and inevitable. This is a very young field and a critical mass of investigators is still being constituted. Therefore, despite prob-lems, collective progress is impressive, with profi-ciency demonstrated in an increasing number of species and with different cell types. Ultimately, selection of a particular cell line or primary culture for somatic cell cloning based on karyotype, cell cycle stage, telomere length, and in vitro blastocyst development rates of NT embryos may become feasible, not to mention the possibility of specific molecular markers, such as α-fetoprotein expres-sion driven by a G_0-specific promoter (Colman, 2000). Underlying this selection process will be knowledge of whether or not the cell type is suitable for NT based on its history, the occurrence of random genetic damage, or the ability to repro-gram epigenetic changes that have occurred during development (Colman, 2000).

Pregnancy maintenance and intervention strate-gies must be improved, especially in sheep and cattle where high fetal and neonatal losses are seen. We also need to know if these undesirable outcomes are unique or whether they apply to other species. An understanding of the causes for these high losses will hopefully lead to strategies to circumvent them.

Improved efficiencies in producing healthy off-spring by somatic cell cloning will allow commercial, agricultural, and medical use. Applications have already emerged with the creation and propagation of transgenic clones wherein the transgenes were randomly integrated into the donor cells used for NT (Cibelli et al., 1998). Coupled with gene targeting, however, NT will be increasingly employed in the creation of transgenics. Success with targeted trans-genesis in mouse ES cells (Rideout et al., 2000) has recently been extended to primary cultures of ovine fetal fibroblasts (McCreath et al., 2000). These results on targeted mutagenesis also carry important implications for the creation of human disease models where the first choice of mammalian models, the mouse, might not be appropriate or precise because of differences between the two species. Cystic fibrosis and ataxia telangiectasia are two examples that might benefit from research in a ruminant or non-human primate model.

Somatic cell cloning has been proposed as an approach for preserving rare or endangered species, for example pandas or Siberian tigers, or for bringing back extinct species, for example wooly mammoth or Tasmanian devils. However, increased experience and proficiency will be required before such an approach can be realistically employed (Wells et al., 1998; Oikawa et al., 2000). Notwithstanding this caveat, tissue that could support future cloning efforts might well be prepared accordingly (derive primary cultures) and maintained at low temperature. Efforts to clone humans, while promoted by some (Clonad; www.Clonaid.com) and arguably inevitable, is still much too risky to the embryo/fetus to be feasible, the ethical concerns notwithstanding (Wolf, 2000).

At a basic level, understanding of reprogramming is likely to come from invertebrates or the mouse, where imprinting studies are underway. The use of differential display technology to follow patterns of gene expression in individual embryos will catalyze these activities (Holding et al., 2000; Kelly and Rizzino, 2000; see also Ch. 12). This knowledge will allow a definition, indeed even laboratory duplication, of the cytoplasmic components required for reprogramming in the absence of an intact cytoplast (Kikyo et al., 2000). The implications for therapeutic cloning alone are immense since it may become possible to reprogram adult cells for therapeutic use, given that they are normal (McLaren, 2000). Federal support for human stem cell research should accelerate progress in therapeutic cloning and we can anticipate progress in the propagation and directed differentiation of primate stem cells, including human, and in tissue engineering in preparation for an anticipated revolution in transplantation medicine.

REFERENCES

Annas, G.J. (2000). Ulysses and the fate of frozen embryos – reproduction, research, or destruction? *The New England Journal of Medicine*, **343**, 373–6.

Baguisi, A. and Overstrom, E.W. (2000). Induced enucleation in nuclear transfer procedures to produce cloned animals. *Theriogenology*, **53**, 209.

Baguisi, A., Behboodi, E., Melican, D.T., et al. (1999). Production of goats by somatic cell nuclear transfer. *Nature Biotechnology*, **17**, 456–61.

Bartolomei, M.S., Thorvaldsen, J.L., Mann, M.R.W., Doherty, A.S., and Schultz, R.M. (2000). Genomic imprinting in mice – in vivo vs. in vitro control. In: *Proceedings of a Meeting on Genetically Engineering and Cloning Animals: Science, Society and Industry*, June, Park City/Deer Valley, UT. Utah State University, Park City, Speakers' Paper 4.

Behboodi, E., Anderson, G.B., BonDurant, R.H., et al. (1995). Birth of large calves that developed from in vitro-derived bovine embryos. *Theriogenology*, **44**, 227–32.

Betthauser, J., Forsberg, E., Augenstein, M., et al. (2000). Production of cloned pigs from in vitro systems. *Nature Biotechnology*, **18**, 1055–9.

Bondioli, K.R., Westhusin, M.E., and Loony, C.R. (1990). Production of identical bovine offspring by nuclear transfer. *Theriogenology*, **33**, 165–74.

Campbell, K.H.S. (1999). Nuclear equivalence, nuclear transfer, and the cell cycle. *Cloning*, **1**, 3–15.

Campbell, K.H.S., McWhir, J., Ritchie, W.A., and Wilmut, I. (1996). Sheep cloned by nuclear transfer from a cultured cell line. *Nature*, **380**, 64–6.

Cheong, H.T., Takahashi, Y., and Kanagawa, H. (1993). Birth of mice after transplantation of early cell-cycle-stage embryonic nuclei into enucleated oocytes. *Biology of Reproduction*, **48**, 958–63.

Cibelli, J.B., Stice, S.L., Golueke, P.J., et al. (1998). Cloned transgenic calves produced from nonquiescent fetal fibroblasts. *Science*, **280**, 1256–8.

Collas, P. and Robl, J.M. (1990). Factors affecting the efficiency of nuclear transplantation in the rabbit embryo. *Biology of Reproduction*, **43**, 877–84.

Colman, A. (2000). Somatic cell nuclear transfer in mammals: progress and applications. *Cloning*, **4**, 185–200.

Doherty, A.S., Mann, M.R.W., Tremblay, K.D., Bartolomei, M.S., and Schultz, R.M. (2000). Differential effects of culture on imprinted *H19* expression in the preimplantation mouse embryo. *Biology of Reproduction*, **62**, 1526–35.

Evans, M.J, Gurer, C., Loike, J.D., Wilmut, I., Schnieke, A.E., and Schon, E.A. (1999). Mitochondrial DNA genotypes in nuclear transfer-derived cloned sheep. *Nature Genetics*, **23**, 90–3.

Hodes, R.J. (1999). Telomere length, aging, and somatic cell turnover. *Journal of Experimental Medicine*, **190**, 153–6.

Holding, C., Bolton, V., and Monk, M. (2000). Detection of human novel developmental genes in cDNA derived from replicate individual preimplantation embryos. *Molecular Human Reproduction*, **6**, 801–9.

Keefer, C.L., Keyston, R., Bhatia, B., et al. (2000). Efficient production of viable goat offspring following nuclear transfer using adult somatic cells. *Biology of Reproduction*, **62**(Suppl. 1), 192.

Kelly, D.L. and Rizzino, A. (2000). DNA microarray analyses of genes regulated during the differentiation of embryonic stem cells. *Molecular Reproduction and Development*, **56**, 113–23.

Kikyo, N. and Wolffe, A.P. (2000). Reprogramming nuclei: insights from cloning, nuclear transfer and heterokaryons. *Journal of Cell Science*, **113**, 11–20.

Kikyo, N., Wade, P.A., Guschin, D., Ge, H., and Wolffe, A.P. (2000). Active remodeling of somatic nuclei in egg cytoplasm by the nucleosomal ATPase ISWI. *Science*, **289**, 2360–3.

Kwon, O.Y. and Kono, T. (1996). Production of identical sextuplet mice by transferring metaphase nuclei from four-cell embryos. *Proceedings of the National Academy of Sciences USA*, **93**, 13010–13.

Lanza, R.P., Cibelli, J.B, Blackwell, C., et al. (2000). Extension of cell life-span and telomere length in animals cloned from senescent somatic cells. *Science*, **288**, 665–9.

McCreath, K.J., Howcroft, J., Campbell, K.H.S., Colman, A., Schnieke, A.E., and Kind, A.J. (2000). Production of gene-targeted sheep by nuclear transfer from cultured somatic cells. *Nature*, **405**, 1066–9.

McLaren, A. (2000). Cloning: pathways to a pluripotent future. *Science*, **288**, 1775–80.

Meng, L., Ely, J.J., Stouffer, R.L., and Wolf, D.P. (1997). Rhesus monkeys produced by nuclear transfer. *Biology of Reproduction*, **57**, 454–9.

Mitalipov, S.M. and Wolf, D.P. (2000). Mammalian cloning: possibilities and threats. *Annals of Medicine*, **32**, 462–8.

Nicholas, J.S. and Hall, B.V. (1942). Experiments on developing rats: II. The development of isolated blastomeres and fused eggs. *Journal of Experimental Zoology*, **90**, 441–59.

Nurse, P. (1990). Universal control mechanism regulating onset of M-phase. *Nature*, **344**, 503–8.

Oikawa, T., Numabe, T., Kikuchi, T., Takada, N., and Izaike, Y. (2000). Production of somatic cell clone calves from cumulus cells of a 20 years old Japanese black cow. *Theriogenology*, **53**, 236.

Onishi, A., Iwamoto, M., Akita, T., et al. (2000). Pig cloning by microinjection of fetal fibroblast nuclei. *Science*, **289**, 1188–90.

Perry, A.C.F. (2000). Hijacking oocyte DNA repair machinery in transgenesis? *Molecular Reproduction and Development*, **56**, 319–24.

Polejaeva, I.A., Chen, S.H., Vaught, T.D., et al. (2000). Cloned pigs produced by nuclear transfer from adult somatic cells. *Nature*, **407**, 86–90.

Prather, R.S., Sims, M.M., and First, N.L. (1989). Nuclear transplantation in early pig embryos. *Biology of Reproduction*, **41**, 414–18.

Rideout III, W.M., Wakayama, T., Wutz, A., et al. (2000). Generation of mice from wild-type and targeted ES cells by nuclear cloning. *Nature Genetics*, **24**, 109–10.

Seidel, G.E., Jr. (1983). Production of genetically identical sets of mammals: cloning? *Journal of Experimental Zoology*, **228**, 347–54.

Shiels, P.G., Kind, A.J., Campbell, K.H., et al. (1999). Analysis of telomere lengths in cloned sheep. *Nature*, **399**, 316–17.

Sims, M. and First, N.L. (1994). Production of calves by transfer of nuclei from cultured inner cell mass cells. *Proceedings of the National Academy of Sciences USA*, **91**, 6143–7.

Spemann, H. (1938). *Embryonic Development and Induction*. Hafner, New York, pp. 210–11.

Stice, S.L. and Robl, J.M. (1988). Nuclear reprogramming in nuclear transplant rabbit embryos. *Biology of Reproduction*, **39**, 657–64.

Stice, S.L., Strelchenko, N.S, Keefer, C.L., and Matthews, L. (1996). Pluripotent bovine embryonic cell lines direct embryonic development following nuclear transfer. *Biology of Reproduction*, **54**, 100–10.

Sutovsky, P., Moreno, R.D., Ramalho-Santos, J., Dominko, T., Simerly, C., and Schatten, G. (1999). Ubiquitin tag for sperm mitochondria. *Nature*, **402**, 371–2.

Takeuchi, T., Raffaelli, R., Rosenwaks, Z., and Palermo, G.D. (2000). Construction of viable mammalian oocytes. *Human Reproduction*, **15**(Suppl. 1), 24.

Tamashiro, K.L.K., Wakayama, T., Blanchard, R.J., Blanchard, D.C., and Yanagimachi, R. (2000). Postnatal growth and behavioral development of mice cloned from adult cumulus cells. *Biology of Reproduction*, **63**, 328–34.

Tarkowski, A.K. (1959). Experiments on the development of isolated blastomeres of mouse eggs. *Nature*, **184**, 1286–7.

Thomson, J.A., Itskovitz-Eldor, J., Shapiro, S.S., et al. (1998). Embryonic stem cell lines derived from human blastocysts. *Science*, **282**, 1145–7.

Wakayama, T. and Yanagimachi, R. (1999). Cloning of male mice from adult tail-tip cells. *Nature Genetics*, **22**, 127–8.

Wakayama, T., Perry, A.C., Zuccotti, M., Johnson, K.R., and

Yanagimachi, R. (1998). Full-term development of mice from enucleated oocytes injected with cumulus cell nuclei. *Nature*, **394**, 369–74.

Wakayama, T., Rodriguez, I., Perry, A.C., Yanagimachi, R., and Mombaerts, P. (1999). Mice cloned from embryonic stem cells. *Proceedings of the National Academy of Sciences USA*, **96**, 14984–9.

Wells, D.N., Misica, P.M., Day, T.A., and Tervit, H.R. (1997). Production of cloned lambs from an established embryonic cell line: a comparison between in vivo- and in vitro-matured cytoplasts. *Biology of Reproduction*, **57**, 385–93.

Wells, D.N., Misica, P.M., Tervit, H.R., and Vivanco, W.H. (1998). Adult somatic cell nuclear transfer is used to preserve the last surviving cow of the Enderby Island cattle breed. *Reproduction, Fertility and Development*, **10**, 369–78.

Willadsen, S.M. (1979). A method for culture of micromanipulated sheep embryos and its use to produce monozygotic twins. *Nature*, **277**, 298–300.

Willadsen, S.M. (1986). Nuclear transplantation in sheep embryos. *Nature*, **320**, 63–5.

Wilmut, I., Schnieke, A.E., McWhir, J., Kind, A.J., and Campbell, K.H. (1997). Viable offspring derived from fetal and adult mammalian cells. *Nature*, **385**, 810–13.

Wilson, J.M., Williams, J.D., Bondioli, K.R., Looney, C.R., Westusin, M.E., and McCalla, D.F. (1995). Comparison of birth weight and growth characteristics of bovine calves produced by nuclear transfer (cloning), embryo transfer and natural mating. *Animal Reproduction Science*, **38**, 73–83.

Wolf, D.P. (2000). Cloning and nuclear transfer in humans. In: *Assisted Fertilization and Nuclear Transfer in Mammals*, Wolf, D.P. and Zelinski-Wooten, M., eds. Humana Press, Totowa, NJ, pp. 285–97.

Wolffe, A.P. and Matzke, M.A. (1999). Epigenetics: regulation through repression. *Science*, **286**, 481–6.

Yang, X., Jiang, S., Kovacs, A., and Foote, R.H. (1992). Nuclear totipotency of cultured rabbit morulae to support full-term development following nuclear transfer. *Biology of Reproduction*, **47**, 636–43.

Yong, Z. and Yuqiang, L. (1998). Nuclear–cytoplasmic interaction and development of goat embryos reconstructed by nuclear transplantation: production of goats by serially cloning embryos. *Biology of Reproduction*, **58**, 266–9.

14

Fluorescence imaging: gamete selection and intracytoplasmic sperm injection

Laura Hewitson, Cal Simerly, and Gerald Schatten

Pittsburgh Development Center (PDC) of the Magee Women's Research Institute, Pittsburgh and the
Department of Obstetrics, Gynecology and Reproductive Sciences, University of Pittsburgh, USA

Introduction

The clinical application of intracytoplasmic sperm injection (ICSI; Palermo et al., 1992; Van Steirteghem et al., 1993) has revolutionized the field of assisted reproduction (ART). While originally introduced to treat oligozoospermic men, ICSI has more recently been applied in those with severe asthenozoospermia and/or teratozoospermia. However, using ICSI to facilitate the introduction of suboptimal sperm into the oocyte may pose a long-term risk to offspring (In't Veld et al., 1995; Silber et al., 1995; Kent-First et al., 1996; reviewed by Vogt, 1995). In some extreme cases, sperm showing spermatogenic impairment have been used to achieve fertilization by ICSI (Mulhall et al., 1997; von Zumbusch et al., 1998; Stone et al., 2000) and there are concerns that the offspring conceived by couples with severe male factor infertility may also suffer from fertility problems, thereby perpetuating infertility in the next generation (Patrizio, 1995; Silber et al., 1995; Cummins, 1997; Schatten et al., 1998). Additionally, there is some indication that babies conceived through ICSI may be at higher risk of increased genetic abnormalities (In't Veld et al., 1995). Recently, Nudell and colleagues reported that there was a higher rate of mutations in the genes necessary for DNA repair in testicular DNA samples from some men demonstrating meiotic arrest than in samples from fertile men with normal spermatogenesis. The same DNA repair problem was also found in malignant tumor cells of some cancer patients, suggesting that ICSI offspring produced from the sperm from these patients may also be infertile and, more important, at a higher risk for certain cancers (Nudell et al., 2000). These risks certainly raise concerns about the widespread use of ICSI (Shoukir et al., 1998; Aytoz et al.,1999; Griffiths et al., 2000).

Possible long-term consequences of ICSI are unknown for two reasons. First, the oldest children conceived in this way are only about 8 years old. Second, ICSI does not work well in most species (Uehara and Yanagimachi, 1976; Westhusin and Kraemer, 1986; Iritani, 1988; Younis et al., 1989; Goto et al., 1990; Kimura and Yanagimachi, 1995; Ron-El et al., 1995; Hewitson et al., 1996a). While the mouse is often preferred for reproductive studies because of its fast generational time, fertilization in rodents is dependent on maternal centrosome (Schatten et al., 1985); in most other species, including humans, the centrosome is paternally derived (Simerly et al., 1995; reviewed by Schatten, 1994). This difference is critical for fertilization studies since sperm from the two species behave very differently during fertilization. More recently, nonhuman primates have emerged as an excellent model for understanding human fertilization and represent a valuable resource for ICSI. Gamete maturation, fertilization, embryonic development, embryo transfer, and implantation have been well documented (Bavister et al., 1983; Boatman, 1987; Lopata et al., 1988; Lanzendorf et al., 1990; VandeVoort and Tarantal, 1991; Hewitson et al., 1998, 1999) and since centrosomal inheritance and the cytoskeletal events of fertilization are very similar to humans (Simerly et al., 1995; Wu et al., 1996), comparisons between the two species are well justified (Schatten et al., 1998).

Fluorescence microscopy for studying fertilization

Understanding cytoskeletal motility during fertilization is paramount for designing and enhancing novel methods of ART. Recording these events requires the use of sophisticated digital imaging tools including conventional epifluorescence microscopy, laser-scanning confocal microscopy, and time-lapse video microscopy. These techniques have been particularly useful in determining the cytoskeletal and nuclear architectural structures of gamete interactions during fertilization. Conventional epifluorescence microscopy provides two-dimensional, static images of sperm incorporation, oocyte activation, pronuclear formation, etc., although the large size of oocytes can affect image clarity, especially when trying to visualize smaller structures such as centrosomes (Simerly and Schatten, 1993). This can often be overcome by employing confocal microscopy, which images thin sections through an oocyte thereby eliminating out-of-focus fluorescence typically seen with conventional epifluorescence microscopy. The sections can then be reconstructed to produce a three-dimensional image, preserving spatial integrity (Wright et al., 1993). Ideally, living oocytes and embryos should be studied to appreciate fully the enormous number of dynamic processes occurring during fertilization. For example, fluorescently labeled tubulin microinjected into unfertilized mouse oocytes is quickly incorporated into the microtubules of the meiotic spindle, demonstrating rapid cycles of assembly and disassembly (Gorbsky et al., 1990). As more sensitive dyes and probes for use in fluorescence microscopy become available and more powerful microscopes and imaging software are designed, fluorescence imaging techniques will play a vital role in reproductive biology as tools for analyzing cellular structure, physiology, and function.

Fluorescence imaging of gametes

Oocytes

ICSI has met with phenomenal success during the 1990s with thousands of ICSI babies being born to couples who might otherwise have been unable to conceive their own biological children. However, questions still remain about the dangers of passing traits responsible for male infertility, sex and autosomal chromosome aberrations (In't Veld et al., 1995), and genes responsible for mental, physical and reproductive abnormalities (Bonduelle et al., 1998; Bowen et al., 1998).

Whether the ICSI technique itself could pose a risk for offspring has yet to be determined, but certainly the physical insertion of a micropipette into the oocyte not only leaves microscopic blemishes on the oocyte's surface for several hours postinjection (Hewitson et al., 1996a) but may also damage the second meiotic spindle (Hewitson et al., 1999). Typically, the spindle region is avoided during ICSI by aligning the first polar body at right angles to the site of injection, since it is assumed that the first polar body resides close to the spindle. However, rhodamine-labeled bovine brain tubulin microinjected into rhesus oocytes imaged with low-light video microscopy demonstrated that the first polar body can be as much as 68° displaced from the cortical positioning of the meiotic spindle (Fig. 14.1a). In donated human oocytes, the mean displacement between the polar body and the meiotic spindle was $12.0 \pm 7.8°$ for in vitro matured (IVM) oocytes and $10.8 \pm 7.6°$ for in vitro fertilization (IVF) failures. In contrast, oocytes undergoing ICSI, which are first mechanically stripped of surrounding cumulus cells in the presence of hyaluronidase, showed higher angles of displacement between the second meiotic spindle and the first polar body $(56.0 \pm 27.5°)$. In mature oocytes, the first meiotic mid-body does not persist after extrusion of the first polar body. This mid-body, the remnant of the first meiotic spindle, bridges the first polar body with the oocyte at the site of the second meiotic spindle. Since the first polar body is not anchored firmly, mechanical manipula-

Fig. 14.1. Live imaging of gametes. (a) Dynamic labeling of a metaphase II arrested Rhesus oocyte showing meiotic spindle positioning. Arcs denoted by asterisks demonstrate the greatest displacement between the polar body (PB) and spindle. (b,c) A bovine sperm pre-incubated with the vital mitochondrion-specific dye Mito Tracker prior to in vitro fertilization (b) and at 16 hours after, showing the male pronucleus (c). Labeled mitochondria are shown by arrowheads. (d,e) On-stage identification of live rhesus monkey round spermatids labeled with Mito Tracker based on differential interference contrast (d) and epifluorescence (e) microscopy. Mito Tracker labeling reveals the onset of mitochondrial polarization (arrowheads), at this stage seen near the apex of the nucleus. Bar indicates 10 μm (a); 18 μm (b,c) and 6 μm (d,e). (Reprinted with permission from Hewitson et al., 1999 (a); Sutovsky et al., 1996a (b,c) and Sutovsky et al., 1999 (d,e), European Society of Human Reproduction and Embryology; reproduced by permission of Oxford University Press/ Human Reproduction.)

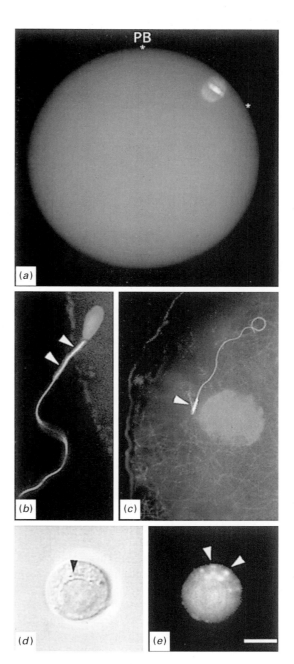

tions may result in its lateral displacement within the perivitelline space. Therefore, polar body positioning may be an unreliable indicator of the position of the meiotic spindle (Hewitson et al., 1999; Silva et al., 1999; Hardarson et al., 2000).

Sperm

Fluorescence microscopy has been invaluable for assessing the quality of populations of sperm. However, the use of sperm prelabeled with vital dyes prior to fertilization for the purpose of initiating pregnancy is restricted because of the possible detrimental effects on the offspring. Nevertheless, fluorescent probes have been very useful for determining the fate of sperm components during fertilization in animal species. Probes with higher excitation and emission wavelengths, such as SYBR 14[R] (membrane-permeant nucleic acid stain), are considered less harmful to DNA than Hoechst 33342 (bisbenzimide dyes) or DAPI (4′,6-diamidino-2-phenylindole), which have much lower wavelengths (Dominko et al., 2000). For example, when sperm mitochondria were prelabeled with the vital probe MitoTracker, prior to bovine fertilization, paternal mitochondria were found to persist throughout several cleavage divisions of the resultant embryo (Sutovsky et al., 1996a). One of the advantages of using this probe prior to fertilization is that the male pronucleus can be easily distinguished from the female pronucleus within the fertilized zygote by its association with paternal mitochondria (Fig. 14.1*b*). Furthermore, confirming the presence of a male pronucleus after fertilization (Fig. 14.1*c*) also prevents the misidentification of parthenogenotes, which look morphologically similar to normally fertilized zygotes.

The low number of sperm available in an ejaculate or testicular biopsy often hampers the selection of sperm for ICSI. Now that ICSI has been extended to include immature sperm (Devroey et al., 1994; Bourne et al., 1995; Palermo et al., 1999) or sperm with abnormal morphology (Harari et al., 1995; Liu et al., 1995; Nagy et al., 1995; Tournaye et al., 1996), the selection process is almost bypassed. Meanwhile, little is done to monitor the use of such abnormal sperm for ICSI (Moutel et al., 1999). While concerns about the long-term health of children conceived using poor-quality sperm for ICSI need to be addressed, the application of ICSI as the treatment of choice for all cases of in vitro conception is also currently being examined (Fishel et al., 2000).

The use of ICSI as a model for understanding human ART has enabled researchers to begin to assess some of the concerns about this method of fertilization. ICSI in the rhesus monkey is very successful and has recently been exploited as a method to produce transgenic animals (Chan et al., 2000). Using live dynamic imaging, sperm prelabeled with a rhodamine-tagged, plasmid encoding the green fluorescent protein (GFP) can be selected using fluorescence microscopy prior to ICSI to enhance the rate of transgenesis in ICSI embryos. After ICSI, the transgene (GFP) can be observed from the 4-cell to the blastocyst stage of rhesus embryo development (Chan et al., 2000). The ability to prelabel sperm prior to selection for ICSI without compromising their DNA will enable studies examining sperm function and structure during fertilization.

Spermatids

The introduction of a single round spermatid into a metaphase II-arrested oocyte (round spermatid injection, ROSI) to achieve fertilization is technically feasible. However, a major obstacle hindering the success of this technique is the questionable ability of the operator to identify and select the appropriate cell unambiguously (Fishel et al., 1996; Tesarik, 1997; Silber et al., 1998, 2000). Cell identification is usually based on size ($\sim$8 μm) and the presence of an acrosomal vesicle, a structure typical of round spermatids. While cell selection based on size alone is a challenging task because of the presence of Sertoli cells, Leydig cells, spermatogonia, blood cells, and other testicular components (Silber et al., 2000), the presence of an acrosomal vesicle is often difficult to discern owing to the low resolution of light microscopy. Although several new methods to distinguish round spermatids in testicular biopsies have been recently proposed (Angelopoulos et al., 1997; Reyes et al., 1997; Vanderzwalmen et al., 1997; Yamanaka et al., 1997; Aslam et al., 1998; Lassalle et al., 1999), cell size and morphology remain the criteria by which round spermatids are usually selected.

During spermatogenesis, round spermatids undergo a polarization of mitochondria, which localize close to the acrosomal vesicle. Mitochondrial polarization has been recently exploited as a criterion for selecting round spermatids for ROSI (Sutovsky et al., 1999). Using the mitochondrion-specific fluorescent vital dye MitoTracker to label spermatid mitochondria, round spermatids can be selected from a heterogeneous population of testicular cells based on their mitochondrial polarization (Fig. 14.1*d,e* and Sutovsky et al., 1999). Since paternal mitochondria are selectively destroyed after fertilization (Cummins et al., 1998), one could argue that the labeling of paternal mitochondria prior to fertilization would not interfere with embryo viability. However, since the dye also weakly labels the cell's nucleus, it could be harmful if these prelabeled cells were used for ROSI and a pregnancy was subsequently established. Certainly this technology would be suitable for training new technicians in the correct identification of round spermatids (when combined with size and morphological assessment), provided that the selection of cells to be used for ROSI was made in the absence of the dye (Sutovsky et al., 1999).

Imaging cytoskeletal dynamics following intracytoplasmic sperm injection

Fluorescence microscopy has been invaluable for determining the fates of sperm and oocyte components during fertilization. The first study on cytoskeletal dynamics in rhesus macaques ICSI zygotes (Fig. 14.2; Hewitson et al., 1996b) reported that sperm microinjected into rhesus oocytes (Fig. 14.2a) nucleated microtubules (Fig. 14.2b) and completed the repositioning of the maternal and paternal pronuclei (Fig. 14.2c) in a manner similar to that seen in rhesus oocytes fertilized by IVF (Wu et al., 1996). After pronuclear apposition, the sperm centrosome duplicated and split to establish a bipolar microtubule array (Fig. 14.2d,e). The sperm tail remained attached to the centrosome that was introduced by the sperm during ICSI and constituted one of the poles of the mitotic spindle (Fig. 14.2f). Since this study used IVM oocytes obtained from older, unstimulated animals, a number of fertilization failures were also noted. These included (i) the inability to resume meiosis, shown by metaphase II arrest and premature chromosome condensation and; (ii) centrosomal defects characterized by microtubule nucleation arrest, premature detachment of the sperm axoneme and aster from the paternal pronucleus, and sperm aster microtubule growth defects. Similar cytoskeletal anomalies have been seen in human IVF failures (Asch et al., 1995; Simerly et al., 1995).

The similarities between IVF- and ICSI-derived rhesus oocytes in terms of their cytoskeletal dynamics suggest that an injected sperm behaves similarly to a noninjected sperm that has bound to and fused with the oolemma. However, analysis of rhesus ICSI zygotes using transmission electron microscopy revealed that the pattern of sperm decondensation

is altered after the injection of sperm (Fig. 14.2g,h; Hewitson et al., 1996b; Sutovsky et al., 1996b). The persistence of the acrosome overlying the apical region of the injected sperm caused delayed chromatin decondensation in this region (Hewitson et al., 1996b). Removal of the acrosome did not alleviate this problem, suggesting the involvement of other structures. The perinuclear theca, which is found on the inner acrosomal membrane of the sperm, is typically removed during mammalian fertilization at either the zona pellucida or the oocyte's plasma membrane (Sutovsky et al., 1997). However, during ICSI, the persistence of the perinuclear theca on the injected sperm head prevented the underlying chromatin from undergoing decondensation until this structure is finally shed, approximately 12–16 hours post-ICSI (Fig. 14.3a).

Additional differences between ICSI-fertilized oocytes and those fertilized via in vitro insemination have recently been reported (Hewitson et al., 1999; Ramalho-Santos et al., 2000). For example, vesicle-associated membrane protein (VAMP; Conner et al., 1997), a constituent of the sperm acrosome typically lost at the cell surface during sperm penetration (Ramalho-Santos et al., 2000), is detected as a constriction around the forming paternal pronucleus in rhesus ICSI zygotes (Fig. 14.3b). The retention of VAMP following ICSI serves to separate the condensed and decondensing chromatin, persisting until paternal pronucleus formation is completed. Asynchronous chromatin decondensation also prevents the import of maternal nuclear proteins during sperm decondensation. For example, NuMA (nuclear mitotic apparatus), a nuclear protein important during interphase and in maintaining spindle architecture (Compton and Cleveland, 1994), typically enters the sperm nucleus as it decondenses during fertilization. However, after ICSI, NuMA is initially excluded from the regions of paternal chromatin that remain condensed, perhaps because of the physical constraints imposed by the still-intact acrosome and perinuclear theca (Fig. 14.3c; Hewitson et al., 1999). The significance of asynchronous decondensation is not completely understood but it may result in diminished ability of the oocyte to express, or be

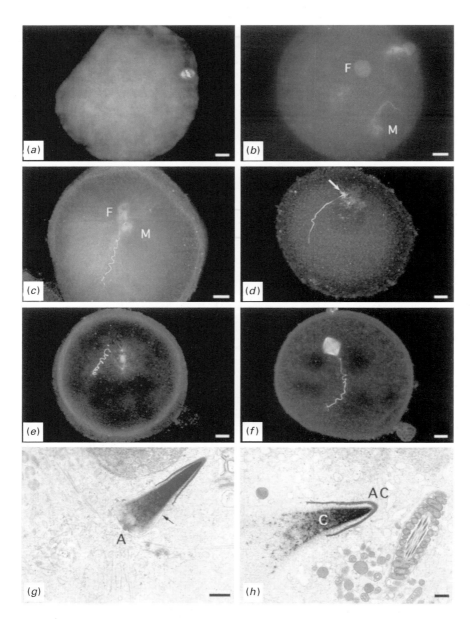

Fig. 14.2. Microtubule patterns in rhesus intracytoplasmic sperm injection (ICSI) zygotes. (*a*) The meiotic spindle in a mature rhesus oocyte is anastral, barrel shaped and eccentrically positioned near the cortex. (*b,c*) Microtubules assemble near the decondensing, injected sperm (*b*) and elongate to fill the cytoplasm during pronuclear formation and apposition (*c*). (*d*) By prophase, most of the cytoplasmic microtubules disassemble leaving a small tuft of microtubules associated with the introduced centrosome (arrow). (*e*) The centrosome duplicates and separates to form a bipolar array. (*f*) The chromosomes align across the metaphase spindle. (*g,h*) Asynchronous decondensation of sperm chromatin. M, male; F, female; A, aster; C, chromatin; AC, acrosome. Bars indicates 15 μm (*a–f*) and 500 nm (*g, h*). (Reprinted with permission from Hewitson et al., 1996b.)

Fig. 14.3. Unusual nuclear remodeling after intracytoplasmic sperm injection (ICSI). (*a*) The perinuclear theca (arrows) persists for up to 12 hours after ICSI, constricting the apical DNA. (*b*) Membrane vesicle-associated membrane protein is detected as a constricting ring (inset, arrow and outline) around the paternal pronucleus. (*c*) The nuclear mitotic apparatus is excluded from the condensed, apical region of the paternal pronucleus; there is asynchronous chromatin decondensation (inset, arrow and outline). M, male; F, female. Bar indicates 10 μm (*a,c*) and 8 μm (*b*). (Reprinted with permission from Hewitson et al., 1999.)

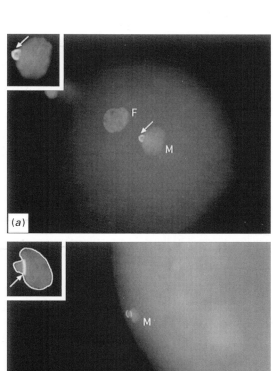

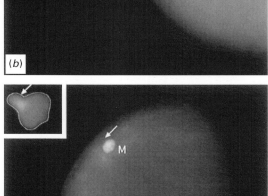

exposed to, important paternal genes or gene products, thus leading to improper embryo formation (reviewed by Schatten et al., 1998).

Furthermore, DNA synthesis, as detected by bromodeoxyuridine incorporation, and pronuclear migration can be delayed by several hours after ICSI in both pronuclei when the paternal pronucleus is still undergoing decondensation in the apical region, identifying a unique G_1/S cell cycle checkpoint (Hewitson et al., 1999). Conversely, pronuclear migration has been completed and DNA synthesis is detected in both pronuclei by 12 hours after in vitro insemination of oocytes. These unique differences between IVF- and ICSI-fertilized oocytes raise concern about the increasing use of ICSI in fertility clinics and demonstrate the need for further animal research in an attempt to improve the safety of this procedure. Furthermore, since the X chromosome appears to be preferentially located in the human sperm head apex when decondensed in *Xenopus laevis* cell-free extracts (Luetjens et al., 1999), delayed decondensation of sperm chromatin in this region after ICSI could lead to chromatin damage. The role, if any, that asynchronous sperm nuclear decondensation after ICSI plays in increased chromosomal anomalies will be an exciting new avenue of research for future investigations.

Conclusions

The use of fluorescence microscopy and dynamic imaging has been invaluable for evaluating the safety of ICSI. Not only can we image the cytoskeletal events during normal ICSI fertilization but we can also evaluate causes of fertilization failure in arrested oocytes. This might aid in the design and testing of other emerging methods of ART. Dynamic imaging of rhesus and human oocytes demonstrated that the position of the second meiotic spindle in relation to the first polar body is often variable. Consequently, this could lead to the sperm being placed in, or in close proximity to, the meiotic spindle, which could have disastrous consequences. ICSI results in abnormal sperm decondensation, with the unusual retention of VAMP and the perinuclear theca, and the exclusion of NuMA from the decondensing sperm nuclear apex. In addition, male pronuclear remodeling in ICSI oocytes is required prior to replication of either parental genomes indicating a unique G_1 to S phase transition checkpoint during zygotic interphase, i.e. the first cell cycle. These unusual deviations during ICSI fertilization raise concerns that the ICSI procedure itself may lead to chromatin damage in the male pronucleus through asynchronous chromatin decondensation. Continued research efforts using both nonhuman primate oocytes and discarded human oocytes (donated by consenting patients) will facilitate the development of safer methods for the selection and injection of sperm and spermatids, as well as providing a more rigorous assessment of methods for ART in humans and prior to their global application.

Acknowledgements

The authors would like to thank Drs. Anthony Chan, Tanja Dominko, John Fanton, David Hess, Marc Luetjens, Martha Neuringer, João Ramalho-Santos and Peter Sutovsky; and Kevin Muller, Darla Jacob, Crista Martinovich, Ethan Jacoby, Christopher Payne, Tonya Swanson and Diana Takahashi. Hormones for oocyte stimulations were gratefully provided by Ares Serono, Inc. and Organon, Inc. Funding for animal studies was provided by the National Institute of Health (NICHD and NCRR), the US Department of Agriculture, and the Mellon Foundation. Animal protocols were approved by the Oregon Health Sciences University's Institutional Animal Care and Use Committee (IACUC).

REFERENCES

Angelopoulos, T., Krey, L., McCullough, A., Adler, A., and Grifo, J.A. (1997). A simple and objective approach to identifying human round spermatids. *Human Reproduction*, **12**, 2208–16.

Asch, R., Simerly, C., Ord, T., Ord, V.A., and Schatten, G. (1995). The stages at which human fertilization arrests: microtubule and chromosome configurations in inseminated oocytes which fail to complete fertilization and development in humans. *Human Reproduction*, **10**, 1897–1906.

Aslam, I., Robins, A., Dowell, K., and Fishel, S. (1998). Isolation, purification and assessment of viability of spermatogenic cells from testicular biopsies of azoospermic men. *Human Reproduction*, **13**, 639–45.

Aytoz, A., Van den Abbeel, E., Bonduelle, M., et al. (1999). Obstetric outcome of pregnancies after transfer of cryopreserved and fresh embryos obtained by conventional in-vitro fertilization and intracytoplasmic sperm injection. *Human Reproduction*, **14**, 2619–24.

Bavister, B.D., Boatman, D.E., Leibfried, L., Loose, M., and Vernon, M.W. (1983). Fertilization and cleavage of rhesus monkey oocytes in vitro. *Biology of Reproduction*, **28**, 983–99.

Boatman, D.E. (1987). In vitro growth of non-human primate pre- and peri-implantation embryos. In: *The Mammalian Preimplantation Embryo*, Bavister, B.D., ed., Plenum Press, New York, pp. 273–85.

Bonduelle, M., Joris, H., Hofmans, K., Liebaers, I., and Van Steirteghem, A. (1998). Mental development of 201 ICSI children at 2 years of age. *Lancet*, **351**, 1553.

Bourne, H., Richings, N., Liu, D.Y., Clarke, G.N., Harari, O., and Baker, H.W. (1995). The use of intracytoplasmic sperm injection for the treatment of severe and extreme male infertility. *Reproduction, Fertility and Development*, **7**, 237–45.

Bowen, J.R., Gibson, F.L., Leslie, G.I., and Saunders, D.M. (1998). Medical and developmental outcome at 1 year for children conceived by intracytoplasmic sperm injection. *Lancet*, **351**, 1529–34.

Chan, A.W.S., Luetjens, C.M., Dominko, T., et al. (2000). TransgenICSI: foreign DNA transmission by intracytoplasmic sperm injection. Injection of sperm bound with exogenous DNA results in embryonic GFP expression and live rhesus births. *Molecular Human Reproduction*, **6**, 26–33.

Compton, D.A. and D.W. Cleveland (1994). NuMA, a nuclear

protein involved in mitosis and nuclear reformation. *Current Opinions in Cell Biology*, **6**, 343–6.

Conner, S., Leaf, D., and Wessel, G. (1997). Members of the SNARE hypothesis are associated with cortical granule exocytosis in the sea urchin egg. *Molecular Reproduction and Development*, **48**, 106–18.

Cummins, J.M. (1997). Controversies in science: ICSI may foster birth defects. *Journal of NIH Research*, **9**, 36–40.

Cummins, J.M., Wakayama, T., and Yanagimachi, R. (1998) Fate of microinjected spermatid mitochondria in the mouse oocyte and embryo. *Zygote*, **6**, 213–22.

Devroey, P., Liu, J., Nagy, Z., Tournaye, H., Silber, S.J., and Van Steirteghem, A.C. (1994). Normal fertilization of human oocytes after testicular sperm extraction and intracytoplasmic sperm injection. *Fertility and Sterility*, **62**, 639–41.

Dominko, T., Chan, A., Simerly, C., et al. (2000). Dynamic imaging of the metaphase II spindle and maternal chromosomes in bovine oocytes: implications for enucleation efficiency verification, avoidance of parthenogenesis, and successful embryogenesis. *Biology of Reproduction*, **62**, 150–4.

Fishel, S., Aslam, I., and Tesarik, J. (1996). Spermatid conception: a stage too early, or a time too soon? *Human Reproduction*, **11**, 1371–5.

Fishel, S., Aslam, I., Lisi, F., et al. (2000). Should ICSI be the treatment of choice for all cases of in-vitro conception? *Human Reproduction*, **15**, 1278–83.

Gorbsky, G.J., Simerly, C., Schatten, G., and Borisy, G.G. (1990). Microtubules in the metaphase-arrested mouse oocyte turn over rapidly. *Proceedings of the National Academy of Sciences USA*, **87**, 6049–53.

Goto, K., Kinoshita, A., Takuma, T.Y., et al. (1990). Fertilization by sperm injection in cattle. *Theriogenology*, **33**, 238.

Griffiths, T.A., Murdoch, A.P., and Herbert, M. (2000). Embryonic development in vitro is compromised by the ICSI procedure. *Human Reproduction*, **15**, 1592–6.

Harari, O., Bourne, H., Baker, G., Gronow, M., and Johnston, I. (1995). High fertilization rate with intracytoplasmic sperm injection in mosaic Klinefelter's syndrome. *Fertility and Sterility*, **63**, 182–4.

Hardarson, T., Lundin, K., and Hamberger, L. (2000). The position of the metaphase II spindle cannot be predicted by the location of the first polar body in the human oocyte. *Human Reproduction*, **15**, 1372–6.

Hewitson, L., Simerly, C., Tengowski, M., et al. (1996a). The cell biological basis of intracytoplasmic sperm injection: microtubule, chromatin and membrane dynamics. *Molecular Biology of the Cell*, **7**(Suppl.), 3717.

Hewitson, L., Simerly, C., Tengowski, M., et al. (1996b). Microtubule and chromatin configurations during rhesus intracytoplasmic sperm injection: successes and failures. *Biology of Reproduction*, **55**, 271–80.

Hewitson, L., Takahashi, D., Dominko, T., Simerly, C., and Schatten, G. (1998). Fertilization and embryo development to blastocysts by intracytoplasmic sperm injection in the rhesus monkey. *Human Reproduction*, **13**, 2786–90.

Hewitson, L., Dominko, T., Takahashi, D., et al. (1999). Unique checkpoints during the first cell cycle of fertilization after intracytoplasmic sperm injection in rhesus monkeys. *Nature Medicine*, **5**, 431–3.

In't Veld, P., Brandenburg, H., Verhoeff, A., Dhont, M., and Los, F. (1995). Sex chromosomal abnormalities and intracytoplasmic sperm injection. *Human Reproduction*, **773**, 346.

Iritani, A. (1988). Current status of biotechnological studies in mammalian reproduction. *Fertility and Sterility*, **50**, 543–51.

Kent-First, M. G., Kol, S., Muallem, A., et al. (1996). The incidence and possible relevance of Y-linked microdeletions in babies born after intracytoplasmic sperm injection and their infertile fathers. *Molecular Human Reproduction*, **2**, 943–50.

Kimura, Y. and Yanagimachi, R. (1995). Intracytoplasmic sperm injection in the mouse. *Biology of Reproduction*, **52**, 709–20.

Lanzendorf, S.E., Zelinski-Wooten, M.B., Stouffer, R.L., and Wolf, D.P. (1990). Maturity at collection and the developmental potential of rhesus monkey oocytes. *Biology of Reproduction*, **42**, 703–11.

Lassalle, B., Ziyyat, A., Testart, J., Finaz, C., and Lefevre A. (1999). Flow cytometric method to isolate round spermatids from mouse testis. *Human Reproduction*, **14**, 388–94.

Liu, J., Nagy, Z., Joris, H., Tournaye, H., Devroey, P., and Van Steirteghem, A. (1995). Successful fertilization and establishment of pregnancies after intracytoplasmic sperm injection in patients with globozoospermia. *Human Reproduction*, **10**, 626–9.

Lopata, A., Summers, P.M., and Hearn, J.P. (1988). Births following the transfer of cultured embryos obtained by in vitro and in vivo fertilization in the marmoset monkey (*Callithrix jacchus*). *Fertility and Sterility*, **50**, 503–9.

Luetjens, C.M., Payne, C., and Schatten, G. (1999). Non-random chromosome positioning in human sperm and sex chromosome anomalies following intracytoplasmic sperm injection. *Lancet*, **353**, 1240.

Moutel, G., Leroux, N., and Herve, C. (1999). Keeping an eye on ICSI. *Nature Medicine*, **5**, 593.

Mulhall, J. P., Reijo, R., Alagappan, R., et al. (1997). Azoospermic men with deletion of the DAZ gene cluster are capable of completing spermatogenesis: fertilization, normal embryonic development and pregnancy occur when retrieved testicular spermatozoa are used for intracytoplasmic sperm injection. *Human Reproduction*, **12**, 503–8.

Nagy, Z. P., Liu, J., Joris, H., et al. (1995). The result of intracytoplasmic sperm injection is not related to any of the three basic sperm parameters. *Human Reproduction*, **10**, 1123–9.

Nudell, D., Castillo, M., Turek, P.J., and Pera, R.R. (2000). Increased frequency of mutations in DNA from infertile men with meiotic arrest. *Human Reproduction*, **15**, 1289–94.

Palermo, G., Joris, H., Devroey, P., and Van Steirteghem, A. (1992). Pregnancies after intracytoplasmic sperm injection of single spermatozoon into an oocyte. *Human Reproduction*, **340**, 17–18.

Palermo, G.D., Schlegel, P.N., Hariprashad, J.J., et al. (1999). Fertilization and pregnancy outcome with intracytoplasmic sperm injection for azoospermic men. *Human Reproduction*, **14**, 741–8.

Patrizio, P. (1995). Intracytoplasmic sperm injection (ICSI): potential genetic concerns. *Human Reproduction*, **10**, 2520–3.

Ramalho-Santos, J., Sutovsky, P., Oko, R., et al. (2000). ICSI choreography: fate of sperm structures after monospermic ICSI and first cell cycle implications. *Human Reproduction*, **15**, 2610–20.

Reyes, J.G., Diaz, A., Osses, N., Opazo, C., and Benos, D.J. (1997). One stage single cell identification of rat spermatogenic cells. *Biology of the Cell*, **89**, 53–66.

Ron-El, R., Liu, J., Nagy, Z., et al. (1995). Intracytoplasmic sperm injection in the mouse. *Human Reproduction*, **10**, 2831–4.

Schatten, G. (1994). The centrosome and its mode of inheritance: the reduction of the centrosome during gametogenesis and its restoration during fertilization. *Developmental Biology*, **165**, 299–335.

Schatten, G., Simerly, C., and Schatten, H. (1985). Microtubule configurations during fertilization, mitosis, and early development in the mouse and the requirement for egg microtubule-mediated motility during mammalian fertilization. *Proceedings of the National Academy of Sciences USA*, **82**, 4152–6.

Schatten, G., Hewitson, L., Simerly, C., and Huszar, G. (1998). Cell and molecular biological challenges of ICSI: A.R.T. before science? *Journal of Law, Medicine and Ethics*, **26**, 29–37.

Shoukir, Y., Chardonnens, D., Campana, A., and Sakkas, D. (1998). Blastocyst development from supernumerary embryos after intracytoplasmic sperm injection: a paternal influence? *Human Reproduction*, **13**, 1632–7.

Silber, S.J., Nagy, Z., Liu, J., et al. (1995). The use of epididymal and testicular spermatozoa for intracytoplasmic sperm injection: the genetic implications for male infertility. *Human Reproduction*, **10**, 2031–43.

Silber, S.J., Verheyen, G., and Van Steirteghem, A.C. (1998). Spermatid conception. *Human Reproduction*, **13**, 2976–9.

Silber, S.J., Johnson, L., Verheyen, G., and Van Steirteghem, A. (2000). Round spermatid injection. *Fertility and Sterility*, **73**, 897–900.

Silva, C.P., Kommineni, K., Oldenbourg, R., and Keefe, D.L. (1999). The first polar body does not predict accurately the location of the metaphase II meiotic spindle in mammalian oocytes. *Fertility and Sterility*, **71**, 719–21.

Simerly, C. and Schatten, G. (1993). Techniques for localization of specific molecules in oocytes and embryos. *Methods in Enzymology*, **225**, 516–52.

Simerly, C., Wu, G., Zoran, S., et al. (1995). The paternal inheritance of the centrosome, the cell's microtubule-organizing center, in humans and the implications for infertility. *Nature Medicine*, **1**, 47–53.

Stone, S., O'Mahony, F., Khalaf, Y., Taylor, A., and Braude, P. (2000). A normal livebirth after intracytoplasmic sperm injection for globozoospermia without assisted oocyte activation: case report. *Human Reproduction*, **15**, 139–41.

Sutovsky, P., Navara, C.S., and Schatten, G. (1996a). Fate of the sperm mitochondria, and the incorporation, conversion, and disassembly of the sperm tail structures during bovine fertilization. *Biology of Reproduction*, 55, 1195–205.

Sutovsky, P., Hewitson, L., Simerly, C.R., et al. (1996b). Intracytoplasmic sperm injection for Rhesus monkey fertilization results in unusual chromatin, cytoskeletal, and membrane events, but eventually leads to pronuclear development and sperm aster assembly. *Human Reproduction*, **11**, 1703–12.

Sutovsky, P., Oko, R., Hewitson, L., and Schatten, G. (1997). Binding of oocyte microvilli to the perinuclear theca of fertilizing sperm and subsequent theca removal constitute a previously unrecognized step in mammalian fertilization. *Developmental Biology*, **188**, 75–84.

Sutovsky, P., Ramalho-Santos, J., Moreno, R.D., Oko, R., Hewitson, L., and Schatten G. (1999). On-stage selection of single round spermatids using a vital, mitochondrion-specific fluorescent probe MitoTracker$^{(TM)}$ and high resolution differential interference contrast microscopy. *Human Reproduction*, **14**, 2301–12.

Tesarik, J. (1997). Sperm or spermatid conception? *Fertility and Sterility*, **68**, 214–16.

Tournaye, H., Liu, J., Nagy, Z., et al. (1996). Correlation between testicular histology and outcome after intracytoplasmic sperm injection using testicular spermatozoa. *Human Reproduction*, **11**, 127–32.

Uehara, T. and Yanagimachi, R. (1976). Microsurgical injection of spermatozoa into hamster eggs with subsequent transformation of sperm nuclei into male pronuclei. *Biology of Reproduction*, **15**, 467–70.

Vanderzwalmen, P., Zech, H., Birkenfeld, A., et al. (1997). Intracytoplasmic injection of spermatids retrieved from testicular tissue: influence of testicular pathology, type of selected spermatids and oocyte activation. *Human Reproduction*, **12**, 1203–13.

VandeVoort, C.A. and Tarantal, A.F. (1991). The macaque model for in vitro fertilization: superovulation techniques and ultrasound-guided follicular aspiration. *Journal of Medical Primatology*, **20**, 110–16.

Van Steirteghem, A.C., Nagy, Z., Joris, H., et al. (1993). High fertilization and implantation rates after intracytoplasmic sperm injection. *Human Reproduction*, **8**, 1061–6.

Vogt, P.H. (1995). Genetic aspects of artificial fertilization. *Human Reproduction*, **10**(Suppl. 1), 128–37.

von Zumbusch, A., Fiedler, K., Mayerhofer, A., Jessberger, B., Ring, J., and Vogt, H.J. (1998). Birth of healthy children after intracytoplasmic sperm injection in two couples with male Kartagener's syndrome. *Fertility and Sterility*, **70**, 643–6.

Westhusin, M.E. and Kraemer, D.C. (1986). Fertilization of hamster ova by sperm injection: the effect of sperm placement on sperm decondensation and pronuclear formation. *Theriogenology*, **25**, 215.

Wright, S.J., Centonze, V.E., Stricker, S.A., De Vries, P.J., Paddock, S.W., and Schatten, G. (1993). Introduction to confocal microscopy and three-dimensional reconstruction. *Methods in Cell Biology*, **38**, 1–45.

Wu, G., Simerly, C., Zoran, S., Funte, L.R., and Schatten, G. (1996). Microtubule and chromatin configurations during fertilization and early development in rhesus monkeys, and regulation by intracellular calcium ions. *Biology of Reproduction*, **55**, 269–71.

Yamanaka, K., Sofikitis, N.V., Miyagawa, I., et al. (1997). Ooplasmic round spermatid nuclear injection procedures as an experimental treatment for nonobstructive azoospermia. *Journal of Assisted Reproduction and Genetics*, **14**, 55–62.

Younis, A.I., Keefer, C.L., and Brackett, B.G. (1989). Fertilization of bovine oocytes by sperm injection. *Theriogenology*, **31**, 276.

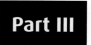

Part III

The clinic

15

Diagnosis and treatment of male infertility

Axel Kamischke and Eberhard Nieschlag

Institute of Reproductive Medicine of the University, Münster, Germany

Introduction

This chapter focuses on the diagnosis of male infertility. Special diagnostic and therapeutic aspects of infertility and hypogonadism are covered in Nieschlag and Behre (2000). The following procedures are widely used for the diagnosis of male infertility. Special examinations are discussed together with the relevant diseases.

Anamnesis

Male fertility and infertility are strongly dependent on female fertility/infertility and, therefore, the anamnesis of male infertility should also provide information about the female partner (e.g., duration of unprotected intercourse, menstrual cycle anamnesis, earlier pregnancies). Special andrological medical history includes information about any testicular maldescent, the age at therapy, and the kind of therapy (none, medical, surgical). Infectious diseases, with or without clinically manifest orchitis or epididymitis, and sexually transmitted diseases and their respective treatments must be recorded. In some cases, the family history provides information for a possible genetic cause of infertility. As infertility is a frequent sequela of general diseases (e.g., diabetes mellitus, liver or kidney diseases) and a common side-effect of some drug therapies (e.g., sulfasalazine, cytostatic agents, anabolic hormones), the relevant symptoms and substances should be recorded.

Physical examination

Suspicion of infertility associated with androgen deficiency may arise from eunuchoid tall stature, lumbago, female fat distribution, a straight frontal hairline combined with reduced beard growth, and a horizontal upper pubic hairline (Behre et al., 2000). Gynecomastia can be present in primary hypogonadism (e.g., Klinefelter's syndrome), diseases of androgen target organs, hyperprolactinemia or may indicate an endocrinologically active testicular tumor (Braunstein, 1993).

Palpation of the testes is performed with the patient standing. Ultrasonography is useful for confirming a missing testis, and magnetic resonance tomography may help to determine the location in suspected intraabdominal testes. The normal testes have a firm consistency. Soft testes are indicative of absent gonadotropin stimulation, while very firm testes are typical for Klinefelter's syndrome. Differences in testicular consistency between the two sides, a very hard testis, or an uneven surface raise suspicion of a testicular tumor. As testicular volume correlates grossly with sperm production (Behre et al., 2000), testicular size should be determined by palpation (Prader orchidometer) or better by ultrasonography (Behre et al., 1989) and should range between 12 and 30 ml for Caucasians. Common pathology of the epididymis includes smooth cystic distensions or indurations indicative of an obstruction as well as spermatoceles; painful swelling of the epididymis may point to an acute or chronic inflammation. The venous pampiniform plexus should be examined for the presence of a varicocele by palpation or preferably by ultrasonography. The presence of both deferent ducts must be documented. Apart from erectile dysfunction, hypospadias and epispadias, as well as phimosis and deviations of the penis during erection, can lead to infertility. A small prostate gland can be a symptom of hypogonadism-related infertility, while a doughy, soft consistency points to prostatitis.

Ultrasonography of scrotal content and transrectal ultrasonography

Because the incidence of testicular tumors and carcinoma in situ (CIS) in infertile patients is markedly higher than in the general population (Pierik et al., 1999), ultrasonography should be mandatory in the diagnostic work-up of infertile patients as even unpalpable, intratesticular tumors can be recognized (Behre et al., 2000). In addition, ultrasonography provides important diagnostic clues to other conditions leading to infertility. A normal testis (Fig. 15.1a) and epididymis displays homogeneous parenchymal echogenicity. Testicular tumors appear as hyperechogenic or, mostly, as hypoechogenic or mixed areas. CIS often shows focal single or multiple hyperechogenicity (Fig. 15.1b). The maldescended testis frequently displays diminished echogenicity. Varicoceles show an enlargement of the venous diameter of the pampiniform plexus, and the increase in the diameter of individual veins can be measured during the Valsalva maneuver. Acute epididymitis results in a hypoechogenic and enlarged sonographical picture of the epididymis, often in combination with an accompanying hydrocele. Chronic epididymitis causes hyperechogenicity, while spermatoceles appear as an echo-free, round area within the epididymis. Transrectal sonography of the prostate can be applied for diagnosis of prostatitis, benign prostatic hyperplasia, and prostate carcinoma. It allows intraprostatic cysts and dilatations of the ejaculatory duct to be ascertained as the cause or result of obstructions. Transrectal ultrasonography of the seminal vesicles may reveal agenesis or aplasia, as

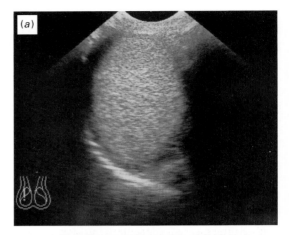

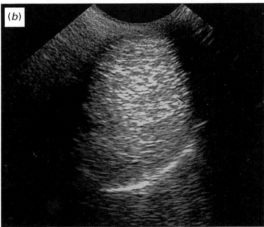

Fig. 15.1. Scrotal sonography performed with a 7.5 MHz sector scanner of a normal (*a*) and inhomogeneous parenchyma with numerous small hyperechogenic areas (*b*). Histology of the testis with inhomogeneous parenchyma revealed a carcinoma in situ of the testis.

well as dysfunction of the seminal vesicles as possible causes of male infertility (von Eckardstein et al., 2000).

Endocrine laboratory diagnosis

The main constituent of endocrine laboratory diagnosis of testicular disorders is the determination of the gonadotropins luteinizing hormone (LH; normal range 2–10 IU/l) and follicle-stimulating hormone (FSH; normal range 1–7 IU/l). High gonadotropin levels in serum combined with low testosterone levels indicate testicular origin of hypogonadism (primary hypogonadism); low gonadotropin levels point to a central cause (secondary hypogonadism). Within wide margins, the extent of FSH elevation (>7 IU/l) is correlated with the number of seminiferous tubules lacking germ cells (Sertoli cell-only tubules) (Bergmann et al., 1994; von Eckardstein et al., 1999).

Testosterone is the most important secretion of the Leydig cells. When interpreting testosterone values, diurnal variations should be considered, with morning serum concentrations lying approximately 20–40% higher than evening values. Normal serum testosterone concentrations in the adult male fall between 12 and 40 nmol/l during the first half of the day. For estimating testosterone bioactivity, free testosterone can be calculated from the serum concentration of total testosterone plus that of steroid hormone-binding globulin using a standardized formula (Vermeulen et al., 1999).

Inhibin B is produced by the Sertoli cells in the testes and shows a marked diurnal rhythm parallel to testosterone (Anderson et al., 1998; Carlsen et al., 1999). Evidence exists that germ cells (Andersson et al., 1998; Foppiani et al., 1999; Foresta et al., 1999) are important modulators of inhibin B secretion. In combination with FSH, inhibin B adds useful information concerning the possible presence of sperm in testicular tissue in patients prior to testicular sperm extraction (TESE) for intracytoplasmic sperm injection (ICSI) (von Eckardstein et al., 1999; Ballesca et al., 2000).

When hypothalamic or pituitary diseases are suspected, a gonadotropin-releasing hormone (GnRH) stimulation test should be performed to determine the gonadotropin reserve capacity of the pituitary (Behre et al., 2000). Prolactin should be measured in patients with unclear fertility disturbances and symptoms that indicate a pituitary disorder or a pituitary tumor. The human chorionic gonadotropin (hCG) test evaluates the endocrine reserve capacity of the testes. The test is predominantly used for differentiation between anorchia and cryptorchidism or ectopy of the testis.

Semen analysis

The investigation of ejaculate parameters plays a central role in the evaluation of male fertility. However, since semen parameters have value only in relation to the underlying disorder on the one side and to female reproductive functions on the other (with the exception of azoospermia), isolated examination of only the ejaculate parameters is of limited value for prognosis of the couple's fertility. For evaluation of male fertility, standardized semen analysis according to the guidelines of the World Health Organization (WHO) *Laboratory Manual for the Examination of Human Semen and Sperm–Cervical Mucus Interaction* (1999) is mandatory. In addition to the need for standardization, semen analysis must be performed under rigid internal and external quality control to avoid systematic bias and assure interlaboratory comparability (Cooper et al., 1992, 1999). As the WHO *Laboratory Manual* should be a requisite of all andrology laboratories, the essential aspects of semen analysis are mentioned only briefly here. For sperm function tests, we refer to Chapter 17 in this volume. Normal values and classifications of ejaculate parameters are given in Tables 15.1 and 15.2.

The estimation of fertility potential after abstinence of 48 hours to 7 days should be based on at least two semen analyses performed at an interval of 4 to 12 weeks. The ejaculate should be obtained at the clinic by masturbation into a wide-mouthed, clean glass container with a graduated cylinder to avoid transfer into other vials.

Physical examination

In contrast to the normal gray-opalescent appearance, a yellowish color, a prolonged liquefaction time, a pH >8 and purulent smell is indicative for infections of the genital tract. Hemospermia (reddish-brown appearance) indicates the presence of red blood cells and is often seen in infections of the seminal vesicles and the prostate. Obstructions and malformations of the genital tract can be suspected if

Table 15.1. Normal values of semen variables according to WHO Guidelines (1999)

Variable	Normal values
Ejaculate volume	≥2.0 ml
Ejaculate appearance	Gray-opalescent
Ejaculate liquefication	<60 minutes
pH	7.2–8.0
Sperm concentration	≥20 × 10⁶ spermatozoa/ml
Total sperm count	≥40 × 10⁶ spermatozoa/ejaculate
Motility (within 60 minutes of ejaculation)	Category a+b: ≥50% spermatozoa with forward progression Category a: ≥25% spermatozoa with rapid progression
Morphology	≥30% spermatozoa with normal forms[a]
Vitality	≥75% vital spermatozoa, e.g., sperm excluding the dye eosin
Mixed antiglobulin reaction (MAR) test	<50% of spermatozoa with adherent particles or erythrocytes
Leukocytes	<1 × 10⁶/ml
α-Glucosidase (neutral)	≥11 mU/ejaculate
Citric acid	≥52 μmol/ejaculate
Acid phosphatase	≥200 U/ejaculate
Fructose	≥13 μmol/ejaculate
Zinc	≥2.4 μmol/ejaculate

Notes:
[a] The 4th edition of the WHO Guidelines (1999) provides no reference values for normal sperm morphology, so the percentage value of the 3rd edition (1992) is maintained here. Currently, multicenter studies are underway to determine new reference values. Data from assisted reproduction indicate that fertility rates in vitro decrease if normal sperm morphology falls below 15%.
Source: World Health Organization (1992c, 1999).

Table 15.2. Descriptive terminology for the semen variables according to WHO Guidelines (1999)

Term	Definition
Normozoospermia	Normal ejaculate as defined in Table 15.1
Oligozoospermia	<20 million spermatozoa/ml
Asthenozoospermia	Categories a and b: <50% spermatozoa with forward progression Category a: <25% spermatozoa with rapid progression
Teratozoospermia	<30% spermatozoa with normal morphology (see Table 6.3 in WHO, 1999)
Oligoasthenoterato-zoospermia (OAT)	Signifies disturbance of all three variables (combinations of only two prefixes may also be used)
Azoospermia	No spermatozoa in the ejaculate
Parvisemia	Ejaculate volume <2 ml
Aspermia	No ejaculate

Source: World Health Organization (1999).

pH values are <7.2 (von Eckardstein et al., 2000) and are commonly seen in combination with azoospermia in patients with congenital bilateral aplasia of the vas deferens (CBAVD).

Microscopic examination

After liquefaction at room temperature, microscopic examination can begin, preferably with a phase contrast microscope. Sperm motility (normal values Table 15.1) is examined at 37 °C or at room temperature in the fresh sample at a magnification of ×400 to ×600. The quality of motility is expressed according to the WHO *Laboratory Manual* (1999) as:
a. Rapid progressive motility (>25 μm/s)
b. Slow or sluggish progressive motility (5–25 μm/s)
c. Nonprogressive motility (<5 μm/s)
d. Immotility.
Among the various methods for objective measurements of sperm motility, the tracking of video images of individual sperm cells by computer-aided sperm analysis (CASA) is the best developed and has

shown predictive value for fertility (Barratt et al., 1993; Irvine et al., 1994; De Geyter et al., 1998). Selective impairment of sperm motility is often seen in patients with infections or immunological infertility. Selective complete immotility is rarely seen and indicates disturbances of the flagellar structure (Neugebauer et al., 1990; Zamboni, 1992; Chemes et al., 1998).

Sperm concentration is determined in a counting chamber after dilution with a fixative solution (World Health Organization, 1999). Azoospermia must be confirmed in the sediment after high-speed centrifugation of the ejaculate. Objective and precise determination of sperm concentration can be performed by DNA flow cytometry (Hacker-Klom et al., 1999) and, with lower accuracy, also by modern (CASA) systems. Azoospermia with elevated FSH is indicative for tubular defects. Azoospermia with normal gonadotropins and decreased biochemical semen markers raises the suspicion of occlusions of the deferent ducts or epididymis (von Eckardstein et al., 2000). Azoospermia with decreased or absent gonadotropins is seen in men with pituitary or hypothalamic disturbances.

Sperm morphology is examined in a fixed microscopic preparation of a portion of a well-mixed semen sample, best stained according to Papanicolaou (World Health Organization, 1999). Normal sperm have a regular oval-shaped head with an intact mid-piece and an intact tail. The acrosome should be clearly visible and cover 40–70% of the sperm head area. Objective methods for sperm morphology do not exist. However, computer-aided video techniques are under investigation (Steigerwald and Krause, 1998). Abnormal forms of spermatozoa are manifold. In general, various forms of unspecific head defects are the main defects. However, in the rare case of all sperm without acrosomes and globular heads, the morphology is classified as globozoospermia. Besides sperm cells, the semen contains epithelial cells of the urogenital tract and so-called round cells. A distinction between white blood cells and spermatogenic cells is achieved by specific staining (World Health Organization, 1999).

Biochemical analysis

The determination of substances secreted by specific organs or compartments of the reproductive system allows a rough localization of the disorder. However, it should be considered that in the case of bilateral organs only bilateral dysfunction will cause significant changes of the biochemical markers derived from bilateral organs. Prostate function can be gauged by the measurement of zinc, citric acid, and (prostatic) acid phosphatase. Seminal vesicle function can be estimated by the measurement of fructose. Low levels of seminal markers for prostate function are often seen in acute or chronic prostatitis. Low fructose concentrations in the seminal plasma may indicate bilateral agenesis, severe dysfunction of the seminal vesicles, or obstruction of the ejaculatory ducts. Disturbances of prostate or seminal vesicle function can be further investigated by transrectal ultrasonography. Neutral α-glucosidase has a high specificity and sensitivity for evaluation of epididymal function. Severely diminished or undetectable neutral α-glucosidase is indicative for bilateral obstruction or dysgenesis of the epididymis or efferent ducts.

Immunological tests

If more than 10% of sperm are agglutinated in the fresh semen sample, the presence of specific sperm antibodies can be suspected. For the determination of antibodies of the IgA or IgG class in semen directed against sperm surface antigens, the mixed antiglobulin reaction test (MAR test) has proven to be useful (World Health Organization, 1999). If more than 50% of the spermatozoa are coated with IgG or IgA antibodies, immunological infertility is likely (Abshagen et al., 1998). Determination of sperm antibodies in serum has no diagnostic value in the infertility workup (Behre et al., 2000).

Microbiology

The predominant microorganisms found are *Chlamydia trachomatis* or *Ureaplasma urealyticum*, as well as Gram-negative bacteria typical of urogenital infections (Purvis and Christiansen, 1993). Leukocyte concentrations higher than 1×10^6 cells/ml and/or a significant growth of microorganisms in the ejaculate culture indicate an infection of the efferent seminal system (World Health Organization, 1999). Whereas the determination of different microorganisms in an aerobic ejaculate culture is unproblematic, proof of chlamydia infection in the ejaculate is best achieved by the polymerase chain reaction (PCR).

Electron microscopy

In a minority of infertile patients, specific anomalies of sperm cells can be found only by electron microscopy. This allows head defects with and without defects of the nucleus (e.g., globozoospermia) and tail defects (e.g., immotile cilia syndrome) to be differentiated from each other.

Testicular biopsy

The importance of testicular biopsy as part of routine diagnostics in the male infertility workup has decreased continually. However, in azoospermia, only testicular biopsy can determine whether haploid germ cells are present. At present, the main indications for testicular biopsy are the retrieval of testicular tissue for TESE in conjunction with ICSI (Schulze et al., 1999) and the exclusion of a CIS and tumors of the testis in those with sonographic inhomogeneities or contralateral testicular tumor (Bamberg et al., 1997).

Diagnostic testicular biopsy

Because of the increased incidence of CIS and testicular tumors in infertile patients, the testicular biopsy should be always performed bilaterally. Testicular biopsy can be performed under local anesthesia. After scrotal incision, testicular tissue of the size of a rice kernel should be retrieved (Schulze and Knuth, 2000) to allow analysis of at least 30 cross-sections of testicular tubules. For correct evaluation of testicular tissue, it should be fixed in 5.5% glutaraldehyde for light microscopy in semi-thin sections (Laczkó and Lévai, 1975) or in Bouin's solution (Böck, 1989). Fixation of testicular tissue in the usual formalin solution is not suitable. Semi-thin section histology

is the optimal method for routine diagnosis of testicular biopsies because of excellent tissue preservation and the possibility of later investigation using a transmission electron microscope (Holstein et al., 1988; Behre et al., 2000). Alternatively, Bouin's solution-fixed paraffin section histology can be used, especially when additional immunocytochemical investigations are planned. Of particular clinical importance is the immunocytochemical demonstration of placental alkaline phosphatase for the detection of CIS. Approximately 90% of tumor cells can be found with this method (Heidenreich et al., 1998).

The quality of spermatogenesis can be evaluated using histological scoring systems (for review see Doerr and Seifert, 1991). In our institute, we use the Holstein score (Behre et al., 2000). These are of importance as histological examination of testicular biopsies from infertility patients often reveal areas of intact spermatogenesis alongside tubules containing only Sertoli cells or various forms of spermatogenic arrest (mixed atrophy). In the case of complete Sertoli-cell-only syndrome (germinal cell aplasia), no spermatogenic cells aside from Sertoli cells can be detected. Spermatogenic arrest is defined as an interruption in the development of spermatogonia to mature sperm at the level of spermatogonia, primary or secondary spermatocytes, or round spermatids. As the incidence of testicular tumors and CIS is increased in infertile patients (approximately 0.7%), every testicular biopsy should be checked for exclusion of these malignant lesions (Schulze et al., 1999). For more detailed information on diagnostic testicular biopsy we refer to Behre et al. (2000).

Therapeutic testicular biopsy

In azoospermic patients, the diagnostic testicular biopsy should be combined with a therapeutic testicular biopsy. For this procedure, further samples the size of a rice grain are retrieved and directly cryopreserved (two biopsies from each side in addition to the diagnostic specimen). If histological analysis (one biopsy each side) reveals elongated spermatids, these samples can be thawed later for use in combination with ICSI (Fischer et al., 1996). In general, elongated spermatids can be expected in 77% of testicular biopsies (Schulze et al., 1999). However, in nonobstructive azoospermia, sperm retrieval may be possible only in 40–50% of patients (De Geyter et al., 2000). For TESE, the thawed testicular samples are enzymatically digested or mechanically minced and vital motile sperm are then identified for ICSI using the inverted microscope (Salzbrunn et al. 1996). Recent studies have shown that retrieval of testicular tissue on the day prior to designated ICSI and incubation in FSH-containing culture medium can increase sperm retrieval rates as well as pregnancy rates (Balaban et al., 1999). To improve the prognostic accuracy of later sperm retrieval for ICSI, some centers take further testicular samples (one from each side) for direct mechanical mincing or enzymatic digestion on the day of biopsy.

Cytogenetics and molecular genetics

The prevalence of chromosomal abnormalities increases with decreasing semen quality and can be expected in up to 10% of infertile couples (Meschede and Horst, 1997). Relatively frequent among infertile patients are males with Klinefelter's syndrome (47XXY), CBAVD, and microdeletions of the gene for the azoospermia factor (*AZF*) on the long arm of the Y chromosome. Klinefelter's syndrome can be suspected in patients with very firm, small testes (usually <5 ml) and hypergonadotropic azoospermia. Evaluation of buccal mucosa cell smears provides a simple and quick diagnostic screening method for detection of Barr bodies (sex chromatin). However, definite diagnosis requires karyotyping of peripheral lymphocytes. A mutation in the gene for the cystic fibrosis transmembrane conductance regulator (CFTR) has to be excluded in azoospermic patients with CBAVD and aplasia or dysplasia of the seminal vesicles or epididymis. Analysis of the *AZF* region is indicated in severely oligo- or azoospermic patients with often otherwise unexplained infertility.

Fertility prognosis of untreated infertile couples

There are few patients (e.g., those with anorchia or complete Sertoli-cell-only syndrome) for whom no treatment option is available to achieve paternity. In some infertile patients with severe impairments of semen parameters it is clearly evident that fertility can be achieved only by substitution of gonadotropin secretion (e.g., Kallmann syndrome) or assisted reproductive techniques (ART). However, most infertile patients present with impairments of fertility that do not generally exclude spontaneous induction of pregnancy. Therefore, in these patients, any infertility treatment has to be considered with respect to the chances of a couple conceiving spontaneously.

The best evidence concerning the prognosis of well-diagnosed, unselected, untreated infertile couples for spontaneous pregnancies is provided by two independent cohort studies. The Walcheren Island study (Snick et al., 1997) was carried out at a primary care infertility center. When the observations of all 726 untreated couples enrolled were considered, the cumulative rate of conceptions leading to livebirth 36 months after registration for the trial was 52.5% (95% confidence interval (CI) 44.7–60.2%). The CITES study (Collins et al., 1995) was performed at a secondary and tertiary care infertility center. When all 2198 untreated couples enrolled were analyzed, the cumulative rate of conceptions leading to livebirth 36 months after registration for the trial was 25.2% (95% CI 21.8–28.6%). Factors that significantly influence pregnancy prognosis positively in both studies were female age less than 30 years, prior pregnancy in partnership, and duration of infertility <24 (Walcheren study) or <36 (CITES study) months. Factors that significantly negatively influenced pregnancy prognosis in both studies were tubal defects, sperm defects, and endometriosis. With the help of the identified prognostic factors, the accuracy for prediction scores for livebirths in untreated infertile couples were 62% (CITES study) and 76% (Walcheren study). With the help of these predictions it is also possible to estimate the effect of treatment in a given couple (Collins et al., 1995).

Treatment of male fertility

This section will focus solely on medical or surgical treatment options for the restoration of fertility. For cases where only symptomatic treatment by assisted reproduction techniques (ARTs) or no therapies to achieve fertility are available (e.g., spermatogenic arrest, anorchia, complete androgen resistance or Klinefelter's syndrome), we refer to the other chapters of this volume and to Nieschlag and Behre (2000).

Preventive treatment of male fertility

Testicular maldescent

At birth, maldescended testes are estimated to occur in 2–3% of full term males and about 30% of premature newborns. However, the gonads will descend to assume a scrotal position within a few months in around 60% of these children (Nieschlag et al., 2000). The incidence of testicular maldescent is increased in patients with hypopthalamic–pituitary disturbances, disorders of testosterone synthesis or testosterone action, reduced abdominal wall tension, and primary testicular disorders. Maldescended testes can be diagnosed by anamnesis and genital examination. In some cases, imaging procedures (especially sonography) and endocrine procedures (hCG test) support diagnosis when the testis is in a high position.

Since germ cell degeneration and dysplasia start in early infancy, the position of maldescended testes should be corrected by the end of the first year of life or earlier because of the five- to tenfold fold higher risk for testicular tumors (Huff et al., 1991). However, whether early treatment of maldescent, as practiced today, prevents infertility and testicular cancer has not yet been resolved. Therapy of maldescended testes in childhood by GnRH or hCG has only been successful in 10–20% in randomized clinical trials (de Muinck Keizer-Schrama et al., 1986; Rajfer et al., 1986; Hoorweg-Nijman et al., 1994); therefore, if

endocrine therapy fails, orchidopexy should be performed (Deutsche Gesellschaft für Endokrinologie, 1991).

Apart from relatively frequent retractile testes (the testis alternates its position from the scrotum and the inguinal channel), maldescended testes occur in about 0.5% of adult men. In our infertility clinic, 8% of patients have successfully treated or still existing maldescended testes, which is significantly higher than the prevalence of 0.5% in the general male population (Nieschlag et al., 2000). However, in a recent large observational cohort study, only patients with previously bilaterally maldescended testes were afflicted by infertility compared with controls and with patients with previously unilaterally maldescended testes (Coughlin et al., 1997). From this study, it can be further suspected that the contralateral descended testis may compensate for damage of a unilaterally maldescended testis (Coughlin, et al., 1997). Apart from preventive therapy, maldescent-related infertility has the same treatment options as idiopathic infertility.

Infections of the testis and seminal ducts

Major acute symptomatic bacterial infections or venereal diseases of the genital tract should be treated with antibiotics in order to prevent occlusions of the efferent ducts. Acute epididymitis is characterized by scrotal pain, painful palpation of the epididymis, as well as local swelling and tenderness. Suspicion of an infection of the male reproductive tract can be clarified by microbiological investigations. Viral orchitis is known to lead to possible profound impairment of spermatogenesis and infertility but can only be treated symptomatically in the acute phase or preventively by vaccination, as in the case of mumps.

The biological significance of increased white blood cells in semen and asymptomatic subclinical genital tract infections, as well as the role of antibiotic treatment in these cases, remains unclear (Wolff, 1995; Eggert-Kruse et al., 1997). Only a very limited number of randomized controlled studies dealing with asymptomatic genital tract infections have been performed so far. In three randomized placebo-controlled trials, antibiotic treatment led to a higher resolution of leukocytospermia (Branigan and Muller, 1994) or bacteria (Harrison et al., 1975; Hinton et al., 1979) while in the other three studies no treatment effect could be achieved (Comhaire et al., 1986; Yanushpolsky et al., 1995; Erel et al., 1997). No significant differences were seen in semen parameters between treatment and control groups in these randomized controlled clinical trials. One study suggested an improved pregnancy rate compared with the no-treatment group (Branigan and Muller, 1994) while the other studies with pregnancy as an outcome parameter showed no benefit on pregnancy rates (Harrison et al., 1975; Hinton et al., 1979; Comhaire et al., 1986). Meta-analysis of these studies involving 187 patients reveals no significant influence (odds ratio 1.76; 95% CI 0.70–4.46) of antibiotic treatment on pregnancy rates in asymptomatic genital tract infections (Kamischke and Nieschlag, 1999a). Therefore, in contrast to acute epididymitis and in view of the possible side-effects, antibiotic treatment of asymptomatic genital tract infections cannot be recommended by the criteria of evidence-based medicine.

Rational treatment of male infertility

Secondary hypogonadism/ gonadotropin deficiency

Disturbances of GnRH secretion (e.g., idiopathic hypogonadotropic hypogonadism; Kallmann syndrome) or gonadotropin secretion (e.g., hypopituitarism, pituitary surgery) can be congenital or acquired. Symptoms of related androgen deficiency and infertility can be variable, depending on the onset and magnitude of the secretion disturbances. In general, the testes have a soft consistency and ejaculate analysis reveals severe oligo- or azoospermia. Serum gonadotropins are decreased or not measurable. Depending on the origin and duration of hypogonadism, a GnRH test reveals normal or nonstimulatable gonadotropins. For detailed diagnosis we refer to Behre et al. (2000).

In patients with hypothalamic or pituitary dysfunction, GnRH and/or gonadotropin treatment has been applied successfully for decades. Therapy should be adjusted according to serum testosterone levels, testicular growth, appearance of sperm in the ejaculate, and induction of pregnancy. The hCG dose should be adjusted to the testosterone and estradiol serum levels, which should not exceed normal values. Doses commonly used are 1000–2500 IU hCG twice a week combined with human menopausal gonadotropin (hMG) 150 IU three times weekly (Burgues and Calderon, 1997; Büchter et al., 1998). Pulsatile GnRH therapy consists of 5–20 μg GnRH pulses every 120 minutes delivered through a portable pump and should be adjusted to reproductive hormone levels (Büchter et al., 1998). Treatment efficacy for both therapies is similar although GnRH treatment has a tendency for higher success in some studies (Schopohl et al., 1991; Schopohl, 1993). In most cases, induction of spermatogenesis and paternity can be expected in 80–88% within one year (Burgues and Calderon, 1997; Büchter et al., 1998). Interestingly, patients usually become fertile with sperm concentrations far below the normal limit (Burris et al., 1988; Büchter et al., 1998). In consecutive treatment courses, time to induction of spermatogenesis is shorter than in the first stimulation cycle. Therefore, it is advisable to induce spermatogenesis even before paternity is desired, to assure the patient that paternity is possible and to reduce time to pregnancy when desired (Kliesch et al., 1994). Recent studies suggested comparable efficacy of stimulation using recombinant FSH (Kliesch et al., 1995; Liu et al., 1999) and the urinary preparations. However, appropriate prospective, randomized controlled multicenter trials to compare urinary and recombinant FSH preparations have not been performed.

Carcinoma in situ and testicular tumors

CIS is considered an obligatory precancerous stage of a testicular tumor (seminoma or nonseminoma). Germ cell tumors account for 95% of all testicular tumors (Bosl and Motzer, 1997) and reach their peak in the main reproductive phase of life. The remaining testicular tumors consist largely of stromal tumors (Leydig cell and Sertoli cell tumors). The risk of developing a testicular germ cell tumor or a CIS is four to five times higher in men with maldescended testes than in the general male population.

Leading symptoms of all malignant transformations may be decreased seminal parameters, and any sudden decline of semen parameters should always prompt thorough investigation of the testes. In addition, patients with seminoma and nonseminoma may present with testicular pain and swelling, very firm testicular consistency, and gynecomastia. Large tumors may be palpable. However, early intratesticular tumors and CIS are generally discovered only with the aid of ultrasonography. In ultrasound imaging, testicular tumors appear mostly inhomogeneous with areas of increased or reduced echodensity, while an inhomogeneous sonographic appearance of the testis is often seen in CIS (Parra et al., 1996). The tumor markers α-fetoprotein and β-hCG represent further important tools for diagnosis of germ cell tumors (sometimes also of CIS). Diagnostic certainty is achieved by testicular biopsy followed by histological and immunohistological stainings. Moreover, in case of unilateral alterations, biopsies should always be performed bilaterally.

Therapy of CIS and germ cell tumors according to the International Germ Cell Cancer Classification Group greatly depends on histology results and stages (for review see Bosl and Motzer, 1997). Generally (with the exception of bilateral CIS) the affected testis is removed. Further treatment of germ cell tumors may involve retroperitoneal lymphadenectomy, chemotherapy, and irradiation. Germ cell tumors have now become a largely curable disease. On a long-term basis, tumor treatment may restore the patient's often-impaired semen parameters. However, chemotherapy and irradiation at higher doses may also lead to persistent azoospermia. Therefore, prior to bilateral orchidectomy, chemotherapy, testicular irradiation, or retroperitoneal lymphadenectomy, patients must be given the possibility of cryopreserving their sperm to preserve fertility.

Obstructions of the seminal ducts

Obstructions of the male reproductive tract can be congenital (e.g., CBAVD, Young's syndrome, intra-prostatic cysts), acquired (e.g., acute or chronic inflammations of the genital tract), iatrogenic (e.g., complications arising from herniotomy, vasography, surgery, or puncture of the epididymis), or intended (vasectomy). Obstructive azoospermia can be suspected where there is normal testicular volume with normal or slightly elevated FSH in combination with azoospermia and decreased marker substances in seminal plasma for the epididymis and/or seminal vesicle and/or prostate gland. A distal obstruction can lead to parvisemia (ejaculate volume <2ml), while ejaculate volume generally remains normal when the obstruction is proximal to the ejaculatory ducts. Partial obstructions or unilateral obstruction can be compensated completely by the contralateral side and thus may remain asymptomatic. Frequent findings are further thickening and induration of the epididymis, aplasia or hypoplasia of the deferent ducts, and infectious alterations, anomalies, or cysts in the prostate gland or seminal vesicles. These can be verified, preferably by ultrasonography.

A bilateral testicular biopsy for the evaluation of spermatogenesis is recommended before any interventional therapy to allow the identification of other conditions leading to azoospermia (e.g., spermatogenetic arrest). In patients with an obstruction of the reproductive tract and at least qualitatively normal spermatogenesis, rational therapy is to restore reproductive duct system patency (epididymo- or vasovasostomy). However, the success of the operation is dependent on the primary cause of obstruction, its duration, and the surgical technique employed (Belker et al., 1991). In general, short-term obstructions with clearly definable lesions showed best results, while infectious or long-standing lesions (e.g., in most cases of CBAVD) showed lower patency rates. Of the various surgical methods, microsurgical techniques performed in specialized centers showed the highest patency rates (Schlegel and Goldstein, 1993). However, even if patency is re-established, fertility can remain reduced because of antisperm antibodies or a secondary obstruction. To avoid further operations, spermatozoa should be aspirated microsurgically from the epididymis or extracted from the testis for cryopreservation in parallel with the reconstructive surgery. If patency of the male reproductive tract cannot be achieved or high numbers of antisperm antibodies are present after surgery, these cryopreserved specimens can then be used for ICSI.

Anatomical penile alterations

Congenital or acquired penile abnormalities can lead to functional and anatomical disturbances of semen deposition. Among the most common anatomical penile alterations are hypospadias, epispadias, penile deviations, and phimosis (for review see van Ahlen and Hertle, 2000). In congenital hypospadias and epispadias, the urethra does not extend to the glans and the meatus is situated on the ventral or the dorsum of the penis, respectively. In hypospadias, surgical distal advancement of the meatus, within the first two years of life, will in the vast majority allow normal sperm deposition. In general, hypospadias represent more of a cosmetic than a functional problem. In contrast, epispadias are often part of a major genital abnormality (especially bladder dystrophy) and, in the majority, lead to severe dorsal deviation of the penis, making intercourse and sperm deposition very difficult or even impossible. Satisfactory surgical correction of epispadias is difficult to achieve and should be performed in specialized centres. However, even after successful surgical correction, the often-accompanying retrograde ejaculation or anejaculation may persist. If surgery fails, ART techniques appear to be the method of choice.

Congenital penile deviations are caused by asymmetric corpora cavernosa or their bony fixation. Acquired penile deviations can result from blunt trauma, penile fractures, from urethral strictures and their treatment by urethrotomy, or as a result of long-term cavernosal autoinjection therapy. However, the majority of acquired penile deviations result from induratio penis plastica (Peyronie's disease). The spontaneous course of induratio penis plastica is highly variable. The disease is characterized by localized and often progressive fibrosis at the borderline between cavernosal tissue and the tunica, with an initial phase of pain during erection over a period of approximately three months. In a secondary phase, a penile plaque formation mostly in dorsal position is evident, which can lead to penile deviation. Lateral and ventral deviations, particularly, can severely impair capability for copulation and may prevent intercourse. For diagnosis of penile deviations, polaroid autophotographs of the penis in erectile status taken at three levels have proven most useful. Surgical therapy for penile deviations is only indicated when copulation is mechanically impaired, regardless of the deviation's cause, or when pain occurs at erection or during intercourse. Generally, the progression of penile deviation should come to a clinical standstill at least three to six months before surgery. The most popular surgical method is the Nesbit operation (Nesbit, 1954). Postoperative results are good and major complications are not observed. For induratio penis plastica, first-line treatment may involve symptomatic antiphlogistic treatment to relieve pain, as in up to 30–50% of the patients spontaneous remission can be observed. The efficacy of oral vitamin E or potassium-*para*-aminobenzoate therapy is not definitely proven in view of high spontaneous remission rates of induratio penis plastica (van Ahlen and Hertle, 2000).

Empirical treatment of male infertility

Varicocele

Apart from idiopathic infertility, varicoceles are the most frequent physical finding in infertile men (Behre et al., 2000; World Health Organization, 1992b). Varicoceles are believed to cause testicular and epididymal damage via hypoxia and stasis, increased testicular pressure, elevated spermatic vein catecholamines, and/or increased testicular temperature (Fujisawa et al., 1989; Comhaire, 1991; Sweeney et al., 1995; Wright et al., 1997). However, to-date, there is no indisputable evidence that varicocele reduces fertility.

Varicoceles may be associated with various degrees of decreased sperm parameters and increased FSH values. Some patients mention feelings of pressure or sometimes pain in the afflicted testis or in the scrotum, which can worsen after longer periods of standing or sitting in unchanged position. Careful palpation of the pampiniform plexus, provoking engorgement with the Valsalva maneuver, is an important diagnostic measure. Depending on results from palpation, the varicocele can be classified into three degrees of severity:

grade I: enlargement of the pampiniform plexus, only palpable following Valsalva maneuver

grade II: clearly palpable enlargement of the pampiniform plexus

grade III: visible enlargement of the pampiniform plexus.

While grade III varicoceles are clinically easily identifiable, small varicoceles may be diagnosed with the help of sonography.

Ligation, embolization, or sclerosing of the spermatic vein have long been accepted as the treatment of choice (Takihara et al., 1991). Treatment of varicoceles became the most empirical common treatment for male infertility (Marsman and Schats, 1994). Nowadays, treatment is suggested even in azoospermic men with varicocele (Matthews et al., 1998; Kim et al., 1999). Applying the principles of evidence-based andrology to the treatment of varicocele, it is surprising that only a few and mainly recent randomized controlled clinical trials with relevant outcome parameters (induction of pregnancy, improvement in sperm parameters) have been published (Nilsson et al., 1979; Breznik et al., 1993; Madgar et al., 1995; Yamamoto et al., 1996; Hargreave, 1997; Nieschlag et al., 1998; Grasso et al., 2000).

Two trials suggested significant benefits (Madgar et al., 1995; Hargreave, 1997). However, the control groups remained completely untreated and were not even counseled, ignoring the existence of unspecific (placebo) effects. The other four randomized clinical trials, including the largest single-center study (Nieschlag et al., 1998), suggested no significant benefits (Nilsson et al., 1979; Breznik et al., 1993; Grasso et al., 2000). However, in two of these studies, the integrity of female reproductive functions was doubtful and in one study only subclinical varicoceles were investigated (Yamamoto et al.,

1996). In agreement with the majority of randomized controlled clinical trials and in contrast to the majority of uncontrolled studies on varicocelectomy, meta-analysis of all randomized controlled clinical studies involving 587 patients showed no significant treatment benefit and questions the common practice of varicocelectomy (Fig. 15.2). However, as even the high-quality studies show conflicting results, the topic of varicocele treatment will remain controversial. Further randomized clinical trials should readdress this issue, preferably in patients with third-grade varicocele where the presumed treatment effect should be highest. However, for the time being, there are no convincing reasons indicating that interventive treatment is superior to counseling combined with optimization of female reproductive functions (RCOG Study Group, 1998; Kamischke and Nieschlag, 2001).

Immunological male infertility

The clinical significance of antisperm antibodies in semen is yet not well established. Associations of antisperm antibodies with leukocytospermia and subclinical infection or other autoantibodies have been described and further complicate the concept of immunological infertility. Prospective, controlled studies showed negative influences of more than 30% antisperm antibodies on fertility (Eggert-Kruse et al., 1991, 1995; Mahmoud et al., 1996) while others showed no effects (Collins et al., 1993). The uncertain clinical significance is also reflected by the WHO Guidelines (1999), which currently set the threshold for a positive MAR test above 50% (formerly 10%), in agreement with a previous study showing that antisperm IgG or IgA antibodies above a concentration of 50% lead to significantly reduced pregnancy rates and concentrations above 90% almost exclude the chance for a spontaneous pregnancy (Abshagen et al., 1998).

Glucocorticoids have been used in an attempt to reduce antisperm antibodies. Treating patients with antisperm antibody levels above 10% had no effect on these levels or semen characteristics (De Almeida et al., 1985). In contrast, a marked decrease in the proportion of spermatozoa positive for IgG and IgA antibodies (Rasanen et al., 1996) has also

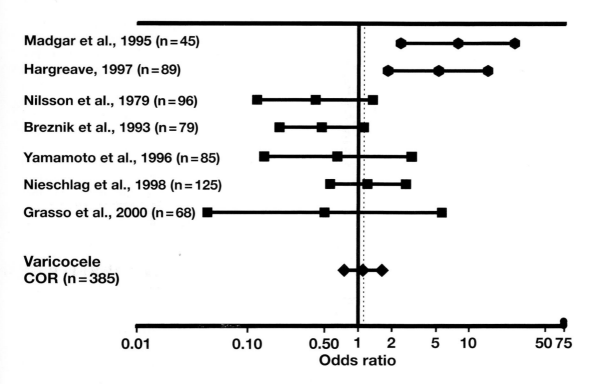

Fig. 15.2. Individual (squares) or combined odds ratios (COR; diamonds) of induced pregnancies based on analysis of randomized, controlled clinical trials on varicocele treatment. Results are presented as odds ratio with 95% confidence interval. The dashed line represents the COR of all included studies, indicating that two randomized controlled trials (hexagons) showing inhomogeneity with the other trials (squares).

been described. For pregnancy analysis, four randomized placebo-controlled studies (two crossover studies) (Haas and Manganiello, 1987; Hendry et al., 1990; Bals-Pratsch et al., 1992; Lahteenmaki et al., 1995) and two randomized controlled studies (one cross-over study) (Gregoriou et al., 1996; Omu et al., 1996) having pregnancies as outcome parameter were analyzed. Two studies (Hendry et al., 1990; Omu et al., 1996) claimed a beneficial effect of corticosteroid therapy on the conception rate, while the other authors found no beneficial effect of corticosteroid therapy.

Studies that contained detailed pregnancy analysis (in crossover studies only the first treatment phase before crossing over was considered) were grouped together for pregnancy analysis in a meta-analysis on corticosteroid treatment (Haas and Manganiello, 1987; Bals-Pratsch et al., 1992; Lahteenmaki et al., 1995; Omu et al., 1996). Meta-analysis revealed no significant influence (odds ratio 2.02; 95% CI 0.88–4.61) of corticosteroid treatment on pregnancy rates in 190 patients presenting with immunological infertility (Kamischke and Nieschlag, 1999a). However, despite an overall odds ratio bordering on the 5% significance level, meta-analysis in this case might be misleading. Only low numbers of patients with antisperm antibodies clearly were included in the studies; moreover, a considerable proportion of these patients can be suspected to have antisperm antibody titers below 50%. Also, in view of the possibly severe side-effects of corticosteroid treatment, well-designed clinical studies should readdress this issue before drawing further conclusions. For the

Idiopathic male infertility

Patients with "idiopathic male infertility" represent the largest group of men consulting for infertility. The diagnosis can be established only after all other possible causes for infertility have been eliminated. Seminal parameters are frequently subnormal and may be associated with elevated serum FSH and histological disturbances. Despite uncertain diagnosis, in the past, many empirical therapies were applied (O'Donovan et al., 1993; Vandekerckhove et al., 1993; Kamischke and Nieschlag, 1999a).

Hormonal treatment

GnRH and hCG/hMG treatments were used for many years and many uncontrolled studies have been published. For GnRH treatment, only uncontrolled trials showing opposing results are available and no valid conclusion for treatment efficacy can be drawn. Uncontrolled studies with hCG/hMG have been summarized in a review of 39 uncontrolled studies reporting pregnancy rates of 8–14% on average (Schill, 1986). However, the only available randomized, placebo-controlled study of hCG/hMG treatment in idiopathic infertility could not demonstrate any beneficial effect on sperm parameters or pregnancy rates (Knuth et al., 1987), questioning the efficacy of the approach.

The availability of purified hMG and recombinant FSH has led to a reconsideration of FSH treatment in male infertility. So far, four randomized controlled clinical trials using highly purified hMG or recombinant FSH and with pregnancy as an outcome parameter have been published (Comodo et al., 1996; Matorras et al., 1997; Kamischke et al., 1998). None of these randomized, placebo-controlled (Comodo et al., 1996; Kamischke et al., 1998) or randomized controlled (Matorras et al., 1997) trials showed any significant improvements of conventional semen parameters compared with placebo or baseline values. This was confirmed by another randomized placebo-controlled clinical trial with no

pregnancy as an outcome parameter (Foresta et al., 1998). In addition, in this study, a detailed subgroup analysis based on testicular histology showed some significant improvements of semen parameters and testicular histology (Foresta et al., 1998). In contrast to the majority of uncontrolled studies, none of the controlled studies nor the meta-analysis (odds ratio 1.45; 95% CI 0.78–2.70) of all 233 patients enrolled in the randomized studies could detect a significant increase in pregnancy rates (Kamischke and Nieschlag, 1999a). In view of the high costs of FSH therapy and the questionable minor benefits, FSH treatment, as practiced today, cannot be recommended.

Since the 1970s, administration of exogenous testosterone (especially mesterolone) has been proposed as a therapy for idiopathic infertility on the basis of uncontrolled studies. Nine randomized placebo-controlled, double-blind studies (Mauss, 1974; Aafjes et al., 1983; Scottish Infertility Group, 1984; Pusch, 1989; World Health Organization Task Force on the Diagnosis and Treatment of Infertility, 1989; Comhaire, 1990; Gerris et al., 1991; Gregoriou et al., 1993; Comhaire et al., 1995) with pregnancy as outcome parameter could be identified. Five of these studies proposed a beneficial effect of treatment. However, meta-analysis of all randomized, placebo-controlled trials revealed no significant influence of androgens on pregnancy rates in 1025 patients (odds ratio 1.02; 95% CI 0.72–1.44) (Kamischke and Nieschlag, 1999a). Therefore, androgens can be considered ineffective for therapy (Vandekerckhove et al., 1988; O'Donovan et al., 1993; Kamischke and Nieschlag, 1999a).

Antiestrogenic compounds might lead to elevation of gonadotropin and testosterone serum levels. Six randomized, placebo-controlled studies (Ronnberg, 1980; Scottish Infertility Group, 1982; Török, 1985; Ainmelk et al., 1987; Sokol et al., 1988; World Health Organization, 1992a) could be identified. Neither treatment with tamoxifen nor clomiphene showed any significant therapeutic effect on pregnancy rates in a single study. Meta-analysis of all the above mentioned randomized placebo-controlled trials showed no significant influence (odds ratio 1.33; 95% CI 0.78–2.28) of antiestrogens on pregnancy rates in 449 patients analyzed (Kamischke and Nieschlag, 1999a). If controlled studies without placebo treatment are also included in the analysis, only a small beneficial effect of anti-estrogens remains plausible (Vandekerckhove et al., 1998b), which has to be counterbalanced by their potentially toxic side-effects (for review see Rolf et al., 1996).

Nonhormonal therapies

Kallikrein has been widely used for idiopathic male infertility in andrological practice in continental Europe and Japan. Four randomized, double-blinded, placebo-controlled trials having pregnancy as an outcome have been published (Bedford and Elstein, 1981; Izzo et al., 1984; Keck et al., 1994; Schill et al., 1994). None of these studies alone nor the combined odds ratio (odds ratio 0.92; 95% CI 0.40–2.08) of these 200 patients showed a significant effect of kallikrein or angiotensin-converting enzyme inhibitors on sperm parameters or pregnancy rates (Kamischke and Nieschlag, 1999a). However, a less-restrictive analysis, also including studies that were not truly randomized, showed weak beneficial effects, mostly because of the lack of pregnancies in the control groups. In view of the high-quality studies and the meta-analysis, kinin-enhancing agents should only be used in the context of clinical trials, if at all (Vandekerckhove et al., 1998a).

Based on a vague pathophysiological concept, antioxidants have been applied to infertile men, mainly in uncontrolled clinical trials. Of the five randomized controlled clinical trials, two studies failed to find any significant improvements in semen characteristics (Moilanen and Hovatta, 1995; Rolf et al., 1999), while the other three found improvements in sperm function with antioxidants (Lenzi et al., 1993; Suleiman et al., 1996; Kessopoulou et al., 1995). In the studies with pregnancy as an outcome parameter, one study showed a marked effect of vitamin E treatment on pregnancy rates (Suleiman et al., 1996) while the other studies showed no effect (Kessopoulou et al., 1995; Rolf et al., 1999). Meta-analysis (Fig. 15.3) of these three trials showed a sig-

nificant effect of antioxidative vitamins on pregnancy rates (odds ratio 4.53, 95% CI 1.25–16.48). However, the meta-analysis was markedly biased by the one study showing a significant effect on pregnancy rates; this effect was mainly a consequence of the missing pregnancies in the placebo group despite a six-month follow-up. Further evidence concerning the efficacy of vitamin E in infertile men should be evaluated in good-quality trials before it can be recommended.

Three randomized placebo-controlled and double-blinded trials using bromocriptine have been published (Hovatta et al., 1979; Glatthaar et al., 1980; Ainmelk et al., 1982;). No beneficial effects of the treatment were reported in terms of sperm parameters or pregnancy rates, suggesting that bromocriptine treatment promises no benefit.

Ejaculation problems

Retrograde ejaculation

Retrograde ejaculation accounts for around 0.3% of male infertility (Yavetz et al., 1994). It is mainly caused by injury to the lumbar sympathetic nerves (e.g., retroperitoneal lymphadenectomy, aortofemoral bypass, sympathectomies) or by surgery (especially prostate and bladder neck) that damages the neck of the bladder. Common additional reasons include idiopathic and pharmacological causes (alpha-blockers) and neurological diseases (especially diabetic polyneuropathy). Retrograde ejaculation must be differentiated from anejaculation, insufficient production of seminal plasma, and obstructive problems of emission. Diagnostically, transrectal sonography and microscopic investigations of the postcoital or postmasturbatory urine are most important. Diagnosis is confirmed when more than 15 spermatozoa per field or fructose can be detected in the urine after ejaculation (Kamischke and Nieschlag, 1999b).

Evidence concerning efficacy of reversal of retrograde ejaculation mostly comes from small cohort studies (less than 20 participants) or case reports and suggests a considerable publication bias in the papers (for review see Kamischke and Nieschlag,

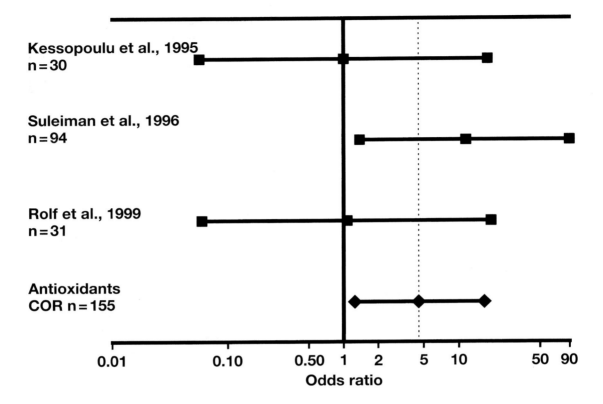

Fig. 15.3. Individual (squares) or combined odds ratios (COR; diamonds) of induced pregnancies based on analysis of randomized, controlled clinical trials with antioxidant treatment of idiopathic male infertility. The dashed line represents the COR of all included studies, indicating homogeneity. Results are presented as odds ratio with 95% confidence interval.

1999b). Medical treatment for reversal of retrograde ejaculation has to be considered the first choice as it offers the opportunity to conceive offspring naturally. Although not significantly different from other drugs, 50 mg orally per day of the commercially distributed combination of chlorphenamine plus phenylpropanolamine (79% success rate), 25–75 mg orally per day imipramine (64% success rate) or 5–40 mg intravenous milodrin (56% success rate) seem to offer the best treatment, especially with respect to spontaneous and ART pregnancy rates

(Kamischke and Nieschlag, 1999b). Sperm recovery from the bladder should be the second approach to retrieve sperm for artificial procedures in men with retrograde ejaculation. As urinary pH and osmolarity are important for sperm quality, alkalinization of the urinary pH with sodium bicarbonate (oral dose 1.2–16 g) given a few hours and up to three days prior to ejaculation should be performed. Osmolarity of the urine can be manipulated via fluid intake. Medium instillation seems to offer no benefit over noninvasive procedures (Kamischke and Nieschlag, 1999b). Most studies have performed inseminations with sperm recovered from urine. However, ICSI has been shown to be superior to other ART in severe male infertility. Therefore, the choice whether to perform intrauterine insemination or to use IVF or ICSI should be made on the basis of the sperm criteria, as is the case when applying ART to ejaculated semen with disturbed characteristics. If no viable sperm can be retrieved, TESE should be considered as a last resort.

Anejaculation

Anejaculation is defined as the total failure of seminal emission into the posterior urethra. Anejaculation is mainly observed in patients with spinal cord injuries, with ejaculations being reported in only 14% of these patients (Otani et al., 1986). Other causes of anejaculation include retroperitoneal lymph node dissection, diabetes mellitus, idiopathic conditions, and secondary obstructions (congenital or postinfectious) of the ejaculatory ducts, which may be visualized by transrectal sonography. Diagnostic clues are the complete absence of an antegrade ejaculation combined with a nonviscous, fructose-negative and sperm-negative postorgasmic urinanalysis (Murphy and Lipshultz, 1987). Differential diagnosis of men with anejaculation includes retarded ejaculation and primary anorgasmia or aspermia owing to androgen deficiency.

Medical treatment of anejaculation with alpha agonists generally has a low (19%) success rate. The more effective (51% overall success) parasympathomimetica suffer from potentially severe side-effects and should only be applied in a clinical setting after pretreatment with hyocine butyl bromide. Consequently, medical treatment of anejaculation cannot be recommended generally as treatment of first choice and warrants further investigation. Although no spontaneous pregnancies could be achieved, electrovibration stimulation together with auto-intrauterine insemination offers the couple the possibility of achieving a pregnancy in the privacy of their home. Evidence from controlled clinical trials indicates that sperm obtained with vibratory stimulation had better quality, better patient acceptance, and higher pregnancy rates in ART than that obtained through electroejaculation (Kamischke and Nieschlag 1999b). Therefore, penile vibratory stimulation should be attempted first to induce ejaculation in patients with anejaculation (Brackett et al. 1997; Ohl et al. 1997). Prognostic factors for overall success of electrovibration

therapy include high vibrator amplitude (≥ 2.5 mm) in patients with high spinal lesions ($\geq$ T11). Patients with lesions above T6 should be treated with caution to prevent autonomic dysreflexia; for these patients pretreatment with nifedipine or prazosin and careful monitoring should be performed. Electroejaculation can be used when electrovibration stimulation is not successful (Kamischke and Nieschlag, 1999b). As in treatment by electrovibration, pretreatment is required and those with spinal cord injuries and unpredictable tolerance plus all patients without such injuries require general anesthesia. After sperm retrieval, IVF and ICSI are the treatment of choice in patients with poor sperm quality. If no viable sperm can be retrieved with the other treatment modalities, surgical sperm retrieval together with ICSI provides a good alternative for anejaculatory men (Hovatta and von Smitten, 1993). Most studies have applied the relatively easy, microsurgical vas deferens aspiration to retrieve sperm in anejaculatory patients. If no sperm can be aspirated from the vas deferens or epididymis, TESE in combination with ICSI offers the final possibility for treatment.

Premature ejaculation

Premature ejaculation as a functional disturbance is characterized by the inability of the patient to control the time of ejaculation so as to allow both partners to reach orgasm. Ejaculation may occur even before intromission of the penis into the vagina. The pathogenesis of this disturbance is largely unknown and in the vast majority of cases an underlying functional problem exists. As premature ejaculation is a problem of the couple, the female partner should be included in diagnosis and treatment of the disease. Because of the acceptable success rates combined with no costs and neglectable side-effects, the "squeeze technique" and the desensitization by two ejaculates in sequence offer the first non-invasive treatment alternatives. In the squeeze technique, a firm squeeze in the region of the frenulum is applied for 3–4 seconds just prior to the onset of ejaculation. With increasing practice, this manipulation leads to a slightly reduced erection and the man will learn to control the time of ejaculation much better (Masters and Johnson, 1970). Medical treatment involves the use of local anesthesia and systemic drugs. Local anesthetics are applied to the glans penis prior to sexual intercourse. However, they are only partially effective and often desensitize the female genitalia if used without a condom (van Ahlen and Hertle, 2000). Systemic pharmacological treatment includes serotonin reuptake inhibitors (sertraline, fluoxetine, paroxetine), tricyclic antidepressant drugs (clomipramine) and alpha-1 blockers. Randomized placebo-controlled studies using fluoxetine (20 mg orally daily), sertraline (50 mg orally daily) or paroxetine (20 mg orally daily), have shown consistently significant improvements of the latent period of intravaginal ejaculation in over 70% of patients (Waldinger et al., 1994; Mendels et al., 1995; Kara et al., 1996; Biri et al., 1998; McMahon, 1998; Murat Baser et al., 1999; Yilmaz et al., 1999). Clomipramine (10–50 mg per day or up to 4–6 hours prior to ejaculation) and alpha-1 blockers have shown slightly lower success rates (around 50%) in some studies (Goodman, 1980; Segraves et al., 1993; Montorsi et al., 1995; Strassberg et al., 1999). However, apart from one study showing similar efficacy of two serotonin reuptake inhibitors, no comparative studies of the different treatment modalities have been performed (Murat Basar et al., 1999) judging treatment efficacy of the different drugs. Until such comparative studies are achieved, the serotonin reuptake inhibitors seem to offer the best medical treatment for premature ejaculation.

Symptomatic treatment of male infertility

If fertility cannot be achieved by other treatments, ART offers possibilities for symptomatic treatment of male infertility. The severity of male fertility impairments often mainly determines the ART possible. However, there are no definite guidelines indicating which ART modality is suited to which level of impairment. Notwithstanding the great success, especially of the ICSI technique, in this as in other areas of male infertility, therapeutic options have to show their effectiveness in controlled clinical studies. In view of the spontaneous pregnancy rates in couples where the men have mild semen disturbances, trials comparing the success of insemination or IVF with counseling appear mandatory. In the ideal case, clear-cut limits for the different ARTs can be established.

REFERENCES

Aafjes, J.H., van der Vijver, J.C., Brugman, F.W., and Schenck, P.E. (1983). Double-blind cross over treatment with mesterolone and placebo of subfertile oligozoospermic men: value of testicular biopsy. *Andrologia*, **15**, 531–5.

Abshagen, K., Behre, H.M., Cooper, T.G., and Nieschlag, E. (1998). Influence of sperm surface antibodies on spontaneous pregnancy rates. *Fertility and Sterility*, **70**, 355–6.

Ainmelk, Y., Belisle, S., Kandalaft, N., McClure, D., Tetreault, L., and Elhilali, M. (1982). Bromocriptine therapy in oligozoospermic infertile men. *Archives of Andrology*, **8**, 135–41.

Ainmelk, Y., Belisle, S., Carmel, M., and Jean-Pierre, T. (1987). Tamoxifen citrate therapy in male infertility. *Fertility Sterility*, **48**, 113–17.

Anderson, R.A., Irvine, D.S., Balfour, C., Groome, N.P., and Riley, S.C. (1998). Inhibin B in seminal plasma: testicular origin and relationship to spermatogenesis. *Human Reproduction*, **13**, 920–6.

Andersson, A.M., Muller, J., and Skakkebaek, N.E. (1998). Different roles of prepubertal and postpubertal germ cells and Sertoli cells in the regulation of serum inhibin B levels. *Journal of Clinical Endocrinology and Metabolism*, **83**, 4451–8.

Balaban, B., Urman, B., Sertac, A., et al. (1999). In-vitro culture of spermatozoa induces motility and increases implantation and pregnancy rates after testicular sperm extraction and intracytoplasmic sperm injection. *Human Reproduction*, **14**, 2808–11.

Ballesca, J.L., Balasch, J., Calafell, J.M., et al. (2000). Serum inhibin B determination is predictive of successful testicular sperm extraction in men with non-obstructive azoospermia *Human Reproduction*, **15**, 1734–8.

Bals-Pratsch, M., Doren, M., Karbowski, B., Schneider, H.P., and Nieschlag, E. (1992). Cyclic corticosteroid immunosuppression is unsuccessful in the treatment of sperm antibody-related male infertility: a controlled study. *Human Reproduction*, **7**, 99–104.

Bamberg, M., Schmoll, H.-J., and Weißbach, L. (1997). Diagnostik und Therapie von Hodentumoren. *Deutsches Ärzteblatt*, **94**, c-2050–6.

Barratt, C.L.R., Tomlinson, M.J., and Cooke, I.D. (1993). Prognostic significance of computerized motility analysis for in vivo fertility. *Fertility Sterility*, **60**, 520–5.

Bedford, N. and Elstein, M. (1981). Effects of kallikrein on male subfertility – a double blind cross-over study. In: *Advances in Diagnosis and Treatment of Infertility*, Insler, V. and Bettendorf, G., eds. Elsevier, New York, pp. 339–43.

Behre, H.M., Nashan, D., and Nieschlag, E. (1989). Objective measurement of testicular volume by ultrasonography: evaluation of the technique and comparison with orchidometer estimates. *International Journal of Andrology*, **12**, 395–403.

Behre, H.M., Yeung, C.H., Holstein, A.F., Weinbauer, G.F., Gassner, P., and Nieschlag, E. (2000). Diagnosis of male infertility and hypogonadism. In: *Andrology: Male Reproductive Health and Dysfunction*, Nieschlag, E. and Behre, H.M., eds. Springer-Verlag, Heidelberg, pp. 90–124.

Belker, A.M., Thomas, A.J., and Fuchs, E.F. (1991). Results of 1469 microsurgical reversals by vasovasostomy study group. *Journal of Urology*, **145**, 505–11.

Bergmann, M., Behre, H.M., and Nieschlag, E. (1994). Serum FSH and testicular morphology in male infertility. *Clinical Endocrinology (Oxford)*, **40**, 133–6.

Biri, H., Isen, K., Sinik, Z., Onaran, M., Kupeli, B., and Bozkirli, I. (1998). Sertraline in the treatment of premature ejaculation: a double-blind placebo controlled study. *International Urology and Nephrology*, **30**, 611–15.

Böck, P. (1989). *Romeis Mikroskopische Technik*. Urban & Schwarzenberg, Munich.

Bosl, G.J. and Motzer, R.J. (1997). Testicular germ-cell cancer. *New England Journal of Medicine*, **337**, 242–53.

Brackett, N.L., Padron, O.F., and Lynne, C.M. (1997). Semen quality of spinal cord injured men is better when obtained by vibratory stimulation versus electroejaculation. *Journal of Urology*, **157**, 151–7.

Branigan, E.F. and Muller, C.H. (1994). Efficacy of treatment and recurrence rate of leukocytospermia in infertile men with prostatitis. *Fertility Sterility*, **62**, 580–4.

Braunstein, G.D. (1993). Gynecomastia. *New England Journal of Medicine*, **328**, 490–5.

Breznik, R., Vlaisavljevic, V., and Borko, E. (1993). Treatment of varicocele and male fertility. *Archives of Andrology*, **30**, 157–60.

Büchter, D., Behre, H.M., Kliesch, S., and Nieschlag, E. (1998). Pulsatile GnRH or human chorionic gonadotropin/human menopausal gonadotropin as effective treatment for men with hypogonadotropic hypogonadism: a review of 42 cases. *European Journal of Endocrinology*, **139**, 298–303.

Burgues, S. and Calderon, M.D. (1997). Subcutaneous self-administration of highly purified follicle stimulating hormone and human chorionic gonadotrophin for the treatment of male hypogonadotrophic hypogonadism. Spanish Collaborative Group on Male Hypogonadotropic Hypogonadism. *Human Reproduction*, **12**, 980–6.

Burris, A. S., Clark, R.V., Vantman, D.J., and Sherins, R.J. (1988). A low sperm concentration does not preclude fertility in men with isolated hypogonadotropic hypogonadism after gonadotropin therapy. *Fertility Sterility*, **50**, 343–7.

Carlsen, E., Olsson, C., Petersen, J.H., Andersson, A.M., and Skakkebaek, N. E. (1999). Diurnal rhythm in serum levels of inhibin B in normal men: relation to testicular steroids and gonadotropins. *Journal of Clinical Endocrinology and Metabolism*, **84**, 1664–9.

Cavallini, G. (1995). Alpha-1 blockade pharmacotherapy in primitive psychogenic premature ejaculation resistant to psychotherapy. *European Urology*, **28**, 126–30.

Chemes, H.E., Olmedo, S.B., Carrere, C., et al. (1998). Ultrastructural pathology of the sperm flagellum: association between flagellar pathology and fertility prognosis in severely asthenozoospermic men. *Human Reproduction*, **13**, 2521–6.

Collins, J.A., Burrows, E.A., Yeo, J., and Young Lai, E.V. (1993). Frequency and predictive value of antisperm antibodies among infertile couples. *Human Reproduction*, **8**, 592–8.

Collins, J.A., Burrows, E.A., and Wilan, A.R. (1995). The prognosis for live birth among untreated infertile couples. *Fertility Sterility*, **64**, 22–8.

Comhaire, F. (1990). Treatment of idiopathic testicular failure with high-dose testosterone undecanoate: a double-blind pilot study. *Fertility Sterility*, **54**, 689–93.

Comhaire, F. (1991). The pathogenesis of epididymo-testicular dysfunction in varicocele: factors other than temperature. *Advances in Experimental Medicine and Biology*, **286**, 281–7.

Comhaire, F.H., Rowe, P.J., and Farley, T.M. (1986). The effect of doxycycline in infertile couples with male accessory gland infection: a double blind prospective study. *International Journal of Andrology*, **9**, 91–8.

Comhaire, F., Schoonjans, F., Abdelmassih, R., et al. (1995). Does treatment with testosterone undecanoate improve the in-vitro fertilizing capacity of spermatozoa in patients with idiopathic testicular failure? (Results of a double blind study.) *Human Reproduction*, **10**, 2600–2.

Comodo, F., Vargiu, N., and Farina, M. (1996). Double-blind FSH-HP/placebo treatment of severe male factor related infertility: effect on sperm parameters and IVF/ICSI outcome. In: *Annual Meeting of the European Society of Human Reproduction and Embryology*. Oxford University Press for ESHRE, Oxford, Poster S41.

Cooper, T.G., Neuwinger, J., Bahrs, S., and Nieschlag, E. (1992). Internal quality control of semen analysis. *Fertility Sterility*, **58**, 172–8.

Cooper, T.G., Atkinson, A.D., and Nieschlag, E. (1999). Experience with external quality control in spermatology. *Human Reproduction*, **14**, 765–9.

Coughlin, M.T., O'Leary, L.A., Songer, N.J., Bellinger, M.F., LaPorte, R.E., and Lee, P.A. (1997). Time to conception after orchidopexy: evidence for subfertility? *Fertility Sterility*, **67**, 742–6.

De Almeida, M., Feneux, D., Rigaud, C., and Jouannet, P. (1985). Steroid therapy for male infertility associated with antisperm antibodies. Results of a small randomized clinical trial. *International Journal of Andrology*, **8**, 111–17.

De Geyter, C., De Geyter, M., Koppers, B., and Nieschlag, E. (1998). Diagnostic accuracy of computer-assisted sperm motion analysis. *Human Reproduction*, **13**, 2512–20.

De Geyter, C., De Geyter, M., Meschede, M., and Behre, H. M. (2000). Assisted fertilization. In: *Andrology: Male Reproductive Health and Dysfunction*, Springer-Verlag, Heidelberg, pp. 337–65.

de Muinck Keizer-Schrama, S.M., Hazebroek, F.W., Matroos, A.W., Drop, S.L., Molenaar, J.C., and Visser, H.K. (1986). Double-blind, placebo-controlled study of luteinising-hormone-releasing-hormone nasal spray in treatment of undescended testes. *Lancet*, **i**, 876–80.

Deutsche Gesellschaft für Endokrinologie (1991). Zur Therapie des Hodenhochstandes. *Endokrinologie-Information*, **15**, 20–22.

Doerr, W. and Seifert, G. (1991). *Pathologie des männlichen Genitales*. Springer-Verlag, Heidelberg.

Eggert-Kruse, W., Hofsass, A., Haury, E., Tilgen, W., Gerhard, I., and Runnebaum, B. (1991). Relationship between local anti-sperm antibodies and sperm-mucus interaction in vitro and in vivo. *Human Reproduction*, **6**, 267–76.

Eggert-Kruse, W., Rohr, G., Bockem-Hellwig, S., Huber, K., Christmann-Edoga, M., and Runnebaum, B. (1995). Immunological aspects of subfertility. *International Journal of Andrology*, **18**(Suppl. 2), 43–52.

Eggert-Kruse, W., Rohr, G., Demirakca, T., et al. (1997). Chlamydial serology in 1303 asymptomatic subfertile couples. *Human Reproduction*, **12**, 1464–75.

Erel, C.T., Senturk, L.M., Demir, F., Irez, T., and Ertungealp, E. (1997). Antibiotic therapy in men with leukocytospermia. *International Journal of Fertility and Women's Medicine*, **42**, 206–10.

Fischer, R., Baukloh, V., Naether, O.G., Schulze, W., Salzbrunn, A., and Benson, D.M. (1996). Pregnancy after intracytoplasmic sperm injection of spermatozoa extracted from frozen-thawed testicular biopsy. *Human Reproduction*, **11**, 2197–9.

Foppiani, L., Schlatt, S., Simoni, M., Weinbauer, G.F., Hacker-Klom, U., and Nieschlag, E. (1999). Inhibin B is a more sensi-tive marker of spermatogenetic damage than FSH in the irradiated non-human primate model. *Journal of Endocrinology*, **162**, 393–400.

Foresta, C., Bettella, A., Ferlin, A., Garolla, A., and Rossato, M. (1998). Evidence for a stimulatory role of follicle-stimulating hormone on the spermatogonial population in adult males. *Fertility Sterility*, **69**, 636–42.

Foresta, C., Bettella, A., Petraglia, F., Pistorello, M., Luisi, S., and Rossato, M. (1999). Inhibin B levels in azoospermic subjects with cytologically characterized testicular pathology. *Clinical Endocrinology (Oxford)*, **50**, 695–701.

Fujisawa, M., Yoshida, S., Kojima, K., and Kamidono, S. (1989). Biochemical changes in testicular varicocele. *Archives of Andrology*, **22**, 149–59.

Gerris, J., Comhaire, F., Hellemans, P., Peeters, K., and Schoonjans, F. (1991). Placebo-controlled trial of high-dose mesterolone treatment of idiopathic male infertility. *Fertility Sterility*, **55**, 603–7.

Glatthaar, C., Donald, R.A., Smith, R., and McRae, C.U. (1980). Pituitary function in normoprolactinaemic infertile men receiving bromocriptine. *Clinical Endocrinology (Oxford)*, **13**, 455–9.

Goodman, R.E. (1980). An assessment of clomipramine (Anafranil) in the treatment of premature ejaculation. *Journal of International Medical Research*, **8**, 53–9.

Grasso, M., Lania, C., Castelli, M., Galli, L., Franzoso, F., and Rigatti, P. (2000). Low-grade left varicocele in patients over 30 years old: the effect of spermatic vein ligation on fertility. *British Journal of Urology*, **85**, 305–7.

Gregoriou, O., Papadias, C., Konidaris, S., Gargaropoulos, A., and Kalampokas, E. (1993). A randomized comparison of intrauterine and intraperitoneal insemination in the treatment of infertility. *International Journal of Gynaecology and Obstetrics*, **42**, 33–6.

Gregoriou, O., Konidaris, S., Antonaki, V., Papadias, C., Antoniou, G., and Gargaropoulos, A. (1996). Corticosteroid treatment does not improve the results of intrauterine insemination in male subfertility caused by antisperm antibodies. *European Journal of Obstetrics, Gynaecology and Reproductive Biology*, **65**, 227–30.

Haas, G.G., Jr. and Manganiello, P. (1987). A double-blind, placebo-controlled study of the use of methylprednisolone in infertile men with sperm-associated immunoglobulins. *Fertility Sterility*, **47**, 295–301.

Hacker-Klom, U.B., Gohde, W., Nieschlag, E., and Behre, H.M. (1999). DNA flow cytometry of human semen. *Human Reproduction*, **14**, 2506–12.

Hargreave, T.B. (1997). Varicocele: overview and commentary on the results of the World Health Organization varicocele trial. In: *Current Advances in Andrology (Proceedings of the VIth International Congress of Andrology)*, Waites, G.M.H., Frick, J. and Baker, G.W.H., eds. Monduzzi Editore, Bologna, Italy, pp. 31–44.

Harrison, R.F., de Louvois, J., Blades, M., and Hurley, R. (1975). Doxycycline treatment and human infertility. *Lancet*, i, 605–7.

Heidenreich, A., Sesterhenn, I.A., Mostofi, F.K., and Moul, J.W. (1998). Immunohistochemical expression of monoclonal antibody 43–9F in testicular germ cell tumors. *International Journal of Andrology*, 21, 283–8.

Hendry, W.F., Hughes, L., Scammell, G., Pryor, J.P., and Hargreave, T.B. (1990). Comparison of prednisolone and placebo in subfertile men with antibodies to spermatozoa. *Lancet*, 335, 85–8.

Hinton, R.A., Egdell, L.M., Andrews, B.E., Clarke, S.K., and Richmond, S.J. (1979). A double-blind cross-over study of the effect of doxycycline on mycoplasma infection and infertility. *British Journal of Obstetrics and Gynaecology*, 86, 379–83.

Holstein, A.F., Roosen-Runge, E.C., and Schirren, C. (1988). *Illustrated Pathology of Human Spermatogenesis*. Grosse-Verlag, Berlin.

Hoorweg-Nijman, J.J., Havers, H.M., and Delemarre-van de Waal, H.A. (1994). Effect of human chorionic gonadotrophin (hCG)/follicle-stimulating hormone treatment versus hCG treatment alone on testicular descent: a double-blind placebo-controlled study. *European Journal of Endocrinology*, 130, 60–4.

Hovatta, O. and von Smitten, K. (1993). Sperm aspiration from vas deferens and in-vitro fertilization in cases of non-treatable anejaculation. *Human Reproduction*, 8, 1689–91.

Hovatta, O., Koskimies, A.I., Ranta, T., Stenman, U.H., and Seppala, M. (1979). Bromocriptine treatment of oligospermia: a double blind study. *Clinical Endocrinology (Oxford)*, 11, 377–82.

Huff, D.S., Hadziselimovic, F., Snyder, H.M., Blythe, B., and Duckett, J.W. (1991). Histologic maldevelopment of unilaterally cryptorchid testes and their descended partners. *European Pediatrics*, 152(Suppl. 2), 10–14.

Irvine, D.S., Macleod, I.C., Templeton, A.A., Masterton, A., and Taylor, A. (1994). A prospective clinical study of the relationship between the computer-assisted assessment of human semen quality and the achievement of pregnancy in vivo. *Human Reproduction*, 9, 2324–34.

Izzo, P.L., Canale, D., Bianchi, B., et al. (1984). The treatment of male subfertility with kallikrein. *Andrologia*, 16, 156–61.

Kamischke, A. and Nieschlag, E. (1999a). Analysis of medical treatment of male infertility. *Human Reproduction*, 14(Suppl. 1), 1–23.

Kamischke, A. and Nieschlag, E. (1999b). Treatment of retrograde ejaculation and anejaculation. *Human Reproduction Update*, 5, 448–74.

Kamischke, A. and Nieschlag, E. (2001). Varicocele treatment in the light of evidence-based andrology. *Human Reproduction Update*, 7, 65–9.

Kamischke, A., Behre, H.M., Bergmann, M., Simoni, M., Schäfer, T., and Nieschlag, E. (1998). Recombinant human follicle stimulating hormone for treatment of male idiopathic infertility: a randomized, double-blind, placebo-controlled, clinical trial. *Human Reproduction*, 13, 596–603.

Kara, H., Aydin, S., Yucel, M., Agargun, M.Y., Odabas, O., and Yilmaz, Y. (1996). The efficacy of fluoxetine in the treatment of premature ejaculation: a double-blind placebo controlled study. *Journal of Urology*, 156, 1631–2.

Keck, C., Behre, H.M., Jockenhövel, F., and Nieschlag, E. (1994). Ineffectiveness of kallikrein in treatment of idiopathic male infertility: a double-blind, randomized, placebo-controlled trial. *Human Reproduction*, 9, 325–9.

Kessopoulou, E., Powers, H.J., Sharma, K.K., et al. (1995). A double-blind randomized placebo cross-over controlled trial using the antioxidant vitamin E to treat reactive oxygen species associated male infertility. *Fertility Sterility*, 64, 825–31.

Kim, E.D., Leibman, B.B., Grinblat, D.M., and Lipshultz, L.I. (1999). Varicocele repair improves semen parameters in azoospermic men with spermatogenic failure. *Journal of Urology*, 162, 737–40.

Kliesch, S., Behre, H.M., and Nieschlag, E. (1994). High efficacy of gonadotropin or pulsatile gonadotropin-releasing hormone treatment in hypogonadotropic hypogonadal men. *European Journal of Endocrinology*, 131, 347–54.

Kliesch, S., Behre, H.M., and Nieschlag, E. (1995). Recombinant human follicle-stimulating hormone and human chorionic gonadotropin for induction of spermatogenesis in a hypogonadotropic male. *Fertility Sterility*, 63, 1326–8.

Knuth, U.A., Hönigl, W., Bals-Pratsch, M., Schleicher, G., and Nieschlag, E. (1987). Treatment of severe oligospermia with human chorionic gonadotropin/human menopausal gonadotropin: a placebo-controlled, double blind trial. *Journal of Clinical Endocrinology and Metabolism*, 65, 1081–7.

Laczkó, J. and Lévai, G. (1975). A simple differential staining method for semi-thin sections of ossifying cartilage and bone tissues embedded in epoxy resin. *Mikroskopie*. 31, 1–4.

Lahteenmaki, A., Veilahti, J., and Hovatta, O. (1995). Intra-uterine insemination versus cyclic, low-dose prednisolone in couples with male antisperm antibodies. *Human Reproduction*, 10, 142–7.

Lenzi, A., Culasso, F., Gandini, L., Lombardo, F., and Dondero, F. (1993). Placebo-controlled, double-blind, cross-over trial of glutathione therapy in male infertility. *Human Reproduction*, **8**, 1657–62.

Liu, P.Y., Turner, L., Rushford, D., et al. (1999). Efficacy and safety of recombinant human follicle stimulating hormone (Gonal-F) with urinary human chorionic gonadotrophin for induction of spermatogenesis and fertility in gonadotrophin-deficient men. *Human Reproduction*, **14**, 1540–5.

Madgar, I., Weissenberg, R., Lunenfeld, B., Karasik, A., and Goldwasser, B. (1995). Controlled trial of high spermatic vein ligation for varicocele in infertile men. *Fertility Sterility*, **63**, 120–4.

Mahmoud, A.M., Tuyttens, C.L., and Comhaire, F.H. (1996). Clinical and biological aspects of male immune infertility: a case-controlled study of 86 cases. *Andrologia*, **28**, 191–6.

Marsman, J.W. and Schats, R. (1994). The subclinical varicocele debate. *Human Reproduction*, **9**, 1–8.

Masters, W.H. and Johnson, V.E. (1970). *Human Sexual Inadequacy*. Little, Brown, Boston, MA.

Matorras, R., Perez, C., Corcostegui, B., et al. (1997). Treatment of the male with follicle-stimulating hormone in intrauterine insemination with husband's spermatozoa: a randomized study. *Human Reproduction*, **12**, 24–8.

Matthews, G.J., Matthews, E.D., and Goldstein, M. (1998). Induction of spermatogenesis and achievement of pregnancy after microsurgical varicocelectomy in men with azoospermia and severe oligoasthenospermia. *Fertility Sterility*, **70**, 71–5.

Mauss, J. (1974). Ergebnisse der Behandlung von Fertilitätsstörungen des Mannes mit Mesterolon oder einem Placebo. *Arzneimittel Forschung*, **24**, 1338–41.

McMahon, C.G. (1998). Treatment of premature ejaculation with sertraline hydrochloride. *International Journal of Impotence Research*, **10**, 181–4; discussion 185.

Mendels, J., Camera, A., and Sikes, C. (1995). Sertraline treatment for premature ejaculation. *Journal of Clinical Psychopharmacology*, **15**, 341–6.

Meschede, D. and Horst, J. (1997). Genetic counselling for infertile male patients. *International Journal of Andrology*, **20**(Suppl. 3), 20–30.

Moilanen, J. and Hovatta, O. (1995). Excretion of alpha-tocopherol into human seminal plasma after oral administration. *Andrologia*, **27**, 133–6.

Montorsi, F., Guazzoni, G., Trimboli, F., Rigatti, P., Pizzini, G., and Miani, A. (1995). Clomipramine for premature ejaculation: a randomized, double blind, placebo controlled study. *Acta Urologica Italia*, **9**, 5–6.

Murat Basar, M., Atan, A., Yildiz, M., Baykam, M., and Aydoganli, L. (1999). Comparison of sertraline to fluoxetine with regard to their efficacy and side effects in the treatment of premature ejaculation. *Archivos Espanoles Urologia*, **52**, 1008–11.

Murphy, J.B. and Lipshultz, L.I. (1987). Abnormalities of ejaculation. *Urologic Clinics of North America*, **14**, 583–96.

Nesbit, R.M. (1954). The surgical treatment of congenital chordee without hypospadias. *Journal of Urology*, **72**, 1178–80.

Neugebauer, D.C., Neuwinger, J., Jockenhövel, F., and Nieschlag, E. (1990). 9 + 0 axoneme in spermatozoa and some nasal cilia of a patient with totally immotile spermatozoa associated with thickened sheath and short midpiece. *Human Reproduction*, **5**, 981–6.

Nieschlag, E. and Behre, H.M., eds. (2000). *Andrology: Male Reproductive Health and Dysfunction*. Springer-Verlag, Heidelberg.

Nieschlag, E., Hertle, L., Fischedick, A., Abshagen, K., and Behre, H.M. (1998). Update on treatment of varicocele: counselling as effective as occlusion of the vena spermatica. *Human Reproduction*, **13**, 2147–50.

Nieschlag, E., Behre, H.M., Meschede, D., and Kamischke, A. (2000). Disorders at the testicular level. In: *Andrology: Male Reproductive Health and Dysfunction*, Nieschlag, E. and Behre, H.M., eds. Springer-Verlag, Heidelberg, pp. 133–59.

Nilsson, S., Edvinsson, A., and Nilsson, B. (1979). Improvement of semen and pregnancy rate after ligation and division of the internal spermatic vein: fact or fiction? *British Journal of Urology*, **51**, 591–6.

O'Donovan, P.A., Vandekerckhove, P., Lilford, R.J., and Hughes, E. (1993). Treatment of male infertility: is it effective? Review and meta-analyses of published randomized controlled trials. *Human Reproduction*, **8**, 1209–22.

Ohl, D.A., Sonksen, J., Menge, A.C., McCabe, M., and Keller, L.M. (1997). Electroejaculation versus vibratory stimulation in spinal cord injured men: sperm quality and patient preference. *Journal of Urology*, **157**, 2147–9.

Omu, A.E., al-Qattan, F., and Abdul Hamada, B. (1996). Effect of low dose continuous corticosteroid therapy in men with antisperm antibodies on spermatozoal quality and conception rate. *European Journal of Obstetrics, Gynecology and Reproductive Biology*, **69**, 129–34.

Otani, T., Kondo, A., and Takita, T. (1986). A paraplegic fathering a child after an intrathecal injection of neostigmine: case report. *Paraplegia*, **24**, 32–7.

Parra, B.L., Venable, D.D., Gonzalez, E., and Eastham, J.A. (1996). Testicular microlithiasis as a predictor of intratubular germ cell neoplasia. *Urology*, **48**, 797–9.

Pierik, F.H., Dohle, G.R., van Muiswinkel, J.M., Vreeburg, J.T., and Weber, R.F. (1999). Is routine scrotal ultrasound advantageous in infertile men? *Journal of Urology*, **162**, 1618–20.

Pusch, H.H. (1989). Oral treatment of oligozoospermia with testosterone-undecanoate: results of a double-blind-placebo-controlled trial. *Andrologia*, **21**, 76–82.

Purvis, K. and Christiansen, E. (1993). Infection in the male reproductive tract. Impact, diagnosis and treatment in relation to male infertility. *International Journal of Andrology*, **16**, 1–13.

Rajfer, J., Handelsman, D.J., Swerdloff, R.S., et al. (1986). Hormonal therapy of cryptorchidism. A randomized, double-blind study comparing human chorionic gonadotropin and gonadotropin-releasing hormone. *New England Journal of Medicine*, **314**, 466–70.

Rasanen, M., Lahteenmaki, A., Agrawal, Y.P., Saarikoski, S., and Hovatta, O. (1996). A placebo-controlled flow cytometric study of the effect of low-dose prednisolone treatment on sperm-bound antibody levels. *International Journal of Andrology*, **19**, 150–4.

RCOG Study Group (1998). Recommendations arising from the 35th RCOG Study Group: evidence based fertility treatment. In: *Evidence Based Infertility Treatment*, Templeton, A., Cooke, I., and O'Brian, P.M.S., eds. RCOG Press, London, pp. 397–403.

Rolf, C., Behre, H.M., and Nieschlag, E. (1996). Tamoxifen in male infertility. Analysis of a questionable therapy. *Deutsche Medizinische Wochenschrift*, **121**, 33–9.

Rolf, C., Cooper, T.G., Yeung, C.H., and Nieschlag, E. (1999). Antioxidant treatment of patients with asthenozoospermia or moderate oligoasthenozoospermia with high-dose vitamin C and vitamin E: a randomized, placebo-controlled, double-blind study. *Human Reproduction*, **14**, 1028–33.

Ronnberg, L. (1980). The effect of clomiphene citrate on different sperm parameters and serum hormone levels in preselected infertile men: a controlled double-blind cross-over study. *International Journal of Andrology*, **3**, 479–86.

Salzbrunn, A., Benson, D.M., Holstein, A.F., and Schulze, W. (1996). A new concept for the extraction of testicular spermatozoa as a tool for assisted fertilization (ICSI). *Human Reproduction*, **11**, 752–5.

Schill, W. (1986). Medical treatment of male infertility. In: *Infertility: Male and Female*, Insler, V. and Lunenfeld, B., eds. Churchill Livingstone, Edinburgh, pp. 533–73.

Schill, W.B., Parsch, E.M., and Miska, W. (1994). Inhibition of angiotensin-converting enzyme—a new concept of medical treatment of male infertility? *Fertility Sterility*, **61**, 1123–8.

Schlegel, P.N. and Goldstein, M. (1993). Microsurgical vasoepididymostomy: refinements and results. *Journal of Urology*, **150**, 1165–8.

Schopohl, J. (1993). Pulsatile gonadotrophin releasing hormone versus gonadotrophin treatment of hypothalamic hypogonadism in males. *Human Reproduction*, **8**(Suppl. 2), 175–9.

Schopohl, J., Mehltretter, G., von Zumbusch, R., Eversmann, T., and von Werder, K. (1991). Comparison of gonadotropin-releasing hormone and gonadotropin therapy in male patients with idiopathic hypothalamic hypogonadism. *Fertility Sterility*, **56**, 1143–50.

Schulze, W. and Knuth, U.A. (2000). Diagnostics of testicular dysfunction: testicular biopsy. In: *Oxford Textbook of Endocrinology*, Shalet, S.M., and Wass, J.A.H. eds. Oxford University Press, Oxford, in press.

Schulze, W., Thoms, F., and Knuth, U.A. (1999). Testicular sperm extraction: comprehensive analysis with simultaneously performed histology in 1418 biopsies from 766 subfertile men. *Human Reproduction*, **14**(Suppl. 1), 82–96

Scottish Infertility Group (1982). Randomised trial of clomiphene citrate treatment and vitamin C for male infertility. *British Journal of Urology*, **54**, 780–4.

Scottish Infertility Group (1984). Randomised trial of mesterolone versus vitamin C for male infertility. *British Journal of Urology*, **56**, 740–4.

Segraves, R.T., Saran, A., Segraves, K., and Maguire, E. (1993). Clomipramine versus placebo in the treatment of premature ejaculation: a pilot study. *Journal of Sex and Marital Therapy*, **19**, 198–200.

Snick, H.K., Snick, T.S., Evers, J.L., and Collins, J.A. (1997). The spontaneous pregnancy prognosis in untreated subfertile couples: the Walcheren primary care study. *Human Reproduction*, **12**, 1582–8.

Sokol, R.Z., Steiner, B.S., Bustillo, M., Petersen, G., and Swerdloff, R.S. (1988). A controlled comparison of the efficacy of clomiphene citrate in male infertility. *Fertility Sterility*, **49**, 865–70.

Steigerwald, P. and Krause, W. (1998). Estimation of sperm morphology using a new CASA system. *Andrologia*, **30**, 23–7.

Strassberg, D.S., de Gouveia Brazao, C.A., Rowland, D.L., Tan, P., and Slob, A.K. (1999). Clomipramine in the treatment of rapid (premature) ejaculation. *Journal of Sex and Marital Therapy*, **25**, 89–101.

Suleiman, S.A., Ali, M.E., Zaki, Z.M., el-Malik, E.M., and Nasr, M.A. (1996). Lipid peroxidation and human sperm motility: protective role of vitamin E. *Journal of Andrology*, **17**, 530–7.

Sweeney, T.E., Rozum, J.S., and Gore, R.W. (1995). Alteration of testicular microvascular pressures during venous pressure elevation. *American Journal of Physiology*, **269**, H37–45.

Takihara, H., Sakatoku, J., and Cockett, A.T. (1991). The pathophysiology of varicocele in male infertility. *Fertility Sterility*, **55**, 861–8.

Torök, L. (1985). Treatment of oligozoospermia with tamoxifen (open and controlled studies). *Andrologia*, **17**, 497–501.

van Ahlen, H. and Hertle, L. (2000). Disorders of sperm disposition. In: *Andrology: Male Reproductive Health and Dysfunction*, Nieschlag, E. and Behre, H.M., eds. Springer-Verlag, Heidelberg, pp. 90–124.

Vandekerckhove, P., O'Donovan, P.A., Lilford, R.J., and Harada, T.W. (1993). Infertility treatment: from cookery to science. The epidemiology of randomised controlled trials. *British Journal of Obstetrics and Gynaecology.*, **100**, 1005–36.

Vandekerckhove, P., Lilford, R., and Hughes, E. (1998a). Kinin enhancing drugs for male infertility. In: *Subfertility Module of the Cochrane Database of Systematic Reviews*, Lilford, E., Hughes, P. and Vandekerckhove, P. eds. The Cochrane Collaboration, Update Software, Oxford.

Vandekerckhove, P., Lilford, R., and Hughes, E. (1998b). The medical treatment of idiopathic oligo/asthenozoospermia: anti-oestrogens (clomiphene or tamoxifen) versus placebo or no treatment. In: *Subfertility Module of the Cochrane Database of Systematic Reviews.*, Lilford, E., Hughes, P. and Vandekerckhove, P. eds. The Cochrane Collaboration, Issue 2, Update Software, Oxford.

von Eckardstein, S., Simoni, M., Bergmann, M., et al. (1999). Serum inhibin B in combination with serum follicle-stimulating hormone (FSH) is a more sensitive marker than serum FSH alone for impaired spermatogenesis in men, but cannot predict the presence of sperm in testicular tissue samples. *Journal of Clinical Endocrinology and Metabolism*, **84**, 2496–501.

von Eckardstein, S., Cooper, T.G., Rutscha, K., Meschede, D., Horst, J., and Nieschlag, E. (2000). Seminal plasma characteristics as indicators of cystic fibrosis transmembrane conductance regulator (CFTR) gene mutations in men with obstructive azoospermia. *Fertility Sterility*, **73**, 1226–31.

Vermeulen, A., Verdonck, L., and Kaufman, J.M. (1999). A critical evaluation of simple methods for the estimation of free testosterone in serum. *Journal of Clinical Endocrinology and Metabolism*, **84**, 3666–72.

Waldinger, M.D., Hengeveld, M.W., and Zwinderman, A.H. (1994). Paroxetine treatment of premature ejaculation: a double-blind, randomized, placebo-controlled study. *American Journal of Psychiatry*, **151**, 1377–9.

Wolff, H. (1995). The biologic significance of white blood cells in semen. *Fertility Sterility*, **63**, 1143–57.

World Health Organization (1992a). A double-blind trial of clomiphene citrate for the treatment of idiopathic male infertility. *International Journal of Andrology*, **15**, 299–307.

World Health Organization (1992b). The influence of varicocele on parameters of fertility in a large group of men presenting to infertility clinics. *Fertility Sterility*, **57**, 1289–93.

World Health Organization (1992c). *WHO Laboratory Manual for the Examination of Human Semen and Sperm–Cervical Mucus Interaction*, 3rd edn. Cambridge University Press, Cambridge, UK.

World Health Organization (1999). *WHO Laboratory Manual for the Examination of Human Semen and Sperm-Cervical Mucus Interaction*, 4th edn. Cambridge University Press, Cambridge, UK.

World Health Organization Task Force on the Diagnosis and Treatment of Infertility (1989). Mesterolone and idiopathic male infertility: a double-blind study. *International Journal of Andrology*, **12**, 254–64.

Wright, E.J., Young, G.P., and Goldstein, M. (1997). Reduction in testicular temperature after varicocelectomy in infertile men. *Urology*, **50**, 257–9.

Yamamoto, M., Hibi, H., Hirata, Y., Miyake, K., and Ishigaki, T. (1996). Effect of varicocelectomy on sperm parameters and pregnancy rate in patients with subclinical varicocele: a randomized prospective controlled study. *Journal of Urology*, **155**, 1636–8.

Yanushpolsky, E.H., Politch, J.A., Hill, J.A., and Anderson, D.J. (1995). Antibiotic therapy and leukocytospermia: a prospective, randomized, controlled study. *Fertility Sterility*, **63**, 142–7.

Yavetz, H., Yogev, L., Hauser, R., Lessing, J.B., Paz, G., and Homonnai, Z.T. (1994). Retrograde ejaculation. *Human Reproduction*, **9**, 381–6.

Yilmaz, U., Tatlisen, A., Turan, H., Arman, F., and Ekmekcioglu, O. (1999). The effects of fluoxetine on several neurophysiological variables in patients with premature ejaculation. *Journal of Urology*, **161**, 107–11.

Zamboni, L. (1992) Sperm structure and its relevance to infertility. An electron microscopic study. *Archives in Pathology and Laboratory Medicine*, **116**, 325–44.

16

Tests of male fertility

R. John Aitken

School of Biological and Chemical Sciences, University of Newcastle, Australia.

Introduction

Defective sperm function has long been recognized as a major cause of human infertility (Hull et al., 1985). Notwithstanding the importance of this condition, we have little understanding of the causes of male infertility and, as a consequence, little capacity to generate true diagnoses in this field. For many years, the only analytical tool available to andrologists was a descriptive analysis of semen quality (MacLoed and Gold, 1951). The initial thrust of such analyses was to place the emphasis on sperm count; infertility being inferred when sperm counts fell below a certain critical threshold. Patients failing to reach this threshold were defined as oligozoospermic. Other descriptive attributes of semen quality that have been linked with male infertility include poor sperm motility (asthenozoospermia), abnormal sperm morphology (teratozoospermia), and the presence of leukocytes (leukocytospermia). The culmination of this descriptive approach towards the assessment of male fertility was the World Health Organization (WHO) manual (World Health Organization, 1999). This monograph described a set of standardized techniques for the preparation of a semen profile together with guidelines for the thresholds of normality for each descriptive criterion (see Table 15.1, p. 234). This publication made an extremely important contribution to the field by facilitating the establishment of global standards. Despite this achievement, it should be recognized that this descriptive approach to semen analysis has taken us no closer to a diagnosis of male infertility. It establishes a set of descriptive criteria that may be loosely correlated with infertility but sheds no light on the causes of male infertility or possible strategies for the effective management of patients. A graphic illustration of the weakness of these conventional criteria of semen quality is afforded by studies on men participating in contraceptive trials. Exposure of men to androgen/gestogen combinations results in a significant reduction in sperm number but no corresponding change in their fertility. Even when sperm counts are suppressed well into the pathological range ($< 5 \times 10^6$ spermatozoa/ml), such men are still fertile (Wallace et al., 1992). It is clear from such studies that fertility is rarely a question of sperm number. It is fundamentally a question of sperm function.

In light of this fact, a second wave of diagnostic tests was developed in the late 1970s and 1980s that sought to generate information on the functional competence of human spermatozoa rather than their appearance. Since fertilization of the human oocyte calls upon many unrelated sperm properties, the development of a single global test of sperm function was never a likely proposition. Instead, emphasis was placed on the development of an integrated battery of tests each of which would reflect a different aspect of sperm function. Thus computerized techniques were introduced for the accurate measurement of sperm motility, while simple bioassays were developed to measure such elements of sperm function as cervical mucus penetration, sperm–zona interaction, and competence to undergo the acrosome reaction. All of these tests provided information of prognostic significance and most yielded diagnostic information that could not have been obtained from the semen profile alone (Aitken et al., 1991). While these bioassays are theoretically valuable, their clinical use has been curtailed by two factors. First, they are too labor intensive, expensive, and technically difficult to be practical. Second, tests of sperm function have been largely rendered redundant by the advent of intracytoplasmic sperm injection (ICSI) therapy, the success of which is largely independent of the functional integrity of the gamete (Twigg et al., 1998).

After the descriptive and functional approaches to male fertility diagnosis, we are now entering an era where emphasis will be on the development of biochemical criteria for the evaluation of male fertility that are simple, inexpensive, and readily standardized. Moreover, these assays should tell us something about the causes of defective sperm function and be helpful in determining the most appropriate avenues of therapeutic intervention.

In this brief review we shall consider examples of diagnostic tests from the descriptive, functional, and biochemical divisions of diagnostic seminology and reflect on how such tests are helping to provide insights into the origins, treatment, and prevention of male infertility.

It should also be emphasized at the outset that male infertility has multiple etiologies and this review is confined to a consideration of those conditions involving primary defects of germ cell differentiation and function. Causes of male infertility that have a primary anatomical, endocrine, or behavioral basis are not discussed since excellent reviews of these topics already exist (Hellstrom, 1997).

The conventional semen profile

Sperm count

Sperm count provides an insensitive, indirect indicator of male fertility. Large numbers of spermatozoa are not required to fertilize the oocyte; however, low sperm counts are frequently symptomatic of an underlying defect in spermatogenesis. A weak rela-

tionship between sperm count and fertility undoubtedly exists (Larson et al., 2000) although fertility only starts to decline significantly when sperm concentrations fall to $<5 \times 10^6$ cells/ml (Joannet et al., 1988). Above this concentration no relationship with fertility is evident. One of the problems with sperm count as a diagnostic criterion is that it is not a very robust variable because it is heavily influenced by both sperm output and seminal plasma volume. The latter can be influenced by a variety of factors such as infection or ejaculation frequency and, as a result, the interejaculate coefficient of variation for this variable can be as high as 45% (Aitken and Irvine, 1998). Another confounding variable in such analyses is the highly significant regional variation in sperm concentration (Auger and Jouannet, 1997), which presumably reflects the impact of local environmental and genetic factors on sperm production without necessarily affecting fertility.

Sperm morphology

A much more sensitive indicator of male fertility than sperm count is sperm morphology. Abnormalities of sperm morphology can affect any compartment of this cell: the acrosome, the head, the mid-piece or the tail. The usual approach is to examine 200 cells and score the percentage that are normal using a hierarchical system whereby the head is examined first, then the mid-piece and then the tail (World Health Organization, 1999). This approach has the disadvantage that it does not take account of the number of structural abnormalities present in each cell. Once a spermatozoon has been classified as abnormal because of some defect in the head region, the remainder of the cell is not examined. This deficiency in the conventional "percentage normal" approach to morphological analysis is accommodated by an alternative strategy that documents the mean number of defects per abnormal cell by calculating a "multiple anomalies index" that appears to be predictive of fertility (Jouannet et al., 1988).

A major difficulty with either of the above approaches to morphology analysis is the definition of "normal". The traditional approach to sperm

Table 16.1. Strict criteria for sperm normality according to the World Health Organization (1999)

Domain	Criteria for normality
Sperm head	
Shape	Oval, acrosome occupying 40–70% of head area
Length	4.0–5.0 μm
Width	2.5–3.5 μm
Aspect ratio	1.5–1.75
Midpiece	
Shape	Slender, attached axially to the head
Length	One and a half times the length of the head
Width	<1 μm
Cytoplasmic droplet	Less than half the size of the head
Tail	

Source: World Health Organization (1999).

morphology assessment was calibrated such that the percentage of abnormal forms was less than 60% in normal fertile men. However, the current trend is to adopt stricter criteria for assessing morphology that give an upper limit of normality at around 15% normal forms (Table 16.1). Such strict criteria have been shown to correlate with in vitro fertilization (IVF) rates according to a number of independent studies (Kruger et al., 1988; Ombelet et al., 1994). However, where strict and traditional criteria for assessing sperm morphology have been compared, the prognostic value of the results appeared to depend as much on the laboratory where the analysis was conducted as the scoring criteria used (Ombelet et al., 1997). Such results emphasize that the evaluation of sperm morphology is purely subjective with very little functional justification for the criteria selected. For example, while a pyriform sperm head may be counted as abnormal according to the conventional scoring system, there are no data to indicate that such a shape is incompatible with normal fertilization. Similarly, while advocates of "strict" criteria may assert that the mid-piece should be one and a half times the length of the sperm tail, there is no

logical basis for such an assertion other than it seems subjectively abnormal to go beyond that length. The problem with morphology is that the functional significance of specific deviations from the normal pattern is, in general, unknown. Like sperm count, the value of this criterion is that it gives a general indication of the underlying status of spermatogenesis.

An exception to this rule may be the presence of a cytoplasmic droplet. It has been appreciated for some time that defective sperm function is correlated with an abnormally high cellular content of enzymes such as lactic acid dehydrogenase (Casano et al., 1991), creatine kinase (Huszar et al., 1988), superoxide dismutase (Aitken et al., 1996a), and glucose 6-phosphate dehydrogenase (Aitken et al., 1994b; Gomez et al., 1996). The feature that all these enzymes possess in common is that they are cytosolic. In keeping with this observation, the cellular contents of these enzymes are highly correlated with the retention of excess residual cytoplasm by human spermatozoa (Gomez et al., 1996). Indeed the retention of excess residual cytoplasm seems to be an extremely important indicator of defective sperm function (Zini et al., 1998). For example, recent studies have demonstrated that the loss of sperm function associated with varicoceles and idiopathic male infertility is associated with the retention of excess residual cytoplasm by the spermatozoa (Zini et al., 1999, 2000). Similarly, the loss of fertility associated with heavy smoking is correlated with the excessive presence of cytoplasmic droplets (Mak et al., 2000). In the case of patients with varicoceles, varicocelectomy has been shown to induce a significant increase in sperm motility in association with a reduction in the percentage of cells carrying excess cytoplasm (Zini et al., 1999). Furthermore, studies of patients undergoing IVF therapy have demonstrated the existence of a strong negative correlation between the presence of residual cytoplasm on the mid-piece of spermatozoa and fertilization rate (Keating et al., 1997). This study also revealed a negative correlation between the presence of cytoplasmic droplets and sperm concentration in the original ejaculate as well as with sperm membrane integrity.

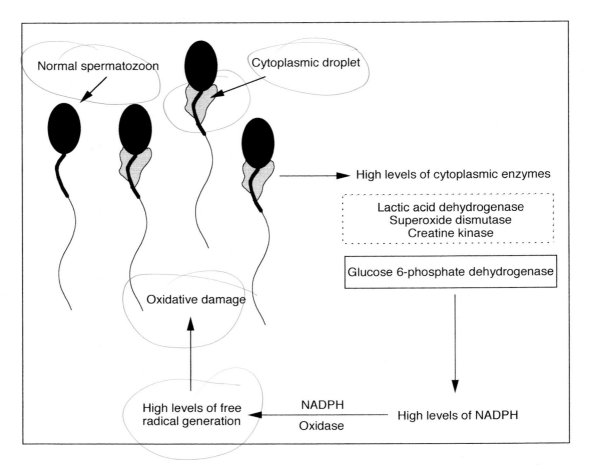

Fig. 16.1. Schematic representation of the possible relationships between the retention of excess residual cytoplasm, oxidative stress and defective sperm function. According to this hypothesis, the presence of glucose 6-phosphate dehydrogenase in the excess cytoplasm fuels the generation of NADPH. The latter then acts as a substrate for the production of a superoxide anion, which dismutates to hydrogen peroxide and damages the cell.

The linkage between defective sperm function and the retention of excess residual cytoplasm is clearly an important one and must shed some light on the mechanisms responsible for the loss of sperm function in subfertility. Normal spermatozoa discharge most of their cytoplasm immediately before spermiation. Since this act deprives these cells of valuable cytosolic enzymes such as creatine kinase, superoxide dismutase, and lactic acid dehydrogenase, the advantage conferred upon spermatozoa by jettisoning their cytoplasm must be considerable. The observed association between the retention of excess residual cytoplasm and the occurrence of oxidative stress provides a rationale for this behavior (Aitken et al., 1994b). If too much cytoplasm is retained by the spermatozoa, they appear to generate excess reactive oxygen species. This may be because the excessive presence of cytosolic enzymes that control the hexose monophosphate pathway, particularly glucose 6-phosphate dehydrogenase, provides additional NADPH to a putative free radical-generating, membrane-bound oxidase (Gomez et al., 1996; Aitken et al., 1997) (Fig. 16.1).

Table 16.2. Prevalence of leukocytospermia

Authors	No. of subjects (prevalence)
Aitken et al. (1994c)	9/120 (7.5%)
Wolff and Anderson (1988)	41/179 (23%)
Tomlinson et al. (1993)	14/512 (2.7%)
Wang et al. (1994)	8/101 (7.9%)

Leucocytospermia

Leukocytospermia (leukocyte counts $> 1 \times 10^6$ cells/ ml) is a relatively rare condition affecting 5–10% of the patient population in locations such as the UK and China, but can rise to $>20\%$ in certain patient groups (Table 16.2). Granulocytes are the most abundant leukocyte species in human semen although occasionally macrophages or lymphocytes predominate, emphasizing that leukocytospermia is a condition with multiple underlying etiologies (Kaleli et al., 2000). The phagocytes present in human semen spontaneously generate reactive oxygen species and yet sperm function does not appear to be significantly altered in most cases (Aitken et al., 1994c). Although this situation seems paradoxical, the preservation of sperm function in the presence of free radical generating-leukocytes is simply a reflection of the powerful antioxidant properties exhibited by seminal plasma. However, when spermatozoa are washed free of seminal plasma they are extremely susceptible to oxidative stress. In the context of assisted reproduction technology (ART), even low levels of leukocyte contamination appear to have a detrimental effect on the fertilizing potential of the spermatozoa (Aitken and Clarkson, 1988). A rational solution to this problem would be to incorporate antioxidants into the culture media used for IVF. In this context, glutathione, *N*-acetylcysteine, hypotaurine, and catalase all appear to offer some promise (Baker et al., 1996).

Functional assays

Sperm–cervical mucus interaction

Penetration of cervical mucus represents such an important barrier to conception that it has been used as a target for novel methods of fertility control. For example, a recent morning-before pill has been developed that relies entirely on the use of a single dose of gestogen to transform the cervical mucus into an impenetrable barrier for spermatozoa (Kovacs et al., 2000). Given the importance of the cervical barrier to conception, it is clearly important to identify male infertility associated with failures of gamete transport to the site of fertilization. In order to address this issue the WHO has attempted to standardize protocols for the assessment of sperm–cervial mucus interaction both in vivo and in vitro (World Health Organization, 1999).

The in vivo assessment of sperm–cervical mucus interaction is achieved with the postcoital test. This procedure involves assessment of the number and motility of spermatozoa in mid-cycle cervical mucus recovered 9 to 24 hours after coitus. The presence of rapid, progressively motile spermatozoa in the endocervix at this time is taken as evidence that cervical factors are not a key contributory factor in a couple's infertility (World Health Organization, 1999). The test is difficult to standardize and interpret but in experienced laboratories has been shown to have some prognostic value. For example, in a recent retrospective study, couples with infertility of less than three years and a positive postcoital test exhibited a 68% conception rate within two years compared with 17% for those with a negative result. However, once the period of infertility extended beyond three years, the conception rate was low, even with a positive test (Glazener et al., 2000). Such results emphasize the multifactorial nature of human infertility and the limitations of the postcoital test. Nevertheless, this test is simple and inexpensive to perform and may indicate patients for whom intrauterine insemination is a rational therapeutic approach (Farhi et al., 1995).

A more controlled approach towards the study of sperm–cervical mucus interaction is possible if appropriate in vitro assays are used (World Health Organization, 1999). There are many different versions of the cervical mucus penetration test involving a range of different scoring strategies (Katz et al., 1980; Mortimer et al., 1986; Aitken et al., 1992a). However, regardless of the detailed assessment criteria used, there is general agreement that cervical mucus penetration is heavily dependent on the movement characteristics of the spermatozoa. (Aitken et al., 1986, 1992a; Mortimer et al., 1986, 1990). The attributes of sperm movement that appear to be particularly important for cervical mucus penetration include the average path velocity and measures of the straightness of individual sperm trajectories (linearity and mean linear index). Another extremely important variable is the lateral displacement of the sperm head. Indeed, this is such an important attribute of sperm movement that infertile men have been identified in which the only defect in the semen profile is a reduced amplitude of lateral sperm head displacement. In such patients, cervical mucus penetration cannot occur (Feneux et al., 1985; Aitken et al., 1986; Mortimer et al., 1986), presumably because the amplitude of lateral sperm head displacement reflects the amplitude of the flagellar wave (David et al., 1981) and it is the latter that determines the propulsive force that can be generated by the spermatozoa as they arrive at the cervical mucus interface.

Clinically, the most difficult aspect of performing cervical mucus penetration assays is the amount of time and effort that has to go into timing the aspiration of cervical mucus from the female partner, which must be performed at mid-cycle if the results are to be meaningful. It would clearly be beneficial if an artificial substitute for cervical mucus could be identified, the penetration of which depended on the same characteristics of sperm movement as the native material. Recent independent studies suggest that hyaluronic acid polymers can serve just such a purpose. The penetration of human spermatozoa into hyaluronic acid polymers has been shown to correlate with their ability to penetrate into both human and bovine cervical mucus and to depend upon the same attributes of semen quality, including sperm number, morphology, and movement (Mortimer et al., 1990; Aitken et al., 1992a). Of the parameters of sperm movement examined, penetration of both cervical mucus and hyaluronate were found to depend upon a similar progressive linear mode of motility associated with a significant amplitude of lateral sperm head displacement.

As a consequence of this dependence on similar criteria of semen quality, the outcome of sperm penetration assays employing either hyaluronic acid polymers or cervical mucus are highly correlated, giving correlation coefficients of 0.7–0.8 depending on the criterion of penetration used (Mortimer et al., 1990; Aitken et al., 1992a). It has been proposed that the ability of long-chain polymers to create channels accounts for their similarity with cervical mucus in terms of sperm penetration (Tang et al., 1999).

Sperm penetration into hyaluronate polymers is so closely dependent on the movement characteristics of human spermatozoa that the outcome of such tests can be used to obtain an extremely accurate assessment of the quality of sperm movement (Aitken et al., 1992a). These observations beg the question as to whether the diagnostic potential of cervical mucus/hyaluronate penetration assays is simply a consequence of their close correlation with sperm movement or whether they are providing additional information of relevance to the fertilizing potential of the spermatozoa. If it is the relationship with sperm movement that is the key to the clinical significance of mucus penetration assays, then it would be simpler and more objective to assess the movement characteristics of human spermatozoa directly, rather than become engaged in the logistical and technical problems of carrying out a cervical mucus penetration assay. The one area where cervical mucus penetration tests might be said to be providing important additional data would be in cases of autoimmunity characterized by the presence of antisperm IgA antibodies. One part of the IgA molecule, the Fc portion, is capable of binding with great tenacity to cervical mucin chains. As a consequence, the spermatozoa become tethered to the cervical mucus in such a way that their struggles to break free give rise to a characteristic shaking phenomenon, which is thought to be indicative of the presence of antisperm IgA on the surface of the spermatozoa or on the cervical mucus itself. If this is the case, then one would expect hyaluronic acid polymers to lack the ability to detect the disruption of sperm–cervical mucus interaction caused by antibodies. However, a recent report suggests that the ability of antisperm antibodies to disrupt sperm–cervical mucus interaction can be detected equally well with hyaluronic acid polymers as with cervical mucus (Tang et al., 1999). Although much might depend on the class and idiotype of the antibody involved, these results suggest that sperm penetration assays involving hyaluronic acid polymers provide a good overall assessment of the functional competence of human spermatozoa. Clearly more studies are required employing such assays in conjunction with tests of the fertilizing potential of human spermatozoa in vivo.

Analysis of sperm movement

The importance of motility in defining the competence of human spermatozoa to penetrate cervical mucus emphasizes the biological significance of this attribute of sperm function. Detailed studies of sperm motion indicate that these cells move in ways that are exquisitely adapted to their functional needs. Consequently, it is important to discern not just the percentage of cells that are motile but the quality of that motility. Computer-aided semen analysis systems have, therefore, been developed that enable the rapid, accurate assessment of the movement characteristics of human spermatozoa (Mortimer et al., 1995; Skakkebaek and Giwercman, 2000).

Freshly ejaculated spermatozoa must use their intrinsic capacity for movement to escape from seminal plasma and penetrate the cervical barrier. In this uncapacitated state, normal human spermatozoa exhibit linear, progressive trajectories characterized by high-frequency, symmetrical flagellar waves of moderate amplitude. As indicated above, this progressive, space-gaining form of movement has been found to be ideally suited to achieving penetration of cervical mucus.

As spermatozoa escape from seminal plasma and capacitate, their movement characteristics change in preparation for the act of fertilization. These capacitation-dependent changes involve increases in curvilinear velocity (VCL) and ALH in association with increases in the amplitude and propagation velocity of the flagellar wave. Capacitation culminates in the expression of a vigorous form of movement known as hyperactivation. This pattern of movement was originally observed in hamster spermatozoa (Yanagimachi, 1994) and first recorded as a feature of human sperm behavior by Burkman (1984). The onset of hyperactivated motility is thought to signal the attainment of a state of capacitation, and its expression has been linked with the ability of spermatozoa to penetrate the zona pellucida. In light of this association, it would seem rational to expect a close correlation between the fertilizing potential of human spermatozoa in vitro and the expression of hyperactivated motion.

Two basic forms of hyperactivated movement have been detected, as described by Mortimer and Mortimer (1990). One form is characterized by high VCL and high ALH and yet retains sufficient beat symmetry to be progressive; this pattern of movement has been termed "transitional" by Robertson et al. (1988). In the second form of hyperactivation, changes in the symmetry and speed of propagation of the flagellar wave give rise to a nonprogressive pattern of hyperactivated movement, frequently characterized by a "star-spin" or whip-lash trajectory. Resolving whether either or both of these patterns should be regarded as "hyperactivated," and the objective criteria by which these patterns might be recognized, is one of the key areas in sperm kinematics requiring consensus.

To-date, the diagnostic significance of hyperactivated movement has only been addressed in the context of predicting the fertilizing potential of human spermatozoa in vitro. Therefore, regression equations have been generated based on the movement characteristics of human spermatozoa that can account for at least half of the variance in IVF rates. The first incorporated and most significant variable in these analyses was a computer-aided semen analysis classification of the incidence of the *nonprogressive* form of hyperactivated movement (Sukcharoen et al., 1995). The threshold criteria used to identify these cells were very similar to those used by Robertson et al. (1988) in that they relied upon measurements of VCL, LIN, and DANCEMEAN. Significantly, none of the alternative algorithms for hyperactivated movement were as effective as those developed by Sukcharoen et al. (1995) for predicting the fertilizing capacity of human spermatozoa in vitro. Clearly this form of movement is predictive of the fertilizing capacity of human spermatozoa in vitro. Additional studies now need to be conducted that will determine which attributes of sperm movement correlate with fertility in vivo.

Sperm–zona interaction

The major problem with developing a diagnostic test for sperm–zona interaction is that this process is extremely species specific. Therefore, if the competence of human spermatozoa to bind to the zona pellucida is to be assessed, human zonae pellucidae must be used. The logistical problems involved in supplying human zonae pellucidae for such a diagnostic purpose have, to some extent, been solved by the discovery that these structures will retain their biological activity when stored in high salt solutions containing magnesium chloride and dextran (Yanagimachi et al., 1979). In order to compensate for differences between individual zonae in their capacity to bind spermatozoa, a hemizona assay has been developed. In this procedure, each zona pellucida is cut into two halves, which are then incubated with patient and donor spermatozoa, respectively. By calculating the ratio of the numbers of spermatozoa bound from the two sources, an indication of the relative binding capacity of the patient's spermatozoa can be obtained (Franken et al., 1989). A large series of clinical studies have been conducted using this assay (Oehninger, 1992) and the general conclusion appears to be that a significant relationship does exist between the outcome of the hemizona assay and the incidence of IVF success.

However, the use of such a complex bioassay to monitor the presence of binding sites on the sperm surface for the zona sperm receptor ZP3 may become a redundant strategy now that biologically active recombinant human ZP3 has been generated (van Duin et al., 1994). With the aid of such material, it should be a relatively straightforward task to devise simple, standardized biochemical assays to monitor the capacity of a human spermatozoon to recognize key components of the zona pellucida.

Even if such assays for sperm–zona interaction are developed, they would not be able to indicate whether a given sperm sample had the capacity to generate the propulsive forces necessary to penetrate the zona pellucida. For this purpose, a bioassay for zona penetration has been developed that appears to show an excellent correlation with fertilization rates in vitro (Liu and Baker, 1994).

Salt-stored human zonae pellucidae can also be used to examine the ability of human spermatozoa to undergo the acrosome reaction on the zona surface. The application of this technique has led to the identification of a group of patients whose spermatozoa have the capacity to bind to the zona pellucida but are unable to exhibit the acrosome reaction (Liu and Baker, 1996). Although such patients can be treated with ICSI (Liu et al., 1997), the finding that failed fertilization can involve a specific defect in the capacity of spermatozoa to undergo the acrosome reaction at the zona surface should be helpful in orientating studies to uncover the underlying etiology.

Sperm–oocyte fusion

One of the most maligned tests of sperm function is the zona-free hamster oocyte penetration test. This test assesses the ability of acrosome reacted spermatozoa to fuse with the vitelline membrane of the oocyte. Although the gametes employed in this test are from two different species, the ultrastructural and, presumably, the molecular details of the fusion process reflect the homologous situation. Thus the plasma membrane overlying the equatorial segment of acrosome-reacted human spermatozoa initiates fusion with the hamster oocyte in exactly the same manner as homologous gametes (Aitken, 1986). Problems with the assay have arisen because it is technically difficult to perform, labor intensive, expensive, and impossible to standardize. The lack of standardization applies particularly to the conditions employed to capacitate the spermatozoa and induce the acrosome reaction. Capacitation conditions have variously employed overnight incubation at 4°C in albumin- or egg yolk-supplemented buffers (Johnson et al., 1984; Aitken, 1986), incubation in albumin-supplemented medium at 37°C for periods ranging from 2 to 24 hours (Yanagimachi et al., 1976; Aitken, 1986), or the use of reagents to enhance capacitation artificially, including NADPH or phosphodiesterase inhibitors such as pentoxifylline (oxpentifylline) (Aitken et al., 1998b).

The methods used to induce the acrosome reaction in this test have been equally variable, including progesterone, sudden temperature changes from 4 to 37°C, electric shock, divalent cation ionophores, and lysophosphatidylcholine (Aitken et al., 1984; Tarin and Trounson, 1993). The WHO (World Health Organization, 1999) has attempted to standardize protocols in this area by describing two different preincubation procedures that can be employed with the zona-free hamster oocyte penetration assay. One involves the prolonged incubation of human spermatozoa for 18 to 24 hours at 37°C in a balanced salt solution supplemented with albumin. The second involves exposure of human spermatozoa to the divalent cation ionophore A23187 (Aitken et al., 1984). This reagent creates channels in the sperm plasma membrane that promote the acrosome reaction by permitting calcium influx from the extracellular space (Aitken et al., 1984). Measurements of sperm–oocyte fusion in the presence of A23187 was significantly correlated with pregnancy rates in couples exhibiting idiopathic infertility for whom the conventional semen profile was of no diagnostic significance (Aitken et al., 1991). Similarly, IVF rates were predicted by the A23187-stimulated assay with an accuracy that could not be achieved with other versions of the hamster oocyte penetration test (Aitken et al., 1987).

The use of A23187 as a stimulant focuses the assay on one particular aspect of sperm function: the ability of acrosome-reacted spermatozoa to fuse with the vitelline membrane of the oocyte. It does not generate any useful data on the ability of spermatozoa to capacitate since the use of the ionophore largely circumvents the capacitation process. Nor does the outcome of this assay correlate well with tests of the acrosome reaction. The reason for this is that the outcome of the hamster–oocyte penetration assay is highly dependent on motility whereas assays of the acrosome reaction are largely independent of the quality of sperm movement (Aitken et al., 1994a). The diagnostic value of the A23187-stimulated version of the hamster oocyte penetration assay, therefore, lies in its association with the movement characteristics of the spermatozoa and the fitness of the sperm plasma membrane for fusion with the oocyte.

The zona-free hamster oocyte penetration assay probably has very little future as a diagnostic test in its own right; nevertheless, it does clearly generate data of diagnostic value. Its greatest use will probably be as a bioassay in fundamental research designed to determine the cellular mechanisms responsible for defective sperm function. Studies conceived along these lines have been instrumental in directing our attention to the importance of oxidative stress as a mediator of pathological damage in populations of human spermatozoa, as discussed below (Jones et al., 1979; Aitken and Clarkson, 1987).

Biochemical assays of male fertility

Diagnostic seminology would be greatly facilitated if it were possible to use biochemical assays to assess the functional competence of human spermatozoa. Biochemical assays are much easier to standardize and perform than bioassays and have the potential to yield information of relevance to the etiology of the infertility. During the 1990s, there were significant advances in this area on two related fronts: oxidative stress and DNA damage, including Y chromosome deletions.

Oxidative stress

Human spermatozoa are particularly vulnerable to oxidative stress. They possess a plasma membrane that is highly enriched in unsaturated fatty acids, which are susceptible to free radical attack (Jones et al., 1979; Aitken et al., 1993a). In addition, these cells are professional generators of reactive oxygen species (Aitken and Clarkson, 1987; Alvarez et al., 1987) and are deficient in antioxidant enzymes by virtue of the limited volume and distribution of the cytoplasmic space. Oxidative stress in the human ejaculate originates from two major sources: seminal leukocytes and defective spermatozoa (Aitken and West, 1990). The problem of leukocytospermia in the human ejaculate has been addressed above. In essence, the leukocytes that infiltrate human semen are spontaneously active in the generation of reactive oxygen species and are potentially capable of creating oxidative stress. In fact, sperm quality is rarely adversely affected by leukocyte infiltration in vivo (Tomlinson et al., 1993); indeed, recent studies have even suggested a positive association between leukocyte contamination and semen quality (Kaleli et al., 2000). Such positive to neutral associations are observed when leukocyte concentrations are $<3 \times 10^6$ cells/ml. Above this level, adverse effects of leukocytospermia on male fertility have been observed (Wolff et al., 1990); however, these may result from the disruption of secondary sexual gland function rather than as a direct effect of oxidative stress on the gamete (Gonzales et al., 1992). The resistance of human spermatozoa to free radical attack from infiltrating leukocytes stems from the powerful antioxidant power of seminal plasma (Jones et al., 1979). As long as the spermatozoa are in contact with seminal plasma they will be protected from the consequences of leukocytospermia. However, as soon as the seminal plasma is removed, as happens with certain sperm preparation protocols when washed spermatozoa are pelleted prior to a swim-up procedure, then oxidative stress will arise and sperm function will suffer as a consequence (Aitken and Clarkson, 1988).

The second source of reactive oxygen species is the spermatozoa themselves. These cells generate low levels of superoxide anion and hydrogen peroxide in order to drive the signal transduction events associated with sperm capacitation (De Lamirande and Gagnon, 1993; Aitken et al., 1995, 1998a). However, under certain circumstances, spermatozoa are capable of overproducing reactive oxygen species, thereby generating a state of oxidative stress. There are many possible mechanisms by which free radical generation by spermatozoa could be raised, including the redox cycling of xenobiotics, defective free radical scavenging systems, enhanced oxidase activity, or cellular immaturity. At present, the major cause of oxidative stress in spermatozoa appears to involve a lack of maturity associated with a failure of these cells to shed their cytoplasm during the terminal stages of spermiogenesis. As a consequence of this defect, the spermatozoa generate higher than normal levels of reactive oxygen species and exhibit signs of oxidative stress (Aitken et al., 1994b; Huszar and Vigue, 1994; Gomez et al., 1996). The mechanism underlying this association is still not understood although one possibility that has been advanced involves the excessive cellular generation of NADPH, as outlined in Fig. 16.1 (Aitken et al., 1993b, 1994b, 1997).

Oxidative stress in the human ejaculate can be measured in a number of ways. First, the cellular generation of reactive oxygen metabolites can be assessed. A major problem in this area is the confounding effect of leukocyte contamination on the levels of reactive oxygen species detected. On a cell-for-cell basis, leukocytes are 100 times more active than spermatozoa in generating these molecules. In order to address the spermatozoa's capacity to generate free radicals, the leukocytes must be selectively removed from the sperm suspension. Although Percoll gradient centrifugation can be helpful in this regard, it is rarely sufficient on its own to remove all traces of contaminating leukocytes (Aitken and West, 1990). The most effective method is to incubate the spermatozoa with paramagnetic beads or ferrofluids coated with a monoclonal antibody against CD45, the common leukocyte antigen

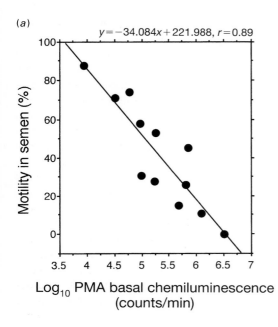

(a) $y = -34.084x + 221.988, r = 0.89$

Motility in semen (%) vs Log$_{10}$ PMA basal chemiluminescence (counts/min)

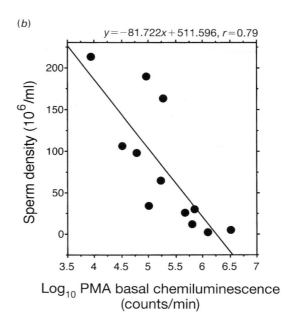

(b) $y = -81.722x + 511.596, r = 0.79$

Sperm density (10^6/ml) vs Log$_{10}$ PMA basal chemiluminescence (counts/min)

Fig. 16.2. Relationship between phorbol myristate acetate (PMA)-induced chemiluminescence in leukocyte-free Percoll-purified sperm suspensions and semen quality. (*a*) Percentage motility; (*b*) sperm concentration in the original semen samples.

(Aitken et al., 1996b). Such treatments can be followed with an FMLP (*N*-formyl-methionyl-leucyl-phenylalanine) provocation test (Krausz et al., 1992) to determine whether leukocyte removal has been complete. Once the leukocytes have been removed, the spermatozoa should be treated with a phorbol ester to stimulate reactive oxygen species generation. This reagent stimulates oxygen radical generation from immature, defective spermatozoa and generates signals that are highly correlated with defective sperm function (Gomez et al., 1998; Fig. 16.2).

Free radical detection can be achieved with chemiluminescent assays involving probes such as luminol and lucigenin (Aitken et al., 1992b). Although there are problems with the use of these probes in terms of their specificity, chemiluminescence has the sensitivity necessary to measure free radical signals from populations of spermatozoa, which will reflect the functional competence of these cells. More specific techniques such as the reduction of acetylated ferricytochrome *c* do not have the sensitivity to be useful in a diagnostic setting.

Alternative biochemical measures of oxidative stress include the thiobarbituric acid test, which may not be specific for the products of lipid peroxidation but does appear to be effective as a criterion for detecting defective sperm function associated with oxidative stress (Jones et al., 1979; Aitken et al., 1993b). An alternative, more specific, spectrophotometric assay for lipid peroxide formation (Gomez et al., 1998) also appears to be very effective as a diagnostic test for male infertility.

DNA damage

Of course, the sperm plasma membrane is not the only component of this cell that is susceptible to oxidative attack. The DNA in the sperm nucleus and mitochondria is also susceptible to this kind of damage. Male infertility is commonly associated with high levels of DNA strand breaks in the sperm nucleus (Irvine et al., 2000), the severity of which is negatively correlated with indices of semen quality, particularly sperm count (Irvine et al., 2000). Moreover, this fragmentation is correlated with the generation of reactive oxygen species by the spermatozoa and with evidence of oxidative DNA base damage (Shen et al., 1999; Irvine et al., 2000). Such oxidatively induced DNA fragmentation is associated with decreased fertilization and pregnancy rates when IVF is used to treat male infertile patients (Host et al., 2000). However, careful comparison of the rates at which sperm function is impaired and DNA damage is induced with increasing levels of oxidative stress have revealed that DNA fragmentation precedes the loss of fertilizing potential (Aitken et al., 1998a). Consequently, there is the potential for oxidative stress to induce DNA damage in the male germline that can then be transmitted to the offspring at fertilization in vitro or in vivo.

Evidence that this phenomenon can occur comes from a recent series of studies focusing on the fertility of male smokers. Men who smoke heavily are known to be under oxidative stress and exhibit a systemic depletion of antioxidants such as vitamin E and C. This depletion results in DNA fragmentation in the germline in association with oxidative base damage to sperm DNA (Fraga et al., 1996). Since one of the consequences of DNA damage in the spermatozoa of heavy smokers is a fourfold increase in the risk of childhood cancer in the offspring (Ji et al., 1997), it will be important to elucidate the factors responsible for the induction of DNA damage in infertile men, most of whom do not smoke. Moreover, because the risk of DNA damage in the germline is inversely correlated with semen quality, we can anticipate that many of the gametes being employed in ICSI are profoundly damaged. Such damage does not appear to alter fertilization rates (Twigg et al., 1998; Host et al., 2000) but, in light of the evidence cited above, might well have long-term consequences for the health and well-being of the offspring.

Assessment of DNA damage in the germline has been achieved with a variety of techniques. The most sensitive appears to be a single-cell electrophoresis (the COMET assay; Fig. 16.3, color plate). However this assay is difficult to control and interpretation of the results requires dedicated software programs (Irvine et al., 2000). Nick translation or TUNEL (terminal transferase-mediated dUTP nick end labeling) assays are easier to perform and produce results that are highly correlated with the COMET assay (Donnelly et al., 2000). One of the advantages of these techniques is that the outcome can be measured by flow cytometry, permitting the sampling of many thousands of cells. Flow cytometry has also been used as the endpoint for an assay of DNA stability in the germline known as the sperm chromatin structure assay. This procedure is a measure of the susceptibility of sperm DNA to low pH-induced denaturation in situ and generates results that correlate well with the outcome of the COMET assay (Aravindan et al., 1997) and are predictive of IVF outcome (Larson et al., 2000).

The consequences of DNA fragmentation in the male germline, therefore, include impaired fertilizing potential in the patient and childhood cancer in the offspring. Another consequence of oxidatively induced DNA fragmentation may be the induction of infertility in the offspring. When breaks in double-stranded DNA are induced the deleted genetic information is recovered by a repair strategy known as homologous recombination. This strategy depends upon the use of the corresponding DNA sequences from the homologous chromosome to recover the lost information. This strategy is effective for every element of the genome except for genes located on the long arm of the Y chromosome, for which there is no homolog. As a consequence, double-stranded DNA deletions on the long arm of the Y chromosome will persist into the next generation. Since many of the genes responsible for the regulation of spermatogenesis are located in this region, such damage will be quickly deleted from the gene pool as a consequence of spermatogenic failure and infertility. Approximately 14% of patients exhibiting nonobstructive oligozoospermia possess deletions on the long arm of the Y chromosome that appear to be causally related to their condition (Pryor et al., 1997;

Roberts, 1998; Plessis et al., 1999). The development of multiplex polymerase chain reaction kits to identify such patients will not only be valuable in the diagnosis of fertility but will also give an indication of the frequency with which DNA fragmentation occurred in the previous generation.

Conclusions

The development of diagnostic tests for male infertility will only be possible once the multifarious etiologies of this complex condition have been resolved. At present, andrology laboratories focus upon a descriptive assessment of the semen in order to predict the fertilizing capacity of the spermatozoa. The criteria assessed have not changed a great deal since the 1960s and still relay heavily on sperm count, motility, and morphology. Through the auspices of the WHO the techniques for conducting a routine semen analysis have been refined and standardized. However, such methods do not yield a diagnosis and have been repeatedly shown to be an insensitive means of assessing fertility. Functional assays certainly augment the conventional semen profile and facilitate the prediction of fertility (Aitken et al., 1991). However, such tests are expensive to perform and provide data of questionable value in terms of managing the patient. Most patients are referred directly for IVF if a male problem is suspected; if fertilization fails, then ICSI is employed in subsequent cycles. Where functional assays have proven useful is in orientating research designed to achieve a better understanding of the causes of male infertility. It was through the analysis of patients exhibiting failed sperm–oocyte fusion, for example, that oxidative stress was identified as a major cause of defective sperm function (Aitken and Clarkson, 1987). Oxidative stress is not only an important cause of male infertility but also has relevance to the health of the offspring in terms of the etiology of childhood cancer and, possibly, Y chromosome deletions responsible for infertility. Clearly oxidative stress is not the only cause of male infertility. The future of this field lies in focusing on the functional phenotypes that have been discovered, such as failed cervical mucus penetration, failed zona-induced acrosome reaction, or failed penetration of the zona matrix, in order to understand the underlying pathophysiology. Such studies will shed light on the etiology of the defects and open the way for the development of logical, effective strategies for the management and prevention of male infertility.

REFERENCES

Aitken, R.J. (ed.) (1986). The zona-free hamster oocyte penetration test and the diagnosis of male fertility. *International Journal of Andrology*, (Suppl.6), 1–199.

Aitken, R.J. and Clarkson, J.S. (1987). Cellular basis of defective sperm function and its association with the genesis of reactive oxygen species by human spermatozoa. *Journal of Reproduction and Fertility*, **83**, 459–69.

Aitken, R.J. and Clarkson, J.S. (1988). Significance of reactive oxygen species and anti-oxidants in defining the efficacy of sperm preparation techniques. *Journal of Andrology*, **9**, 367–76.

Aitken, R.J. and Irvine, D.S. (1998). Reliability of methods for assessing the fertilizing capacity of human spermatozoa. In: *Andrology in the Nineties. Modern ART in the 2000s*, Ombelet, W., Bosmans, E., Vandeput, H., Vereecken, A., Renier, M., and Hoomans, E., eds. Parthenon Press, London, pp. 179–90.

Aitken, R.J. and West, K. (1990). Relationship between reactive oxygen species generation and leucocyte infiltration in fractions isolated from the human ejaculate on Percoll gradients. *International Journal of Andrology*, **13**, 433–51.

Aitken, R.J., Ross, A., Hargreave, T., Richardson, D., and Best, F. (1984). Analysis of human sperm function following exposure to the ionophore A23187: comparison of normospermic and oligozoospermic men. *Journal of Andrology*, **5**, 321–9.

Aitken, R.J., Warner, P., and Reid, C. (1986). Factors influencing the success of sperm–cervical mucus interaction in patients exhibiting unexplained infertility. *Journal of Andrology*, **7**, 3–10.

Aitken, R.J., Thatcher, S., Glasier, A.F., Clarkson, J.S., Wu, F.C.W., and Baird, D.T. (1987). Relative ability of modified versions of the hamster oocyte penetration test, incorporating hyperosmotic medium or the ionophore A23187, to predict IVF outcome. *Human Reproduction*, **2**, 227–31.

Aitken, R.J., Irvine, D.S., and Wu, F.C. (1991). Prospective analysis of sperm–oocyte fusion and reactive oxygen species generation as criteria for the diagnosis of infertility. *American Journal of Obstetrics and Gynecology*, **164**, 542–51.

Aitken, R.J., Bowie, H., Buckingham, D., Harkiss, D., Richardson, D.W., and West, K.M. (1992a). Sperm penetration into a hyaluronic acid polymer as a means of monitoring functional competence. *Journal of Andrology*, **13**, 44–54.

Aitken, R.J., Buckingham, D.W., and West, K.M. (1992b). Reactive oxygen species and human spermatozoa; analysis of the cellular mechanisms involved in luminol- and lucigenin-dependent chemiluminescence. *Journal of Cellular Physiology*, **151**, 466–77.

Aitken, R.J., Buckingham, D., and Harkiss, D. (1993a). Use of a xanthine oxidase oxidant, generating system to investigate the cytotoxic effects of reactive oxygen species on human spermatozoa. *Journal of Reproduction and Fertility*, **97**, 441–50.

Aitken, R.J., Harkiss, D., and Buckingham, D.W. (1993b). Analysis of lipid peroxidation mechanisms in human spermatozoa. *Molecular Reproduction and Development*, **35**, 302–15.

Aitken, R.J., Buckingham, D., and Harkiss, D. (1994a). Analysis of the extent to which sperm movement can predict the results of ionophore-enhanced functional assays of the acrosome reaction and sperm–oocyte fusion. *Human Reproduction*, **9**, 1867–74.

Aitken, R.J., Krausz, C., and Buckingham, D. W. (1994b). Relationships between biochemical markers for residual sperm cytoplasm, reactive oxygen species generation and the presence of leucocytes and precursor germ cells in human sperm suspensions. *Molecular Reproduction and Development*, **39**, 268–79.

Aitken, R.J., West, K., and Buckingham, D. (1994c). Leukocyte infiltration into the human ejaculate and its association with semen quality, oxidative stress and sperm function. *Journal of Andrology*, **15**, 343–52.

Aitken, R.J., Paterson, M., Fisher, H., Buckingham, D.W., and van Duin, M. (1995). Redox regulation of tyrosine phosphorylation in human spermatozoa and its role in the control of human sperm function. *Journal of Cell Science*, **108**, 2017–25.

Aitken, R.J. Buckingham, D.W., Carreras, A., and Irvine, D. S. (1996a). Superoxide dismutase in human sperm suspensions: relationships with cellular composition, oxidative stress and sperm function. *Free Radical Biology and Medicine*, **21**, 495–504.

Aitken, R.J., Buckingham, W., West, K., and Brindle, J. (1996b). On the use of paramagnetic beads and ferrofluids to assess and eliminate the leukocytic contribution to oxygen radical generation by human sperm suspensions. *American Journal of Reproductive Immunology*, **35**, 541–51.

Aitken, R.J., Fisher, H., Fulton, N., Knox, W., and Lewis, B. (1997). Reactive oxygen species generation by human spermatozoa is induced by exogenous NADPH and inhibited by the flavoprotein inhibitors diphenylene iodonium and quinacrine. *Molecular Reproduction and Development*, **47**, 468–82.

Aitken, R.J., Gordon, E., Harkiss, D., et al. (1998a). Relative impact of oxidative stress on the functional competence and genomic integrity of human spermatozoa. *Biology of Reproduction*, **59**, 1037–46.

Aitken, R.J., Harkiss, D., Knox, W., Paterson, M., and Irvine, D.S. (1998b). A novel signal transduction cascade in capacitating human spermatozoa characterised by a redox regulated, cAMP-mediated induction of tyrosine phosphorylation. *Journal of Cell Science*, **111**, 645–56.

Alvarez, J.G., Touchstone, J.C., Blasco, L., and Storey, B.T. (1987). Spontaneous lipid peroxidation and production of hydrogen peroxide and superoxide in human spermatozoa. *Journal of Andrology*, **8**, 338–48.

Aravindan, G.R., Bjordahl, J., Jost, L.K., and Evenson, D.P. (1997). Susceptibility of human sperm to in situ DNA denaturation is strongly correlated with DNA strand breaks identified by single-cell electrophoresis. *Experimental Cell Research*, **236**, 231–7.

Auger, J. and Jouannet, P. (1997). Evidence for regional differences of semen quality among fertile French men. *Human Reproduction*, **12**, 740–5.

Baker, H.W.G., Brindle, J., Irvine, D.S., and Aitken, R.J. (1996). Protective effect of antioxidants on the impairment of sperm motility by activated polymorphonuclear leukocytes. *Fertility and Sterility*, **65**, 411–19.

Burkman, L.J. (1984). Characterization of hyperactivated motility by human sperm during capacitation: comparison of fertile and oligozoospermic sperm populations. *Archives of Andrology*, **13**, 153–65.

Casano, R., Orlando, C., Serio, M., and Forti, G. (1991). LDH and LDH-X activity in sperm from normospermic and oligozoospermic men. *International Journal of Andrology*, **14**, 257–63.

David, G., Serres, C., and Jouannet, P. (1981). Kinematics of human spermatozoa. *Gamete Research*, **4**, 83–6.

De Lamirande, E. and Gagnon, C. (1993). A positive role for superoxide anion in triggering hyperactivation and capacitation of human spermatozoa. *International Journal of Andrology*, **16**, 21–5.

Donnelly, E.T., O'Connell, M., McClure, N., and Lewis, S.E. (2000). Differences in nuclear DNA fragmentation and mitochondrial integrity of semen and prepared human spermatozoa. *Human Reproduction*, **15**, 1552–61.

Farhi, J., Valentine, A., Bahadur, G., Shenfield, F., Steele, S.J., and Jacobs, H.S. (1995). In-vitro cervical mucus–sperm penetration tests and outcome of infertility treatments in couples with repeatedly negative post-coital tests. *Human Reproduction*, **10**, 85–90.

Feneux, D., Serres, C., and Jouannet, P. (1985). Sliding spermatozoa: a dyskinesia responsible for human infertility? *Fertility and Sterility*, **44**, 508–11.

Fraga, C.G., Motchnik, P.A., Wyrobek, A.J., Rempel, D.M., and Ames, B.N. (1996). Smoking and low antioxidant levels increase oxidative damage to DNA. *Mutation Research*, **351**, 199–203.

Franken, D.R., Oehninger, S., Burkman, L.J., et al. (1989). The hemizona assay (HZA): a predictor of human sperm fertilizing potential in in vitro fertilization (IVF) treatment. *Journal of In Vitro Fertilization and Embryo Transfer*, **6**, 44–50.

Glazener, C.M., Ford, W.C., and Hull, M.G. (2000). The prognostic power of the post-coital test for natural conception depends on duration of infertility. *Human Reproduction*, **15**, 1953–7.

Gomez, E., Buckingham, D.W., Brindle, J., Lanzafame, F., Irvine, D.S., and Aitken, R.J. (1996). Development of an image analysis system to monitor the retention of residual cytoplasm by human spermatozoa: correlation with biochemical markers of the cytoplasmic space, oxidative stress and sperm function. *Journal of Andrology*, **17**, 276–87.

Gomez, E., Irvine D.S., and Aitken, R.J. (1998). Evaluation of a spectrophotometric assay for the measurement of malondialdehyde and 4-hydroxyalkenals in human spermatozoa: relationships with semen quality and sperm function. *International Journal of Andrology*, **21**, 81–94.

Gonzales, G.F., Kortebani, G., and Mazzolli, A.B. (1992). Leukocytospermia and function of the seminal vesicles on semen quality. *Fertility and Sterility*, **57**, 1058–65.

Hellstrom, W.J.G. (1997). *Male Infertility and Sexual Dysfunction*. Springer-Verlag, New York.

Host, E., Lindenberg, S., and Smidt-Jensen, S. (2000). The role of DNA strand breaks in human spermatozoa used for IVF and ICSI. *Acta Obstetrica Gynaecologica Scandinavica*, **79**, 559–63.

Hull, M.G.R., Glazener, C.M.A., Kelly, N.J., et al. (1985). Population study of causes, treatment and outcome of infertility. *British Medical Journal*, **291**, 1693–7.

Huszar, G. and Vigue, L. (1994). Correlation between the rate of lipid peroxidation and cellular maturity as measured by creatine kinase activity in human spermatozoa. *Journal of Andrology*, **15**, 71–7.

Huszar, G., Vigue, L., and Corrales, M. (1988). Sperm creatine phosphokinase quality in normospermic, variablespermic and oligospermic men. *Biology of Reproduction*, **38**, 1061–6.

Irvine, D.S., Twigg, J.P., Gordon, E.L., Fulton, N., Milne, P.A., and Aitken, R.J. (2000). DNA integrity in human spermatozoa: relationships with semen quality. *Journal of Andrology*, **21**, 33–44.

Ji, B.T., Shu, X.O., Linet, M.S., et al. (1997). Paternal cigarette smoking and the risk of childhood cancer among offspring of nonsmoking mothers. *Journal of the National Cancer Institute*, **89**, 238–44.

Johnson, A.R., Syms, A.J., Lipshultz, L.I., and Smith, R.G. (1984). Conditions influencing human sperm capacitation and penetration of zona-free hamster ova. *Fertility and Sterility*, **41**, 603–8.

Jones, R., Mann, T., and Sherins, R. (1979). Peroxidative breakdown of phospholipids in human spermatozoa, spermicidal properties of fatty acid peroxides, and protective action of seminal plasma. *Fertility and Sterility*, **31**, 531–7.

Jouannet, P., Ducot, B., Feneux, D., and Spira, A. (1988). Male factors and the likelihood of pregnancy in infertile couples. I. Study of sperm characteristics. *International Journal of Andrology*, **11**, 379–94.

Kaleli, S., Ocer, F., Irez, T., Budak, E., and Aksu,, M.F. (2000). Does leukocytospermia associate with poor semen parameters and sperm functions in male infertility? The role of different seminal leukocyte concentrations. *European Journal of Obsterics, Gynaecology and Reproductive Biology*, **89**, 185–91.

Katz, D.F., Overstreet, J.W., and Hanson, F.W. (1980). A new quantitative test for sperm penetration into cervical mucus. *Fertility and Sterility*, **33**, 179–86.

Kovacs, G.T., Hendricks, J., Summerbell, D., and Baker, H.W. (2000). A pre-coital pill? A preliminary in vitro study. *British Journal of Family Planning*, **26**, 165–6.

Keating, J., Grundy, C.E., Fivey, P.S., Elliott, M., and Robinson, J. (1997). Investigation of the association between the presence of cytoplasmic residues on the human sperm midpiece and defective sperm function. *Journal of Reproduction and Fertility*, **110**, 71–7.

Krausz, C., West, K., Buckingham, D., and Aitken, R.J. (1992). Analysis of the interaction between *N*-formylmethionyl-leucyl phenylalanine and human sperm suspensions: development of a technique for monitoring the contamination of human samples with leukocytes. *Fertility and Sterility*, **57**, 1317–25.

Kruger, T.F., Acosta, A.A., Simmons, K.F., Swanson, R.J., Matta, J.F,. and Oehninger, S. (1988). Predictive value of abnormal sperm morphology in in vitro fertilization. *Fertility and Sterility*, **49**, 112–17.

Larson, L., Scheike, T., Jensen, T.K., Bonde, J.P., Ernst, E., Hjollund, N.H., and Zhou, Y. (2000). Sperm chromatin structure assay parameters as predictors of failed pregnancy following assisted reproductive techniques. *Human Reproduction*, **15**, 1717–22.

Liu, D.Y. and Baker, H.W.G. (1994). A new test for the assessment of sperm–zona pellucida penetration: relationship with results of other sperm tests and fertilization in vitro. *Human Reproduction*, **9**, 489–96.

Liu, D.Y. and Baker, H.W. (1996). A simple method for assessment of the human acrosome reaction of spermatozoa bound to the zona pellucida: lack of relationship with ionophore A23187-induced acrosome reaction. *Human Reproduction*, **11**, 551–7.

Liu, D.Y., Bourne, H., and Baker, H.W.G. (1997). High fertilization and pregnancy rates after intracytoplasmic sperm injection in patients with disordered zona pellucida-induced acrosome reaction. *Fertility and Sterility*, **67**, 955–8.

MacLoed, J. and Gold, R.Z. (1951). The male factor in fertility and infertility. II Spermatozoon counts in 1000 men of known fertility and in 1000 cases of infertile marriage. *Journal of Urology*, **66**, 436–49.

Mak, V., Jarvi, K., Buckspan, M., Freeman, M., Hechter, S., and Zini, A. (2000). Smoking is associated with the retention of cytoplasm by human spermatozoa *Urology*, **56**, 463–6.

Mortimer, S.T. and Mortimer, D. (1990). Kinematics of human sperm incubated under capacitating conditions. *Journal of Andrology*, **11**, 195–203.

Mortimer, D., Pandya, I.J., and Sawers, R.S. (1986). Relationship between human sperm motility characteristics and sperm penetration into human cervical mucus in vitro. *Journal of Reproduction and Fertility*, **78**, 93–102.

Mortimer, D., Mortimer, S.T., Shu, M.A., and Swart, R.A. (1990). Simplified approach to sperm–cervical mucus interaction testing using a hyaluronate migration test. *Human Reproduction*, **5**, 835–41.

Mortimer, D., Aitken, R. J., Mortimer, S.T., and Pacey, A.A. (1995). Clinical CASA: the quest for consensus. *Reproduction, Fertility and Development*, **7**, 951–9.

Oehninger, S. (1992). Diagnostic significance of sperm–zona pellucida interaction. *Reproductive Medicine Reviews*, **1**, 57–81.

Ombelet, W., Fourie, F.L., Vandeput, H., et al. (1994). Teratozoospermia and in-vitro fertilization: a randomized prospective study. *Human Reproduction*, **9**, 1479–84.

Ombelet, W., Wouters, E., Boels, L., et al. (1997). Sperm morphology assessment: diagnostic potential and comparative analysis of strict or World Health Organization criteria in a fertile and a subfertile population. *International Journal of Andrology*, **20**, 367–72.

Plessis, G., Bourgeron, T., Dadoune, J.P., Fellous, M., and McElreavey, K. (1999). A high frequency of Y chromosome deletions in males with nonidiopathic infertility. *Journal of Clinical Endocrinology and Metabolism*, **84**, 3606–12.

Pryor, J.L., Kent-First, M., Muallem, A., et al. (1997). Microdeletions in the Y chromosome of infertile men. *New England Journal of Medicine*, **336**, 534–9.

Roberts, K.P. (1998). Y chromosome deletions and male infertility: state of the art and clinical implications. *Journal of Andrology*, **19**, 255–9.

Robertson, L., Wolfe, D.P., and Tash, J.S. (1988). Temporal changes in motility parameters related to acrosomal status: identification and characterization of populations of hyperactivated human sperm. *Biology of Reproduction*, **39**, 797–805.

Shen, H.M., Chia, S.E., and Ong, C.N. (1999). Evaluation of oxidative DNA damage in human sperm and its association with male infertility. *Journal of Andrology*, **20**, 718–23.

Skakkebaek, N.E. and Giwercman, A. (2000). Computer-assisted semen analysis parameters as predictors for fertility of men from the general population. The Danish First Pregnancy Planner Study Team. *Human Reproduction*, **15**, 1562–7.

Sukcharoen, N., Keith, J. Irvine, D.S., and Aitken, R.J. (1995). Definition of the optimal criteria for identifying hyperactivated spermatozoa at 25 Hz using in vitro fertilization as a functional end-point. *Human Reproduction*, **10**, 2928–37.

Tang, S., Garrett, C., and Baker, H.W. (1999). Comparison of human cervical mucus and artificial sperm penetration media. *Human Reproduction*, **14**, 2812–17.

Tarin, J.J. and Trounson, A.O. (1993). Zona-free sperm penetration assay and inducers of the acrosome reaction: a model for sperm microinjection under the zona pellucida. *Molecular Reproduction and Development*, **35**, 95–104.

Tomlinson, M.J., Barratt, C.L.R., and Cooke, I.D. (1993). Prospective study of leukocytes and leukocyte subpopulations in semen suggests that they are not a cause of male infertility. *Fertility and Sterility*, **60**, 1069–75.

Twigg, J.P., Irvine, D.S., and Aitken, R.J. (1998). Oxidative damage to DNA in human spermatozoa does not preclude pronucleus formation at ICSI. *Human Reproduction*, **13**, 1864–71.

van Duin, M., Polman, J.E.M., De Breet, I.T.M., et al. (1994). Production, purification and biological activity of recombinant human zona pellucida protein, ZP3. *Biology of Reproduction*, **51**, 607–17.

Wallace, E.M., Aitken, R.J., and Wu, F.C. (1992). Residual sperm function in oligozoospermia induced by testosterone enanthate administered as a potential steroid male contraceptive. *International Journal of Andrology*, **15**, 416–24.

Wang, A.W., Politch, J., and Anderson, D. (1994). Leukocytospermia in male infertility patients in China. *Andrologia*, **26**, 167–72.

Wolff, H. and Anderson, D.J. (1988). Immunohistologic characterization and quantification of leukocyte subpopulations in human semen. *Fertility and Sterility*, **49**, 497–504.

Wolff, H., Politch, J.A., Martinez, A., Haimovici, F., Hill, J.A., and Anderson, D.J. (1990). Leukocytospermia is associated with poor semen quality. *Fertility and Sterility*, **53**, 528–36.

World Health Organization (1999). *World Health Organization Laboratory Manual for the Examination of Human Semen and Sperm–Cervical Mucus Interaction*, 4th edn. Cambridge University Press, Cambridge.

Yanagimachi, R. (1994). Mammalian Fertilization. In: *The Physiology of Reproduction*, 2nd edn, Knobil, E. and Neill, J.D., eds. Raven Press, New York, pp. 189–317.

Yanagimachi, R., Yanagimachi, H., and Rogers, B.J. (1976). The use of zona free animal ova as a test system for the assessment of the fertilizing capacity of human spermatozoa. *Biology of Reproduction*, **15**, 471–6.

Yanagimachi, R., Lopata, A., Odom, C.B., Bronson, R.A., Mahi, C.A., and Nicolson, G. (1979). Retention of biologic characteristics of zona pellucida in highly concentrated salt solution: the use of salt stored eggs for assessing the fertilizing capacity of spermatozoa. *Fertility and Sterility*, **31**, 471–6.

Zini, A., O'Bryan, M.K., Israel, L., and Schlegel, P.N. (1998). Human sperm NADH and NADPH diaphorase cytochemistry: correlation with sperm motility. *Urology*, **51**, 464–8.

Zini, A., Buckspan, M., Jamal, M., and Jarvi, K. (1999). Effect of varicocelectomy on the abnormal retention of residual cytoplasm by human spermatozoa. *Human Reproduction*, **14**, 1791–3.

Zini, A., Defreitas, G., Freeman, M., Hechter, S., and Jarvi, K. (2000). Varicocele is associated with abnormal retention of cytoplasmic droplets by human spermatozoa. *Fertility and Sterility*, **74**, 461–4.

17

Diagnosis and treatment for female subfertility

Peter Platteau and Paul Devroey

Center for Reproductive Medicine, Dutch-speaking Brussels Free University, Brussels, Belgium

Introduction

This chapter focuses on the diagnosis and treatment of the main known causes of female infertility. It is clearly important that the infertile couple be investigated together to formulate the most appropriate therapy. Consequently, the reader is also referred to Chapter 16 in which the diagnosis and treatment of the male is discussed.

There is no standard definition of normal fertility. Therefore, evaluating female infertility poses a unique challenge for the clinician. It must be considered with respect to what is normal for a given demographic group and geographical location (Farley and Belsey, 1998). Most of the time there are no clinical somatic complaints or symptoms to help the clinician in the diagnostic process. Female fertility is strongly influenced by age and this has ramifications for treatment: one year of subfertility is acceptable for younger women (below 30 years of age) but could be too long for women over 35 years as fertility diminishes rapidly (Mosher, 1985). Age-related effects include ovulatory dysfunction, impaired egg quality, disturbed endometrial receptivity, and a higher incidence of endometriosis. Advancing maternal age is also associated with a higher risk of miscarriage, fetal chromosomal abnormalities, and maternal illness, which may, in turn, be associated with infertility or increased obstetric risk (Rosene-Montella et al., 2000).

Infertility is classified into primary infertility, where the couple has never achieved a pregnancy, and secondary infertility, where they have achieved a pregnancy in the past even if this did not lead to a livebirth. It has been suggested that around 16% of couples after one year and 9% after two years experience primary infertility; a further 16% of couples after one year and 5% after two years experience secondary infertility (Gunnell and Ewing, 1994).

Infertility is a common problem. The long-term prognosis is good, and many will achieve their desire to have a child. Fertility treatment has advanced at a rapid pace over recent years, providing new effective treatment for women who previously would have been considered sterile. Despite this, prevention is a better option than cure and it is, therefore, essential to educate the public concerning the hazards of smoking to fertility, the sexual health risks that may lead to tubal disease, and the already mentioned declining fertility with advancing female age.

The welfare of any offspring who may result from treatment should be of overriding concern. However, it is very difficult to evaluate the patients' psychosocial status and her ability to care for a child and to withstand the hormonal and emotional effects associated with assisted reproductive technology (ART) during two 30 minute consultations (or less). Any hint that she or the couple are likely to have difficulties caring for a child should alert the clinician to involve or contact the patients' general practitioner, psychiatrist, or counsellor. A team evaluation should then decide the options for future fertility treatment.

The risk to the offspring caused by fertility treatment should also be minimized. The main risk is from prematurity as a result of multiple pregnancy.

Patients should be clearly informed of the possible medical complications before embarking on any treatment, such as the antiestrogen side-effects of clomiphene citrate, the adverse effects of superovulation, and ART, which include ovarian hyperstimulation syndrome, pelvic infection, intraperitoneal bleeding, and adnexal torsion (Govaerts et al., 1998).

Diagnosis of infertility

Infertility patients are a unique population for preconception counseling. All women should be advised on the benefits of stopping smoking (active and passive), reduction of weekly alcohol intake, and the importance of folic acid (0.4 mg/day) for reduction of neural tube defects. They should be screened for rubella, toxoplasmosis, hepatitis B and C, syphilis and human immunodeficiency virus (and immunized, treated, or counseled if necessary) and questioned about family history of genetic disorders and thrombophilia. Diabetic women should be informed of the importance of normalizing hemoglobin A1c levels before conception to prevent congenital anomalies. If possible, all potentially teratogenic medication should be eliminated or substituted with safer ones. If the body mass index is either too low ($<19\,\mathrm{kg/m^2}$) or too high ($>25\,\mathrm{kg/m^2}$) a further discussion regarding diet and exercise should be held; if the body mass index is very high ($>30\,\mathrm{kg/m^2}$) a dietician should be consulted.

Clinical history and examination

It is unusual for couples to seek assistance for infertility if the duration of no conception is less than a year. For these circumstances, unless there is a clear indication on the basis of history or examination, an outline of their excellent potential fertility over the next year may be all that is required. However, more urgency is necessary in women over 35 years of age. Points of particular attention in the history and examination are shown in Table 17.1. A comprehensive history should exclude the possibility of endocrinopathies, major clotting disorders, and major

Table 17.1. History and clinical features in the diagnosis of infertility

Assessment	Features
History	
Infertility	Duration
	Length and type of previous birth control
	Fertility in previous relationships
	Subsequent fertility of any former partners
	Previous investigations and treatment
Menstrual	Cyclicity
	Dysmenorrhea
	Duration and amount of flow
	Intermenstrual bleeding
	Menarche
Obstetrical	Number of previous pregnancies, including miscarriages, terminations, and ectopic pregnancies
	Time to initiate previous pregnancies
Surgical	Especially abdominal and pelvic surgery
Sexual	Coital frequency/timing/dyspareunia
Medical	General health/medication/allergies (especially penicillin, which is present in certain embryo culture media) and serious illnesses
Social	Alcohol/smoking/occupation
Family	Any possible hereditary diseases
Gynecological	Cervical smear, breast pathology, sexually transmitted diseases, and pelvic infections
Examination	
General	Fat and hair distribution; signs of virilism, acne, and galactorrhea; thyroid disease, secondary sexual characteristics
Pelvis	Assess external genitalia to exclude congenital abnormalities or infection
	Assess accessibility of the cervix for insemination or embryo transfer
	Record uterine size, position, mobility, and tenderness

autoimmune disorders. Clinical history must elicit factors indicative of a major cause of infertility, such as anovulation, hyperprolactinemia, endometriosis, and pelvic adhesive disease. A subsequent clinical examination should confirm or reject suspicion from the patient's history and exclude any congenital abnormalities.

Clinical workup

The preliminary clinical investigation centers on the need to demonstrate that the woman is ovulating. Normal ovulation is defined as rupture of the follicle with release of an oocyte (ESHRE Capri Workshop Group, 1995). Regrettably, there is no method to confirm completion of ovulation, as the only true evidence of ovulation is a subsequent pregnancy. However, women with a regular menstrual cycle, defined as not varying each month by more than two days within a cycle range of 23 to 35 days, are likely to be ovulating. The use of temperature charts, cervical mucus recordings and urine luteinising hormone (LH) testing kits are not recommended as they not only incur additional costs but place even more stress on the couple at a time when stress levels may already be high. Midluteal serum progesterone levels (approximately seven days before the onset of the next menstrual period) should preferably be >30 nmol/l. If the level is less than this, the test should be repeated and combined with an ultrasound-monitored cycle. If there is a history of irregular menstruation, in particular associated with galactorrhea, hirsutism, or obesity, additional biochemical tests are appropriate (see below).

Measurements of follicle-stimulating hormone (FSH), LH, and estradiol (within three days of day 1 of menses) serum concentrations should be determined during the early follicular phase of the menstrual cycle. This will give an indication as to whether there is any major problem with ovarian function. The reduction of ovarian "reserve" is apparently caused by reduced numbers of ovarian primordial follicles, which occurs over a woman's reproductive life. This loss accelerates around the age of 37 years and precedes the menopause by

Table 17.2. Initial investigations for infertility

Investigation	Normal value
Mean serum concentration	
Follicle-stimulating hormone (days 1–4)	<10 IU/l
Luteinizing hormone (days 1–4)	<10 IU/l
Progesterone (7 days before menses)	>30 nmol/l
Estradiol (days 1–4)	<80 pg/ml (<80 ng/l)
Transvaginal ultrasound	
Prolactin and thyroid function (if irregular period or symptoms of thyroid disease/hyperprolactinemia)	
Semen analysis	See Table 15.1 (p. 234)

10–12 years (Faddy and Gosden, 1995). Age and regularity of menses alone are unreliable ways of predicting ovarian reserve. An FSH level <10 IU/l and an estradiol level of <80 pg/ml are good markers of normal ovarian reserve. (However, owing to lack of cut-off point and monthly variations, these are only of limited value.) Other tests not so widely used are ovarian volume assessment by ultrasound, basal inhibin B levels, the clomiphene citrate and gonadotropin-releasing hormone (GnRH) agonist challenge test and ovarian biopsy (Navot et al., 1989; Syrop et al., 1995; Lass et al., 1997; Seifer et al., 1997). The recommended initial investigations are listed in Table 17.2.

A transvaginal ultrasound is the preferred method to assess the pelvis. The scan should look at the size and position of the uterus and the presence of fibroids, paying particular attention to their size and location and whether they distort the endometrial cavity. The endometrial thickness should also be measured. The ovaries should then be assessed both for their morphology and for the presence of any cysts. Cysts are evaluated as to their size, configuration, and echogenicity.

When preliminary investigations suggest that the patient is ovulating (and sperm production is satisfactory), a test of tubal patency should be undertaken. It is debatable whether assessment of tubal status is necessary in women with long-standing otherwise unexplained infertility, as in vitro fertilization (IVF) would be the optimal treatment. There are several tests that can be performed, each with advantages and disadvantages. The hysterosalpingogram gives a wealth of information: the uterine cavity can be fully demonstrated and any congenital abnormalities, distortions or intrauterine synechiae are illustrated. It also provides a measure of tubal diameter, locates tubal occlusions, and identifies pathologies such as hydrosalpinx, salpingitis isthmica nodasa, and tubal polyps. Tubal filling pressures can be measured at the same time and can point to dysfunction if the pressures are very high as a result of fibrotic changes in the tube. Hysterosalpingogram cannot, however, distinguish between genuine occlusion and tubal spasm neither can it evaluate peritubal adhesions.

A laparoscopy (which should always go together with a hysteroscopy to evaluate the uterine cavity) is performed under general anesthesia and is a more invasive investigation. It provides information about the normality of the tubal–ovarian relationships, especially tubal motility and the status of the fimbriae. It is the only accurate way of detecting and staging endometriosis and pelvic inflammatory disease; if appropriate, surgical treatment can often occur during the same procedure. The upper abdomen should also be inspected, paying particular attention to the liver surface to exclude the Fitz–Hugh–Curtis syndrome.

Hystero contrast sonography (Hycosy) is the assessment of the uterus and fallopian tubes by the instillation of saline or an echogenic contrast medium, performed under direct ultrasound observation.

Falloposcopy, which is the introduction of a fiberoptic scope of approximately 0.5 mm into the fallopian tube via a transcervical route, and salpingoscopy, where the lumen of the tube is examined from its distal end via a laparoscope, should be considered research tools. They can provide more information about the lumen and the mucosa of the tube and, therefore, assess if the fallopian tubes are not only open but also functional. Prior to any invasive procedure, endocervical swabs should be taken to determine the presence of infection and, if detected, antibiotic prophylaxis should be provided.

If there is any concern about the uterine cavity, then an ambulant hysteroscopy should be performed to exclude uterine anomalies, submucous fibroids, intrauterine synechiae, and endometrial polyps. Other indications for hysteroscopy are a history of instrumental uterine intervention (dilatation and curettage), infection (endometritis), or recurrent miscarriages and multiple implantation failures after IVF cycles (Golan et al., 1992).

Historically, cervical mucus hostile to spermatozoa was usually diagnosed after evaluating results from the postcoital test. Recent studies have shown that this test leads to more infertility investigations and treatments but has no significant effect on the pregnancy rate (Oei et al., 1998).

The preliminary assessment of egg and sperm availability, together with a determination that the gametes can meet, should provide the diagnosis for most couples. Various other more specific tests can be performed if appropriate at a second visit, and appropriate therapeutic strategies can be instituted where required.

Treatment for infertility

Before embarking on treatment, it is essential that an accurate diagnosis has been made. Once investigations are completed, one is left with the following major diagnostic criteria:
- disorders of ovulation
- tubal disease
- endometriosis
- uterine abnormalities
- semen and/or sperm abnormalities
- unexplained infertility.

The choice of therapy depends on a balance of known factors: the duration of the couple's infertility and the woman's age, the chance of pregnancy without treatment, the chance with simple but only modestly effective treatment, and the chance with more successful but more complex and costly treatment.

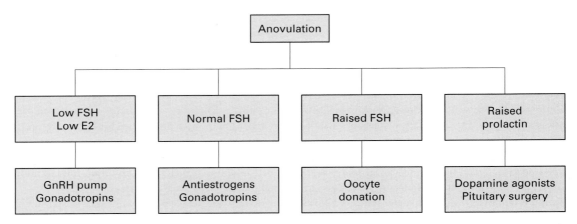

Fig. 17.1. Summary of the diagnosis and treatment of ovulatory disorders. FSH, follicle-stimulating hormone; E2, estradiol; GnRH, gonadotropin-releasing hormone.

Disorders of ovulation

Four conditions are found with relatively high frequency in women with suspected ovulatory failure. A summary of the diagnosis and treatment of ovulatory disorders is outlined in Fig. 17.1.

Normogonadotropic anovulation

The patients have normal FSH but LH may be elevated. The majority of these women have polycystic ovaries and a smaller subgroup of women have multifollicular ovaries. After weight reduction for overweight patients, the treatment of choice is an antiestrogen such as clomiphene citrate or tamoxifen. These drugs act by binding hypothalamic estrogen receptors to cause an increase in FSH and LH concentrations, which, in turn, stimulates the ovaries to ovulate. Side-effects include multiple gestation (7–10%); adverse changes in cervical mucus (mucus hostility from the the antiestrogen effect); vasomotor system effects such as nausea, headache, and hot flushes; and occasionally weight gain or hair loss (reversible). Clomiphene citrate also has a mydriatic action and some patients have blurred vision and scotomas, all of which are reversible.

Patients with high levels of androgens originating from the adrenal glands (elevated dehydroepian-drosterone sulfate are more resistant to antiestrogen treatment. Dexamethasone 0.5 mg at night throughout the cycle is found to decrease circulating androgens and may result in better ovulation. If a patient still does not ovulate, gonadotropin therapy is indicated. This has a higher risk of multiple pregnancies and ovarian hyperstimulation syndrome. However, full-blown development of this syndrome is rare.

An alternative treatment for patients with polycystic ovaries and resistance to antiestrogens is laparoscopic ovarian electrocautery. The mechanism of action of this therapy is still obscure and the efficacy has yet to be evaluated in a prospective randomized study. Possible complications are postoperative adhesions and (rare) ovarian failure as a result of excessive burning.

Hypogonadotropic anovulation

FSH is low, serum estradiol is <40 pg/ml and there is no withdrawal bleeding after a progesterone challenge. Hypogonadotropic anovulation is mostly idiopathic; other causes include under weight (anorexia nervosa) and excessive exercise. If one of these latter conditions is present, the patient should be adequately counseled. If the cause is primary pituitary failure then ovulation can be induced with gonadotropins. If pituitary failure is secondary to hypothalamic dysfunction, the treatment of choice is pulsatile GnRH. The advantages of pulsatile GnRH compared with gonadotropins include minimal risks of hyperstimulation and for multiple pregnancies. Use of pure preparations of FSH is not indicated for this group of patients because some LH is required for ovulation (Couzinet et al., 1988).

Hypergonadotropic anovulation

Plasma concentrations of FSH should be >20 mIU/ml on repeated occasions (Baird, 1995). The patient is usually hypoestrogenic. If the patient is under 35 years of age, a karyotype should be done to exclude the presence of a Y chromosome; if this is present, surgical removal of the gonads is recommended because there is a risk of malignant transformation (Layman and Reindollar, 1994). Although FSH concentrations may fluctuate for months and some patients may occasionally (and unpredictably) ovulate, for all practical purposes these women cannot be treated (Van Kasteren and Schoemaker, 1999). These women have either the so-called resistant ovary syndrome (Falsetti et al., 1999), a rare condition where the ovarian failure is probably caused by an immunological factor, or incipient ovarian failure. A differential diagnosis can only be done after ovarian biopsy, which is obsolete as the histological findings have little influence on the clinical management. These women should, apart from a karyotype (which could, if abnormal have consequences for younger sisters of the patient), have a thorough assessment to exclude associated autoimmune endocrine disorders such as hypothyroidism, adrenal insufficiency, and diabetes mellitus (Kalamtaridou et al., 1998). We perform a full blood count, test for rheumatoid factor and antinuclear antibodies, do a complete thyroid screen with autoantibody testing, and test for adrenal function. Hormone replacement therapy should be started to prevent osteoporosis, decrease the risk of cardiovascular disease, and improve general well-being. The only realistic option for pregnancy is the use of donated oocytes.

Hyperprolactinemic anovulation

Hyperprolactinemia disturbs normal ovulation by negative feedback on the hypothalamic pulsatile secretion of GnRH, resulting in gonadotropin deficiency and secondary ovarian failure. The maximal normal prolactin concentration is 600–800 mIU/ml. If elevated, the measurement should be repeated as stress and drugs are known to raise prolactin levels (phenothiazines and other psychopharmacologic drugs). If possible, such drug treatment should be stopped. Thyroid-stimulating hormone should be measured to exclude hypothyroidism. Thyroid-releasing hormone should also be checked because it acts to stimulate prolactin secretion; renal and liver function should also be checked. If prolactin levels are confirmed to be elevated, some type of pituitary imaging should be carried out (radiography, computered tomography, nuclear magnetic resonance) to exclude a micro- or macroadenoma.

The drug treatment of choice for hyperprolactinemia is a dopamine agonist, such as bromocriptine or carbergoline, to suppress pituitary secretion of prolactin to normal levels. Surgery is sometimes necessary for patients with large tumors, which may be causing specific local dangers, or for patients who have too many side-effects from the medication (rare). Because of these side-effects (nausea, postural hypotension), medication is usually started at a low dose at bedtime. Bromocriptine can also be administered intravaginally and then has fewer associated side-effects. If the hyperprolactinemia cannot be suppressed fully, additional treatment with clomiphene citrate or gonadotropins might be necessary to achieve ovulation.

Summary

In conclusion, the treatment of anovulatory infertility can be successful in many cases but it is not without risk. Relevant investigation and appropriate treatment are necessary. Ovulation induction should be performed with adequate monitoring to avoid the risks of ovarian hyperstimulation syndrome and multiple gestation.

Tubal disease

The fallopian tube is necessary for egg pick-up (tubal fimbriae guiding the egg into the tube), fertilization and embryo transfer (through the unidirectional beating of the tubal cilia coupled with peristaltic contractions of the muscular tubal wall), and nourishing the embryo with secretions originating from the tubal epithelium. Tubal disease includes an array of disorders affecting one or more of the above components, such as peritubal adhesions, proximal or distal tubal blockage, and hydrosalpinx. Several scoring systems for tubal damage have been developed but none has gained universal acceptance (British Fertility Society classification of pelvic disease; scoring system of Wu and Gocial (Wu and Gocial, 1998)). The aim of these classifications is to predict those women who would benefit most from surgery and allow for objective comparison of different surgical approaches. Substantial benefit can be gained from surgery for patients with milder disease, but surgery for severe or extensive disease is not likely to be beneficial, except perhaps for patients where the alternative of IVF treatment is unaffordable or unavailable. Adequate tubal assessment is, therefore, essential prior to tubal surgery.

The main advantage of surgery in properly selected patients is that the chance of success is continuous. However, this needs to be weighed against a higher ectopic pregnancy rate and the associated risks of the surgery. Current methods of surgery are predominantly laparoscopic. The main indication for open surgery is tubal anastomosis, using microsurgical techniques to bypass proximal tubal occlusion, and for the reversal of sterilization. The reversal of a previous sterilisation should be considered separately from other forms of tubal surgery because of previous proven fertility and the absence of previous pelvic inflammatory disease. Success rates are usually high, depending on the experience of the surgeon and the type of previous sterilization (clips and rings give the best prognosis) even in women over 40 years of age. In order to minimize surgical intervention, efforts have been made to achieve tubal recanalization in women with proximal occlusion by applying transcervical tubal catheterization. First, a selective salpingography is performed; if unsuccessful, this is followed by a transcervical balloon tuboplasty. No prospective randomized studies have been performed to document subsequent pregnancy rates. Patients with distal tubal disease appear to benefit by laparoscopic adhesiolysis or salpingostomy. The results are again directly correlated with the tubal disease score and no prospective studies are available. There is now an increasing trend to remove moderate and severely damaged fallopian tubes prior to attempting IVF, particularly in the presence of hydrosalpinges, as the latter are associated with a poorer outcome and there is a higher risk of ectopic pregnancy after IVF in women with tubal damage.

Endometriosis

It is accepted that patients with endometriosis have reduced fecundity. This is easily extended to patients where severe disease has caused damage to their fallopian tubes and/or ovaries. However, the relationship to fertility is less certain for patients with minimal disease, although several mechanisms have been proposed. The fact that several different mechanisms have been proposed casts doubt on a direct link between the visual diagnosis of endometriosis and the cause of infertility. As a consequence, this doubt creates uncertainty regarding the most appropriate treatment for infertility.

It is logical to correct surgically any distortion of the pelvic anatomy caused by moderate-to-severe endometriosis. However, it should be noted that the disease process, unlike pelvic inflammatory disease, does not affect the tubal mucosa. Since laparoscopy has reduced morbidity, it has been suggested as the best treatment option for the patient. The addition of medical treatment as an adjunct either pre- or postoperatively appears to offer no benefit (Vercellini et al., 1998). A more contentious issue is the management of minimal and mild disease. In these cases, there is enough evidence to suggest that medical treatment provides no benefit. Medical treatment only delays potential conception and does not lead to higher fecundity following treatment (ESHRE Capri Workshop Group, 2000). However, a multicenter, randomized controlled trial demonstrated the efficacy of endometrial ablation in increasing the pregnancy rate in infertile women (Marcoux et al., 1997). It might, therefore, be considered unethical to refrain from surgery in the presence of laparoscopic diagnosis of endometriosis.

It is appropriate to utilize ART (superovulation plus intrauterine insemination (IUI), IVF, gamete intrafallopian transfer (GIFT)) when other treatments or managements have been unsuccessful. However, which technique to use is still debatable. Large randomized controlled studies are needed to answer this question. For patients with endometriosis who require ART for other reasons, the pretreatment of endometriosis by surgical excision, in particular of endometriomata, is recommended for two reasons. First, ovarian response to stimulation may be improved. Second, attempted drainage of endometrioma at the time of egg collection is unsatisfactory and it also increases the risk for pelvic sepsis.

Uterine abnormalities

Sound evidence that uterine abnormalities interfere with the chance of natural conception has been difficult to gain. Congenital uterine abnormalities, including the effects of fetal exposure to maternal diethylstilbestrol, and their need for treatment are of doubtful relevance for conception except for rare occlusive types. Surgical correction is mostly of unproven benefit. The value of hysteroscopic resection of an intrauterine septum in the treatment of infertility remains speculative. Small endometrial or tubocornual polyps and minor endometrial adhesions seem to be of no importance. Severe symptomatic adhesions obliterating the cavity are probably significant and can be easily treated by hysteroscopic resection.

Fibroids are the most common uterine abnormality. Their contribution to infertility and the indication that treatment is needed (beneficial) has yet to be proven in prospective studies. Recent studies of IVF treatment have shown only marginal reduction of implantation unless there is evident distortion of the uterine cavity (Elder-Geva et al., 1998). The relevance of a single large subserous fibroid to impairing fertility remains uncertain. Myomectomy (by hysteroscopic resection) should be reserved for fibroids distorting the uterine cavity. Intramural fibroids causing menorrhagia or clinical symptoms because of their size should be removed laparoscopically if smaller than 8 cm in diameter or by a conventional open approach if larger.

Unexplained infertility

Unexplained infertility is a term applied to an infertile couple for whom standard investigations (ovulation disorders, tubal disease, endometriosis, uterine abnormalities, and semen analysis) yield normal results. The clinical approach to investigating unexplained infertility has undergone a major shift in emphasis in the 1990s. Unexplained infertility was traditionally associated with a plethora of tests, few of which contributed significantly to either the choice or the success of the treatment. With the availability of ART, many of the old diagnostic exercises are no longer seen as crucial to the management of the condition. Instead, there is an increasing reliance on evidence-based medicine.

Possible causes of infertility that appear to have no practical relevance but that are still of interest to researchers are luteal phase deficiency, luteinized unruptured follicle syndrome, hyperprolactinemia with normal ovulation, subclinical pregnancy loss, occult infection, sperm dysfunction, immunological causes, and psychological factors. It must be appreciated that the management of unexplained infertility is by definition empirical and that there is always a chance of spontaneous pregnancy, which must be taken into account when treatment is considered.

In addition to duration of infertility, the female partner's age and previous pregnancy history have a major effect on spontaneous conception rates as well as on treatment outcome. In women under 30 years, conservative treatment for up to three years should be considered, since spontaneous conception rates only start to decline significantly after this period. Advancing age (over 30) and no previous pregnancy are associated with lower chances of success and require quicker treatment. Clomiphene citrate has been shown to increase the number of follicles produced per cycle, thus increasing the odds of a fertilized embryo reaching the uterine cavity. While undoubtedly effective in anovulatory cycles, its use in unexplained infertility is still open to debate. Superovulation with gonadotropins with IUI has been a recognized treatment for unexplained infertility for a number of years. However, while less invasive than IVF, this approach puts the patient at significant risk for ovarian hyperstimulation syndrome and multiple pregnancy (Hughes, 1997). The likelihood of pregnancy is approximately twofold higher with FSH and nearly threefold higher with IUI. The combination of the two treatments has a cumulative effect, increasing the odds by a factor of five. This implies that superovulation with IUI should be offered to couples with unexplained infertility prior to embarking on IVF.

If the pelvis is normal, treatment of prolonged or refractory unexplained infertility is best accomplished using IVF or GIFT. The latter obviates the need for a sophisticated embryology laboratory but provides less diagnostic information regarding fertilization and subjects the patient to the risk of using a general anesthetic and laparoscopy. We usually offer our patients intracytoplasmic sperm injection (ICSI) with half of their retrieved ooyctes to avoid failed fertilization. This method is not only diagnostic but also avoids an extra IVF/ICSI cycle.

Conclusions

The practical objectives of infertility treatment are to assist couples with a likely cause of infertility or prolonged unexplained infertility to reach a conclusive solution and within a proper framework of safety for all involved. It may not always be possible to achieve a pregnancy and care must extend to help in other ways. The choice of treatment is seldom absolute but usually depends on a balance of factors to meet each couple's needs. Such factors include the relative effectiveness, complexity, and cost of alternative methods; the woman's age; and personal and emotional preferences. In addition, the choice may be restricted by public or insurance-covered resource limitations. Couples will usually start with simple treatment, although it may be relatively ineffective, before taking up IVF. Some couples need no interventionist treatment – only information and advice.

REFERENCES

Baird, D.T. (1995). Amenorrhoea, anovulation and dysfunctional uterine bleeding. In: *Endocrinology*, De Groot, L.J., ed. Saunders, London, pp. 2059–79.

Couzinet, B., Lestrat, N., Brouilly, S., et al. (1988). Stimulation of ovarian follicular maturation with pure follicle-stimulating hormone in women with gonadotrophin deficiency. *Journal of Clinical Endocrinology and Metabolism*, **66**, 552–6.

Elder-Geva, T., Meagher, S., Healy, D.L., et al. (1998). Effect of intramural, subserosal and submucosal uterine fibroids on the outcome of assisted reproductive technology treatment. *Fertility and Sterility*, **70**, 687–91.

ESHRE Capri Workshop Group (1995). Anovulatory infertility. *Human Reproduction*, **10**, 549–53.

ESHRE Capri Workshop Group (2000). Optimal use of infertility diagnostic tests and treatments. *Human Reproduction*, **15**, 723–32.

Faddy M.J., and Gosden R.G. (1995). A mathematical model of follicle dynamics in the human ovary. *Human Reproduction* **10**, 770–5.

Falsetti, L., Scalchi, S., Villani, M.T., and Bugari, G. (1999). Premature ovarian failure. *Gynecological Endocrinology*, **13**, 189–95.

Farley, T.M. and Belsey, F.H. (1998). The prevalence and etiology of infertility. In: *Biological Components of Fertility. (Proceedings of the African Population Conference*, Dakar, Senegal, November 1998.) International Union for the Scientific Study of Population, Liège, Belgium, Vol. 1, 2.1.15–2.1.30.

Golan, A., Ron-El, R., Herman, A., et al. (1992). Diagnostic hysteroscopy: its value in an in-vitro fertilisation/embryo transfer unit. *Human Reproduction*, **7**, 1433–4.

Govaerts, I., Devreker, F., Delbaere, A., Revelard, P., and Englert, Y. (1998). Short term medical complications of 1500 oocyte retrievals for in-vitro fertilisation and embryo transfer. *European Journal of Obstetrics, Gynaecology and Reproductive Biology*, **77**, 239–43.

Gunnell, D.J. & Ewings, P. (1994). Infertility prevalence, needs assessment and purchasing. *Journal of Public Health Medicine*, **16**, 29–36.

Hughes, E.G. (1997). The effectiveness of ovulation induction and intrauterine insemination in the treatment of unexplained infertility: a meta-analysis. *Human Reproduction*, 12, 1865–72.

Kalamtaridou, S.N., Davis, S.R., and Nelson, L.M (1998). Premature ovarian failure. *Endocrinology and Metabolism Clinics of North America*, 27, 989–1006.

Lass, A., Silye, R., Abrams, D.C., et al. (1997). Follicular density in ovarian biopsy of infertile women: a novel method to assess ovarian reserve. *Human Reproduction*, 12, 1028–31.

Layman, L.C. and Reindollar, R.H. (1994). The genetics of hypogonadism. *Infertility and Reproductive Medicine Clinics of North America*, 1, 53–68.

Marcoux, S., Maheux, R., Berube, S., et al. (1997). Laparoscopic surgery in fertile women with minimal or mild endometriosis. *New England Journal of Medicine*, 337, 217–22.

Mosher, W.D. (1985). Reproductive impairments in the United States, 1965–1982. *Demography*, 22, 415.

Navot, D., Rosenwaks, Z., and Margaliot, E. (1989). Prognostic assessment of female fecundity. *Lancet*, ii, 645–7.

Oei, S.G., Helmerhorst, F.M., Bloemenkamp, K.W., et al. (1998). Effectiveness of the post-coital test. *British Medical Journal*, 317, 502–5.

Rosene-Montella, K., Keely, E., Laifer, S.A., and Lee, R.V. (2000). Evaluation and management of infertility in women: the internists' role. *Annals of Internal Medicine*, 132, 973–81.

Seifer, D.B., Labert-Masserlian, G., Hogan J.W., et al. (1997). Day 3 serum inhibin-B is predictive of assisted reproductive technologies outcome. *Fertility and Sterility*, 67, 110–14.

Syrop, C.H., Wilhoite, A., and Van-Voorkis, B.J. (1995). Ovarian volume: a novel outcome predictor for assisted reproduction. *Fertility and Sterility*, 64, 1167–71.

Templeton, A., Fraser, C., and Thompson, B. (1990). The epidemiology of infertility in Aberdeen. *British Medical Journal*, 301, 148–52.

Van Kasteren, Y.M. and Schoemaker, J. (1999). Premature ovarian failure: a systematic review on therapeutic interventions to restore ovarian function and achieve pregnancy. *Human Reproduction Update*, 5, 483–92.

Vercellini, P., De Giorgi, O., Pesole A., et al. (1998). Endometriosis. Drugs and adjuvant therapy. In: *Evidence-based Fertility Treatment*, Templeton, A.A., Cooke I.D., and O'Brien, P.M.S., eds. Royal College of Obstetricians and Gynaecologists Press, London, pp. 225–45.

Wu, C.H. and Gocial, B. (1998). A pelvic scoring system for infertility surgery. *International Journal of Fertility*, 33, 341–6.

18

Ultrasound imaging at the beginning of the second millennium

Richard P. Dickey[1,2] and Ellen Matulich[1]

[1]Fertility Institute of New Orleans, New Orleans, USA
[2]Department Obstetrics and Gynecology, Louisiana State University School of Medicine, New Orleans, USA

Introduction

Ultrasound is now in universal use for monitoring follicular development during ovulation induction, for guiding oocyte retrieval during in vitro fertilization (IVF), and for evaluation of the uterus and ovaries in infertility. The first use of ultrasound to examine the ovaries and uterus was reported in 1958 (Donald et al., 1958). The first vaginal ultrasound was reported in 1969 (Kratochwil, 1969). Gray scale technique, which enables depiction of pelvic structures in detail, was reported in 1974 (Kossoff et al., 1974). The Graffian follicle was first visualized by ultrasound in 1972 (Kratochwil et al., 1972). Follicular changes throughout a complete menstrual cycle were first described by Hackeloer and colleagues (1979).

Doppler ultrasound has been used to examine the heart and peripheral vessels since the 1960s, and duplex Doppler has been used to examine systemic vessels since 1974 (Barber et al., 1974), but application of Doppler ultrasound to infertility and to IVF is of recent origin. The seminal papers on the use of Doppler ultrasound to examine uterine vessels in spontaneous cycles and in IVF by Goswamy and coworkers appeared in 1988 (Goswamy and Steptoe, 1988; Goswamy et al., 1988). The first articles on the use of three-dimensional ultrasound to evaluate ovarian and endometrial volume appeared in 1996 (Kyei-Mensah et al., 1996).

This chapter will examine how these techniques are being used to evaluate and manage infertility and IVF now, and how they may be used in the future.

Types of ultrasound

Gray scale, B mode, fast B scan, and real-time are descriptive terms assigned to progressively complex ultrasound methods that use a pulse-echo technique. In real-time ultrasound, images are generated at a rate of up to 30 per second, allowing observation of anatomical movement. Linear scan transducers, used for abdominal ultrasound, have 64 or more transducer elements mounted in a linear array that emit parallel beams and produce a rectangular image. Sector scan transducers, used for vaginal ultrasound, emit beams in a fan-shape pattern, usually with an aperture angle of 90°, allowing lateral organs to be visualized. Three-dimensional ultrasound is a refinement of pulse-echo technique that acquires volume data, either by moving the transducer head from side to side manually or by electronic evaluation of pulses emitted sequentially across the face of the transducer.

In Doppler ultrasound, the change in frequency of the returning echo caused by movement results in a Doppler shift. In color flow Doppler, two-dimensional, color-coded Doppler information is superimposed on a real-time anatomical display. Pulsed Doppler systems have the ability to select the depth from which Doppler information is received, thus allowing analysis of blood flow through a single vessel. To do this, the vessel to be studied is first located with real-time ultrasound. A gate is then placed over the vessel that only allows signals to pass that are returned within a defined time. The width of the gate (also called the volume box) is adjusted to the diameter of the vessel.

Measurement and analysis

Gray scale ultrasound

The frequency range most commonly used in obstetrics and gynecology is 3.5–7.5 MHz (1 MHz = 1 000 000 cycles). As frequency is increased, imaging depth decreases and ambiguity occurs because of attenuation and because the next pulse is emitted before all the echoes from the previous pulse have returned. Attenuation is the decrease in amplitude and intensity that occurs through absorption (conversion to heat), reflection, and scattering as sound travels through tissue. For soft tissue, attenuation in decibels (dB) is approximately 0.5 dB/cm for each MHz of frequency. At a pulse repetition frequency of 5 kHz, ambiguity begins at depths beyond 15 cm. At a pulse repetition frequency of 20 KHz, ambiguity begins at depths beyond 4 cm.

Follicle size

The technique for measuring follicle size is not standardized. Radiology-trained ultrasonographers customarily measure follicle dimensions from the outer edge on one side to the inner edge on the opposite side and take measurements in the most rounded configuration. Ultrasonographers trained in gynecology and reproductive endocrinology customarily measure from the inner or outer edge on both sides and record the maximum dimension. Follicles are rarely spherical so the examiner must subjectively decide where to take measurements. For these reasons, recording three dimensions offers little advantage over recording two dimensions and is impractical when large numbers of follicles are present. Differences in how measurements are taken can account for 1–2 mm differences in recorded follicle size (Nitschke-Dabelstein, 1983).

Endometrial thickness and pattern

Endometrial thickness is customarily measured from outside to outside in an anterior–posterior view at the widest point. Smith et al. (1984) were the first to use the appearance and thickness of the endometrium to decide when to administer human chorionic gonadotropin (hCG). They classified endometrial patterns as type A, a multilayered "triple-line" endometrium consisting of a prominent outer and central hyperechogenic line and inner hypoechogenic or black regions; type B, an intermediate isoechogenic pattern, with the same reflectivity as the surrounding myometrium and a nonprominent or absent central echogenic line; or type C, an entirely homogeneous endometrium without a central echogenic line. Subsequently, Gonen and Casper (1990) reversed the A B C order employed by Smith et al. (1984). Descriptions of endometrial pattern in the medical literature may follow either classification system. Most authors now only use the terms triple-line and homogeneous and report only the two most common endometrial patterns; they may include a third term postovulation to describe the bright pattern seen during the midluteal phase (Fig. 18.1).

Doppler ultrasound

The Doppler shift is dependent on the speed of blood flow (usually between 10 and 100 cm/s), the angle between the transducer and the vessel being measured, and the operating frequency of the Doppler instrument. Higher operating frequencies, greater flow speeds, and smaller Doppler angles produce larger Doppler shifts.

Doppler blood flow may be analyzed in three ways: waveform, resistance indices, and flow volume or velocity. Waveform analysis provides the most accurate estimate of blood flow in conditions where flow is not continuous throughout the cardiac cycle, as occurs normally in the uterine and spiral arteries during the proliferative phase of the cycle. Because it is not subject to statistical analysis, waveform analysis is often omitted in reports of infertility investigations. Resistance indices measure downstream impedance to blood flow and are independent of the angle of insonation but are only indirect estimates of flow volume. They are most useful for estimating blood flow in vessels distal to the point of examination. Resistance indices may be highly inaccurate when blood flow in the vessel being measured

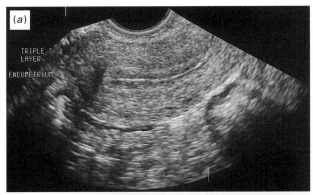

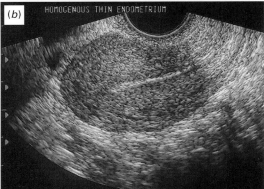

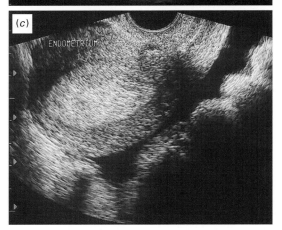

Fig. 18.1. Sonographs of endometrial thickness pattern. (*a*) The triple-line endometrial pattern; this is the day used for human chorionic gonadotropin administration in in vitro fertilization treatments. (*b*) Homogeneous endometrial pattern, seen on cycle day 3. (*c*) The postovulation pattern seen on cycle day 21.

Table 18.1. Common abbreviations used when reporting blood flow measurement

Abbreviation	Term
PI	Pulsatility index
RI	Resistance index, Pourcelot's index/ratio
S/D ratio	Systolic/diastolic ratio
V_{max}	Velocity maximum (same as PSV and MPSV)
MDV	Minimum diastolic velocity
PPI	Peak-to-peak pulsatility index
PSV	Peak systolic velocity (same as MPSV and V_{max})
MPSV	Maximum peak systolic velocity (same as PSV and V_{max})
TAMV	Time-averaged maximum velocity (same as TAMX and TAPV)
TAMX	Time-averaged maximum velocity (same as TAMV and TAPV)
TAPV	Time-averaged peak velocity (same as TAMV and TAMX)

Source: Reprinted with permission from Dickey (1997).

is not continuous. Flow volume analysis is the closest to true blood flow but the most difficult to perform. Flow volume analysis can only be used for vessels 2 mm or larger that are straight for at least 1 cm, such as the ascending uterine arteries. Velocity, a component of flow volume, is used to estimate flow volume in small vessels in the uterus and ovaries when flow volume cannot be measured. Table 18.1 lists common abbreviations used for blood flow measurements.

Waveform analysis

The Doppler waveform represents changes in the velocity of blood flow during the cardiac cycle. Flow conditions at the site of measurement are indicated by the width of the velocity spectrum, with spectral broadening indicative of disturbed and turbulent flow. Flow condition downstream, particularly distal flow impedance, is indicated by the relationship between peak systolic velocity (PSV) and end-

Table 18.2. Waveform classification

Original classification	Revised classification	Present description	Find classification
Type C	Type C	Diastolic component continuous with previous systolic component and present throughout the cardiac cycle	Type C
Type B	Type D-I	Diastolic component continuous with the previous systolic component but not present at the end of the cardiac cycle	Type B
Type A	Type D-II	Diastolic component present at the end of the cardiac cycle, but not continuous with the systolic component	Type A
Not covered	Type D-III	Diastolic component present but neither continuous with the systolic component nor present at the end of the cardiac cycle	Type D
Type 0	Type D-IV	No diastolic component present	Type 0
Not covered	Type N	No systolic or diastolic component present	Type N

Notes:
[a] Goswamy and Steptoe (1988).
[b] Dickey and Hower (1994).
Source: Reprinted with permission from Dickey.

diastolic flow speeds. Goswamy and Steptoe (1988) developed a classification of flow velocity waveforms for use in nonpregnant patients (Table 18.2). In their classification, the term type C was used for waveforms in which diastolic flow was present throughout the cardiac cycle (Fig. 18.2). In type A, diastolic flow was present in mid-diastole, but was absent in early diastole and might or might not be present in late diastole (Fig. 18.3). They considered type A to be a sign of poor perfusion and the result of distal impedance to blood flow. In type B, diastolic flow was continuous with the preceding systolic component but did not extend to the systolic component in the next cardiac cycle (Fig. 18.4). They considered this to be a sign of low impedance but adequate perfusion. In type 0, no diastolic flow was present at any time. They considered type 0 an indication of high distal impedance and low perfusion (Fig. 18.5). Dickey and Hower (1994) published a revised form of this classification but subsequently reverted to Goswamy and Steptoe's original classification with two additions: type D, when flow was present in mid-diastole but absent in both early and late diastole, and type N when no flow was undetect-

able in either systole and diastole. In Goswamy and Steptoe's original classification, type D would be included with type A.

Resistance indices
Resistance indices are based on the ratio of PSV to some measure of diastolic flow and are, therefore, independent of the angle of insonance. When waveforms are continuous resistance indices help to define the magnitude of downstream resistance. Resistance indices commonly used in infertility and obstetrics are illustrated in Fig. 18.6.

Peak-to-peak pulsatility index
The peak-to-peak pulsatility index (PPI) measures the total distance from the top to the bottom of the systolic peak and divides this by the mean velocity over the cardiac cycle. It is expressed by S/V_{max}, where S is PSV and V_{max} is the time-average maximum velocity (TAMV) over the cardiac cycle. This index is used primarily in cardiovascular disease for measurement of high-resistance vascular beds where flow is reversed in early diastole (triphasic flow).

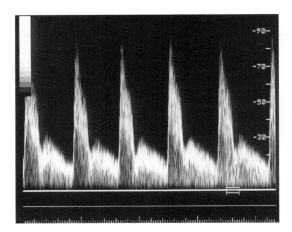

Fig. 18.2. Doppler waveform type C. Uterine flow velocity waveform showing high systolic flow and diastolic wave extending to the next cardiac cycle. This indicates good uterine perfusion. (Reprinted with permission from Dickey, 1997.)

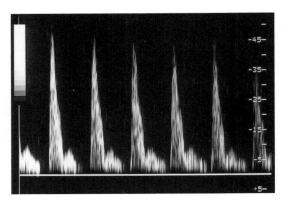

Fig. 18.4. Doppler waveform type B. Uterine flow velocity waveform showing diastolic wave continuous with systole, but not extending to the next cardiac cycle. This indicates good uterine perfusion. (Reprinted with permission from Dickey, 1997.)

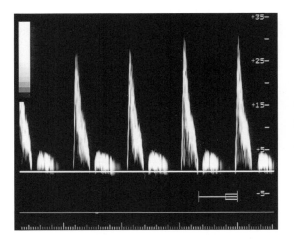

Fig. 18.3. Doppler waveform type A. Uterine flow velocity waveform showing high systolic flow and absence of early diastolic flow. This indicates poor uterine perfusion. (Reprinted with permission from Dickey, 1997.)

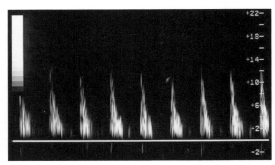

Fig. 18.5. Doppler waveform type 0. Uterine flow velocity waveform showing absence of any diastolic flow. This indicates very high impendence. (Reprinted with permission from Dickey, 1997.)

Resistance index

The resistance index (RI) is also called Pourcelot's ratio (Pourcelot, 1974) and examines the difference between PSV and end-diastolic velocity. It is expressed by $(S-D)/S$ where and D is the minimum or end-diastolic velocity. If D goes to zero, the ratio converges to one. The RI is used for low-resistance vascular beds with continuous flow throughout diastole.

Pulsatility index

The pulsatility index (PI) is also called the mean pulsatility index to distinguish it from PPI. It is expressed by $S-D/V_{max}$. (Gosling et al., 1971). Because it does not go to 1.0 if early or end-diastolic flow is absent, the PI may be recorded when flow is absent during all or part of diastole but is inaccurate in all such cases.

Systolic/diastolic ratio

The systolic/diastolic ratio (S/D) is the simplest of all indices; it is the ratio of the peak systolic frequency to the end-diastolic frequency. Errors in the S/D ratio increase as diastolic velocity becomes small. When flow is reduced in a stepwise fashion, PI and RI are increased in linear fashion, whereas the S/D ratio increases exponentially (Spencer et al., 1991).

Blood flow volume and velocity

Flow volume measures the actual volume of blood utilized by an organ, unlike resistance indices and waveforms, which indicate the state of smaller vessels downstream from the vessel being analyzed.

Flow volume

Flow volume is the only true measurement of blood flow and is expressed by $V_t A$, where V_t is the time-averaged mean velocity throughout the cardiac cycle and A is the cross-sectional area of the vessel. Flow volume measurements (in milliliters per minute) are dependent on the operator's accuracy in aligning the angle of insonation and in measuring diameter.

Time-averaged maximum velocity

TAMV is determined by measuring the average maximum velocity over a minimum of three cardiac

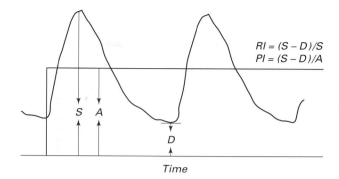

$$RI = (S-D)/S$$
$$PI = (S-D)/A$$

Time

Fig. 18.6. Common resistance indices. *S*, peak systolic velocity; *D*, end-diastolic velocity; *A*, time-average maximum velocity; *RI*, resistance index; *PI*, pulsatility index; *S/D*, systolic to diastolic velocity ratio. (Reprinted with permission from Dickey, 1997.)

cycles. TAMV is used when analyzing blood flow through small vessels with no collateral circulation, such as the ovarian arteries, when diameter cannot be accurately measured. Velocity is dependent on the angle of isonation. In many cases, TAMV mirrors flow volume; however, at points of vessel narrowing, velocity increases to compensate for the decrease in vessel diameter. Therefore, TAMV may give a false impression of blood flow in vessels narrowed by disease or stretching.

Other measurements of velocity

Maximum peak systolic velocity (MPSV), or simply PSV or V_{max} and minimum diastolic velocity (MDV), are sometimes reported. These expressions of velocity are highly unreliable. They are dependent on the angle of insonation and do not describe blood flow over the entire cardiac cycle. They display a high degree of variability on repeat examination (Tekay and Jouppila, 1996).

Relationship of waveforms to flow volume and resistance indices

The relationship of uterine artery waveforms to resistance indices was initially reported by Goswamy and Steptoe (1988) and subsequently by Dickey et al. (1994) and Tekay et al. (1996b). Dickey et al. (1994) established that uterine artery flow

Table 18.3. Relationship of flow volume and resistance indices to uterine artery and spiral artery waveforms in subjects who are recumbent or standing

Waveform classification	Recumbent uterine artery values				Uterine artery values			
	Number	Minute volume (ml/min)	PI	RI	Number	Minute volume (ml/min)	PI	RI
Uterine artery waveforms								
C	115	40.8 ± 2.3	2.47 ± 0.05	0.86 ± 0.01	98	37.9 ± 2.6	2.47 ± 0.05	0.87 ± 0.01
D-I (B)	9	$27.0 \pm 4.8*$	$3.47 \pm 0.17***$	–	0	–	–	–
D-II (A)	7	$19.7 \pm 3.3***$	$3.59 \pm 0.13***$	–	31	$19.4 \pm 1.9***$	$3.59 \pm 0.13***$	–
D-III (D)	17	$22.0 \pm 1.6***$	$3.36 \pm 0.09***$	–	17	$15.2 \pm 2.8***$	$4.45 \pm 0.41***$	–
D-IV (0)	0	–	–	–	2	$3.0 \pm 0.90***$	$9.95 \pm 0.05***$	–
Spiral artery waveforms								
C	59	74.4 ± 5.8	2.63 ± 0.08	0.88 ± 0.01	59	65.4 ± 6.1	2.67 ± 0.15	0.87 ± 0.01
D-I (B)	14	72.8 ± 11.6	2.90 ± 0.11	0.92 ± 0.02	5	80.4 ± 13.9	2.77 ± 0.18	0.93 ± 0.02
D-II (A)	0	–	–	–	1	45.0	3.31	0.92
D-III (D)	1	46.0	2.79	0.88	3	$22.3 \pm 3.0***$	4.30 ± 64.0	1.00 ± 0.015
D-IV (0)	0	–	–	–	0	–	–	–
D-V (N)	0	–	–	–	6	40.0 ± 15.8	$4.24 \pm 1.18**$	0.94 ± 0.04

Notes:

PI, pulsatility index; RI, resistance index.

All values given as means $\pm$ standard error; significance levels (t-test), compared with C (continuous flow): $*p < 0.05$; $**p < 0.01$; $***p < 0.001$.

Source: From Dickey et al. (1994) with permission.

volume was significantly lower and PI was significantly higher when waveforms were not continuous (Table 18.3). Absence of early diastolic flow and absence of any visible flow in spiral arteries was associated with notably lower uterine artery flow volume and higher uterine artery PI. Discontinuous (types A, B, D, or 0) spiral artery waveforms did not occur unless flow volume was markedly decreased in both uterine arteries. Slightly less than 50% of uterine artery PI and RI values were related to flow volume, underscoring the fact that downstream resistance significantly influences PI and RI.

Sources of error in Doppler blood flow measurement

The most important source of error in analysis of uterine and ovarian blood flow is the ultrasonographer's judgement in selecting the part of the vessel on which to place the Doppler gate. The gate may be placed over a portion of the vessel where waveforms have the highest peak systolic or diastolic velocity, the least velocity, or "average" velocity. Doppler blood flow studies have been published that have used each of these choices.

Analysis of blood flow in a single uterine artery, as is sometimes reported, instead of both arteries can lead to a false estimation of uterine perfusion because of the considerable cross-circulation in the uterus.

There is an upper limit to the Doppler shift that can be detected by present instruments. If the Doppler shift frequency exceeds one half the pulse repetition frequency, aliasing occurs. Aliasing is a phenomenon in which the peak of the velocity waveform appears below the base line; it is the most common artefact encountered in Doppler ultrasound. Aliasing can be eliminated by increasing pulse repetition frequency, by increasing the Doppler angle, or by base line shifting. However, increasing the Doppler angle to eliminate aliasing increases the chance of error in detecting flow velocity.

The width of the Doppler ultrasound volume box, compared with the width of the vessel wall, may affect velocity estimation. In small vessels, the average velocity may be only one half the velocity at the center of the stream because of turbulence caused by friction from the vessel wall. Volume box widths that are too small in relation to vessel size and those aimed at the center of the stream may result in overestimation of velocity.

Measurement of vessel diameter from frozen images can cause an error in determining flow volume because vessel diameter changes during the cardiac cycle. However, the normal distensibility of arteries in adults is less than 5% for a 40 mmHg pulse pressure differential (Gosling et al., 1991).

A source of error for measurements of flow volume, TAMV, and PI is the number of discrete velocity points or columns that an instrument generates and is capable of analyzing. With the instruments now available, this varies from 60 to 540 points per cardiac cycle. Depending on where the points fall over the cardiac cycle, analysis of a smaller number of points may overestimate or underestimate velocity compared with analysis of a greater number of points. The number of points analyzed over a cardiac cycle varies with scroll speed and heart rate. A faster scroll speed or slower heart rate will result in more points being analyzed per cardiac cycle. Errors owing to infrequent point analyses decrease when downstream resistance is low and the difference between systole and diastole is small. As better instruments are developed, the measurement of velocity and blood flow volume will become more accurate and may replace indices.

Relationship of ultrasound findings to outcome

Gray-scale ultrasound

Follicle size

In spontaneous cycles, several 3–4 mm follicles can normally be seen in each ovary on cycle day 3.

Follicles that are not atretic grow at a linear rate of 1 mm a day until about day 10 when a single follicle becomes dominant. The dominant follicle continues to grow at a rate of 2 to 3 mm a day for four to five days (Hackeloer et al., 1979; O'Herlihy et al., 1980; Queenan et al., 1980; Smith et al., 1980) reaching a diameter of 13–33 mm (De Cherney et al., 1982; Hamilton et al., 1987) immediately before ovulation. In controlled ovarian hyperstimulation (COH) cycles stimulated with human menopausal gonadotropin hMG) or follicle-stimulating hormone (FSH), the follicular size at ovulation is smaller, 16–20 mm (Ylostalo et al., 1979; Marrs et al., 1983). When gonadotropin-releasing hormone (GnRH) antagonists rather than agonists are used with hMG or FSH for IVF stimulation, follicles are larger and more numerous on stimulation day 6, but the number of follicles ≥17 mm are identical on stimulation day 10 (Borm and Mannaerts, 2000). The number of preovulatory follicles can be used to predict ovarian hyperstimulation syndrome (Blankstein et al., 1997). Silverberg et al. (1991) found that 0.5, 37.4, 72.5, 81.5, and 95.5% of follicles ≤14 mm, 15–16 mm, 17–18 mm, 19–20 mm, and >20 mm, respectively, on the day of hCG administration ovulated in COH cycles. In COH cycles when hMG is used either alone or combined with clomiphene in sequential and concurrent regimens, pregnancy rates are highest if hCG is given before the lead follicle is 18 mm (Dickey et al., 1991, 1993c). All follicles ≥12 mm must be counted when estimating the risk of multiple pregnancy in COH cycles (Dickey et al., 1991).

Size for in vitro fertilization

In IVF cycles, hCG must be given before spontaneous ovulation. Therefore, hCG is customarily administered when two or more follicles are 16–18 mm and at least four follicles are ≥14 mm. Follicular size at the time hCG is administered predicts oocyte quality (Scott et al., 1989; Haines and Emes, 1991; Silverberg et al., 1991; Dubey et al., 1995). Mature oocytes that produce top-quality embryos can be retrieved from follicles 9–10 mm at the time of hCG administration (Pryzak et al., 1999b). There is no difference in embryo quality or pregnancy rates when follicle volume is ≤1 ml which corresponds to a follicular diameter ≤12 mm, compared with >1 ml, despite a higher fertilization rate when volume is >1 ml (Salha et al., 1998). Pregnancy rates are higher when lead follicles are 15–16 mm than when they are 17–18 mm or larger in with high responses patients (Pryzak et al., 1999a).

Bergh et al. (1998) found a difference in fertilization and pregnancy rates between follicles above or below 16 mm in conventional IVF but no difference when intracytoplasmic sperm injection (ICSI) was performed, suggesting that any disadvantages of oocytes from small follicles might be overcome by means of ICSI. In 1109 IVF cycles, the oocyte recovery rate was highest when volume was 3–4 ml; the cleavage rate was highest when volume was 6–7 ml, but embryo quality was not influenced by follicular volume (Wittmaack et al., 1994). Top-quality embryos developed from 60% of oocytes when volume was 2–6 ml, corresponding to a follicle size of 16–23 mm, compared with 50% when volumes were below this level (Ectors et al., 1997). Miller et al. (1996) found that embryo quality, as reflected by decreased fragmentation, increased cleavage, and increased implantation rates, was improved when hCG was delayed until two or more follicles were ≥20 mm in diameter, but Shoham et al. (1991) found no difference in the size of the largest follicle between IVF cycles leading to conception and failing.

Size on cycle day three
The number of follicles 2–8 mm present on cycle day 3 predicts the number of preovulatory follicles >14 mm and the outcome of pregnancy (Chang et al., 1998). No relationship between cysts, 10–45 mm at the start of stimulation, and cancellation or pregnancy rates was found by Hornstein et al. (1989). Nonfunctional ovarian cysts decrease the number of preovulatory follicles on the ipsilateral side but do not affect the number of mature oocytes recovered (Karande et al., 1990). Aspiration of baseline ovarian cysts 20 mm and larger before gonadotropin stimulation does not affect the outcome of IVF (Rizk et al., 1990). However, patients with ovarian cysts 16–60 mm when gonadotropin stimulation is started are more likely to have the procedure canceled because of a premature surge in luteinizing hormone (LH) and low estradiol levels (Thatcher et al., 1989).

Endometrial pattern and thickness
Endometrial thickness measured by transvaginal ultrasound correlates well with histological endometrial maturation according to Hofmann et al. (1996); however, endometrial biopsies, judged at day 17 by histopathology, may have very different ultrasound appearances (Rogers et al., 1991), and Sterzik et al. (2000) found no relationship between histological dating and endometrial thickness or uterine artery PI and RI. Endometrial thickness was ≤6 mm in 92% when estradiol levels were <55 pg/ml in patients with GnRH downregulation (Barash et al., 1998). In spontaneous cycles, endometrial thickness increases from a mean of 4.6 mm 9 to 13 days before the LH surge to 12.4 mm the day of the LH surge (Bakos et al., 1993). The endometrial pattern develops a triple-line appearance from six days before the LH surge until seven days after, when the triple-line pattern becomes obscured by the increasingly hyperechogenic pattern of the endometrium although endometrial thickness remains unchanged (Bakos et al., 1993).

During stimulation cycles for IVF, the mean length of the endometrial cavity increases by 3.8 mm and the length of the cervical canal increases by 1.9 mm; these changes are correlated with changes in endometrial thickness (Strohmer et al., 1994). Endometrial and uterine volume have been measured by three-dimensional ultrasound, but the clinical impact of this technique has not been established (Kyei-Mensah et al., 1996; Lee et al., 1997).

Implantation does not occur, or is reduced, following IVF if the endometrial lacks a triple-line pattern on the day of or one day before ovum retrieval (Smith et al., 1984; Glissant et al., 1985; Gonen et al., 1989; Welker et al., 1989; Gonen and Casper, 1990; Ueno et al., 1991; Sher et al., 1991; Dickey et al., 1992, 1993a; Serafini et al., 1994; Sharara et al., 1999; Fanchin et al., 2000), on day 15 of estrogen administration in donor oocyte cycles

(Coulam et al., 1994), or on the day of hCG administration in COH cycles (Bohrer et al., 1996; Tsai et al., 2000).

Implantation does not occur if endometrial thickness is too thin on the day of hCG administration in IVF cycles (Smith et al., 1984; Gonen and Casper, 1990; Check et al., 1991; Dickey et al., 1992; Strohmer et al., 1994; Noyes et al., 1995; Oliveira et al., 1997), in COH cycles (Shoham et al., 1991, Dickey et al., 1993b; Bohrer et al., 1996; Isaacs et al., 1996), or on the day of embryo transfer in oocyte donation cycles (Antinori et al., 1993; Check et al., 1993; Abdalla et al., 1994; Hofmann et al., 1996). Rinaldi et al. (1996) reported that a thickness <10 mm was prognostic of pregnancy failure when IVF was performed for female indications but not when ICSI was performed. In most studies, 6 mm is the critical value below which no pregnancies occur, but the range is from 4 mm (Sundstrom, 1998) to 7 mm (Shoham et al., 1991).

The highest pregnancy rates occur when endometrial thickness is ≥9 mm (Sher et al., 1991; Dickey et al., 1992; Antinori et al., 1993; Noyes et al., 1995) or ≥10 mm (Check et al., 1991, 1993; Isaacs et al., 1996) the day of hCG administration. However, Weissman et al. (1999) reported that pregnancy rates were reduced when thickness was >14 mm, and Dickey et al. (1992) reported that biochemical pregnancies were increased when thickness was >12 mm the day of hCG administration. Others found no relationship between endometrial thickness and IVF outcome (Glissant et al., 1985; Fleischer et al., 1986; Rabinowitz et al., 1986; Welker et al., 1989; Ueno et al., 1991; Serafini et al., 1994; De Geyter et al., 2000) or biochemical pregnancy following IVF (Krampl and Feichtinger, 1993).

Endometrial thickness changes by up to 3 mm in a single day; consequently the criteria used for hCG administration may affect results. Uterine pathology may also affect results of endometrial studies. Sher et al. (1991) discovered uterine pathology (multiple leiomyomas, severe uterine synechiae, anomalies from material diethylstilbestrol therapy, adenomyosis) in 93.8% of patients with homogeneous endometrial patterns compared with 30% of patients with triple-line pattern and endometrial thickness <9

mm and 5.8% of patients with triple-line pattern and thickness ≥9 mm.

Endometrial waves

Endometrial wavelike activity is detectable by ultrasound throughout spontaneous and COH cycles (Abramowicz and Archer, 1990; De Vries et al., 1990; Lyons et al., 1991; Chalubinski et al., 1993; Ijland et al., 1996, 1998). The highest rate of activity is seen during the periovulatory period when opposing waves from the fundus to the cervix, and from the cervix to the fundus, occur in 30 to 40% of spontaneous cycles at a rate of 3–4 waves/min (Ijland et al., 1996). Endometrial wavelike activity occurred in 100% of COH cycles at the time of ovulation. No waves from the fundus to the cervix occurred during the midluteal phase in COH cycles. A relationship between IVF outcome and the presence or absence of endometrial waves has not been reported.

Embryo transfer

Embryo transfer under ultrasound guidance is advocated by a number of authors, although the difference in success compared with conventional transfer technique is rarely significant (Strickler et al., 1985; Leong et al., 1986; Hurley et al., 1991; Prapas et al., 1995; Woolcott and Stanger, 1997; Kan et al., 1999).

Pregnancy rates are significantly lower when hydrosalpinges are present at the time of transfer (Nackley and Muasher, 1998; Camus et al., 1999). Pregnancy rates doubled when hydrosalpinges are removed before IVF (Nackley and Muasher, 1998) and when they are aspirated at the time of oocyte retrieval (Van Voorhis et al., 1998). Implantation does not occur when endometrial fluid is present on ultrasound the day of embryo transfer, even when the fluid is aspirated (Mansour et al., 1991). Endometrial polyps <2 cm do not decrease pregnancy rates, but there is a trend toward increased pregnancy loss (Lass et al., 1999).

Treatment of suboptimal endometrium

Postponing administration of hCG is the simplest method for increasing endometrial thickness

(Randall and Templeton, 1991; Dickey et al., 1993b). In unstimulated cycles, endometrial thickness increases throughout the proliferative and early secretory phase until a plateau is reached five days after the LH surge (Randall et al., 1989). The benefit of delaying hCG must be balanced against the possibility of premature luteinization.

Administration of gonadotropins to women with poor endometrial linings in natural cycles and use of estradiol valerate in subsequent cycles of cryopreserved embryo transfer were successful in converting endometrial to optimal patterns and increasing its thickness in 40% of patients (Sher et al., 1993). Low-dose aspirin increased pregnancy rates (Wada et al., 1994; Weckstein et al., 1997; Rubinstein et al., 1999; Hsieh et al., 2000) and the incidence of triple-line pattern (Hsieh et al., 2000), but increases in endometrial thickness were not significant (Weckstein et al., 1997; Hsieh et al., 2000).

Doppler ultrasound of uterine blood flow

Normal spontaneous cycles and infertility
Uterine artery PI and RI decrease progressively, and flow volume and velocity increase progressively, during the follicular phase up to the day of ovulation (Sladkevicius et al., 1993; Weiner et al., 1993). After ovulation, a rise in PI and RI and a decrease in velocity is apparent by day 2 of the postovulatory phase (Kupesic and Kurjak, 1993). After day 2, PI and RI decrease again and velocity increases during the remainder of the luteal phase until two days before menstruation (Sladkevicius et al., 1993). Similar changes occur in the internal iliac arteries but not in the common or external iliac arteries (Deichert and Buurman, 1995). There are moderate differences in the values of PI and RI and also in velocity between the uterine artery on the side of the dominant follicle and the contralateral artery in spontaneous cycles (Sladkevicius et al., 1993; Tan et al., 1996). Blood flow increases in the luteal phase are related to increased progesterone levels (Dickey and Hower, 1994; Tan et al., 1996), while blood flow increases in the proliferative phase may be related to estradiol

levels (Steer et al., 1990; Weiner et al., 1993; Tan et al., 1996). There is a circadian rhythm to uterine artery blood flow, with a nadir in PI and a peak in TAMV at 6:00 a.m. (Zaidi et al., 1995c).

Increased uterine artery resistance indices and decreased velocity are present in up to 45% of women with unexplained infertility or repeated spontaneous abortion (Kurjak et al., 1991; Bonilla-Musoles, 1995). The average PI is increased, indicating decreased blood flow in the midluteal phase, in groups of patients with chronic anovulation, endometriosis, tubal infertility, and unexplained infertility compared with that in fertile women (Steer et al., 1994). Absence of diastolic flow in midluteal waveforms is associated with infertility (Goswamy et al., 1988; Serefini et al., 1994) and spontaneous abortion (Serefini et al., 1994).

Outcome in in vitro fertilization
An RI value >0.79 before starting ovarian stimulation is associated with poor uterine blood flow at the time of hCG administration (Bassil et al. (1995). Tekay et al. (1996a) considered that a PI >4.0 or absence of end-diastolic flow in the uterine arteries was inconsistent with implantation. Dickey (1997) reviewed Doppler ultrasound in infertility and early pregnancy and concluded that conception in IVF cycles is decreased when uterine artery PI is ≥3.3–3.5, when RI is ≥0.95, and when waveforms show absence of early or end-diastolic flow at the time of hCG administration (Strohmer et al., 1991; Levi-Setti et al., 1995; Zaidi et al., 1996c), at the time of oocyte retrieval (Stezik et al., 1989), at the time of embryo transfer in IVF cycles (Steer et al., 1992; Favre et al., 1993; Tekay et al., 1995a; Cacciatore et al., 1996; Tekay et al., 1996b), or transfer of cryopreserved embryos in spontaneous cycles (Coulam et al., 1994). No term pregnancies occurred in waveforms studies when end-diastolic flow was absent from both uterine arteries at the time of oocyte retrieval (Sterzik et al., 1989), or embryo transfer (Tekay et al., 1995a, 1996b; Cacciatore et al., 1996). Abnormal uterine artery waveforms, in which diastolic flow was absent or not continuous with preceding systolic flow (type 0 or A), in the midluteal phase were

present in 43% of 153 patients with repeated implantation failure (Goswamy et al., 1988).

Uterine artery PI correlates with immunohistochemical markers of endometrial receptivity (Steer et al., 1995) and with endometrial thickness in the midluteal phase (Steer et al., 1994) but not on the day of embryo transfer (Cacciatore et al., 1996). Sterzik et al. (2000) noted that midluteal phase uterine artery PI was significantly higher in patients whose endometrial biopsy was in phase but concluded that Doppler ultrasound alone was not able to predict endometrial receptivity.

Doppler ultrasound of ovarian blood flow

Normal spontaneous cycles and infertility

Taylor et al. (1985), in a classic study, measured ovarian artery blood flow simultaneously by Doppler ultrasound, using an abdominal transducer, and by invasive technique employing waveflow meters applied directly to the ovarian, iliac, and uterine arteries. Waveforms and PI were identical for both techniques. Ovarian artery blood flow on the side of the dominant follicle and corpus luteum increased progressively throughout the cycle, as shown by decreased RI (Taylor et al., 1985; Kurjak et al., 1991), decreased PI (Deutinger et al., 1989; Scholtes et al., 1989; Sladkevicius et al., 1993; Weiner et al., 1993), and increased PSV (Sladkevicius et al., 1993; Tan et al., 1996). Vascular changes in the wall of the dominant follicle can be detected as early as day 4 or 5 of the cycle (Kurjak et al., 1991; Bonilla-Musoles et al., 1995). In fully developed preovulatory follicles, the RI of perifollicular vessels is below 0.53 (Kurjak et al., 1991). Beginning 12 hours after the LH surge or 29 hours before follicular rupture, there is a marked increase in PSV, but PI remains relatively constant (Bourne et al., 1991; Collins et al., 1991; Campbell et al., 1993; Balakier and Stronell, 1994). The RI of the corpus luteum is never above 0.50 (Kurjak et al., 1991). Blood flow changes in the hilum and stroma of the dominant ovary parallel changes in the dominant follicle and corpus luteum but are less marked (Merce et al., 1989; Sladkevicius et al., 1993).

The PI of ovarian vessels supplying the dominant follicle and corpus luteum is negatively correlated with the number of follicles ≥ 15 mm and with serum estradiol levels (Weiner et al., 1993). Intraovarian RI and PSV are related to serum progesterone levels during the midluteal phase of the cycle in some studies (Glock and Brumsted, 1995; Bourne et al., 1996). However, PI was not related to progesterone levels in the midluteal phase of hMG cycles in one study (Weiner et al., 1993). No significant circadian rhythm occurs in ovarian follicular or stromal PI or PSV (Zaidi et al., 1996b).

Luteal phase defect is associated with higher RI and lower TAMV, but no difference in PSV during the late proliferative to midluteal phase, compared with women with in-phase endometrium. In luteinized unruptured follicle syndrome, PSV is low before and after the LH surge compared with the dominant follicle in normal women (Zaidi et al., 1995b).

In one report of patients with polycystic ovaries, PSV and TAMV of ovarian stromal vessels were significantly higher than in patients with normal ovaries on cycle day 2 or 3 but there was no difference in PI (Zaidi et al., 1995a). In another report of patients with polycystic ovaries, PI and RI were significantly lower on cycle days 3–8, and PSV was lower on days 15–22 compared with patients with normal ovaries (Aleem and Predanic, 1996). Average intraovarian PI was lower and MPSV was higher in patients with ovarian hyperstimulation syndrome than in asymptomatic patients following IVF (Tekay et al., 1995b). However, after resolution of symptoms, only MPSV was different.

Outcome in in vitro fertilization

Doppler ultrasound can be used during oocyte retrieval to identify and avoid ovarian and pelvic vessels. The iliac artery and vein may appear to be similar to medium-sized preovulatory follicles on Gray-scale ultrasound (Fig. 18.7, color plate).

There are very few studies of ovarian blood flow during IVF cycles. Changes in PSV did not correlate with oocyte quality according to Balakier and Stronell (1994). However, good-quality embryo developed from 70% of oocytes when PSV was

$\geq$10cm/s in the perifollicular vessels immediately before oocyte retrieval, compared with 14% if PSV was $\leq$10cm/s (Nargund et al., 1996). Failure to retrieve an oocyte is highly correlated with absence or diminished perifollicular blood flow (Nargund et al., 1996; Oyesanya et al., 1996). Retrieval of less than three oocytes occurs when stromal PI fails to fall during hMG stimulation (Weiner et al., 1993). Low intrastromal PSV on cycle day 3 was associated with retrieval of fewer than six follicles, but no association with PI was seen (Zaidi et al., 1996a). No pregnancies occurred when the stromal RI was greater than 0.5 on day 3 after embryo transfer (Barber et al., 1988).

New areas of investigation

Postural studies

Blood flow measurements while standing may differ significantly from recumbent measurements. Dickey et al. (1994) found that uterine artery blood flow volume fell in 70% of nonpregnant patients while standing, by an average 11% after 3 to 8 minutes, and 34% after 9 to 14 minutes. Decreases in standing blood flow volume were accompanied by significant decreases in uterine artery diameter and significant increases in mean uterine artery PI, with no change in uterine artery RI or in spiral artery PI and RI. Decreases in blood flow volume could be entirely accounted for by the decreases in uterine artery diameter. In patients with unchanged or increased blood flow volume while standing, uterine artery diameter was unchanged, but uterine artery PI and RI were decreased. The effect of standing on uterine and spiral artery blood flow in IVF patients during critical periods for completion of oocyte meiosis and embryo implantation remains to be investigated.

Effect of drugs on uterine and ovarian blood flow

There is limited information about the effect of drugs, other than estrogen and progesterone, on

human uterine and ovarian blood flow in infertility. In nonpregnant women of reproductive age, circulating levels of nitric oxide metabolites are higher in the proliferative phase of the menstrual cycle than in the luteal phase, and these peak at mid-cycle (Cicinelli et al., 1996). In patients undergoing IVF, nitrite and nitrate levels in follicles $\geq$4mm were related to ovarian artery PI (Anteby et al., 1996). Sildenafil, a type 5-specific phosphodiesterase inhibitor that augments the vasodilatory effects of nitrous oxide donor, improved uterine artery PI and endometrial thickness in three of four patients with previous IVF failure, who became pregnant (Sher and Fisch, 2000). Xanthine-type vasodilators increase uterine artery blood flow (Bonilla-Musoles et al., 1995).

Aspirin significantly decreased uterine and ovarian artery PI and increased follicle numbers, estradiol levels, and pregnancy rates in a randomized double-blind study (Rubinstein et al., 1999). Waveforms became continuous and RI and PI were notably reduced 1 hour after acetylsalicylic acid administration in 80% of patients with abnormal waveforms prior to IVF cycles (Dickey, 1997). Acetaminophen (paracetamol), an anti-inflammatory agent, causes disappearance of ovarian blood flow for up to 4 hours (Bonilla-Musoles et al., 1995).

The effect of the beta-adrenergic agents fenoterol and isoxsuprine was studied with intervenous xenon-133 (Kauppila et al., 1978). Fenoterol, but not isoxsuprine, significantly increased myometrial blood flow. Doppler ultrasound studies with the vasodilators nifedipine (Lindow et al., 1988) and atenolol (Montan et al., 1987) have shown that these drugs do not increase uterine blood flow significantly.

Conclusions

Since the early 1980s, gray-scale ultrasound has increased enormously the ability to monitor follicular and endometrial development during spontaneous and ovulation induction cycles to the point of replacing hormonal monitoring in some IVF programs. Doppler ultrasound evaluation of uterine and ovarian blood flow holds the promise of being helpful for investigation of infertility and IVF outcome and for selection of follicles with the greatest potential to produce high-quality embryos. This promise has only partially been fulfilled as yet because of difficulties in interpreting blood flow measurements in small vessels when vessel diameter is <2 mm and in large and small vessels when diastolic flow is not continuous. This difficulty may be overcome as better instrumentation and computer analysis become available.

Additional Doppler investigations of pharmacological methods to improve uterine and ovarian blood flow and of the effect of posture are clearly needed. A role for three-dimensional ultrasound has yet to be established. Doppler ultrasound measurement of uterine and ovarian blood flow is a relatively new technique. Its role in diagnosis and management of infertility and IVF is still being established. As more investigations are performed, as more clinicians become familiar with its use, and as instrumentation is improved, Doppler ultrasound may assume an increasingly important role in IVF.

REFERENCES

Abdalla, H.I., Brooks, A.A., Johnson, M.R., Kirkland, A., Thomas, A., and Studd, J.W.W. (1994). Endometrial thickness: a predictor of implantation in ovum recipients. *Human Reproduction*, **9**, 363–5.

Abramowicz, J. and Archer, D.F. (1990). Uterine endometrial peristalsis – a transvaginal ultrasound study. *Fertility and Sterility*, **54**, 451–4.

Aleem, F.A. and Predanic, M. (1996). Transvaginal color Doppler determination of the ovarian and uterine blood flow characteristics in polycystic ovary disease. *Fertility and Sterility*, **65**, 510–16.

Anteby, E.Y., Hurwitz, A., Korach, O., et al. (1996). Human follicular nitric oxide pathway: relationship to follicular size, estradiol concentrations, and ovarian blood flow. *Human Reproduction*, **11**, 1947–51.

Antinori, S., Versaci, C., Gholami, G.H., Panci, C., and Caffa, B. (1993). Oocyte donation in menopausal women. *Human Reproduction*, **8**, 1487–90.

Bakos, O., Lundkvist, O., and Bergh, T. (1993). Transvaginal sonographic evaluation of endometrial growth and texture in spontaneous ovulatory cycles – a descriptive study. *Human Reproduction*, **8**, 799–806.

Balakier, H. and Stronell, R.D. (1994). Color Doppler assessment of folliculogenesis in in vitro fertilization patients. *Fertility and Sterility*, **62**, 1211–16.

Barash, A., Weissman, A., Manor, M., Millman, D., Ben-Arie, A., and Shoham, Z. (1998). Prospective evaluation of endometrial thickness as a predictor of pituitary down-regulation after gonadotropin-releasing hormone analogue administration in an in vitro fertilization program. *Fertility and Sterility*, **69**, 496–9.

Barber, F.E., Baker, D.W., Nation, A.W.C., et al. (1974). Ultrasonic duplex echo-Doppler scanner. *IEEE Transactions on Biomedical Engineering*, **21**, 109.

Barber, R.J., McSweeney, M.B., Gill, R.W., et al. (1988). Transvaginal pulsed Doppler ultrasound assessment of blood flow to the corpus luteum in IVF patients following embryo transfer. *British Journal of Obstetrics and Gynaecology*, **95**, 1226–30.

Bassil, S., Magritte, J.P., Roth, J., Nisolle, M., Donnez, J., and Gordts, S. (1995). Uterine vascularity during stimulation and its correlation with implantation in in vitro fertilization. *Human Reproduction*, **10**, 1497–501.

Bergh, C., Broden, H., Lundin, K., and Hamberger, L. (1998). Comparison of fertilization, cleavage, and pregnancy rates of oocytes from large and small follicles. *Human Reproduction*, **13**, 1912–15.

Blankstein, J., Shalev, J., Saadon, T., et al. (1997). Ovarian hyperstimulation syndrome: prediction by number and size of preovulatory follicles. *Fertility and Sterility*, **47**, 597–602.

Bohrer, M.K., Hock, D.L., Rhoads, G.G., and Kemmann, E. (1996). Sonographic assessment of endometrial pattern and thickness in patients treated with human menopausal gonadotropins. *Fertility and Sterility*, **66**, 244–7.

Bonilla-Musoles, F., Ballester, M.J., Raga, R., Blanes, J., Osborne, N.G., and Pellicer, A. (1995). Transvaginal color Doppler sonography from folliculogenesis to implantation: normal and abnormal evolution. *Assisted Reproduction Reviews*, **5**, 158–69.

Borm, G. and Mannaerts, B. (2000). Treatment with the gonadotrophin-releasing hormone antagonist ganirelix in women undergoing ovarian stimulation with recombinant follicle stimulating hormone is effective, safe and convenient: results of a controlled, randomized, multicenter trial. *Human Reproduction*, **15**, 1490–8.

Bourne, T.H., Jurkovic, D., Waterstone, J., Campbell, S., and Collins, P. (1991). Intrafollicular, blood flow during human ovulation. *Ultrasound in Obstetrics and Gynecology*, **1**, 53–9.

Bourne, T.H., Hagstrom, H.G., Hahlin, M., et al. (1996). Ultrasound studies of vascular and morphological changes in the human corpus luteum during the menstrual cycle. *Fertility and Sterility*, **65**, 753–8.

Cacciatore, B., Simberg, N., Fusaro, P., and Titinen, A. (1996). Transvaginal Doppler study of uterine artery blood flow in in vitro fertilization–embryo transfer cycles. *Fertility and Sterility*, **66**, 130–4.

Campbell, S., Bourne, T.H., Waterstone, J., et al. (1993). Transvaginal color blood flow imaging of the periovulatory follicle. *Fertility and Sterility*, **60**, 433–8.

Camus, E., Poncelet, C., Goffinet, F.G., et al. (1999). Pregnancy rates after in-vitro fertilization in cases of tubal infertility with and without hydrosalpinx: a meta-analysis of published comparative studies. *Human Reproduction*, **14**, 1243–9.

Chalubinski, K., Deutinger, J., and Bernaschek, G. (1993). Vaginosonography for recording of cycle-related myometrial contractions. *Fertility and Sterility*, **59**, 225–8.

Chang, M.Y., Chiang, C.H., Hsieh, T.T., Soong, Y.K., and Hsu, K.H. (1998). Use of the antral follicle count to predict the outcome of assisted reproductive technologies. *Fertility and Sterility*, **69**, 505–10.

Check, J.H., Nowroozi, K., Choe, J., and Dietterich, C. (1991). Influence of endometrial thickness and echo patterns on pregnancy rates during in vitro fertilization. *Fertility and Sterility*, **56**, 1173–5.

Check, J.H., Nowroozi, K., Choe, J., Lurie, D., and Dietterich, C. (1993). The effect of endometrial thickness and echo pattern on in vitro fertilization outcome in donor oocyte–embryo transfer cycle. *Fertility and Sterility*, **59**, 72–5.

Cicinelli, E., Ignarro, L.J., Lograno, M., Galantino, P., Balzano, G., and Schonauer, L.M. (1996). Circulating levels of nitric oxide in fertility women in relation to the menstrual cycle. *Fertility and Sterility*, **66**, 1036–8.

Collins, W., Jurkovic, D., Bourne, T., Kurjak, A., and Campbell, S. (1991). Ovarian morphology, endocrine function, and intrafollicular blood flow during the periovulatory period. *Human Reproduction*, **6**, 319–24.

Coulam, C.B., Bustillo, M., Soenksen, D.M., and Britten, S.T. (1994). Ultrasonographic predictors of implantation after assisted reproduction. *Fertility and Sterility*, **62**, 1004–10.

De Cherney, A.H., Romero, R., and Polan, M.L. (1982). Ultrasound in reproductive endocrinology. *Fertility and Sterility*, **37**, 25–35.

De Geyter, C., Schmitter, M., De Geyter, M., Nieschlag, E., Holzgreve, W., and Schneider, H.P.G. (2000). Prospective evaluation of the ultrasound appearance of the endometrium in a cohort of 1186 infertile women. *Fertility and Sterility*, **73**, 106–13.

De Vries, K., Lyons, E.A., Ballard, G., Levi, C.S., and Lindsay, D. (1990). Contraction of the inner third of the myometrium. *American Journal of Obstetrics and Gynecology*, **162**, 679–82.

Deichert, U. and Buurman, C. (1995). Transabdominal Doppler sonographic measurements of blood flow differences in the main pelvic arteries during physiological spontaneous ovarian cycles. *Human Reproduction*, **10**, 1531–6.

Deutinger, J., Reinthaller, A., and Bernaschek, G. (1989). Transvaginal pulsed Doppler measures of blood flow velocity in the ovarian arteries during cycle stimulation and after follicle puncture. *Fertility and Sterility*, **51**, 466–70.

Dickey, R.P. (1997). Doppler ultrasound investigation of uterine and ovarian blood flow in infertility and early pregnancy. *Human Reproduction*, **3**, 467–503.

Dickey, R.P. and Hower, J.F. (1994). Effect of ovulation induction on uterine blood flow and oestradiol and progesterone concentrations in early pregnancy. *Human Reproduction*, **10**, 2875–9.

Dickey, R.P., Olar, T.T., Taylor, S.N., Curole, D.N., Rye, P.H., and Matulich, E.M. (1991). Relationship of follicle number, serum estradiol, and other factors to birth rate and multiparity in human menopausal gonadotropin-induced intrauterine insemination cycles. *Fertility and Sterility*, **56**, 89–92.

Dickey, R.P., Olar, T.T., Curole, D.N., Taylor, S.N., and Rye, P.H. (1992). Endometrial pattern and thickness associated with pregnancy outcome after assisted reproduction technologies. *Human Reproduction*, **7**, 418–21.

Dickey, R.P., Olar, T.T., Taylor, S.N., Curole, D.N., and Harrigill, K. (1993a). Relationship of biochemical pregnancy to preovulatory endometrial thickness and pattern in patients undergoing ovulation induction. *Human Reproduction*, **8**, 327–30.

Dickey, R.P., Olar, T.T., Taylor, S.N., Curole, D.N., and Matulich, E.M. (1993b). Relationship of endometrial thickness and pattern to fecundity in ovulation induction cycles: effect of clomiphene citrate alone and with human menopausal gonadotropin. *Fertility and Sterility*, **59**, 756–60.

Dickey, R.P., Olar, T.T., Taylor, S.N., Curole, D.N., and Rye, P.H. (1993c). Sequential clomiphene citrate and human menopausal gonadotropin for ovulation induction: comparison to clomiphene citrate alone and human menopausal gonadotropin alone. *Human Reproduction*, **8**, 56–9.

Dickey, R.P., Hower, J.F., Matulich, E.M., and Brown, G.T. (1994). Effect of standing on non-pregnant uterine blood flow. *Ultrasound in Obstetrics and Gynecology*, **4**, 480–7.

Donald, I., MacVicar, J., and Brown, T.G. (1958). Investigation of abdominal masses by pulsed ultrasound. *Lancet*, **i**, 1188.

Dubey, A.K., Wang, H.A., Duffy, P., and Penzias, A.S. (1995). The correlation between follicular measurements, oocyte morphology, and fertilization rates in an in vitro fertilization program. *Fertility and Sterility*, **64**, 787–90.

Ectors, F.J., Vanderzwalmen, P., Van Hoeck, J., et al. (1997). Relationship of human follicular diameter with oocyte fertilization and development after in-vitro fertilization or intracytoplasmic sperm injection. *Human Reproduction*, **12**, 2002–5.

Fanchin, R., Righini, C., Ayoubi, J.M., Olivennes, F., de Ziegler, D., and Frydman, R. (2000). New look at endometrial echogenicity: objective computer-assisted measurements predict endometrial receptivity in in vitro fertilization-embryo transfer. *Fertility and Sterility*, **74**, 274–81.

Favre, R., Bettahar, K., Grange, G., et al. (1993). Predictive value of transvaginal uterine Doppler assessment in an in vitro fertilization program. *Ultrasound in Obstetrics and Gynecology*, **3**, 350–3.

Fleischer, A.C., Herbert, C.M., Sacks, G.A., Wentz, A.C., Entman, S.S., and Jeames, A.E. (1986). Sonography of the endometrium during conception and nonconception cycles of in vitro fertilization and embryo transfer. *Fertility and Sterility*, **46**, 442–7.

Fujino, Y., Ito, F., Matuoka, I., Kojima, T., Koh, B., and Ogita, S. (1993). Pulsatility index of uterine artery in pregnancy and non-pregnant women. *Human Reproduction*, **8**, 1126–8.

Glissant, A., de Mouzon, J., and Frydman, R. (1985). Ultrasound study of the endometrium during in vitro fertilization cycles. *Fertility and Sterility*, **44**, 786–90.

Glock, J.L. and Brumsted, J.R. (1995). Color flow pulsed Doppler ultrasound in diagnosing luteal phase defect. *Fertility and Sterility*, **64**, 500–4.

Gonen, Y. and Casper, R. (1990). Prediction of implantation by the sonographic appearance of the endometrium during controlled ovarian stimulation for in vitro fertilization. *Journal of In Vitro Fertilization and Embryo Transfer*, **7**, 146–52.

Gonen, Y., Casper, R.F., Jacobson, W., and Blankier, J. (1989). Endometrial thickness and growth during ovarian stimulation: a possible predictor of implantation in in vitro fertilization. *Fertility and Sterility*, **52**, 466–50.

Gosling, R.G., Dunbar, G., King, D.H., et al. (1971). The quantitative analysis of occlusive peripheral arterial disease by a non-intrusive ultrasonic technique. *Angiology*, **22**, 52–5.

Gosling, R.G., Lo, P.T.S., and Taylor, M.G. (1991). Interpretation of pulsatility index in feeder arteries to low impedance vascular beds. *Ultrasound in Obstetrics and Gynecology*, **1**, 175–9.

Goswamy, R.K. and Steptoe, R.P. (1988). Doppler ultrasound studies of the uterine artery in spontaneous ovarian cycles. *Human Reproduction*, **3**, 721–6.

Goswamy, R.K., Williams, G., and Steptoe, P.C. (1988). Decreased uterine perfusion – a cause of infertility. *Human Reproduction*, **3**, 955–9.

Hackeloer, B.J., Fleming, R., Robinson, H.P., Adam, A.H., and Coutts, J.R.T. (1979). Correlation of ultrasonic and endocrinologic assessment of human follicular development. *American Journal of Obstetrics and Gynecology*, **135**, 122–8.

Haines, C.J. and Emes, A.L. (1991). The relationship between follicle diameter, fertilization rate, and microscopic embryo quality. *Fertility and Sterility*, **55**, 205–7.

Hamilton, C.J.C.M., Evers, J.L.H., Tan, F.E.S., and Hoogland, H.J. (1987). The reliability of ovulation prediction by a single ultrasonographic follicle measurement. *Human Reproduction*, **2**, 103–7.

Hofmann, G.E., Thie, J., Scott, R.T., and Navot, D. (1996). Endometrial thickness is predictive of histologic endometrial maturation in women undergoing hormone replacement for ovum donation. *Fertility and Sterility*, **66**, 380–3.

Hornstein, M.D., Barbieri, R.L., Ravnikar, V.A., and McShane, P.M. (1989). The effects of baseline ovarian cysts on the clinical response to controlled ovarian hyperstimulation in an in vitro fertilization program. *Fertility and Sterility*, **52**, 437–40.

Hsieh, Y.Y., Tsal, H.D., Chang, C.C., Lo, H.Y., and Chen, C.L. (2000). Low-dose aspirin for infertile women with thin endometrium receiving intrauterine insemination: a prospective randomized study. *Journal of Assisted Reproduction and Genetics*, **17**, 174–7.

Hurley, V.A., Osborn, J.C., and Leoni, M.A. (1991). Ultrasound-guided embryo transfer: a controlled trial. *Fertility and Sterility*, **55**, 559–62.

Ijland, M.M., Evers, J.L.H., Dunselman, G.A.J., van Katwijk, C., Lo, C.R., and Hoogland, H.J. (1996). Endometrial wavelike movements during the menstrual cycle. *Fertility and Sterility*, **65**, 746–9.

Ijland, M.M., Evers, J.L.H., Dunselman, G.A.J., and Hoogland, H.J. (1998). Endometrial wavelike activity, endometrial thickness, and ultrasound texture in controlled ovarian hyperstimulation cycles. *Fertility and Sterility*, **70**, 279–83.

Isaacs, J.D., Wells, C.S., Williams, D.B., Odem, R.R., Gast, M.J., and Strickler, R.C. (1996). Endometrial thickness is a valid monitoring parameter in cycles of ovulation induction with menotropins alone. *Fertility and Sterility*, **65**, 262–6.

Kan, A.K.S., Abdalla, H.I., Gafar, A.H., et al. (1999). Embryo transfer: ultrasound-guided versus clinical touch. *Human Reproduction*, **14**, 1259–61.

Karande, V.C., Scott, R.T., Jones, G.S., and Muasher, S.J. (1990). Non-functional ovarian cysts do not affect ipsilateral or contralateral ovarian performance during in-vitro fertilization. *Human Reproduction*, **5**, 431–3.

Kauppila, A., Kuikka, J., and Tuimala, R. (1978). Effect of fenoterol and isoxsuprine on myometrial and intervillous blood flow during late pregnancy. *Obstetrics and Gynecology*, **52**, 558–62.

Kossoff, G., Garrett, W.J., and Radovabovich, G. (1974). Gray scale echography in obstetrics and gynecology. *Australian Radiology*, **18**, 662.

Krampl, E. and Feichtinger, W. (1993). Endometrial thickness and echo patterns. *Human Reproduction*, **8**, 1339.

Kratochwil, A. (1969). Ein neus vaginales Schnittbildverfahren. *Geburtshilfe Frauenheilkd*, **29**, 379–85.

Kratochwil, A., Urbab, G.V., and Friedrich, F. (1972). Ultrasonic tomography of the ovaries. *Annales de Chirurgie et Gynaecologiae (Helsinki)*, **61**, 211–14.

Kupesic, S. and Kurjak, A. (1993). Uterine and ovarian perfusion during the periovulatory period assessed by transvaginal color Doppler. *Fertility and Sterility*, **60**, 439–43.

Kurjak, A., Kupesic-Urek, S., Schulman, H., and Zalud, I. (1991). Transvaginal color flow Doppler in the assessment of ovarian and uterine blood flow in infertile women. *Fertility and Sterility*, **56**, 870–3.

Kyei-Mensah, A., Maconochie, N., Zaidi, J., Pittrof, R., Campbell, S., and Tan, S.L. (1996). Transvaginal three-dimensional ultrasound: reproducibility of ovarian and endometrial volume measurements. *Fertility and Sterility*, **66**, 718–22.

Lass, A., Williams, G., Abusheikha, N., and Brinsden, P. (1999). The effect of endometrial polyps on outcomes of in vitro fertilization cycles. *Journal of Assisted Reproduction and Genetics*, **16**, 410–15.

Lee, A., Sator, M., Kratochwil, A., Deutinger, J., Binsdorfer, E.V., and Bernaschek, G. (1997). Endometrial volume change during spontaneous menstrual cycles: volumetry by transvaginal three-dimensional ultrasound. *Fertility and Sterility*, **68**, 831–5.

Leong, M., Leung, C., and Tucker, M. (1986). Ultrasound-assisted embryo transfer. *Journal of In Vitro Fertilization and Embryo Transfer*, **3**, 383–5.

Levi-Setti, P.E., Rognoni, G., Bozzo, M., et al. (1995). Color Doppler velocimetry of uterine arteries in pregnant and non-pregnant patients during multiovulation induction for IVF. *Journal of Assisted Reproduction and Genetics*, **12**, 413–17.

Lindow, S.W., Davies, N., Davey, D.A., and Smith, J.A. (1988). The effect of sublingual nifedipine on uteroplacental blood flow in hypertensive pregnancy. *British Journal of Obstetrics and Gynaecology*, **95**, 1276–81.

Lyons, E.A., Taylor, P.J., Zheng, X.H., Ballard, G., Levi, C.S., and Kredentser, J.V. (1991). Characterization of subendometrial myometrial contractions throughout the menstrual cycles in normal fertile women. *Fertility and Sterility*, **55**, 771–4.

Mansour, R.T., Aboulghar, M.A., Serour, G.I., and Riad, R. (1991). Fluid accumulation of the uterine cavity before transfer: a possible hindrance for implantation. *Journal of In Vitro Fertilization and Embryo Transfer*, **8**, 157–9.

Marrs, R.P., Vargyas, J.M., and March, C.M. (1983). Correlation of ultrasonic and endocrinologic measurements in human menopausal gonadotropin therapy. *American Journal of Obstetrics and Gynecology*, **145**, 417–21.

Merce, L., Garces, D., and de la Fuente, F. (1989). Luteal conversion of the ovarian flow velocity-time wave form: new ultrasonographic parameter of ovulation and luteal function. *Acta Obstetrica et Gynecologica Scandinavica*, **82**, 113–14.

Miller, K.F., Goldberg, J.M., and Falcone, T. (1996). Follicle size and implantation of embryos from in vitro fertilization. *Obstetrics and Gynecology*, **88**, 583–6.

Montan, S., Liedholm, H., Lingman, G., Marsal, K., Sjoberg, N.O., and Solum, T. (1987). Fetal and uteroplacental haemodynamics during short term atenolol treatment of hypertension in pregnancy. *British Journal of Obstetrics and Gynaecology*, **94**, 312–17.

Nackley, A.C. and Muasher, S.J. (1998). The significance of hydrosalpinx in in vitro fertilization. *Fertility and Sterility*, **69**, 373–84.

Nargund, G., Bourne, T., Doyle, P., et al. (1996). Associations between ultrasound indices of follicular blood flow, oocyte recovery, and preimplantation embryo quality. *Human Reproduction*, **11**, 109–13.

Nitschke-Dabelstein, S. (1983). Monitoring of follicular development using ultrasonography. In *Infertility – Male and Female*, Insler, V. and Lunenfeld, B., eds. Churchill-Livingstone, Edinburgh.

Noyes, N., Liu, H.C., Sultan, K., Schattman, G., and Rosenwaks, Z. (1995). Endometrial thickness appears to be a significant factor in embryo implantation in in-vitro fertilization. *Human Reproduction*, **10**, 919–22.

O'Herlihy, C., de Crespigny, L.Ch., Lopata, A., Johnston, I., Hoult, I., and Robinson, H. (1980). Preovulatory follicular size: a comparison of ultrasound and laparoscopic measurement. *Fertility and Sterility*, **34**, 24–6.

Oliveira, J.B.A., Baruffi, R.L.R., Mauri, A.L., Petersen, C.G., Borges, M.C., and Franco, J.G. (1997). Endometrial ultrasonography as a predictor of pregnancy in an in-vitro fertilization programme after ovarian stimulation and gonadotropin-releasing hormone and gonadotropin. *Human Reproduction*, **12**, 2515–18.

Oyesanya, O.A., Parsons, J.H., Collins, W.P., and Campbell, S. (1996). Prediction of oocyte recovery rate by transvaginal ultrasonography and color Doppler imaging before human chorionic gonadotropin administration in in vitro fertilization cycles. *Fertility and Sterility*, **65**, 806–9.

Pourcelot, L. (1974). Applications clinique de pexamen Doppler transcutane. In *Beclocimetric Ultrasonore Doppler*, Pourcelot L., ed. INSERM, Paris, p. 213.

Prapas, T., Prapas, N., and Hatziparasidou, A. (1995). The echo-guide embryo transfer maximizes the IVF results. *Acta Europaea Fertilitatis*, **26**, 113–15.

Pyrzak, R., Dickey, R.P., Sartor, S., Lu, P.Y., Taylor, S.N., and Rye, P.H. (1999a). Multiple pregnancy outcome in IVF–ET can be predicted by size of lead follicle at the time of hCG administration. *Fertility and Sterility*, **72**, S38.

Pyrzak, R., Dickey, R.P., Sartor, S., Lu, P.Y., Taylor, S.N., and Rye, P.H. (1999b). Relationship between lead follicular size and oocyte maturity in the cohort at the time of hCG administration. *Fertility and Sterility*, **72**, S98.

Queenan, J.T., O'Brien, G.D., Bains, L.M., Simpson, J., Collins, W.P., and Campbell, S. (1980). Ultrasound scanning of ovaries to detect ovulation in women. *Fertility and Sterility*, **34**, 99–105.

Rabinowitz, R., Laufer, N., Lewin, A., Navot, D., Bar, I., and Margalioth, E.J. (1986). The value of ultrasonographic endometrial measurement in the prediction of pregnancy following in vitro fertilization. *Fertility and Sterility*, **45**, 824–8.

Randall, J.M. and Templeton, A. (1991). Transvaginal sonographic assessment of follicular and endometrial growth in spontaneous and clomiphene citrate cycles. *Fertility and Sterility*, **56**, 208–12.

Randall, J.M., Fisk, M.M., McTavish, A., and Templeton, A.A. (1989). Transvaginal ultrasonic assessment of endometrial growth in spontaneous and hyperstimulated menstrual cycles. *British Journal of Obstetrics and Gynaecology*, **96**, 954–9.

Rinaldi, L., Lisi, F., Floccari, A., Lisi, R., Pepe, G., and Fishel, S. (1996). Endometrial thickness as a predictor of pregnancy after in-vitro fertilization but not after intracytoplasmic sperm injection. *Human Reproduction*, **11**, 1538–41.

Rizk, B., Tan, S.L., Kingsland, C., Steer, C., Mason, B.A., and Campbell, S. (1990). Ovarian cyst aspiration and the outcome of in vitro fertilization. *Fertility and Sterility*, **54**, 661–4.

Rogers, P.A.W., Polson, D., Murphy, C.R., Hosie, M., Susil, B., and Leoni, M. (1991). Correlation of endometrial histology, morphometry, and ultrasound appearance after different stimulation protocols for in vitro fertilization. *Fertility and Sterility*, **55**, 583–7.

Rubinstein, M., Marazzi, A., and de Fried, E.P. (1999). Low-dose aspirin treatment improves ovarian responsiveness, uterine and ovarian blood flow velocity, implantation, and pregnancy rates in patients undergoing in vitro fertilization: a prospective, randomized double-blind placebo-controlled assay. *Fertility and Sterility*, **71**, 825–9.

Salha, O., Nugent, D., Dada, T., et al. (1998). The relationship between follicular fluid aspirate volume and oocyte maturity in in-vitro fertilization cycles. *Human Reproduction*, **13**, 1901–6.

Scholtes, M.C.W., Wladimiroff, J.W., van Rijen, H.J.M., and Hop, W.C.J. (1989). Uterine and ovarian flow velocity waveforms in the normal menstrual cycle: a transvaginal study. *Fertility and Sterility*, **52**, 981–5.

Scott, R.T., Hofmann, G.E., Muasher, S.J., Acosta, A.A., Kreiner, D.K., and Rosenwaks, Z. (1989). Correlation of follicular diameter with oocyte recovery and maturity at the time of transvaginal follicular aspiration. *Journal of In Vitro Fertilization and Embryo Transfer*, **6**, 73–5.

Serafini, P., Batzofin, J., Nelson, J., and Olive, D. (1994). Sonographic uterine predictors of pregnancy in women undergoing ovulation induction for assisted reproductive treatments. *Fertility and Sterility*, **62**, 815–22.

Sharara, F.I., Lim, J., and McClamrock, D. (1999). Endometrial pattern on the day of oocyte retrieval is more predictive of implantation success than the pattern or thickness on the day of hCG administration. *Journal of Assisted Reproduction and Genetics*, **16**, 523–8.

Sher, G. and Fisch, J.D. (2000). Vaginal sildenafil (Viagra): a preliminary report of a novel method to improve uterine artery blood flow and endometrial development in patients undergoing IVF. *Human Reproduction*, **13**, 806–9.

Sher, G., Herbert, C., Maassarani, G., and Jacobs, M.H. (1991). Assessment of the late proliferative phase endometrium by ultrasonography in patients undergoing in-vitro fertilization and embryo transfer. *Human Reproduction*, **6**, 232–7.

Sher, G., Dodge, S., Maassarani, G., Knutzen, V., Zouves, C., and Feinman, M. (1993). Management of suboptimal sonographic endometrial patterns in patients undergoing in-vitro fertilization and embryo transfer. *Human Reproduction*, **8**, 347–9.

Shoham, Z., De Carlo, C., Patel, A., Conway, G.S., and Jacobs, H.S. (1991). Is it possible to run a successful ovulation induction program based solely on ultrasound monitoring? The importance of endometrial measurements. *Fertility and Sterility*, **56**, 836–41.

Silverberg, K.M., Olive, D.L., Burns, W.N., Johnson, J.V., Groff, T.R., and Schenken, R.S. (1991). Follicular size at the time of hCG administration predicts ovulation outcome in human menopausal gonadotropin-stimulated cycles. *Fertility and Sterility*, **56**, 296–300.

Sladkevicius, P., Valentin, L., and Marsal, K. (1993). Blood flow velocity in the uterine and ovarian arteries during the normal menstrual cycle. *Ultrasound in Obstetrics and Gynecology*, **3**, 199–208.

Smith, B., Porter, R., Ahuja, K., and Craft, I. (1984). Ultrasonic assessment of endometrial changes in stimulated cycles in an in vitro fertilization and embryo transfer program. *Journal of In Vitro Fertilization and Embryo Transfer*, **1**, 233–8.

Smith, D.H., Picker, R.H., Sinosich, M., and Saunders, D.M. (1980). Assessment of ovulation by ultrasound and estradiol levels during spontaneous and induced cycles. *Fertility and Sterility*, **33**, 387–90.

Spencer, J.A.D., Giussani, D.A., Moore, P.D., and Hanson, M.A. (1991). In vitro validation of Doppler indices using blood and water. *Journal of Ultrasound Medicine*, **10**, 305–8.

Steer, C.V., Campbell, S., Pampiglione, J., Mason, B.A., and Collins, W.P. (1990). Transvaginal colour flow imaging of the uterine arteries during the ovarian and menstrual cycles. *Human Reproduction*, **5**, 391–5.

Steer, C.V., Campbell, S., Tan, S.L., et al. (1992). The use of transvaginal color flow imaging after in vitro fertilization to identify optimum uterine conditions before embryo transfer. *Fertility and Sterility*, **57**, 372–6.

Steer, C.V., Tan, S.L., Mason, B.A., and Campbell, S. (1994). Midluteal phase vaginal color Doppler assessment of uterine artery impedance in a subfertile population. *Fertility and Sterility*, **61**, 53–8.

Steer, C.V., Tan, S.L., Dillon, D., Mason, B.A., and Campbell, S. (1995). Vaginal color Doppler assessment of uterine artery impedance correlates with immunohistochemical markers of endometrial receptivity required for the implantation of an embryo. *Fertility and Sterility*, **63**, 101–8.

Sterzik, K., Hutter, W., Grab, D., Rosenbusch, B., Sasse, V., and Terinde, R. (1989). Doppler sonographic findings and their correlation with implantation in an in vitro fertilization program. *Fertility and Sterility*, **52**, 825–8.

Sterzik, K., Abt, M., Grab, D., Schneider, V., and Strehler, E. (2000). Predicting the histologic dating of an endometrial biopsy specimen with the use of Doppler ultrasonography and hormone measurements in patients undergoing spontaneous ovulatory cycles. *Fertility and Sterility*, **73**, 94–8.

Strickler, R.C., Christianson, C., and Crane, J.P. (1985). Ultrasound guidance for human embryo transfer. *Fertility and Sterility*, **43**, 54–61.

Strohmer, H., Herczeg, C., Plockinger, B., Kemeter, P., and Feichtinger, W. (1991). Prognostic appraisal of success and failure in an in vitro fertilization program by transvaginal Doppler ultrasound at the time of ovulation induction. *Ultrasound in Obstetrics and Gynecology*, **1**, 272–4.

Strohmer, H., Obruca, A., Radner, K.M., and Feichtinger, W. (1994). Relationship of the individual uterine size and the endometrial thickness in stimulated cycles. *Fertility and Sterility*, **61**, 972–5.

Sundstrom, P. (1998). Establishment of a successful pregnancy following in-vitro fertilization with an endometrial thickness of no more than 4 mm. *Human Reproduction*, **13**, 1550–2.

Tan, S.L., Zaidi, J., Campbell, S., Doyle, P., and Collins, W. (1996). Blood flow changes in the ovarian and uterine arteries during the normal menstrual cycle. *American Journal of Obstetrics and Gynaecology*, **175**, 625–31.

Taylor, K.J.M., Burns, P.N., Wells, P.N.T., Conway, D.I., and Hull, N.G.R. (1985). Ultrasound Doppler flow studies of the ovarian and uterine arteries. *British Journal of Obstetrics and Gynaecology*, **92**, 240–6.

Tekay, A. and Jouppila, P. (1996). Intraobserver reproducibility of transvaginal Doppler measurements in uterine and intra-ovarian arteries in regularly menstruating women. *Ultrasound in Obstetrics and Gynaecology*, **7**, 129–34.

Tekay, A., Martikainen, H. and Jouppila, P. (1995a). Blood flow changes in uterine and ovarian vasculature, and predictive value of transvaginal pulsed colour Doppler ultrasonography in an in vitro fertilization programme. *Human Reproduction*, **10**, 688–93.

Tekay, A., Martikainen, H., and Jouppila, P. (1995b). Doppler parameters of the ovarian and uterine blood circulation in ovarian hyperstimulation syndrome. *Ultrasound in Obstetrics and Gynaecology*, **6**, 50–3.

Tekay, A., Martikainen, H., and Jouppila, P. (1996a). The clinical value of Doppler ultrasound. *Human Reproduction*, **11**, 1589–93.

Tekay, A., Martikainen, H., and Jouppila, P. (1996b). Comparison of uterine blood flow characteristics between spontaneous and stimulated cycles before embryo transfer. *Human Reproduction*, **11**, 364–8.

Thatcher, S.S., Jones, E., and de Cherney, A.H. (1989). Ovarian cysts decrease the success of controlled ovarian stimulation and in vitro fertilization. *Fertility and Sterility*, **52**, 812–16.

Tsai, H.D., Chang, C.C., Hsieh, Y.Y., Lee, C.C., and Lo, H.Y. (2000). Role of endometrial thickness and pattern, of vascular impedance of the spiral and uterine arteries, and of the dominant follicle. *Journal of Reproductive Medicine*, **44**, 195–200.

Ueno, J., Oehninger, S., Bryzski, R.G., Acosta, A.A., Philput, B., and Muasher, S.J. (1991). Ultrasonographic appearance of the endometrium in natural and stimulated in-vitro fertilization cycles and its correlation with outcome. *Human Reproduction*, **6**, 901–4.

Van Voorhis, B.J., Sparks, E.T., Syrop, C.H., and Stovall, D.W. (1998). Ultrasound-guided aspiration of hydrosalpinges is associated with improved pregnancy and implantation rates after in-vitro fertilization cycles. *Human Reproduction*, **13**, 736–9.

Wada, I., Hs, C.C., Williams, G., Macnamee, M.C., and Brinsden, P.R. (1994). The benefits of low-dose aspirin therapy in women with impaired uterine perfusion during assisted conception. *Human Reproduction*, **9**, 1954–7.

Weckstein, L.N., Jacobson, A., Galen, D., Hampton, K., and Hammel, J. (1997). Low-dose aspirin or oocyte donation recipients with a thin endometrium: prospective, randomized study. *Fertility and Sterility*, **68**, 927–30.

Weiner, Z., Thaler, I., Levron, J., Lewit, N., and Itskovitz-Eldor, J. (1993). Assessment of ovarian and uterine blood flow by transvaginal color Doppler in ovarian-stimulated women: correlation with the number of follicles and steroid hormone levels. *Fertility and Sterility*, **59**, 743–9.

Weissman, A., Gotlieb, L., and Casper, R.F. (1999). The detrimental effect of increased endometrial thickness on implantation and pregnancy rates and outcome in an in vitro fertilization program. *Fertility and Sterility*, **71**, 147–9.

Welker, B.G., Gembruch, U., Diedrich, K., Al-Hasani, S., and Krebs, D. (1989). Transvaginal sonography of the endometrium during ovum pickup in stimulated cycles for in vitro fertilization. *Journal of Ultrasound Medicine*, **8**, 549–53.

Wittmaack, F.M., Kreger, D.O., Blasco, L., Tureck, R.W., Mastroianni, L., and Lessey, B.A. (1994). Effect of follicular size on oocyte retrieval, fertilization, cleavage, and embryo quality in in vitro fertilization cycles: a 6-year data collection. *Fertility and Sterility*, **62**, 1205–10.

Woolcott, R. and Stanger, J. (1997). Potentially important variables identified by transvaginal ultrasound-guided embryo transfer. *Human Reproduction*, **12**, 963–6.

Ylostalo, P., Ronnberg, L., and Jouppila, P. (1979). Measurement of the ovarian follicle by ultrasound in ovulation induction. *Fertility and Sterility*, **31**, 651–5.

Zaidi, J., Campbell, S., Pittrof, R., et al. (1995a). Ovarian stromal blood flow in women with polycystic ovaries – a possible new marker for diagnosis. *Human Reproduction*, **10**, 1992–6.

Zaidi, J., Jurkovic, D., Campbell, S., Collins, W., McGregor, A., and Tan, S.L. (1995b). Luteinized unruptured follicles: morphology, endocrine function and blood flow changes during the menstrual cycle. *Human Reproduction*, **10**, 44–9.

Zaidi, J., Jurkovic, D., Campbell, S., Pittrof, R., McGregor, A., and Tan, S.L. (1995c). Description of circadian rhythm in uterine artery blood flow during the periovulatory period. *Human Reproduction*, **10**, 1642–6.

Zaidi, J., Barber, J., Kyei-Mensah, A., Bekir, J., Campbell, S., and Tan, S.L. (1996a). Relationship of ovarian stromal blood flow at the baseline ultrasound scan to subsequent follicular response in an in vitro fertilization program. *Obstetrics and Gynaecology*, **88**, 779–84.

Zaidi, J., Collins, W., Campbell, S., Pittrof, R., and Tan, S.L. (1996b). Blood flow changes in the intraovarian arteries during the periovulatory period: relationship to the time of day. *Ultrasound Obstetrics and Gynaecology*, **7**, 135–40.

Zaidi, J., Pittrof, R., Shaker, A., Kyei-Mensah, A., Campbell, S., and Tan, S.L. (1996c). Assessment of uterine artery blood flow on the day of human chorionic gonadotropin administration by transvaginal color Doppler ultrasound in an in vitro fertilization program. *Fertility and Sterility*, **65**, 377–81.

19

The natural and the stimulated cycle

Ian D. Cooke

University of Sheffield, Sheffield, UK

Introduction

The natural cycle seemed the obvious starting point to Edwards et al. (1980) in their attempts to bring in vitro fertilization (IVF) into clinical use. However, they soon abandoned it in favor of a more controllable endocrine program. Ovarian hyperstimulation, which replaced it, resulted in multiple follicular development and a greater yield of oocytes; it led to a larger number of embryos being available. To overcome poor pregnancy rates, larger numbers of embryos were transferred and higher order multiple pregnancies resulted. The high mortality and morbidity rates and the socioeconomic cost of higher order multiple pregnancies raised many questions about the wisdom of transferring large numbers of embryos. This led to the regulation in some countries, e.g. the Human Fertilization and Embryology Authority (HFEA) in the UK, that not more than three embryos could be transferred after IVF.

More recently, with improvements in culture techniques, there have been attempts to transfer single embryos, but there has been reluctance on the part of clinics to accept any reduction in pregnancy rates. The natural cycle remains the choice of those patients who cannot accept the multiple pregnancy risk, the potential complications, or the cost of stimulated IVF. They must accept a very reduced livebirth rate, repeated attempts, or even failure. However, there is considerable pressure on scientists and clinicians to move toward single livebirths. The natural cycle has been disappointing, but the end-point of a single livebirth cannot only be reached from that approach to treatment.

This chapter reviews the background of natural cycle IVF in relation to the stimulated cycle. Further, it will indicate the future direction of developments in the field of IVF that attempt to achieve the objective of a single livebirth.

The natural cycle

The early years of natural cycle IVF (i.e., completely natural, without using human chorionic gonadotropin (hCG)) were reviewed by Lenton et al. (1992, 1995). In their 1991–3 program, 676 treatment cycles (including women over 40 years) resulted in a livebirth rate of 6.8% (46/676). This was made up of an 82% egg collection rate, a 72% normal fertilization rate of oocytes collected, and a 53% embryo transfer (ET)/cycle started. There was a 19% implantation rate of those embryos transferred and the clinical pregnancy rate was 15.8%/ET.

Foulot et al. (1989) had reported 26 unstimulated cycles with a luteinizing hormone (LH) surge, but 19 of them had received a "reinforcing" dose of 3000 IU hCG. There was an ongoing pregnancy rate of 11.5% (3/26).

Svalander et al. (1991) also described 51 unstimulated cycles in 44 patients, but they routinely used 5000 IU hCG. They achieved six ongoing pregnancies (12%). In the same period, they had 121 patients treated in stimulated cycles and made the comparison that 71% of stimulated cycles achieved ET whereas only 39% of natural cycles did so.

From 101 cycles started, Paulson et al. (1992) achieved 78 aspirations after 10 000 IU hCG was used to trigger ovulation. Of the oocytes obtained, 66 were from dominant follicles and 61 from secondary follicles, 82 embryos being transferred in 63 procedures. Nevertheless there were only 9% (9/100) clinical pregnancies with no difference between single and multiple transfers.

A comparison was made by Claman et al. (1993) between 75 unstimulated cycles, supplemented with 2500 or 5000 IU hCG, and 450 superovulated cycles. There were 47% (37/75) cancellations before oocyte recovery in the natural cycles and 25% (112/450) in the superovulated group. One or more oocytes were aspirated in 60% (24/40) and 99% (336/338) of natural and stimulated cycles, respectively. These led to 11% and 22% pregnancies/ET, respectively. The numbers of term pregnancies per oocyte recovery were 5% (2/40) and 14% (48/338) and the numbers of pregnancies per cycle started 2.7 (2/75) and 14.4% (65/450), respectively. These authors concluded that since procedure and laboratory costs had been incurred in spite of cancellations and because of failed retrievals, "natural cycle" IVF (which should more accurately be termed "unstimulated" IVF) was too inefficient to be used compared with superovulation IVF.

Fahy et al. (1995) also reported on their completely natural cycle experience, i.e., *not* using supplementary hCG. They described a 7.6% clinical pregnancy rate per cycle. They noted that much more intensive monitoring was required, but therein lay an opportunity for clinical research into unexplained infertility or that associated with endometriosis. There were also hints that patient selection, such as choosing women of less than 40 years with normal follicle-stimulating hormone (FSH) concentrations and having partners with normal semen parameters, could provide suitable candidates for natural cycle IVF.

The reason for using hCG to trigger ovulation is that intensive monitoring of serum LH is avoided. Lenton (1993) described the relationship between particular concentrations of serum LH at 08.00 and the variable, but corresponding, time of ovulation on the following day. hCG has been used to overcome this superficial unpredictability in an attempt to program the cycle more efficiently to create a clinical service. Fahy et al. (1995) described how the patients themselves collected the serial blood samples for the assays. Lindheim et al. (1998) described the potential use of serum progesterone and inhibin A on the day of hCG administration as the concentrations were lower in those cycles where ET was achieved.

Using hCG, Daya et al. (1995) described the results of 240 unstimulated cycles resulting in nine livebirths (3.75%). However, when the data were re-expressed as 12% clinical pregnancies/ET or 10% livebirths/ET, these data were claimed as a "suitable alternative" to stimulated cycles for IVF. This conclusion was reached after pooling all the outcome data from the studies described above to yield 6.8% (56/828) livebirths/cycle. These data were compared with 16.1% livebirths/cycle with stimulated IVF (American Fertility Society and the Society for Assisted Reproductive Technology, 1994). The cost of natural cycle IVF was calculated to be $1200 versus $5680 for stimulated IVF, which included the cost of drugs, embryo cryopreservation and one ET using thawed oocytes. The 16.1% was made up of 14.3% from the initial stimulated cycle and 18% frozen/thawed cycles, each of which has an 11.6% livebirth rate. From these calculations the cost of IVF/livebirth was US$17 647 for an unstimulated cycle and $35 280 for a stimulated cycle. In other words, the difference in cost (incremental cost) in treating 100 couples by each method would be that the stimulated regimen would be $48 172 more expensive, a figure of some importance in a nationalized or managed care system.

Further arguments against stimulated IVF are the greater discomfort, the greater frequency of general anesthesia, the slower recovery period before another attempt can be made, and the seemingly larger emotional toll. The risk of occurrence of ovarian hyperstimulation syndrome and the possible increased risk of malignancy, although not yet clear, relating to ovarian cancer, but more likely breast and uterine corpus cancer, may further increase anxiety (Venn et al., 1995). Additional points are that there may be a need for embryo cryo-preservation (not permitted in Germany) or fetal reduction, which to some is abhorrent.

Although natural cycle IVF was initially used for treating tubal disease, patients with endometriosis could also be treated, but with a lower success rate. Reduced semen quality is inimical to success, but the use of stimulated cycles and intracytoplasmic sperm injection (ICSI) has superseded its use in male factor infertility. ICSI could, however, potentially increase the fertilization rate and extend the indications for natural cycle use.

In natural cycle IVF, repeat cycles provide acceptable results. Lenton et al. (1995) described 13.5% livebirths/ET in a first cycle and 11.8% in a second. Janssens et al. (2000) reported a 5.3% ongoing pregnancy/cycle started in 75 unstimulated cycles with hCG. There were six patients who had second attempts, yielding a cumulative ongoing pregnancy rate of 9.8% (8/81). Paulson et al. (1992) had reported a cumulative clinical pregnancy rate of 43% from 46 initial cycles, nine reaching the third attempt.

Lenton et al. (1995) showed that in the under 31 year age group natural cycle IVF yielded 7.3% livebirths/cycle and stimulated IVF resulted in 33.6% livebirths/cycle. In contrast, in those aged 40 years and over, the natural cycle group resulted in 6.3% livebirths/cycle against 6.0% livebirths/cycle in stimulated cycles. Bar-Hava et al. (2000) described using unstimulated cycle IVF ($\pm$ hCG) in women aged 44–47 years, since stimulated IVF and oocyte donation was refused to this age group. Twenty women were treated in 48 cycles, oocyte retrieval being 46% and fertilization 48%. Only one clinical and one ongoing pregnancy were achieved in spite of 9 of 12 embryos being grade A (highest quality). Ron-El et al. (2000) described a mean of 5.3% (17/320) births/oocyte retrieval procedure in women aged 41–43 years (ranging from 2 to 7% at each age), but there were no pregnancies beyond 43 years of age.

"Proper patient selection" in unstimulated cycles using hCG to trigger ovulation was discussed by Seibel et al. (1995). They described a clinical pregnancy rate of 9.4% (6/64), but by restricting age to 26–34 years, there were seven pregnancies from 17 ET after one or two attempts. They suggested that an unstimulated IVF cycle could be used to identify those patients more likely to succeed at IVF. Lenton and Woodward (1993) took this much further, classifying couples according to cause (male factor or unexplained infertility) and whether fertilization occurred normally, abnormally, or not at all. The results of subsequent stimulated IVF cycles were then correlated. They showed that there was a substantial difference at the subsequent stimulated IVF between male factor and unexplained infertility as cause. After normal fertilization had occurred in natural cycle IVF, there was always embryo replacement at stimulated IVF. The delivery rate/cycle with ET was 38% (3/8) and 9% (2/23), respectively. As spare embryos developed to blastocysts in 62% (8/13) and 96% (22/23) respectively, the problem could be failure of in vivo fertilization and an endometrial problem respectively. In the two categories of male and unexplained infertility, those cases where abnormal fertilization occurred resulted in 25% and 22% of stimulated cycles without any ET, but there were excellent delivery rates/ET where normal fertilization did occur (44 and 36%, respectively). In those cycles where no oocyte was obtained or the cycle was cancelled before oocyte recovery, there were very poor delivery rates/ET (7 and 6%) respectively. They postulated that natural cycle IVF could be used as a screening program, particularly for male factor infertility and unexplained infertility.

Of course male factor cases would now more likely be treated by ICSI, but cost could militate against this. Malpani and Malpani (1992), because of the lower cost, felt that natural cycle IVF could have a place in the developing world. A screening natural cycle would result in much higher delivery rates in those selected to proceed to stimulated IVF, making the cost per maternity much lower.

Unusual clinical conditions may suggest a role for unstimulated IVF. Brown et al. (1996) reported using an unstimulated cycle (with hCG) in a patient after surgery for carcinoma of the breast, as they wished

Table 19.1. Pregnancy outcomes

Pregnancies	Livebirths	Perinatal mortality rate (per 1000)[a]
Singletons	3902	10.5
Twins	1526	41.3
Triplets	256	74.2
Quadruplets	2	500

Notes:
[a]Stillbirths and neonatal deaths.
Source: Data from Human Fertilization and Embryology Authority (1999).

to avoid substantial endocrine stimulation prior to combination chemotherapy. One follicle yielded a mature oocyte, which was fertilized and the embryo cryopreserved. A second immature oocyte was successfully re-inseminated and ultimately a second embryo was cryopreserved. The embryos had not been thawed at the time of the report.

Multiple pregnancy

The HFEA Annual Report (Human Fertilization and Embryology Authority, 1999) for the UK, covering the period from April 1997 to March 1998, indicated that 31.4% (1784/5686) of all births from IVF and frozen embryo transfers were multiple. The perinatal mortality rate following multiple pregnancy is markedly increased and it is well documented (Petterson et al., 1993) that the morbidity and long-term handicap(s) are high with the higher order pregnancies (Table 19.1). From these data, it was apparent that unstimulated cycles constituted only 0.003% (77/26163) of the cycles. In US data published by the Society for Assisted Reproductive Technology and the American Society for Reproductive Medicine (2000), it was evident that the multiple pregnancy rate from stimulated IVF in 1997 was 39% and this rose to 44.7% in women of 34 years or more who had no male factor cause for infertility. About 6.8% of all deliveries were triplet or of a higher order.

Much attention has recently been drawn to the risks to the children and the mothers (Elster et al., 2000; Olivennes, 2000). Vilska et al. (1999) compared a single ET after stimulated IVF when there was only *one* embryo available and when there were *two or more* available. The clinical pregnancy rates/ET were 20.2% and 29.7% respectively, but in the latter group there were 24% twins. In women 35 years old or less, the pregnancy rate following elective transfer of one embryo was 32.8%. The cumulative pregnancy rates were subsequently increased by the use of frozen/thawed embryos. Gerris et al. (1999) carried out a prospective, randomized, controlled trial of single and two ETs after IVF or ICSI in women of less than 34 years of age. Criteria for top-quality embryos had been decided (van Royen et al., 1999) and such embryos, when available, were transferred to randomized patients. There was no difference in implantation rates of 42.3% for single and 48.1% for two ETs. There were no dizygotic twins in the single ET group (n=26). Hazecamp et al. (2000) have recommended that data be reported as *birth rates per embryo transferred* to reflect the value of single ET and to compromise figures when larger numbers of embryos are transferred.

The European Society of Human Reproduction and Embryology (ESHRE Capri Workshop Group, 2000) has strongly recommended reducing the number of embryos transferred and has suggested that embryo reduction should be used only as a last resort. They point out that currently the average hospital cost per multiple gestation is greater than the average cost of IVF and ICSI cycles, highlighting the need for prevention.

Improvements in stage-specific embryo culture media have led to extended culture to the blastocyst stage. Certainly transferred blastocysts can yield excellent results; however, it is not easy to calculate, from the data provided, the proportion of cycles started that ultimately reach the blastocyst stage. A recent randomized controlled trial of a broad spectrum of eligible patients (201) using culture in appropriate media compared subsequent transfer on day 3 with transfer on day 5 (Coskun et al., 2000). Eligible patients still required four or more fertilized oocytes to have a chance of reaching the blastocyst stage. Pregnancy rates/ET were the same in each group (39%), but on day 5 there were one or more blastocysts available in only 48% of patients. The triplet pregnancy rates were low (no ongoing pregnancy) by transfer of only two embryos, but the twin rates were high (33 and 38%, respectively), leading the authors to state that "further efforts should be made towards reducing multiple pregnancies as far as possible by transferring a single embryo . . . or blastocyst."

The practice of transferring multiple embryos is now experiencing a strong backlash. Education of clinic staff, the patients, and public health providers will inexorably push practitioners to single embryo/blastocyst transfer. Staff will need to learn to cope with the problem of not having an embryo to transfer, a problem that was common in natural cycle management.

Additional physiological data

Some interesting data have come from the more intensive study of natural cycles. The geometric mean serum estradiol concentration was 1279 pmol/l in cycles that lead to fertilization of the oocyte, whereas it was 1055 pmol/l in cycles where the oocyte was not fertilized. Functional oocyte competence was not related to follicle diameter (Cahill et al., 2000). The preovulatory LH surge begins between midnight and 08.00, but it seems unlikely to occur either before the follicle has reached 15 mm or before the serum estradiol concentration has reached 600 pmol/l (Cahill et al., 1998). Patients with minimal and mild endometriosis and with unexplained infertility had a longer follicular phase, reduced estradiol secretion (as expressed by the median of areas under the curve), and a significantly reduced peak serum LH (Cahill et al., 1995). Ovarian stimulation results in supraphysiological concentrations of progesterone and estrogen in the luteal phase, leading to a reduced implantation rate and a higher pregnancy loss before pregnancies can be detected clinically compared with natural cycle conceptions (Macklon and Fauser, 2000). Junctional zone myometrial activity is more exaggerated in stimulated cycles compared with natural cycles. The increased mobility of the endometrium may impair its receptivity and affect implantation (Lesny et al., 1998). Fukuda et al. (1996) reported that, when ovulation occurred on the opposite side in a succeeding cycle, natural cycle oocyte retrieval, fertilization, cleavage, and ET rates were significantly higher than when ovulation occurred on the same side as the previous cycle.

There is a significant increase in the total number of lymphocytes, B cells, and natural killer cells in the late follicular phase and the T helper/ T suppressor cell ratio declines (Giuliana et al., 1998).

Ultrasonographic appearances of the endometrium are similar in natural and stimulated cycles. A homogeneous, hyperechoic pattern on the day prior to oocyte retrieval was associated with nonconceptual cycles (Ueno et al., 1991). Hassan and Saleh (1996) selected patients with a natural cycle in which the endometrium was not greater than 7 mm thickness. These patients were given estriol 6–8 mg/day from the time that the leading follicle reached a diameter of 12 mm. Those that responded by increasing their endometrial thickness to greater than 7 mm at the time of maximum follicular diameter had a 21.7% (5/23) pregnancy rate in a subsequent stimulated cycle. The authors recommend natural cycle evaluation for prediction of response in a later stimulated cycle. Kliman et al. (1997) described abnormalities in immunohistochemistry of endometrial glandular or Golgi MAG mucin (mouse ascites Golgi epitope) expression in patients of blood groups A and AB in a natural cycle, which was highly predictive of failure in a subsequent stimulated cycle.

Other stimulation regimens

A prospective randomized controlled trial of unstimulated and clomiphene-stimulated IVF (100 mg daily from days 2 to 6), each with hCG, was carried out by MacDougall et al. (1994). There were

2.4 ± 0.3 (standard error (SE)) follicles in the clomiphene group against 0.9 ± 0.2 for the unstimulated group; peak serum estradiol concentrations were 1387 ± 247 and 748 ± 61 pmol/l, respectively. All 16 cycles reached oocyte recovery in the stimulated group, whereas 10 of 14 cycles in the unstimulated group were cancelled. The cancellation figures were more striking than those reported from larger programs where more experience had been gained.

Branigan and Estes (2000) found that oral contraception could prevent or delay the LH surge in the cycle after it was stopped and used this approach to avoid premature LH surges in clomiphene/hCG-stimulated IVF cycles. A monophasic low-dose oral contraceptive was given continuously for 35–42 days. Clomiphene 100 mg daily was given on day 3 of a subsequent cycle for eight days, two follicles being required to proceed. In this mild stimulation regimen, 10% of cycles were cancelled, a mean of 2.5 embryos were transferred, and a clinical pregnancy rate of 32.8% (21/64) was achieved. This compared with 1.1 embryos transferred and a 15.4% clinical pregnancy rate (8/52; $p < 0.05$) in an unstimulated group. A contemporary stimulated group had 3.3 embryos transferred, a clinical pregnancy rate of 44% (33/75; not significant), and 9% (3/33) twin gestations.

Recognizing the importance of single follicle development, Rongieres-Bertrand et al. (1999) gave a gonadotropin-releasing hormone (GnRH) antagonist Cetrorelix (Asta Medica, France) 0.5 or 1 mg subcutaneously when the serum estradiol concentration was 367–551 pmol/l and there was a lead follicle of 12–14 mm. At the same time, human menopausal gonadotropin (hMG; 150 IU daily-mean, 4.7 ampules) was given and repeated daily until hCG administration. There were 4 of 44 cycles cancelled and in 10 cycles no oocyte was obtained. Fertilization failed despite ICSI in six cycles. Seven clinical and five ongoing pregnancies were obtained, giving a 22.7% ongoing pregnancy rate/ET and a 12.5% pregnancy rate/retrieval.

The GnRH antagonist Nal-Glu has been used in natural cycles in five oocyte donors at a daily intramuscular dosage of 75 μg/kg starting at a mean follicle diameter of 14 mm. A step-down hMG regimen was continued until the day after the hCG administration. Two ongoing pregnancies were achieved (Meldrum et al., 1994).

Retrieval of immature oocytes

In 1991, Cha et al. described aspiration of immature unstimulated oocytes. They were cultured in follicular fluid, fertilized in vitro, and ultimately embryos developed. A set of triplets was born to a woman with premature ovarian failure after transfer of five donated embryos from a total of 270 oocytes. Immature oocytes have also been retrieved from patients with polycystic ovaries. The oocytes were matured in vitro and replaced, the patient receiving steroid replacement after ET. A pregnancy and a birth have been recorded (Trounson et al., 1994). A further pregnancy was reported by Russell et al. (1997) in a patient whose endometrium had been primed with 2 mg estradiol twice daily from days 5 to 7 with progressive increase by 1–2 mg/day until oocyte retrieval and in vitro maturation in 0.075 IU FSH or hMG and 0.5 IU hCG and 1 mg estradiol. A mean of 11.1 oocytes were retrieved and 61.5% matured in vitro (48/78), 75% fertilized, 92% cleaved, and a mean of 4.0 embryos were transferred.

Aspiration of immature oocytes before dominant follicle selection has been recommended for poorly responding patients who have more than five early antral follicles (Requena et al., 2000). The group had previously described aspiration of follicles < 10 mm in diameter, which resulted in blastocyst formation in 56.6% (13/23) after in vitro maturation, a mean of 6.8 oocytes being retrieved (Cobo et al., 1999).

Using unstimulated cycles with ovulation triggered by hCG, Thornton et al. (1998) retrieved, after aspiration of the dominant follicle, all visible secondary follicles that were 12 mm or less. Metaphase I oocytes were inseminated at the same time as the dominant oocyte, whereas prophase I oocytes were cultured either in media or follicular fluid. Of the metaphase I oocytes, 44% (25/56) matured to metaphase II within 24 hours. Of the prophase I oocytes,

30% (17/55; no significant difference) matured in vitro. One fresh transfer was undertaken, yielding a livebirth. Six of nine immature oocytes were cryopreserved at the pronuclear stage and also yielded one livebirth.

Priming of immature oocytes by FSH before retrieval was assessed by Mikkelson et al. (1999) in a prospective, randomized, controlled trial, no stimulation being compared with three days of recombinant FSH at 150 IU/day from day 3. Oocytes were aspirated when the follicles were 10 mm and matured in vitro for 36 hours in the presence of FSH and hCG before ICSI. They were replaced after endometrial preparation when the endometrium was not less than 6 mm on the day of aspiration. It was prepared by priming with 2 mg estradiol three times a day and two days later intravaginal progesterone pessaries were begun. Three implantations occurred in the FSH group and two in the unstimulated group; the authors concluding that prior preparation with FSH provided no advantage. They further reported (Mikkelson et al., 2000) that 11 singleton pregnancies were obtained, each with a live fetus after transfer in 63 cycles, leading on to the birth of nine normal babies. Two endocrine parameters were predictive of pregnancy: an increase of 100% in serum estradiol concentrations and an increase of 80% in the serum inhibin A concentration between day 3 and the day of aspiration. They concluded that the development potential of immature oocytes might be improved by timing aspiration appropriately.

Vitrification of oocytes retrieved from unstimulated and stimulated cycles has been compared by Chung et al. (2000). There were no differences in the time of vitrification at, before or after 48 hours in culture from unstimulated cycles, but oocytes from stimulated cycles vitrified after 24–48 hours in culture yielded more morphologically normal oocytes. Nevertheless, high cleavage rates (83–100%), which did not differ between groups, were obtained, and 20–43% of cleaved oocytes developed to the blastocyst stage by six days after fertilization. Three and four blastocysts from each of the unstimulated and stimulated groups, respectively, were karyotyped and all were found to be normal.

The unstimulated cycle has also been used with hCG to recover a single oocyte for later fresh transfer at the time of replacement of thawed embryos cryopreserved from a prior stimulated cycle (Kim et al., 1996). This was particularly useful when the number of cryopreserved embryos was fewer than four and it could avoid the need for a further stimulated cycle, although up to a total of five embryos were replaced. The clinical pregnancy rate/ET was 34.2% (13/40) using the combined approach compared with 16.4% (10/61) in the natural cycle controls.

Conclusions

Although IVF began with natural cycles, they fell from favor when downregulation and hyperstimulation resulted in higher pregnancy rates. However, there is now increasing anxiety about the complications of IVF with controlled ovarian hyperstimulation, multiple pregnancy being rightly regarded as a complication. Alternative approaches to ovarian stimulation and single ET, with or without cryopreservation, seem to be the way forward for most patients. However older women and poor responders could well continue to use natural cycle IVF. The development of in vitro maturation following retrieval in natural cycles may yet lead to a resurgence of interest in the natural cycle.

REFERENCES

American Fertility Society and the Society for Assisted Reproductive Technology (1994). Assisted reproductive technology in the United States and Canada: 1992 results generated from the American Fertility Society/Society for Assisted Reproductive Technology Registry. *Fertility and Sterility*, **62**, 1121–8.

Bar-Hava, I., Ferber, A., Ashkenazi, J., et al. (2000). Natural-cycle in vitro fertilization in women over 44 years. *Gynecological Endocrinology*, **14**, 248–52.

Branigan, E.M. and Estes, M.A. (2000). Minimal stimulation IVF using clomiphene citrate and oral contraceptive pill pretreatment for LH suppression. *Fertility and Sterility*, **73**, 587–90.

Brown, J.R., Modell, E., Obasaju, M., and King, Y.-K. (1996).

Natural cycle in-vitro fertilization with embryo cryopreservation prior to chemotherapy for carcinoma of the breast. *Human Reproduction*, 11, 197–9.

Cahill, D.J., Wardle, P.G., Maile, L.A., et al. (1995). Pituitary dysfunction as a cause for endometriosis-associated and unexplained infertility. *Human Reproduction*, 10, 3142–6.

Cahill, D.J., Wardle, P.G., Harlow, C.R., and Hull, M.G.R. (1998). Onset of the preovulatory luteinizing surge: diurnal timing and critical follicular prerequisites. *Fertility and Sterility*, 70, 56–9.

Cahill, D.J., Wardle, P.G., Harlow, C.R., et al. (2000). Expected contribution to serum estradiol from individual ovarian follicles in unstimulated cycles. *Human Reproduction*, 15, 1909–12.

Cha, K.Y., Koo, J.J., Ko, J.J., et al. (1991). Pregnancy after in vitro fertilization of human follicular oocytes collected from non-stimulated cycles, their culture in vitro and their transfer in a donor oocyte program. *Fertility and Sterility*, 55, 109–13.

Chung, H.M., Hong, S.W., Lim, J.M., et al. (2000). In vitro blastocyst formation of human oocytes obtained from unstimulated and stimulated cycles after vitrification at various maturational stages. *Fertility and Sterility*, 73, 545–51.

Claman, P., Domingo, M., Garner, P., et al. (1993). Natural cycle in vitro fertilization–embryo transfer at the University of Ottawa: an inefficient therapy for tubal infertility. *Fertility and Sterility*, 60, 298–302.

Cobo, A.C., Requena, A., Neuspiller, F., et al. (1999). Maturation *in vitro* of human oocytes from unstimulated cycles: selection of the optimal day for ovum retrieval based on follicular size. *Human Reproduction*, 14, 1864–8.

Coskun, S., Hollanders, J., Al-Hassan, S., et al. (2000). Day 5 versus day 3 embryo transfer: a controlled randomized trial. *Human Reproduction*, 15, 1947–52.

Daya, S., Gunby, J., Hughes, E.G., Collins, J.A., and Sagle, M.A. (1995). Natural cycles for in-vitro fertilization: cost-effectiveness analysis and factors influencing outcome. *Human Reproduction*, 10, 1719–24.

Edwards, R.G., Steptoe, P.C., and Purdy, J.M. (1980). Establishing full-term human pregnancies using cleaving embryos grown in vitro. *British Journal of Obstetrics and Gynaecology*, 87, 737–56.

Elster, N. and the Institute for Science, Law, and Technology Working Group on Reproductive Technology (2000). Less is more: the risks of multiple births. *Fertility and Sterility*, 74, 617–23.

ESHRE Capri Workshop Group (2000). Multiple gestation pregnancy. *Human Reproduction*, 15, 1856–64.

Fahy, U.M., Cahill, D.J., Wardle, P.G., and Hull, M.G.R. (1995). In-vitro fertilization in completely natural cycles. *Human Reproduction*, 10, 572–5.

Foulot, H., Ranoux, C., Dubuisson, J.-B., et al. (1989). In vitro fertilization without ovarian stimulation: a simplified protocol applied in 80 cycles. *Fertility and Sterility*, 52, 617–21.

Fukuda, M., Fukuda, K., Andersen, C.Y., and Byskov, A.G. (1996). Contralateral selection of dominant follicle favours pre-embryo development. *Human Reproduction*, 11, 1958–62.

Gerris, J., de Neubourg, D., Mangelschots, K., et al. (1999). Prevention of twin pregnancy after in-vitro fertilization or intracytoplasmic sperm injection based on strict embryo criteria: a prospective randomized trial. *Human Reproduction*, 14, 2581–7.

Giuliana, A., Schoell, W., Auner, J., and Urdl, W. (1998). Controlled ovarian hyperstimulation in assisted reproduction: effect on the immune system. *Fertility and Sterility*, 70, 831–5.

Hassan, H.-A. and Saleh, H.A. (1996). Endometrial unresponsiveness: a novel approach to assessment and prognosis in in vitro fertilization cycles. *Fertility and Sterility*, 66, 604–7.

Hazecamp, J., Bergh, C., Wennerholm, U.-B., et al. (2000). Avoiding multiple pregnancies in ART. Consideration of new strategies. *Human Reproduction*, 15, 1217–19.

Human Fertilization and Embryology Authority (1999). *Eighth Annual Report*. HMSO, London.

Janssens, R.M., Lambalk, C.B., Vermeiden, J.P.W., et al. (2000). In-vitro fertilization in a spontaneous cycle: easy, cheap and realistic. *Human Reproduction*, 15, 314–18.

Kim, S.H., Kim, C.H., Suh, C.S., et al. (1996). Simultaneous program of natural-cycle in vitro fertilization and cryopreservation-thawed embryo transfer. *Journal of Assisted Reproduction and Genetics*, 13, 716–21.

Kliman, J., Barmat, L.I., and Wang, F.F. (1997). MAG mucin expression abnormalities in natural cycle biopsies predict subsequent IVF failure. *Fertility and Sterility*, Suppl, S156.

Lenton, E.A. (1993). Ovulation timing. In: *Donor Insemination*, Barratt, C.L.R. and Cooke, I.D. eds. Cambridge University Press, Cambridge, UK, pp. 97–110.

Lenton, E.A. and Woodward, B. (1993). Natural-cycle versus stimulated-cycle IVF: is there a role for IVF in the natural cycle? *Journal of Assisted Reproduction and Genetics*, 10, 406–8.

Lenton, E.A., Cooke, I.D., Hooper, M., et al. (1992). In vitro fertilization in the natural cycle. *Baillière's Clinical Obstetrics and Gynaecology*, 2, 229–45.

Lenton, E.A., Kumar, A., Turner, K., et al. (1995). Natural cycle in vitro fertilization: is there a place? In: *Advances in Reproductive Endocrinology*, Ser. 7, *Assisted Reproduction: Progress in Research and Practice*. Shaw, R.W., ed. Parthenon Press, Carnforth, UK, pp. 59–72.

Lesny, P., Killick, S.R., Tetlow, R.L., et al. (1998). Uterine junctional zone contractions during assisted reproduction cycles. VIDEO. *Human Reproduction Update*, **4**, 440–5.

Lindheim, S.R., Chang, P.L., Vidali, A., et al. (1998). The utility of serum progesterone and inhibin A for monitoring natural-cycle IVF-ET. *Journal of Assisted Reproduction and Genetics*, **15**, 538–41.

MacDougall, M.J., Tan, S.L., Hall, V., et al. (1994). Comparison of natural with clomiphene citrate-stimulated cycles in in-vitro fertilization – a prospective randomised trial. *Fertility and Sterility*, **64**, 1141–6.

Macklon, N.S. and Fauser, B.C.J.M. (2000). Impact of ovarian hyperstimulation on the luteal phase. *Journal of Reproduction and Fertility*, **Suppl. 55**, 101–8.

Malpani, A. and Malpani, A. (1992). Simplifying assisted conception techniques to make them universally available – a view from India. *Human Reproduction*, **7**, 49–50.

Meldrum, D.R., Rivier, J., Garzo, G., et al. (1994). Successful pregnancies with unstimulated cycle oocyte donation using an antagonist of gonadotropin releasing hormone. *Fertility and Sterility*, **61**, 556–7.

Mikkelson, A.L., Smith, S.D., and Lindenberg, S. (1999). In-vitro maturation of human oocytes from regularly menstruating women may be successful without stimulating hormone priming. *Human Reproduction*, **14**, 1847–51.

Mikkelson, A.K., Smith, S., and Lindenberg, S. (2000). Impact of oestradiol and inhibin A concentrations on pregnancy rate in in-vitro oocyte maturation. *Human Reproduction*, **15**, 1685–90.

Olivennes, F. (2000). Double trouble: yes, a twin pregnancy is an adverse outcome. *Human Reproduction*, **15**, 1623–5.

Paulson, R.J., Sauer, M.V., Francis, M.M., et al. (1992). In vitro fertilization in unstimulated cycles: the University of Southern California experience. *Fertility and Sterility*, **57**, 290–3.

Petterson, B., Nelson, K.B., Watson, L., and Stanley, F. (1993). Twins, triplets and cerebral palsy in births in Western Australia in the 1980s. *British Medical Journal*, **307**, 1239–43.

Requena, A., Neuspiller, F., Cobo, A.C., et al. (2000). The potential use of maturation in vitro of human oocytes in low responder patients. *Journal of Assisted Reproduction and Genetics*, **17**, 239–44.

Ron-El, R., Raziel, A., Strassburger, D., et al. (2000). Outcome of assisted reproductive technology in women over the age of 41. *Fertility and Sterility*, **74**, 471–5.

Rongieres-Bertrand, C., Olivennes, F., Righini, C., et al. (1999). Revival of the natural cycles in in-vitro fertilization with the use of a new gonadotrophin-releasing hormone antagonist (Cetrorelix): a pilot study with minimal stimulation. *Human Reproduction*, **14**, 683–8.

Russell, J.B., Knezevich, K.M., Fabian, K.F., and Dickson, J.A. (1997). Unstimulated immature oocyte retrieval: early versus midfollicular endometrial priming. *Fertility and Sterility*, **67**, 616–20.

Seibel, M.M., Kearnan, M., and Kiessling, A. (1995). Parameters that predict success for natural cycle in vitro fertilization–embryo transfer. *Fertility and Sterility*, **63**, 1251–4.

Society for Assisted Reproductive Technology and the American Society for Reproductive Medicine (2000). Assisted reproductive technology in the United States: 1997 results generated from the American Society for Reproductive Medicine/Society for Assisted Reproductive Technology Registry. *Fertility and Sterility*, **74**, 641–54.

Svalander, P., Green, B., Haglund, K., et al. (1991). Natural versus stimulated cycles in IVF–ET treatment for tubal factor infertility. (7th World Congress on In Vitro Fertilization and Assisted Procreations, P131.) *Human Reproduction*, **6**, 101–2.

Thornton, M.H., Francis, M.M., and Paulson, R.J. (1998). Immature oocyte retrieval: lessons from unstimulated IVF cycles. *Fertility and Sterility*, **70**, 647–50.

Trounson, A., Wood, C., and Kausche, A. (1994). In vitro maturation and the fertilization and developmental competence of oocytes recovered from untreated polycystic ovarian patients. *Fertility and Sterility*, **62**, 353–62.

Ueno, J., Oehninger, S., Brzyski, R.G., et al. (1991). Ultrasonographic appearance of the endometrium in natural and stimulated in vitro fertilization cycles and its correlation with outcome. *Human Reproduction*, **6**, 901–4.

van Royen, E., Mangelschots, K., De Neubourg, D., et al. (1999). Characterization of a top quality embryo, a step towards single-embryo transfer. *Human Reproduction*, **14**, 2345–9.

Venn, A., Watson, L., Lumley, J., et al. (1995). Breast and ovarian-cancer incidence after infertility and in-vitro fertilization. *Lancet*, **346**, 995–1000.

Vilska, S., Tiitinen, A., Hyden-Granskog, C., and Hovatta, O. (1999). Elective transfer of one embryo results in an acceptable pregnancy rate and eliminates the risk of multiple birth. *Human Reproduction*, **14**, 2392–5.

20

Embryo stage and transfer number

Alan Trounson

Centre for Early Human Development, Monash Institute of Reproduction and Development, Clayton, Australia

Introduction

The increased incidence of multiple gestations associated with multiple embryo transfers leads to an increased risk of perinatal morbidity. The high implantation rates resulting from blastocyst transfer on days 5 or 6 after insemination gives rise to greater chances of pregnancy while decreasing the risk of multiple gestation. When blastocyst transfer is used, there is no increase in probability of conception when three rather than two embryos are transferred, although the risk of multiple pregnancy is significantly higher. With improved culture systems, embryos are grown sequentially, which appears to result in higher implantation rates and facilitates successful conception with the transfer of fewer embryos. Since blastocysts have a higher implantation rate than less-developed cleavage stage embryos, the transfer of more than two blastocysts may no longer be necessary to maintain adequate pregnancy rates. Given that only one or two blastocysts are required for transfer, any that remain can be cryopreserved, increasing the opportunity for pregnancy from subsequent transfers. The new culture media do not necessarily result in the development of more blastocysts. More important, however, is the observation that the viable blastocysts created by this technique provide a means of reducing the number of embryos transferred. This reduces both spontaneous miscarriage and maternal–fetal risks associated with multiple pregnancy. It is logical that there will be an increasing trend to transfer blastocysts on day 5 or 6, instead of transfer of early cleavage stage embryos on day 2 or 3.

Success rates in in vitro fertilization and multiple pregnancy

With an increasing incidence of infertility and delayed child-bearing, the demand for assisted reproductive technology (ART) continues to grow. Rates of multiple pregnancies associated with ART are reportedly as high as between 15 and 36% (Rein et al., 1990; Bollen et al., 1991). During 1990, 55% of the clinics in the USA reporting to the IVF-ET Registry claimed to transfer, on average, 3.5 or more embryos per cycle (Society for Assisted Reproductive Technology and the American Fertility Society, 1992); 7% reported transferring an average of more than five embryos per cycle. In 1995, within Canada and the USA, 41 209 cycles of in vitro fertilization (IVF) were reported. During this year, the delivery rates per cycle of embryo transfer for women of less than 35 years, 35–39 years, and greater than 39 years were 34.3, 27.6, and 11.4%, respectively, for those with a male cause for infertility and 33.2, 26.4, and 12.4%, respectively, without a known male cause. Of these IVF cycles, 31 794 embryo transfer procedures resulted in 9760 clinical pregnancies, where 29.6% were twin gestations, 6.4% were triplets, and 0.6% were higher-order multiple deliveries, despite the apparent use of fetal reduction techniques (Society for Assisted Reproductive Technology and the American Society for Reproductive Medicine, 1999). These percentages can be contrasted with the spontaneous rates of 1.05–1.35% for twins and 0.01–0.017% for triplets (Callahan et al., 1994) in the general community. In Australia and New Zealand, during 1996 and 1997, only 2.7% of clinics reported transferring four or more embryos per cycle of transfer; 17% of clinics reported transferring only three embryos; 62% claimed an average transfer of two embryos; and 8% reported transferring only one embryo (Lancaster et al., 1997).

The increased rate of multiple gestation associated with ART gives rise to an increased incidence of both neonatal and maternal morbidity and mortality (Rizk et al., 1991). Prematurity, low birthweight, pregnancy-induced hypertension, gestational diabetes, postpartum hemorrhage, and cesarean section all more frequently in cases of multiple pregnancy. The higher-order multiple birth rate (the number of births in triplet, quadruplet, and greater deliveries per 100 000 livebirths) rose by 20% in 1996 in the USA, increasing from 127.5 to 152.6, the largest single-year increase in at least 25 years. The 5939 higher-order multiple births occurring in 1996 included 5298 triplets, 560 quadruplets, and 81 quintuplet or greater multiples. Both the number and rate of higher-order multiple births have quadrupled since 1980 (Newman et al., 1989).

Patients' reactions to higher-order multiple pregnancies vary enormously and may depend, in part, on the degree of multiplicity of the pregnancy. The conception of IVF twins are often seen as a bonus by many long-term IVF couples, although even this occurrence can bring about significantly increased obstetric risks. Indeed, Gerris and Van Royen (2000) assert an increasing awareness of the risks, costs, and 'epidemic size' of twin pregnancies after IVF. Higher-order implantations compound the risk of obstetric problems and may intensify certain socioeconomic concerns. The pressure to succeed with IVF therapy and the associated financial burdens (given the commonly poor insurance coverage in the USA) may exacerbate the temptation to transfer greater numbers of embryos in the hope that at least one will implant successfully. The recent decision of the Australian government to remove limits on the number of subsidized IVF cycles for heterosexual couples will accelerate the acceptance of single embryo transfers despite the probable decline in overall IVF success rates.

Callahan et al. (1994) argue that the higher rate of multiple pregnancies arising from the use of ART adds a considerable burden to the costs of health care, considering that multiple gestations are associated with more preterm deliveries and perinatal complications. Nonetheless, several studies, such as those of Petersen et al. (1995), Lipitz et al. (1993), Bernasko et al. (1997), and Olivennes et al. (1996) have shown that there is no difference in hospitalization rates, complication rates, mean gestational age, birthweights, Apgar score, overall morbidity, and perinatal mortality. Brandes et al. (1992) studied the long-term outcomes of infants from ART multiple gestations, matching them with control infants. While they found no significant difference in mental development indexes between control and study groups, both twins and triplets (IVF and controls) had significantly lower physical and mental indices compared with singletons. Perinatal and neonatal morbidity, gestational age at delivery, and birthweight are not affected by ART. Hence there may be no increased risk for infants from multiple births arising from ART, aside from the risks inherent to multiple pregnancy (Fitzsimmons et al., 1998).

Multiple pregnancies are associated with certain major risks quite independently of whether or not ART has been utilized. Complications arising from multiple gestations occur because of the inherent risks of plural gestations and births (Table 20.1), which have medical, social, psychological, ethical and financial dimensions.

The risks, complications, and sequelae in the offspring of high-order multiple pregnancies, and the costs to the parents and community, are much more than several times that of a singleton pregnancy. This is reflected by the fact that approximately one in every six babies received in neonatal intensive care units at the Queen Victoria Hospital in Adelaide, Australia has been part of a multiple gestation.

Table 20.1. Summary of medical complications for multiple pregnancy

Complication	Occurrence
Abortion	Twice as common in multiple, as opposed to singleton, pregnancies
Congenital abnormalities	Twice as common in twins as in singleton infants and four times as common in triplets; monozygotic twins have twice the incidence of fetal abnormalities compared with dizygotic twins
Pregnancy-induced hypertension	Hypertension complicates 60% of triplet pregnancies; in multiple pregnancies, there is, at least, a threefold increase in the incidence of pregnancy-induced hypertension and also an increase in the severity of this condition
Preterm delivery	The incidence of preterm birth in twin gestation varies from 22 to 39%; in triplet gestation it is as high as 75%. The average length of gestation decreases inversely with the number of fetuses present. The critical gestational and birthweight limits, based on current perinatal mortality figures, appear to be between 26 and 32 weeks and 600–1000 g, respectively
Intrauterine growth retardation	Approximately 70% of infants born of multiple births are significantly restricted in terms of growth; both the incidence and degree of growth restriction increase towards term
Neurological damage	Cerebral palsy, microcephaly, porencephaly, and encephalomalacia are more frequent in multiple than singleton pregnancies, and occur at a greater rate when delivery is preterm; necrosis of the cerebral white matter is approximately 14% in multiple gestations delivered at less than 36 weeks of gestation

Financial implications

When considering the cost-effectiveness of IVF, there are several relevant factors that need to be taken into account. In addition to the cost of each treatment cycle, the success rate, measured in terms of women delivered, must also be determined. The latter figure involves the added costs of "successful" IVF pregnancies, which include the antenatal and neonatal hospitalizations that are usually attributable to the high incidence of multiple pregnancies. Neumann et al. (1994) calculated the cost per woman delivered using data from six IVF units, adding estimates of outcome measures such as maternal and neonatal complications. They concluded with an estimate of cost per delivery ranging from US$50 000 for the first cycle of a woman with tubal disease to US$80 000 for the sixth cycle in an older woman where there was also a male cause for infertility present. If the respective costs of the estimated antenatal and neonatal hospitalizations are added, then the medical cost per woman delivered is US$65 872. If time lost from employment, or the ongoing cost for premature neonates once they leave the nursery, is considered, an additional cost of US$18 447 has to be added to each delivery, giving rise to a total of US$84 319 (Goldfarb et al., 1996). These figures are only approximate. Hospital costs, for example, are based on average discount rates. Therefore, actual costs are likely to diverge from these estimates, in part depending on insurance contracts. Despite the approximate nature of the costs suggested, it is evident that triplet and quadruplet pregnancies contribute most prominently to increased expenses. Indeed, in comparison with singleton and twin pregnancies, triplet and quadruplet pregnancies have been estimated to cost more than nine times as much per woman delivered (Callahan et al., 1994).

IVF can become more cost-effective by taking steps to eliminate high-order multiple pregnancies. The increased implantation rates for blastocysts transferred during human IVF procedures should result in both increased pregnancy rates and a decrease in multiple gestations. These changes in outcome measures are expected as a result of the reduced number of embryos apparently required for transfer to achieve an acceptable pregnancy rate.

Blastocyst transfer technology

Embryo transfer in humans has traditionally been performed two days after insemination, at which embryos have developed to the 2- to 4-cell stage (Trounson et al., 1982). The timing of this technique was largely motivated by the fear that prolonged exposure to suboptimal conditions of culture in the laboratory may compromise embryo viability. Premature exposure of embryos to the uterus, however, may act synergistically with the stress already experienced in the artificial in vitro environment. When embryo transfers are performed on day 2 or 3, pregnancy rates of between 10 and 30% are routinely reported. However, these pregnancy rates are usually attained following transfer of multiple embryos, and the resulting implantation rates are low. Although pregnancy rates may increase when up to four embryos are transferred, so does the possibility of a multiple gestation. The analysis of pregnancy data shows no increase in pregnancy rates when three rather than two embryos are transferred, but multiple pregnancies are significantly increased (Tasdemir et al., 1995; Roest et al., 1997). In summary, an increase in the number of embryos transferred invariably results in higher rates of multiple births, without necessarily improving the overall success rates of IVF.

Obtaining greater understanding of the embryo's nutrient requirements and physiology has led to the development of more physiological culture media. These media are capable of supporting acceptable levels of human blastocyst development in vitro, enabling a transfer at day 5 or 6, when the embryo normally resides in the uterus. By delaying embryo transfer until after the developmental hurdle that appears to exist between the 4- and 8-cell stage (Ashwood-Smith et al., 1989), during which the embryonic genome is activated, the selection of embryos for transfer may be less arbitrary than at the 2- to 4-cell stage. Selection may be based, for example, on morphological criteria to increase pregnancy rates (Jones et al., 1998b). The development of embryos to the blastocyst stage is an indicator of their increased viability. Some genetically abnormal embryos will stop development during cleavage in culture; however, chromosomally abnormal blastocysts can still be identified (Magli et al., 2000). Embryo biopsy at the blastocyst stage (Lopata and Hay, 1989) would allow the safe removal of a relatively large number (5–25) of trophectoderm cells from the embryo for genetic and chromosomal analyses. This technique would be unlikely to compromise the subsequent development of the fetus (Tarin and Trounson, 1993).

In the early 1990s, the pregnancy rate following blastocyst transfer was not significantly different from that following the transfer of early cleavage embryos (Bolton et al., 1991). In the next few years, however, the use of co-culture techniques (Menezo et al., 1993; Olivennes et al., 1994; Schillaci et al., 1994) and changes in culture medium alone (Scholtes and Zeilmaker, 1996) have resulted in implantation and pregnancy rates following blastocyst transfer that were comparatively high (Gardner et al., 1998a). Indeed, blastocyst transfer is thought to be so promising that some scientists are advocating the introduction of single embryo transfer in attempt to avoid the risk of twins (Gerris and Van Royen, 2000). Recently, it has been shown that the transfer of one high-quality blastocyst should lead to a pregnancy rate of over 60% (Gardner et al., 2000). Others suggest that blastocyst transfer provides an effective treatment for patients who receive donor oocytes and for whom embryos are not plentiful. Despite the numerous studies claiming that the advantages of transferring blastocysts are clear, there are, however, data to the contrary. Coskun et al. (2000), for example, compared day 3 and day 5 transfers, concluding that the latter have no advantage over the former, a result that stands in marked contrast to other studies in which the increase in blastocyst implantation rate has been significant. Table 20.2 outlines the indications for and advantages/disadvantages of blastocyst culture and transfer.

Table 20.2. Blastocyst culture and transfer

	Factors
Indications	Patients with repeated implantation failure
	Patients with uterine abnormalities that preclude multiple pregnancies, who consequently require more careful selection of the single embryo for transfer
	Patients with suspected defects in oocyte quality whose embryos should be assessed – for an extended period of in vitro development
	Patients needing embryo biopsy for genetic selection
	Patients undergoing replacement of supernumerary embryos frozen at the blastocyst stage
Advantages	The most developmentally competent embryos can be selected for transfer
	Transfer of the appropriate-stage embryo to the uterus; prior to the morula stage, embryos reside in the Fallopian tube: premature entry into the uterus can jeopardize embryo development in other species
	Cryostorage of embryos is rendered more efficient; since the most competent embryos can be preferentially selected for storage, fewer numbers need to be stored, and problems with disposal of unwanted preserved embryos will be lessened
	Sequential, physiologically based serum- and cell-free culture media can be used to produce highly viable human blastocysts; the use of such defined systems should not only reduce the variability of certain markers of success across various IVF programs, but is also expected to increase the efficiency of human IVF in general
Possible disadvantages	Under suboptimal culture conditions in vitro, an embryo that failed to develop in vitro to the blastocyst stage, and was subsequently not transferred, may have been capable of developing into a viable fetus
	Cost/benefit ratios may not be favorable; increased costs may be incurred because (i) culturing embryos to the blastocyst stage requires 3–5 additional days of incubation in the laboratory; (ii) the possible use of cell lines for co-culture carries attendant complications such as the screening for contamination; (iii) the need for subpassaging of cells for co-culture; (iv) requirements for animal serum and, more generally, the preparation and use of cell- and serum-free sequential culture media
	When using co-culture cells, there is a risk of transmitting infectious agents to the embryos from the feeder cell line, particularly from those derived from the human oviduct and those of bovine and primate origin

Day of transfer of embryos

For blastocyst transfer to provide a superior alternative to the transfer of embryos that are two to three days old (2- to 8-cell embryos), a sufficient proportion of embryos must develop into viable blastocysts to enable most patients to receive one embryo. The proportion of embryos that develop to the blastocyst stage is increased by the number of oocytes collected and inseminated, the number of zygotes produced, and the number of embryos showing normal development to at least the 8-cell stage by day 3 after insemination (Jones et al., 1998b). The number and the quality of the blastocysts transferred significantly increases the likelihood of clinical pregnancy, indicating that quality blastocysts may be selected for transfer, based on morphological criteria, to increase pregnancy rates (Jones et al., 1998b).

Cleavage stage embryos, which are chosen for transfer during conventional IVF procedures, have comparatively low implantation rates (Trounson and Bongso, 1996). This motivates the transfer of multiple embryos to raise pregnancy rates, and this accounts for the high number of multiple gestations commonly associated with IVF. It has been suggested that the reported 5–10% embryo implantation rate of early cleavage stage embryos might be explained by premature entry of embryos in the uterus (Croxatto et al., 1978; Buster et al., 1985). Recently, alternative in vitro systems have been developed in which embryos are grown sequentially in media of changing composition in order to respond to their changing metabolic requirements. These techniques have utilized a mixture of simple and complex culture media, facilitating the routine development of pronucleate embryos to the blastocyst stage over four to five days (Gardner et al., 1997, 1998b; Jones et al., 1998a; see also Ch. 8).

Cultivation for five days, as opposed to the normal two to three days, allows more advanced embryos to be transferred to the uterine cavity. The higher implantation rate observed after transferring blastocysts is thought to be a result, in part, of reaching a more appropriate embryonic stage for intrauterine implantation (Buster et al., 1985). Such increased implantation rates are also explained by the ability to select against embryos that fail to develop in culture, indicating negligible developmental potential (Lopata and Hay, 1989; Magli et al., 2000). The concern that embryos should be returned to the uterus as soon as possible to prevent loss of viability in vivo is now seemingly less important than taking the opportunity to select for embryos with increased developmental competence. A strong correlation between blastocyst quality and the success of blastocyst transfer has been demonstrated (Balaban et al., 2000). Since blastocysts have a higher implantation rate than cleavage stage embryos, longer cultivation in vitro allows the transfer of fewer embryos without decreasing pregnancy rates (Jones et al., 1998a; Balaban et al., 2000). Consequently, the use of such culture systems reduces the risk of multiple pregnancy without compromising the success of IVF procedures.

Assisted hatching or zona removal

Finding a means of increasing the implantation rates of embryos after IVF is an important area of research. Higher implantation rates would facilitate the transfer of fewer embryos, lowering the risk of multiple pregnancy, while also increasing the availability of viable blastocysts for cryopreservation. It has been proposed that removing the zona pellucida that surrounds embryos may increase implantation rates (Jones et al., 1998a). The reason for this relates to the trapping of embryos within the zona pellucida. Removal of the zona avoids this possibility. Blastocysts normally hatch from the zona on day 5–6, after which the trophectoderm has direct contact with the uterine endometrial cells, which is essential for implantation.

It was hypothesized that hardening of the zona pellucida impaired hatching after the transferral procedure involved in IVF and culture in vitro (Cohen et al., 1992). Fong et al. (1997) demonstrated that both implantation and pregnancy were possible after Pronase digestion of the blastocyst zona. Jones et al. (1998a) showed that Pronase digestion of the zona pellucida before the transfer of blastocysts developed in vitro increased their implantation rates. However, the action of Pronase is non-specific; consequently, it not only degrades the zona pellucida but may also remove a number of molecules located at the cell surface (Tarone et al., 1982). However, numerous animal embryo experiments have shown no apparent effect of Pronase on either embryo viability or the presence of cell surface antigens (Trounson and Moore, 1974). It has also been shown that 92% of Pronase-treated, zona-free blastocysts are capable of attachment to all various feeder monolayers (Magli et al., 1998). This suggests that the interaction between the trophectoderm and the endometrium is preserved in vitro and almost certainly in vivo.

Blastocyst transfer and cryopreservation

Considering the relatively high implantation rate of blastocysts, it is no longer justifiable to transfer more than two embryos at any one time in the vast majority of women. If the likelihood of one blastocyst successfully implanting was 30%, the transfer of two would predict a pregnancy rate of around 50%. Of course, transferring two blastocysts will not eliminate the risk of conceiving twins, but it will reduce the occurrence of higher-order multiple pregnancies, which are associated with the greatest risks both for pregnant women and fetuses and which incur the greatest costs. Recently, Gardner et al. (2000) have claimed that selecting high-quality blastocysts can allow single embryo transfers to lead to pregnancy rates greater than 60%, which would minimize the complication of twins. One of the interesting complications of blastocyst transfers is the apparent increase in monozygotic twinning (Rijnders et al., 1998; Peramo et al., 1999). The reasons for this are not known.

If it becomes standard practice to transfer only one or two blastocysts to each patient per cycle, there will be an increased need for the cryopreservation of excess embryos for many patients. At present, about 40% of patients who have undergone blastocyst transfer at the Monash IVF program in Melbourne have blastocysts cryopreserved each cycle. Current data from those using sequential culture media approximate the proportion of blastocysts developing from pronuclear stage embryos to be 50–66% (Gardner et al., 1998b; Jones et al., 1998a; Balaban et al., 2000). In the past, glycerol has been the favored agent for cryopreservation (Menezo et al., 1992; Jones et al., 1998a). The use of glycerol enables a relatively large proportion of embryos to survive thawing and develop during the course of pregnancy.

The future of blastocyst transfer in the human: towards single embryo transfers

The viability of blastocysts grown in sequential culture media is demonstrated by their high implantation rates, which are equal to, if not greater than, those observed using co-culture techniques (Gardner et al., 2000). The proportion of embryos able to reach blastocyst stage in culture should increase as further improvements are made to culture media and culture conditions. Even with the expected improvements, however, the maximum percentage of blastocysts formed from human embryos is not expected to exceed 60–70%. Within the Monash IVF program, 48–65% of fertilized embryos currently develop into blastocysts. These figures may be explained by chromosomal abnormalities known to be present in a significant proportion of oocytes and early cleavage stage embryos, most of which would be lethal prior to implantation (Magli et al., 2000).

Conclusions

A review of data shows that the implantation rate of embryos transferred five days after oocyte retrieval and IVF is higher than that of those transferred between two and three days. This observation has several implications. First, delaying embryo transfer until day 5 facilitates the emergence of selective criteria by which the most developmentally competent embryos can be chosen for transfer. Second, embryo biopsy of 5–25 cells at the blastocyst stage could be more reliable than single or twin cell biopsy during cleavage, which would improve the accuracy of preimplantation diagnosis. Third, higher implantation rates mean that only one or two blastocysts need to be transferred in order to maintain comparative pregnancy rates. This enables patients to avoid the risk of high-order multiple gestations, which is not only one of the most common complications of human IVF but also one of the most serious, giving rise to medical, economic, and social concerns. The development of sequential culture media has enabled the routine transfer of human blastocysts to become a reality. Developing embryos into blastocysts in vitro can be achieved by culturing embryos under defined conditions, where quality-controlled, serum-free, cell-free culture media from a number of different sources have been designed for optimal development of embryos.

Acknowledgements

The author would like to acknowledge the editorial assistance of Jacinta Kerin and assistance with manuscript preparation by Alfonso Batiza.

REFERENCES

Ashwood-Smith, M.J., Hollands, P., and Edwards, R.G. (1989). The use of Albuminar 5 as a medium supplement in clinical IVF. *Human Reproduction*, **4**, 702–5.

Balaban, B., Urman, B., Sertac, A., Alatas, C., Aksoy, S., and Mercan, R. (2000). Blastocyst quality affects the success of blastocyst-stage embryo transfer. *Fertility and Sterility*, **74**, 282–7.

Bernasko, J., Lynch, L., Lapinski, R., and Berkowitz, R.L. (1997). Twin pregnancies conceived by assisted reproductive techniques: maternal and neonatal outcomes. *Obstetrics and Gynecology*, **89**, 368–72.

Bollen, N., Camus, M., Staessen, C., et al. (1991). The incidence of multiple pregnancy after in vitro fertilization and embryo transfer, gamete, or zygote intrafallopian transfer. *Fertility and Sterility*, **55**, 314–18.

Bolton, V.N., Wren, M.E., and Parsons, J.H. (1991). Pregnancies after in vitro fertilization and transfer of human blastocysts. *Fertility and Sterility*, **55**, 830–2.

Brandes, J.M., Scher, A., Itzkovits, J., Thaler, I., Sarid, M., and Gershoni-Baruch, R. (1992). Growth and development of children conceived by in vitro fertilization. *Pediatrics*, **90**, 424–9.

Buster, J.E., Bustillo, M., Rodi, I.A., et al. (1985). Biologic and morphologic development of donated human ova recovered by nonsurgical uterine lavage. *American Journal of Obstetrics and Gynecology*, **153**, 211–17.

Callahan, T.L., Hall, J.E., Ettner, S.L., et al. (1994). The economic impact of multiple-gestation pregnancies and the contribution of assisted-reproduction techniques to their incidence. *New England Journal of Medicine*, **331**, 244–9.

Cohen, J., Alikani, M., Trowbridge, J., and Rosenwaks, Z. (1992). Implantation enhancement by selective assisted hatching using zona drilling of human embryos with poor prognosis. *Human Reproduction*, **7**, 685–91.

Coskun, S., Hollanders, J., Al-Hassan, S., Al-Sufyan, H., Al-Mayman, H., and Jaroudi, K. (2000). Day 5 versus day 3 embryo transfer: a controlled randomized trial. *Human Reproduction*, **15**, 1947–52.

Croxatto, H.B., Ortiz, M.E., Diaz, S., Hess, R., Balmaceda, J., and Croxatto, H.D. (1978). Studies on the duration of egg transport by the human oviduct. II. Ovum location at various intervals following luteinizing hormone peak. *American Journal of Obstetrics and Gynecology*, **132**, 629–34.

Fitzsimmons, B.P., Bebbington, M.W., and Fluker, M.R. (1998). Perinatal and neonatal outcomes in multiple gestations: assisted reproduction versus spontaneous conception. *American Journal of Obstetrics and Gynecology*, **179**, 1162–7.

Fong, C.Y., Bongso, A., Ng, S.C., Anandakumar, C., Trounson, A., and Ratnam, S. (1997). Ongoing normal pregnancy after transfer of zona-free blastocysts: implications for embryo transfer in the human. *Human Reproduction*, **12**, 557–60.

Gardner, D.K., Lane, M., Kouridakis, K., and Schoolcraft, W.B. (1997). Complex physiologically based serum-free culture media increase mammalian embryo development. In: *In Vitro Fertilization and Assisted Reproduction*, Gomel, V. and Leune, P.C.H., eds. Monduzzi Editore, Bologne, pp. 187–91.

Gardner, D.K., Schoolcraft, W.B., Wagley, L., Schlenker, T., Stevens, J., and Hesla, J. (1998a). A prospective randomized trial of blastocyst culture and transfer in in-vitro fertilization [see comments]. *Human Reproduction*, **13**, 3434–40.

Gardner, D.K., Vella, P., Lane, M., Wagley, L., Schlenker, T., and Schoolcraft, W.B. (1998b). Culture and transfer of human blastocysts increases implantation rates and reduces the need for multiple embryo transfers. *Fertility and Sterility*, **69**, 84–8.

Gardner, D.K., Lane, M., Stevens, J., Schlenker, T., and Schoolcraft, W.B. (2000). Blastocyst score affects implantation and pregnancy outcome: towards a single blastocyst transfer. *Fertility and Sterility*, **73**, 1155–8.

Gerris, J. and Van Royen, E. (2000). Avoiding multiple pregnancies in ART: a plea for single embryo transfer. *Human Reproduction*, **15**, 1884–8.

Goldfarb, J.M., Austin, C., Lisbona, H., Peskin, B., and Clapp, M. (1996). Cost-effectiveness of in vitro fertilization. *Obstetrics and Gynecology*, **87**, 18–21.

Jones, G.M., Trounson, A.O., Gardner, D.K., Kausche, A., Lolatgis, N., and Wood, C. (1998a). Evolution of a culture protocol for successful blastocyst development and pregnancy. *Human Reproduction*, **13**, 169–77.

Jones, G.M., Trounson, A.O., Lolatgis, N., and Wood, C. (1998b). Factors affecting the success of human blastocyst development and pregnancy following in vitro fertilization and embryo transfer. *Fertility and Sterility*, **70**, 1022–9.

Lancaster, P., Shafir, E., and Huang, J. (1997). *Assisted Conception Australia and New Zealand*. Australian Institute of Health and Welfare, National Perinatal Statistics Unit and the Fertility Society of Australia, Canberra, Australia.

Lipitz, S., Seidman, D.S., Alcalay, M., Achiron, R., Mashiach, S., and Reichman, B. (1993). The effect of fertility drugs and in vitro methods on the outcome of 106 triplet pregnancies. *Fertility and Sterility*, **60**, 1031–4.

Lopata, A. and Hay, D.L. (1989). The potential of early human embryos to form blastocysts, hatch from their zona and secrete HCG in culture. *Human Reproduction*, **4**, 87–94.

Magli, M.C., Gianaroli, L., Ferraretti, A.P., Fortini, D., Aicardi, G., and Montanaro, N. (1998). Rescue of implantation potential in embryos with poor prognosis by assisted zona hatching. *Human Reproduction*, **13**, 1331–5.

Magli, M.C., Jones, G.M., Gras, L., Gianaroli, L., Korman, I., and Trounson, A.O. (2000). Chromosome mosaicism in day 3 aneuploid embryos that develop to morphologically normal blastocysts in vitro. *Human Reproduction*, **15**, 1781–6.

Menezo, Y., Nicollet, B., Herbaut, N., and Andre, D. (1992). Freezing cocultured human blastocysts. *Fertility and Sterility*, **58**, 977–80.

Menezo, Y.J., Nicollet, B., Dumont, M., Hazout, A., and Janny, L. (1993). Factors affecting human blastocyst formation in vitro and freezing at the blastocyst stage. *Acta Europaea Fertilitatis*, **24**, 207–13.

Neumann, P.J., Gharib, S.D., and Weinstein, M.C. (1994). The cost of a successful delivery with in vitro fertilization [see comments]. *New England Journal of Medicine*, **331**, 239–43.

Newman, R.B., Hamer, C., and Miller, M.C. (1989). Outpatient triplet management: a contemporary review. *American Journal of Obstetrics and Gynecology*, **161**, 547–53; discussion 553–5.

Olivennes, F., Hazout, A., Lelaidier, C., et al. (1994). Four indications for embryo transfer at the blastocyst stage. *Human Reproduction*, **9**, 2367–73.

Olivennes, F., Kadhel, P., Rufat, P., Fanchin, R., Fernandez, H., and Frydman, R. (1996). Perinatal outcome of twin pregnancies obtained after in vitro fertilization: comparison with twin pregnancies obtained spontaneously or after ovarian stimulation. *Fertility and Sterility*, **66**, 105–9.

Peramo, B., Ricciarelli, E., Cuadros-Fernandez, J.M., Huguet, E., and Hernandez, E.R. (1999). Blastocyst transfer and monozygotic twinning. *Fertility and Sterility*, **72**, 1116–17.

Petersen, K., Hornnes, P.J., Ellingsen, S., et al. (1995). Perinatal outcome after in vitro fertilisation. *Acta Obstetricia et Gynaecologica Scandinavica*, **74**, 129–31.

Rein, M.S., Barbieri, R.L., and Greene, M.F. (1990). The causes of high-order multiple gestation. *International Journal of Fertility*, **35**, 154–6.

Rijnders, P.M., van Os, H.C., and Jansen, C.A.M. (1998). Increased incidence of monozygotic twining following the transfer of blastocysts in human IVF/ICSI. *Fertility and Sterility*, **70**, 15–16.

Rizk, B., Doyle, P., Tan, S.L., et al. (1991). Perinatal outcome and congenital malformations in in-vitro fertilization babies from the Bourn–Hallam group. *Human Reproduction*, **6**, 1259–64.

Roest, J., van Heusden, A.M., Verhoeff, A., Mous, H.V., and Zeilmaker, G.H. (1997). A triplet pregnancy after in vitro fertilization is a procedure-related complication that should be prevented by replacement of two embryos only [see comments]. *Fertility and Sterility*, **67**, 290–5.

Schillaci, R., Ciriminna, R., and Cefalu, E. (1994). Vero cell effect on in-vitro human blastocyst development: preliminary results. *Human Reproduction*, **9**, 1131–5.

Scholtes, M.C., and Zeilmaker, G.H. (1996). A prospective, randomized study of embryo transfer results after 3 or 5 days of embryo culture in in vitro fertilization. *Fertility and Sterility*, **65**, 1245–8.

Society for Assisted Reproductive Technology and the American Fertility Society (1992). In vitro fertilization–embryo transfer (IVF–ET) in the United States: 1990 results from the IVF–ET Registry. [Published erratum appears in *Fertility and Sterility* (1993) **59**, 250.] *Fertility and Sterility*, **57**, 15–24.

Society for Assisted Reproductive Technology and the American Society for Reproductive Medicine (1999). Assisted reproductive technology in the United States: 1996 results generated from the American Society for Reproductive Medicine/Society for Assisted Reproductive Technology Registry. *Fertility and Sterility*, **71**, 798–807.

Tarin, J. and Trounson, A.O. (1993). Embryo biopsy for preimplantation diagnosis. In: *Handbook of In Vitro Fertilization*, Trounson, A. and Gardner, D.K., eds. CRC Press, Boca Raton, FL, pp. 115–30.

Tarone, G., Galetto, G., Prat, M., and Comoglio, P.M. (1982). Cell surface molecules and fibronectin-mediated cell adhesion: effect of proteolytic digestion of membrane proteins. *Journal of Cell Biology*, **94**, 179–86.

Tasdemir, M., Tasdemir, I., Kodama, H., Fukuda, J., and Tanaka, T. (1995). Two instead of three embryo transfer in in-vitro fertilization. *Human Reproduction*, **10**, 2155–8.

Trounson, A.O. and Bongso, A. (1996). Fertilization and development in humans. In: *Current Topics in Developmental Biology*, Vol. 32, Pedersen, R.A. and Schatten, G.A., eds. Academic Press, New York, pp. 59–101.

Trounson, A.O., and Moore, N.W. (1974). The survival and development of sheep eggs following complete or partial removal of the zona pellucida. *Journal of Reproduction and Fertility*, **41**, 97–105.

Trounson, A.O., Mohr, L.R., Wood, C., and Leeton, J.F. (1982). Effect of delayed insemination on in-vitro fertilization, culture and transfer of human embryos. *Journal of Reproduction and Fertility*, **64**, 285–94.

21

The federal research base in the USA for assisted reproductive technology[1]

Donna L. Vogel

National Cancer Institute, Bethesda, USA

The origin of the US government enterprise in human infertility research is neither human nor infertility. Prevented from directly studying advanced assisted reproductive technology (ART) in humans, federally supported investigators have nonetheless contributed to the knowledge base for infertility treatment. Although the picture is beginning to change, as the twenty-first century opens, much of the experimental work in the USA that will benefit infertile couples remains in the indirect arena of animal models and fundamental reproductive biology.

Early reproductive research was driven by the economic and pragmatic needs of animal breeding. Pioneering ARTs such as artificial insemination and cryopreservation of semen were in widespread use in farm species when treatment of human infertility was little more than an anecdote, and research was not even imagined. Much of the research on reproductive biology in the first half of the twentieth century was supported by nongovernment sources, notably the Rockefeller Foundation.

In the 1950s and 1960s, international concern about global overpopulation brought human reproduction issues into greater visibility. The stated aim of "population control" created a need for knowledge of the economic, behavioral, and biomedical factors contributing to population growth. The Ford Foundation played an active role in funding research during this time. The relationship between family planning, health, and socioeconomic progress began to emerge. At the same time, contraceptive technology underwent a dramatic change from sterilization, barrier methods, and abstinence to reversible methods with greater reliability and ease of use, oral contraceptives, and intrauterine devices.

Several key events for reproductive research occurred in the 1960s at the National Institutes of Health (NIH). Population issues came up during the Congressional hearings which led to the establishment of the National Institute of Child Health and Human Development (NICHD) in 1963. During the early 1960s, concerns emerged about adverse effects of the new contraceptive technologies, which were also drawing religious and political reaction. Even as the new Institute awarded its first grants in reproductive biology, the social and political context developed and has surrounded federal activities in the field ever since. In 1965, reproduction was identified as one of the four program areas of NICHD. The Center for Population Research (CPR) was established within NICHD in 1968 and designated by President Lyndon Johnson as the federal agency with primary responsibility for population research and research training. In 1970, a law was enacted establishing within the Department of Health, Education and Welfare (renamed in 1979 as the Department of

---

[1] The opinions expressed herein are those of the author, and are not necessarily those of the National Institutes of Health or the United States Department of Health and Human Services.

Health and Human Services) the Office of Population Affairs, to be directed by the Deputy Assistant Secretary for Population Affairs. The same law added a new section to the Public Health Service Act, authorizing and defining population research and providing budget authority to award grants and contracts (US Congress, 1970).

The focus in NIH support of human reproductive research remained on contraception in the early 1970s. The CPR was organized into branches: Contraceptive Development, Contraceptive Evaluation, and Reproductive Sciences. The Demographic and Behavioral Sciences Branch was subsequently separated from Reproductive Sciences. In the CPR, infertility was mentioned but initially was not part of any specific plan. (P. A. Corfman, personal communication). Both NIH and the US Department of Agriculture actively supported basic reproductive biology in animal models but, at NIH, leads for better contraception were of greater programmatic interest than infertility (US Department of Health, Education and Welfare, 1973).

Elsewhere in the government, at the National Center for Health Statistics in what is now the Centers for Disease Control and Prevention, efforts to collect data on women's health and pregnancy were part of the first National Survey of Family Growth conducted in 1973. The extent of impaired fecundity, infertility, and use of medical services for infertility have continued to be tracked through five cycles since then, with a sixth conducted in 2001 (Abma et al., 1997). With growing awareness of the magnitude of infertility as a public health problem, NICHD began a series of initiatives to stimulate research on both male and female infertility. In 1977 and 1981, the Reproductive Sciences Branch issued two requests for applications (RFAs) for research grants addressing infertility and reproductive disorders. Three more such requests were issued in 1983, as infertility became increasingly recognized as a priority. These early initiatives highlighted a number of topics that were to have direct bearing on ART, such as ovarian physiology, gonadotropin-releasing hormone analogs, and oocyte development and release (NIH Guide to Grants and Contracts, 1983;

Reproductive Sciences Branch, 1986). From 1977 to 1986, federal funding for research on "Reproductive Processes" grew from US$36 million to $109 million, yet human infertility accounted for only $6 million of the latter figure (US Department of Health and Human Services, 1987).

While NIH-funded research was beginning to create a knowledge base with eventual application to the diagnosis and treatment of human infertility, direct support of in vitro fertilization (IVF) was placed out-of-bounds for federally supported investigation. The 1975 regulations protecting human research subjects included a provision that: "No application or proposal involving human in vitro fertilization may be funded by the Department or any component thereof until the application or proposal has been reviewed by the Ethical Advisory Board and the board has rendered advice as to its acceptability from an ethical standpoint (Code of Federal Regulations 1975)."

The first Ethical Advisory Board (EAB) issued a report in 1979 concluding that research involving human IVF could be ethically acceptable under some circumstances (US Department of Health, Education and Welfare, 1979). This report generated controversy, and the review requirement became a de facto ban on federal support of human IVF research when the EAB was allowed to pass out of existence in 1980. In fact, no applications ever completed this review process. NIH policy at that time was that applications needed first to receive a potentially fundable score in peer review, then be approved by the Institute's Advisory Council, then finally be referred to the EAB. The interpretation of what constituted human IVF research came to encompass not only direct performance of the procedure but also studies of human materials that had IVF as a prerequisite. Human embryos, fertilized ova, and parthogenetically activated eggs were included. Even apparently unfertilized ova that had failed to fertilize after exposure to sperm fell under the de facto ban, since no reliable method existed to prove they had truly not fertilized. In the late 1980s, a grant application using discarded ova from human IVF did receive an outstanding score but languished for years while the hopes for a policy change at the Department of Health and Human Services rose and fell. A report by the US Congressional Office of Technology Assessment criticized the department for failing to carry out it own regulations requiring EAB review of IVF research (Raymond, 1988; US Congress, 1988). NICHD staff have continued to encourage investigators to submit applications that include well-designed IVF research so that, in the event of such change, approved projects will be ready to begin. In reality, the human IVF portions of the projects have remained nonfundable. The de facto ban clearly had a chilling effect on submission of projects with a primary content that was human IVF. As a result, experimentation in this field has been conducted in the private sector, often without the peer review and oversight standards that apply to federally funded research.

Given the limitations placed on human IVF research, investigators and NIH staff worked to find permissible areas of study that would still provide benefits, even indirect, to those seeking to conceive with ART. Both NIH initiatives and investigator-initiated projects took a variety of approaches "around the edges" of IVF. These approaches have included epidemiological and outcomes research on the safety and success of IVF, and improvement of ART methods other than IVF such as therapeutic insemination, sperm cryopreservation, and ovulation induction (Guzick et al., 1999; Cramer et al., 2000). A large multiproject grant on male infertility included the establishment of a registry for, and follow-up of, outcomes in children born as a result of intracytoplasmic sperm injection (ICSI). The Demographic and Behavioral Sciences Branch of CPR supported another large multiproject grant to study the biomedical, psychological, and social consequences of ART. The National Cooperative Multicenter Reproductive Medicine Network, begun in 1990, conducts clinical trials of treatments for infertility and reproductive disorders, including ovulation induction and therapeutic insemination.

One of the most important of these indirect approaches has been the use of nonhuman animal models to study IVF and biology of the early embryo.

In 1985, an RFA was published requesting applications for a Cooperative Multicenter Program on Environmental Conditions for Nonhuman In Vitro Fertilization and Preimplantation Development (NIH Guide to Grants and Contracts, 1985). The investigators supported under this initiative (and its 1990 recompetition) became known as the "Culture Club." This group produced biological findings and new techniques with direct application to human practice, for example the formulation of defined culture media to optimize embryo development and gene expression, and the testing methods that led to those discoveries (e.g., Gardner and Schoolcraft, 1998).

In a different, but related, area, one of the first official acts of President Bill Clinton in 1992 was to rescind the ban on the use of human fetal tissue in federally supported human therapeutic transplantation research. Until that point, spontaneous abortion or ectopic gestation had been the only permissible sources of fetal tissue for human transplantation research, severely limiting access to biologically useful cells. With careful ethical safeguards in place to allow the use of fetal tissue from therapeutic abortion, NIH officials and investigators once again hoped for progress in the support of IVF research. The next year, the President signed into law the NIH Revitalization Act of 1993, which repealed the requirement for EAB approval (US Congress 1993). The very next month, NICHD published a Program Announcement to inform the investigator community of the repeal and to invite grant applications to conduct basic and clinical research studies that would enhance the outcome of IVF in the normal course of treatment for human infertility. According to this announcement, "With the lifting of this requirement, the NIH can now conduct and support research involving human IVF, in accord with the recommendations of the grantee institution's Institutional Review Board, without the need for a special Federal-level Ethical Advisory Board in each case." The announcement even listed examples of research topics invited: "improved patient selection procedures for treatment with IVF, improved ovulation induction in IVF protocols, improved methods for gamete collection, improved conditions for fertilization, improved conditions for embryo transfer, [and] IVF outcome in different racial and ethnic groups" (NIH Guide to Grants and Contracts, 1993).

This invitation, however, did not result in a rush of new grants on human IVF. The announcement also contained the caveat, "It is anticipated that applications involving certain types of research that relate to human IVF will still be subject to special review on a case-by-case basis." In fact, any possibility of funding a project involving human IVF triggered review by senior NICHD and NIH officials. Some operational principles emerged: any IVF in an NIH project must be with the intention of establishing a pregnancy, the clinical and research teams must be separate groups of individuals, and grant funds could not be used to directly support the IVF procedure or the personnel performing it. Projects were considered on a case-by-case basis, with permissible and disallowed activities spelled out in a letter specific for each project. In the mid-1990s, two projects that included IVF were successfully presented for funding consideration: one comparing treatment protocols for infertile women with polycystic ovarian syndrome and one seeking biological and epidemiological predictors of IVF success. In both cases, support for the IVF portion of the projects was delayed significantly while information was weighed and the exact wording of the letters was determined.

At around the same time, in order to get policy guidance prior to funding IVF research projects that could involve the human embryo, at NICHD's request, the NIH convened the Human Embryo Research Panel. In 1994, the Panel issued a report classifying types of research into acceptable, needing further review, and unacceptable for federal funding (NIH, 1994). While viewed as balanced and reasonable (Annas et al., 1996), the report set off a reaction against any human embryo research. One consequence was a presidential order banning the creation of human embryos for research. This ban was expanded and codified into law by a provision known as the "Dickey–Wicker Amendment" to the 1996 law providing funds for NIH, prohibiting the use of federal funds for most human embryo research. According to that law:

None of the funds made available in this Act may be used for:
(1) the creation of a human embryo or embryos for research purposes; or
(2) research in which a human embryo or embryos are destroyed, discarded, or knowingly subjected to risk of injury or death greater than that allowed for research on fetuses in utero under 45 CFR 46.208(a)(2) and section 498 (b) of the Public Health Service Act (42 U.S.C. 289g (b)).
(b) For purposes of this section, the term "human embryo or embryos" includes any organism, not protected as a human subject under 45 CFR 46 as of the date of the enactment of this Act, that is derived by fertilization, parthenogenesis, cloning, or any other means from one or more human gametes or human diploid cells (US Congress 1996)."

Attempts to craft compromise language to allow the use of "spare" embryos no longer needed for transfer, a possibility that had been left open in the presidential directive, have not been successful, and the amendment provisions have been repeatedly renewed (US Congress, 2000). Human embryos, of course, imply human IVF. Thus federal agencies remain constrained from supporting or conducting a large amount of cutting-edge research to improve the use of ART.

NICHD and other components of NIH have continued to promote research to benefit ART within the limits placed upon them. Workshops and conferences have been held on such topics as preimplantation genetic diagnosis and ICSI. RFAs have been issued for research on human gametes. Today there are about two dozen projects supported by NIH that are expected to yield information which will improve the practice of human ART, but they are in the categories described above. Either they have fiscally separate components for treatment and research or they work "around the edges," with studies of gametes, outcomes after the fact, or animal models. While these efforts have merit, they leave serious gaps in knowledge.

In 1998, the US Food and Drug Administration issued a notice that it proposed initially to establish a registry and product listing (Federal Register, 1998) and later to regulate the "manufacture" of human cells and tissues, including reproductive cells, under its authority to prevent transmission of communicable diseases by biologically derived materials used in the practice of medicine (Federal Register, 1999). The notices were available for public comment, and other federal agencies, including NIH, were consulted. Discussions are ongoing in 2001. Reproductive cells, as used in infertility treatment, are very different from somatic cells and tissues such as blood cells or tissue grafts. Because of the small amount of research, and the resulting paucity of reliable published data, knowledge to guide the regulatory process regarding the appropriate use of human gametes and embryos is severely insufficient for informed regulation.

Human IVF has been with us since the 1980s and is increasingly a mainstream treatment for infertility. In 1997, 51 344 cycles of IVF were performed in the USA (Society for Assisted Reproductive Technology and American Society for Reproductive Medicine, 2000). ICSI has brought new possibilities and new risks. Yet practitioners have few criteria beyond "which one looks good" when choosing an embryo to transfer or a sperm to inject. To best promote public health, ARTs, like all therapies, should have their safety and effectiveness demonstrated by published evidence acquired in well-designed, peer-reviewed research studies subject to objective stewardship and oversight, regardless of their source of funding.

REFERENCES

Abma, J.C., Chandra, A., Mosher, W.D., Peterson, L.S., and Piccinino, L.J. (1997). Fertility, family planning, and women's health: new data from the 1995 National Survey of Family Growth. National Center for Health Statistics. *Vital Health Statistics*, **23**, 1–114.

Annas, G.J., Caplan, A., and Elias, S. (1996). The politics of human-embryo research – avoiding ethical gridlock. *New England Journal of Medicine*, **334**, 1329–32.

Code of Federal Regulations (1975). 45 Part 46.204(d).

Cramer, D.W., Liberman, R.F., Powers, D., Hornstein, M.D., McShane, P., and Barbieri, R.L. (2000). Recent trends in assisted reproductive techniques and associated outcomes. *Obstetrics and Gynecology*, **95**, 61–6.

Federal Register (1998). **63** FR 26744.

Federal Register (1999). **64** FR 52696.

Gardner, D.K. and Schoolcraft, W.B. (1998). No longer neglected: the human blastocyst. *Human Reproduction*, **13**, 3289–92.

Guzick, D.S., Carson, S.A., Coutifaris, C., et al. (1999). Efficacy of superovulation and intrauterine insemination in the treatment of infertility. *New England Journal of Medicine*, **340**, 177–83.

NIH (1994). *Report of the Human Embryo Research Panel*, September 27, 1994. US National Institutes of Health, Bethesda, MD.

NIH Guide to Grants and Contracts (1983). *Request for Research Grant Applications National Institute of Child Health and Human Development-CPR-83-3, Human Female Infertility*, Vol. 12, 15 July, 1983. NIH, Washington, DC.

NIH Guide to Grants and Contracts (1985). *Request for Cooperative Agreement Applications 85-HD-13, Cooperative Multicenter Program on Environmental Conditions for Non-human In Vitro Fertilization and Preimplantation Development*, 21 June, 1985. National Institutes of Health, Washington, DC.

NIH Guide to Grants and Contracts (1993). *Program Announcement, Research Involving Human in Vitro Fertilization, PA-93–101*, 23 July, 1993. National Institutes of Health, Washington, DC.

Raymond, C.A. (1988). In vitro fertilization faces 'R & R': (more) research and regulation. *Journal of the American Medical Association*, **260**, 1191–2.

Reproductive Sciences Branch (1986). *Report to the National Advisory Child Health and Human Development Council*. National Institutes of Health, Bethesda, MD.

Society for Assisted Reproductive Technology and American Society for Reproductive Medicine (2000). Assisted reproductive technology in the United States: 1997 results generated from the American Society for Reproductive Medicine/ Society for Assisted Reproductive Technology Registry. *Fertility and Sterility*, **74**, 641–54.

US Congress, Office of Technology Assessment (1988). *Infertility: Medical and Social Choices*. (OTA-BA-358) US Government Printing Office, Washington, DC.

US Congress (1970). Public Law 91–572.

US Congress (1993). Public Law 103–43.

US Congress (1996). Public Law 104–91.

US Congress (2000). Public Law 106–113.

US Department of Health, Education and Welfare (1973). *A Five-year Plan for Population Research and Family Planning Services*. US Government Printing Office, Washington, DC.

US Department of Health, Education and Welfare (1979). *Ethics Advisory Board, Report and Conclusions: HEW Support of Research Involving Human In Vitro Fertilization and Embryo Transfer.* US Government Printing Office, Washington, DC.

US Department of Health and Human Services (1987). *Inventory and Analysis of Federal Population Research, Fiscal Year 1986.* US Government Printing Office, Washington, DC.

Concepts for the global community

22

From conception to contraception

Gustavo F. Doncel[1], Christine Mauck[1], Douglas S. Colvard[1]
and Lourens J. D. Zaneveld[2]

[1]CONRAD Program, Eastern Virginia Medical School, Norfolk, USA
[2]Program for Topical Prevention of Conception and Disease, Rush University, Chicago, USA

Introduction

Fertility is the ability to reproduce, to conceive an offspring. Numerous interconnected factors determine fertility; anatomical, endocrinological, genetic, environmental, and nutritional factors are some of the most important elements determining the degree of fertility (Dzuik, 1998). At a cellular level, adequate fertility implies successful fertilization, an event that culminates with the fusion of sperm and egg but encompasses a multiplicity of processes, from genesis and maturation of germ cells to transport and interaction of gametes. In recent years, we have witnessed a remarkable advance in the knowledge and understanding of these physiological processes, especially regarding genetic, endocrine, and paracrine control of gametogenesis (Mermillod et al., 1999; Weinbauer and Wessels, 1999; Anderson and Sharpe, 2000), sperm maturation and capacitation (Visconti et al., 1998; Yeung et al., 1998), and molecular determinants of fertilization (Evans, 2000). This new information has provided the basis for the development of new diagnostic and therapeutic modalities for infertility as well as novel contraceptive approaches. It is on this latter application of recently acquired knowledge in reproductive biology that we will focus.

Meeting contraceptive needs for the twenty-first century is a critical and an enormous task. According to the World Health Organization (WHO), over 100 million acts of sexual intercourse take place each day (Senanayake, 1994). These result in some 910 000 conceptions and 356 000 sexually transmitted diseases (STDs) including both bacterial and viral infections. About 50% of the conceptions are unplanned and about 25% are definitely unwanted. About 150 000 unwanted pregnancies are terminated every day by induced abortion. About one-third of these abortions are performed under unsafe conditions in an adverse social and legal climate, resulting in some 500 deaths every day. Estimates show almost 1400 women die every day in the course of pregnancy and childbirth (Senanayake, 1994) and 1 in 12 newborns will not reach their first birthday (Khanna et al., 1992).

Family planning not only enables fertility regulation, but it also saves the lives of women and children. This undeniable truth has been reinforced by the interdependency of family planning and reproductive health, and the deadly impact of the sexually disseminated epidemic of human immunodeficiency virus (HIV) and its consequence, the acquired immunodeficiency syndrome (AIDS). (Cates, 2000). More than 30 million people are infected with HIV worldwide. The death toll related to AIDS exceeds 18 million, and the disease represents the third leading cause of death among women of reproductive age. Sexual transmission of HIV is clearly the predominant mode for AIDS transmission. Therefore, a new challenge is the search for innovative contraceptive technologies to help in the battle against an increasing incidence and prevalence of STDs, especially AIDS.

Although the prevalence of contraceptive use is increasing worldwide (World Health Organization, 1988), there is still considerable variation between different countries. Demographic forces, prevalence of disease, and socioeconomic and cultural factors influence not only the use of contraceptives but also the development of new methods (Baird and Glasier, 1998). Access barriers are an important determinant in contraceptive choice and use. However, method acceptability and contraceptive success are not limited to access. If safer, more convenient, efficacious, and economical methods existed, more people would have the choice of using them. This review focuses on the latest developments in contraceptive technology and describes ongoing preclinical and clinical studies in three main areas: vaginal contraception (and interrelated STD prevention), female steroidal contraception, and male contraception.

New developments in vaginal contraception

Vaginal contraception has been practiced for centuries, but with the advent of hormonal methods, the intrauterine device (IUD) and female sterilization are now only used by a comparatively small proportion of women. Vaginal contraceptives can be divided into two general types: formulations and devices. Total revenues for all vaginal contraceptive products in the USA in 1992 was only $52 million compared with a total of $1243 million for all other contraceptive products (Harrison and Rosenfield, 1996). However, vaginal contraception has several advantages over other birth control methods. It only needs to be applied when intercourse actually takes place and it is safe, i.e., is not associated with any major side-effects. Vaginal spermicidal formulations (but not devices) are readily available over the counter and can be purchased in most drug stores. In addition, they can prevent or at least decrease the chances of contracting certain STDs through heterosexual intercourse. The contraceptive efficacy of vaginal methods, however, is usually less than desired and good success requires a highly motivated user. In addition, spermicidal formulations tend to leak from the vagina and may be messy. Finally, such formulations have a rather short effective period, requiring their vaginal insertion just before intercourse, thereby reducing the spontaneity of the sex act. Devices can be inserted well before coitus but some women have difficulty with their placement (therefore, requiring training) and the devices can sometimes be dislodged during intercourse leaving the woman unprotected.

Updates on new developments in vaginal contraceptives have previously been published (Mauck et al., 1994; Zaneveld, 1994; Mauck and Doncel, 2000). Specific references can be found in these publications. Because of the AIDS epidemic, recent emphasis in vaginal contraception has primarily been focused on the development of methods that provide both contraceptive and antimicrobial activity.

Vaginal antimicrobial products with or without contraceptive activity

Until the recent need for methods that prevent transmission of HIV and other STD-causing pathogens, little had been done to improve vaginal contraception techniques in order to make them more effective and consumer friendly. Since the AIDS epidemic is rapidly spreading, especially in sub-Saharan Africa and southeast Asia, countermeasures need to be taken urgently. Other STDs are also a major problem and can potentiate HIV transmission through their disruption of the vaginal epithelium (Laga et al., 1994). In 1995, more than 333 million new cases of chlamydial and trichomonal infections, gonorrhea, and syphilis occurred worldwide (Gerbase et al., 1998). Other STDs, such as hepatitis, are also on the rise. Cervical cancer is now known to be primarily caused by papilloma virus, a sexually transmitted organism.

Recommendations to change sexual behavior or to use condoms, albeit successful in some countries, have proven insufficient to prevent the spread of AIDS and other STDs. Although both the male and female condom can provide an effective block to the transmission of STD-causing organisms, their use is limited primarily because of "loss in feeling" and aesthetic problems. In addition, the cooperation of the male is required and many men refuse to use these devices. In the USA, condom use averages about 30%, and it is lower in many other countries. New prophylactic methods need to be developed to prevent these diseases and to provide additional protection against unplanned pregnancies. Since women are more frequently affected by STDs/AIDS and they are the only ones subject to unplanned pregnancies, it is particularly important to develop women-controlled methods that protect them from pregnancy and disease.

A topical vaginal product is the primary, if not the only, technique whereby a woman can prevent both microbial infections transmitted through vaginal intercourse and pregnancy. To be effective, a vaginal method must establish a barrier between the infectious organisms/spermatozoa and the female reproductive tract. Such a barrier might be physical (contraceptive devices), chemical (vaginal gel or other dosage form), or immunological (exogenous antibodies or a vaginal immune response). While research is ongoing on all these fronts, there is considerable interest in the development of novel vaginal prophylactic formulations (Mauck and Doncel, 2000).

Commercially available products

Commercially available chemical vaginal contraceptives contain an active ingredient capable of immobilizing and killing spermatozoa (a spermicide). The most commonly used active ingredient is nonoxynol-9, a non-ionic detergent. This compound is a surfactant and destroys the sperm membranes (Schill and Wolff, 1981). Other surfactants and detergents such as octoxynol-9, menfegol, and benzalkonium chloride can be found in commercial products, particularly those marketed outside the USA. Most of these surfactants and detergents have approximately the same potency so the main difference among marketed spermicidal preparations is the base (carrier) of the active ingredient.

Nonoxynol-9 and other detergents effectively inactivate HIV and most other STD-causing organisms in vitro, with the exception of the papilloma virus (a nonenveloped virus) (Zaneveld et al., 1996). However, the ability of vaginal contraceptive formulations to prevent gonococcal, trichomonal, and chlamydial infections is limited (Roddy et al., 1998a). Furthermore, in large clinical trials, none of the vaginal contraceptive products tested, including a sponge, a film, and a gel, prevented HIV transmission (Kreiss et al., 1992; Roddy et al., 1998b; Stephenson, 2000). It is not known why nonoxynol-9 can kill spermatozoa and pathogenic microbes in microgram quantities in vitro but is much less spermicidal in vivo at doses that are 500 times higher, such as those used in marketed contraceptive products. Presumably the compound must not be available for contact with spermatozoa or the STD-causing microbes in sufficient quantities or in time to prevent their migration into the cervix or penetration into vaginal tissue.

Protection versus perturbation

The stratified squamous epithelium covering the vagina and part of the ectocervix physically blocks entry of STD-causing pathogens. In addition, lactobacilli, components of the normal vaginal microbial flora, produce lactic acid in sufficient quantities for the normal vaginal fluids to have a pH of 3.5–4.5. At this acidic pH, HIV and many other pathogenic organisms are inactivated (Voeller and Anderson, 1992; Mahmoud et al., 1995). In addition, the vagina and cervix are both capable of producing antibody and cell-mediated immune responses to genital tract infections (Anderson and Quayle, 1996). Finally, cervicovaginal secretions contain a number of nonspecific antibacterial and antiviral defense agents such as lysozyme, polyamines, hydrogen peroxide, and lactoferrin (Cohen et al., 1990). Therefore, the normal vagina is quite protective against transmission of disease-causing organisms. Perturbation of this protective milieu makes transmission more likely.

The vaginal environment can be disturbed by a variety of events. After intercourse, the basic pH (≥ 7.2) and strong buffering activity of the ejaculate causes a rise in the vaginal pH to above 6.0. Although this is of benefit for fertility since spermatozoa are inactivated at the acidic pH of the vagina, the alkaline environment also allows survival of STD-causing pathogens. Furthermore, some vaginal infections cause the pH to rise. Vaginal diseases resulting from STD-causing pathogens induce vaginal inflammation and epithelial lesions, allowing the transmission of other pathogens such as HIV. Menopause and progestin-dominated hormonal therapies can cause thinning of the squamous epithelium and reduce cervical mucus production.

Chemicals can also cause damage. Detergents such as nonoxynol-9 are not only cytocidal towards spermatozoa and STD-causing organisms but also towards lactobacilli and vaginal and cervical cells. As a result, the frequent daily use of formulations containing these compounds can cause vaginal irritation, inflammation and lesions, and consumer complaints of itching, burning, and pain (Roddy et al., 1993). A recently completed study by UNAIDS and World Health Organization showed that a nonoxynol-9-containing vaginal gel was less protective against HIV transmission than its placebo (Stephenson, 2000). Women using the nonoxynol-9-gel showed an increase in vaginal lesions, which may have been one of the reasons for the enhanced transmission of HIV. All these physiological and pathological aspects of the vagina and cervix must be taken into consideration in the design of improved vaginal formulations. In addition, a compound found to be antimicrobial has to be combined with a useful, consumer-friendly delivery vehicle for the formulation to be highly effective. Some discussion has occurred about whether vaginal antimicrobial formulations should also be contraceptive. Most women want to become pregnant at least once or twice in their lives, at which time they would need an antimicrobial product but not a contraceptive one. However, most of the time, they would want to be protected against both pregnancy and disease (with the exception of some cultures where women want to become pregnant as often as possible to maintain their status in society). Therefore, the large majority of women favor an antimicrobial contraceptive product most of the time (Hardy et al., 1998) and an antimicrobial noncontraceptive product some of the time.

New active ingredients

The following is a brief summary of active ingredients and base formulations presently under investigation or development. Because of renewed interest in this subject, potential candidate products are constantly being developed so the summary is by no means all-inclusive. In addition, because of the need for patent protection and other confidentiality issues, the properties and status of development of new products are often not available. Several reviews have recently appeared on this subject (Elias and Coggins, 1996; Pauwels and De Clercq, 1996; Zaneveld et al., 1996; Harrison, 2000; Mauck and Doncel, 2000) and a report was prepared in 2000 (Alliance for Microbicide Development, 2000).

The antimicrobial and/or contraceptive properties of a compound should not be the only criterion in deciding whether an agent should enter clinical trials. Other considerations should include the difficulty and cost of manufacture, the complexity of formulation into an acceptable vaginal product, and any toxicity or irritating effect on the vagina when used frequently.

Active ingredients in proposed vaginal antimicrobial products are listed in Tables 22.1 and 22.2. These ingredients can generally be divided into two classes: those that inactivate spermatozoa and/or microbes through cytotoxic effects (i.e., by killing them: cytocidal agents (Table 22.1)) and those that prevent their migration into tissue or entry into host cells (i.e, are entry inhibitors: noncytocidal agents (Table 22.2)).

Cytocidal agents

Cytocidal agents usually act by destroying the cell membrane and are, therefore, generally effective against bacteria, enveloped viruses, and spermatozoa. Since cell death is normally easier to identify in in vitro tests than inhibition of tissue or cell entry, and since typical cytocidal agents have already been used in vaginal contraceptives and other topical products, these compounds initially have received the most attention. Surfactants and detergents such as nonoxynol-9, octoxynol-9, Triton X-100, benzalkonium chloride, and chlorhexidine were the first to be tested. C31G, a new cytocidal agent, is composed of an equimolar mixture of two synthetic, amphoteric surface-active compounds, alkyl dimethylglycine

Table 22.1. Vaginal antimicrobial products utilizing cytocidal agents

Product name	Description	Company/institution	Stage of development
Surfactants, detergents, and others			
Prevent-X	Octoxynol-9 with benzalkonium chloride		Clinical
TP1	Triton X-100 product, containing octoxynol-9	Novavax	Clinical
SAVVY	Refined C31G amine oxide and an alkyl betain	Biosyn	Clinical
SDS	Sodium dodecyl sulfate	Pennsylvania State College of Medicine	Preclinical
Polybiguanides	Cationic surfactants	Jelling and Associates	Preclinical
N-Doscosanol	22 Carbon straight chain alcohol	Avanir	Preclinical
Z14/Z15	Acylcarnitine analogs	Virginia Polytechnic Institute, Kensa and CONRAD	Preclinical
Protectaid Sponge	Polyurethane foam sponge impregnated with a gel containing sodium cholate, nonoxynol-9, and benzalkonium chlorides	S.S.P.L.-Axcan	Clinical
Avert Sponge	Contains nonoxynol-9	Gynetech Laboratories	Clinical (halted)
N.A.	Lactobacillus-containing formulations	New York Institute for Basic Research/University of Pittsburg	Preclinical
Inner Confidence	Suppository formulation with nonoxynol-9, benzalkonium chloride, microencapsulated lactobacilli, bioadhesives and buffers	Biofem, Inc	Preclinical
N.A.	Octyl-glycerol synthetic milk lipid	University of Pittsburgh/ Magee Women's Hospital	Preclinical
Haloperoxidases		ExOxEmis Inc.	Preclinical
Gossypol	Polyphenolic plant-derived compound originally developed as an oral male contraceptive	Hebron (Brazil)	Clinical
Praneem Polyherbal	Neem oil extracts from *Sapindus citrata* oil	Talwar Research Foundation (India)	Clinical
Peptides, proteins, and related compounds			
Magainin	Amphoteric, cationic peptides	Magainin Pharmaceuticals	Preclinical
Gramicidin	Peptide	Metatron Inc.	Preclinical
Peptidyl MIMs	Peptide antibiotics	Demegen	Unknown
X2371	Low-molecular-weight nonpeptide oligospecific integrin modulator	Billings Pharmaceutical Company	Preclinical
B-367	Protegrin peptide	Licensed to UCLA from Intro Biotech Pharmaceuticals	Preclinical

Note: N.A., not available.

Source: Prepared by D. P. Waller and L. J. D. Zaneveld.

Table 22.2. Vaginal antimicrobial products utilizing noncytotoxic agents

Product name	Description	Company/institution	Stage of development
Polymeric agents, organometallic compounds, and antibodies			
Dextrin sulfate	Sulfated polysaccharide	Medical Research Council and ML Laboratories	Clinical
Carraguard™ (Carrageenan)	Anionic sulfated polysaccharide derived from seaweed	Population Council	Clinical
Cellulose sulfate (CS; Ushercell)	High-molecular-weight sulfated polysaccharide ($M_r > 1000$)	Polydex Inc, TOPCAD	Clinical
Polystyrene sulfonate (PSS)	High-molecular-weight sulfated polymer ($M_r > 500$)	TOPCAD	Clinical
Pro2000	Naphthalene sulfonate polymer	Interneuron	Clinical
B69	Bovine β-lactoglobulin modified by 3-hydroxyphthalic anhydride	New York Blood Center	Preclinical
B195	Cellulose acetate phthalate; USP/NF excipient	New York Blood Center	Preclinical
CTC-96	Doxovir organometallic compound	Redox Pharmaceutical Corporation	Preclinical
Aryl 4-guanidino-benzoates, and acetaminophen		Metatron, Inc	Preclinical
Cyanovirin-N	Protein isolated and sequenced from cultures of freshwater cyanobacteria	National Cancer Institute (NIH)	Preclinical
N.A.	Polymers to modify the properties of mucins	GelTexPharmaceutical	Preclinical
Plantibodies	Monoclonal antibodies from bioengineered plants	Epicyte Pharmaceutical/ Reprotect	Preclinical
Derivatives of systemic antiviral agents			
WHI-05	5-Bromo-6-methoxy-5,6-dihydro-3′-azidothymidine-5′-(*p*-methoxyphenyl) methoxyaninyl phosphate	Hughes Institute	Preclinical
UC-781	Non-nucleoside reverse transcriptase inhibitor	Rega Institute for Medical Research	Preclinical
PMPA	Adenine antiretroviral	Gilead Sciences	Preclinical
N.A.	Antiviral compounds designed for HIV therapy	Aaron Diamond Research Institute	Preclinical

Note: N.A., not available.

Source: Prepared by D. P. Waller and L. J. D. Zaneveld.

and alkyl dimethylamine oxide, with alkyl chain lengths varying from 12 to 16 (Corner et al., 1998). Like other surfactants, C31G has broad-spectrum antimicrobial and spermicidal properties. More recently, sodium dodecyl sulfate has been proposed as a candidate compound (Howett et al., 2000). The advantage of sodium dodecyl sulfate over some other cytocidal agents is its ability to inactivate the non-enveloped papilloma virus. Novel acylcarnitine analogs have proved to be potent spermicidal and anti-HIV compounds (Savle et al., 1999). One of them (Z-15) is a very potent growth inhibitor of *Candida albicans*. Remarkably, the acylcarnitine analogs do not irritate the vaginal mucosa.

A number of products, including a sponge, combine several active ingredients in the hope of offering additional protection. However, it remains to be established whether a mixture of cytocidal agents provides better prophylaxis than a single agent used at the same concentration as all others combined. A more interesting approach is the addition of microencapsulated lactobacilli to a formulation. It is hoped that these lactobacilli can re-establish the normal vaginal flora when there is an infection. In addition, the acid produced by the lactobacilli may aid in maintaining the normal vaginal pH.

Regarding natural products, a number of plant extracts are known to possess microbicidal and spermicidal properties. One of the earliest vaginal antimicrobial formulations to enter clinical trial was Praneem (based on neem oil) (Talwar et al., 1994). Neem oil has antiviral, antibacterial, antifungal, and antifertility activity (Talwar et al., 2000). Gossypol is another plant product that has been tested in clinical trials. Originally proposed as an oral male contraceptive, Gossypol has proven to be spermicidal and antimicrobial. Peptides isolated from animal sources are also evolving as candidate compounds. The most interesting of these compounds are antimicrobial agents that occur naturally in secretions, leukocytes, and tissues. Magainins are amphoteric cationic peptides isolated from frogs; these peptides have broad antimicrobial and spermicidal properties because of their ability to adopt an amphiphilic

α-helix structure in a hydrophobic environment, causing the formation of holes in cell walls (Edelstein et al., 1991; Reddy et al., 1996). Defensins are another example of such broadly active animal peptides. These are complexly folded amphipathic peptides that, while rich in an antiparallel β-sheet, are devoid of α-helical domains (Ganz and Lehrer, 1994). The antimicrobial properties of the defensins result from their ability to insert into target cell membranes and to form voltage-sensitive ion channels. Protegrins are arginine-rich peptides of 16–18 amino acid residues with two intramolecular disulfide bonds; they were originally isolated from leukocytes (Tamamura et al., 1995). Bacteria can also be a source of antimicrobial peptides. Gramicidin, a peptide antibiotic used in the former Soviet Union as an active ingredient in contraceptive formulations, exhibits anti-HIV activity (Bourinbaiar and Lee-Huang, 1994a).

Noncytocidal agents

A potential problem with many cytocidal agents is their tendency to have nonspecific cytotoxic properties. Like nonoxynol-9, they may cause undesired side-effects with frequent use. An alternative approach is the use of agents that do not destroy the cell membrane or kill the organisms but act by preventing their entry through the vaginal epithelium or into the host cell. It was originally thought it would be difficult to find noncytotoxic compounds that are both antimicrobial and contraceptive but several with "dual" activity have now been discovered. For fertilization to occur, spermatozoa must first penetrate the outer layers of the oocyte (the cumulus oophorus, the corona radiata, and the zona pellucida) and subsequently fuse with and pass through the egg membrane (oolemma). Several components of the egg layer, for example hyaluronic acid (a glycosaminoglycan) and proteins, are also found in the subepithelial layers of the vagina. Therefore, spermatozoa and pathogenic microbes are able to utilize conserved (inherent) mechanisms to accomplish entry. For example, hyaluronidase and proteinases (acrosin in the case of spermatozoa) are used by spermatozoa to penetrate the egg vestments and these same enzymes are used by certain microbes to infect tissues such as the cervicovaginal mucosa. Cell fusion and penetration occur when both spermatozoa and microbes enter host cells. Heparin-like ligands on the surface of spermatozoa and certain viral and bacterial microbes (Herold et al., 1997, 2000) may be essential for such fusion. Consequently, similarities in the tissue/cell entry mechanisms of pathogenic microbes and spermatozoa may be utilized to find inhibitors for both types of cell.

Noncytocidal agents for potential vaginal use are listed in Table 22.2. The sulfated polysaccharide cellulose sulfate and the sulfated polymers (e.g., polystyrene sulfonate and a naphthalene sulfonate derivative (Pro2000)) have broad-spectrum antimicrobial and sperm-inhibitory properties (Bourne et al., 1999; Anderson et al., 2000; Herold et al., 2000; Rencher et al., 2000). Cellulose sulfate and polystyrene sulfonate inhibit HIV, herpesvirus, gonococci, chlamydia and the papilloma virus. Further, they have no effect on lactobacilli and are not irritating to the vagina. Both cellulose sulfate and polystyrene sulfonate have a very high molecular mass ($>500\,kDa$), making their vaginal absorption extremely unlikely. All three products have entered clinical trials. Serine proteinase inhibitors, such as 4′-acetamidophenyl 4-guanidinobenzoate, prevent fertilization by inhibiting acrosin (Zaneveld et al., 1988a) and they also inhibit HIV (Bourinbaiar and Lee-Huang, 1994b). Noncytocidal agents with broad-spectrum antimicrobial but no contraceptive properties include the sulfated polysaccharides carrageenan (Maguire et al., 1998) and dextrin sulfate (Stafford et al., 1997). These compounds are also in clinical trials. Cellulose acetate phthalate (Neurath et al., 1999) and bovine β-lactoglobulin (Kokuba et al., 1998) also inhibit a wide array of microbes; their effect on spermatozoa is not known. Cyanovirin, a protein derived from cyanobacteria, was shown to potently inhibit HIV in vitro (Mori et al., 1998).

Antibodies are another group of noncytocidal compounds. The immune system of the vagina and cervix is protective against infection. Any method that enhances the innate vaginal immune defense can be of potential benefit (Anderson and Quayle, 1996). Alternatively, monoclonal antibodies can be used as active ingredients in vaginal products (Cone and Whaley, 1994). Both contraception and prevention of viral STDs with monoclonal antibodies have been demonstrated in animals. Large-scale manufacture of these antibodies used to be a major problem, but the recent development of bioengineering technology has enabled them to be produced by plants rather than animals ("plantibodies"; Zeitlin et al., 1998).

Another group of compounds that have tentatively been placed in this category until their cytotoxic properties are better established are derivatives of systemic antiviral agents. These agents were initially developed for the treatment of AIDS but they may also have application in vaginal products. One of these, a bromomethoxy-substituted phenyl phosphate derivative of zidovudine (WHI-05) has both antimicrobial and sperm-immobilizing activity (D'Cruz et al., 1999).

Delivery systems

Active agents may be delivered intravaginally by sponges or other cervical/vaginal devices. More frequently, though, they are delivered by formulations. These can take the form of a gel, cream, foam, suppository, tablet, or film. Generally, the base makes up about 95–98% of the vaginal formulation. Each base has specific advantages and disadvantages and a woman can select the one she prefers. For instance, tablets, films, and suppositories can be provided in small packages that are easy to store and the formulation can be applied manually. By contrast, gels and foams need to be inserted with an applicator. Foams require a rather large container, whereas gels can be provided in smaller tubes or even within the applicator. Suppositories melt at body temperature, which makes them less desirable in hot climates. Good studies comparing the contraceptive effectiveness of the different bases and spermicidal agents are not available. This is mainly because only marketed products are compared, which vary in a number of aspects, including base composition, type of spermicide, spermicide concentration, etc. In addition, many of the available

Table 22.3. Vaginal antimicrobial delivery systems

Product	Description	Company/institution	Stage of development
BufferGel	Acid-buffering polymer gel	Reprotect	Clinical
LASRS	Bioadhesive suppository	Advanced Care Products; TOPCAD	Clinical
ACIDFORM	Acid-buffering, bioadhesive gel	TOPCAD	Clinical
Q-2	Double substituted hydrophobe-modified cationic polysaccharide	Integra Life Sciences and CONRAD	Preclinical
Novasome cream	Nonphospholipid-based liposome cream	Novavax	Clinical
N.A.	A polyvinyl pyrrolidone bilayered vaginal suppository tablet with nonoxynol-9	University of Kentucky	Preclinical
Sc-036	Food grade monoglyceride cream with nonoxynol-9	Biotek	Preclinical
N.A.	Thermoelastic gel	Laval University	Preclinical
Pharmagel	Amphiphilic polymer combination	Polytherapeutics	Preclinical

Note: N.A., not available.
Source: Prepared by D. P. Waller and L. J. D. Zaneveld.

studies were performed more than a decade ago and the composition of the products may have changed since that time. The failure rate associated with the typical use of vaginal spermicidal formulations is generally reported to be from 15 to 20% (Hatcher et al., 1994)

The formulation base (delivery system) can either "make or break" an effective ingredient; yet, only limited attention has been given so far to their improvement. Ideally, a delivery system should:

1 Be compatible with the active ingredient
2 Spread rapidly and evenly over the vaginal and cervical surfaces
3 Have bioadhesive properties, thereby promoting vaginal retention and forming a layer (film) over the vaginal/cervical epithelia that prevents contact with pathogenic organisms
4 Retain viscosity on dilution with vaginal fluid and semen, allowing better vaginal retention
5 Be acid-buffering, maintaining the vaginal pH in the presence of semen and a vaginal infection
6 Be noncytotoxic towards the normal vaginal microbial flora and vaginal/cervical epithelial cells
7 Encourage healing of the vagina when lesions are present.

New delivery vehicles are under active development (Rencher, 1998) and are listed in Table 22.3. Some compounds, such as BufferGel (Bentley et al., 2000) and ACIDFORM (Amaral et al., 1999), may potentially be useful without an active ingredient because they have potent acid-buffering properties, which make them both antimicrobial and spermicidal. Phase I clinical safety studies have been performed with both formulations. ACIDFORM can form a layer over the vaginal and cervical surfaces through its bioadhesive ingredients (Amaral et al., 1999). Pilot studies with BufferGel showed it to have a beneficial effect in bacterial vaginosis (Cu-Uvin et al., 2000), similar to other acid-buffering formulations (Andersch et al., 1986). Clinical tests of ACIDFORM in combination with nonoxynol-9 revealed that the latter retained its vaginal irritating properties, so this base is no longer considered as a delivery vehicle for such a detergent. LASRS, a bioadhesive suppository, forms a layer over the vaginal and cervical surfaces that cannot be removed by rinsing and, as a result, may possibly reduce some of the vaginal irritating properties of nonoxynol-9 as detected by colposcopy (Ladipo et al., 2000). After nonoxynol-9 was incorporated, high post-coital spermicidal activity was retained for prolonged periods in women (longest period tested between LASRS insertion and intercourse was 8.5 hours (Ladipo et al., 2000)). Another new delivery system, Q-2, utilizes a hydrophobe-modified cationic polysaccharide as the base for the delivery of active ingredients (Brode, 1998). Q-2 is a biocompatible and bioadhesive polymer that impedes sperm penetration in cervical mucus even at very low concentrations (Brode et al., 2000). Polyvinylpyrrolidone was also tested as an improved delivery system for nonoxynol-9 (Digenis et al., 1999). Another approach to a new base is the use of thermoelastic material that is liquid at room temperature but hardens to a gel at body temperature, i.e., when it is placed in the vagina (Gagne et al., 1999). A similar approach based on the hydration (increase in volume and viscosity) of amphiphilic polymers inside the vagina has also been reported (Shah et al., 2000).

Mechanical contraceptive barrier devices

User needs for greater convenience and for prevention of STDs have driven the development of new mechanical contraceptive barriers. Diaphragms and cervical caps used with spermicide are messy, must be fitted, and have been associated with an increased risk of urinary tract infections (in large part caused by the spermicide used with the device rather than the device itself). The Reality® female condom was a breakthrough when it was approved in 1993 as the first and only female-controlled method that reduces the chance of both pregnancy and STDs. However, it is relatively expensive and is unacceptable to some users because of discomfort and/or aesthetics. New devices are being developed that are made of less expensive, durable materials, do not require fitting, are easier to insert and remove, and are more comfortable and attractive. In addition, existing contraceptive barriers are being tested for their ability to prevent STDs.

Lea's Shield®

Lea's Shield® (also called Lea Contraceptive®) is a vaginal barrier device made of silicone rubber that is designed to be used with spermicide for contraception (Fig. 22.1). It comes in one size that fits most

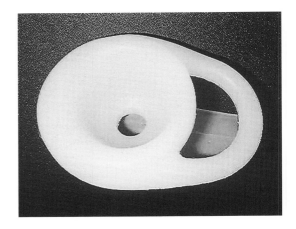

Fig. 22.1. Lea's Shield®.

women. It has a one-way valve leading toward the introitus to permit egress of any trapped air between the cervix and device during insertion, thereby allowing a tight seal.

A phase I study of postcoital testing involving Lea's Shield® showed that the device prevents motile sperm from entering the cervical mucus (Archer et al., 1995). A phase II study of 185 women from six sites located throughout the USA compared the contraceptive efficacy and safety of the device when used with and without a 3% nonoxynol-9 spermicide (Mauck et al., 1996). The six-month probability of pregnancy among the 90 women who used the device with 3% nonoxynol-9 was 8.7%. No serious device-related problems were reported and acceptability of the device was high. Data from these studies were reviewed by a US Food and Drug Administration (FDA) advisory panel in October 1996 and were found to be insufficient for approval because the number of subjects was too small. The device is now in final clinical trials sponsored by the Contraceptive Research and Development (CONRAD) program to determine changes in microflora and epithelial integrity induced by the device and the exact position of the device. Submission to the FDA is expected in early 2002.

FemCap™

The FemCap™ is another silicone device and is shaped like an upside-down sailor's hat. It comes in

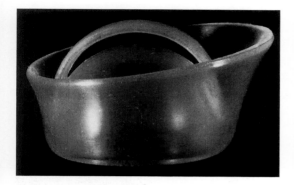

Fig. 22.2. FemCap™.

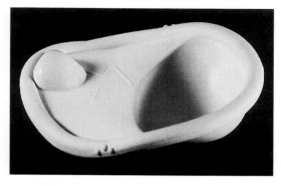

Fig. 22.3. SILCS diaphragm.

three sizes, is meant to be used with spermicide, and, at least initially, will probably require clinician fitting. In a phase II/III contraceptive efficacy trial, users of FemCap™ experienced a 6-month typical-use pregnancy rate of 13.5% compared with users of the Ortho All-Flex™ diaphragm, who experienced a rate of 7.9%. While the two devices were not equivalent in contraceptive efficacy as defined by the study, both devices had pregnancy rates that were within the expected range for barrier methods (Mauck et al., 1999). There were significantly fewer urinary tract infections among FemCap™ users. There was no difference in the incidence of colposcopic findings. However, significantly more FemCap™ users reported problems with removal and dislodgment.

The device has since been modified to have a removal strap and slightly longer brim (Fig. 22.2). The modified device is currently in a CONRAD-sponsored clinical trial aimed at determining whether it reduces removal problems. Submission to the FDA is expected in early 2002.

SILCS diaphragm

The Program for Appropriate Technology in Health (PATH, Seattle, WA) has developed a new one-size-fits-most silicone diaphragm that is in early clinical trials (Fig. 22.3). It was developed through an iterative process involving the production of multiple prototypes based on feedback from women who inserted and removed the device and from couples who used it during intercourse. It has a cup for the cervix, gripping dimples for easier handling, and a flat membrane that holds the device in place by clinging to the vaginal wall. It is currently in a post-coital study sponsored by CONRAD. If results are promising, contraceptive efficacy testing will follow.

Oves™ cervical cap

The Oves™ cervical cap, a disposable cervical cap to be used with spermicide and manufactured by Veos Ltd, UK, has been sold in Europe since 1997. The advantages of the cap, as reported by the manufacturer, are ease of insertion and removal, adherence to the cervix by surface tension rather than suction thereby causing fewer dislodgments, disposability, and reduced partner discomfort because of the thinness of the material used in the dome. Safety and acceptability studies in France, the UK and the USA showed results adequate enough to warrant further acceptability testing by CONRAD. In a study in which 20 couples used the cap for a single act of intercourse, most women reported the cap as being easy to insert and remove but, paradoxically, about three-quarters also reported having problems with insertion and removal. Dislodgement of the device was experienced by 16% and one-quarter of male partners reported pain. Veos Ltd is seeking approval of the Oves™ cap in the USA and is in discussions with the FDA regarding requirements for a phase III study.

New female condoms

The Reddy female condom was developed as a less expensive alternative to the Reality® female condom. It is manufactured in India out of latex and has a V-shaped frame that holds a latex sheath. The sheath contains a sponge that aids insertion and keeps the device in place during intercourse. The condom has undergone acceptability testing during intercourse in comparison with Reality® and with improvements in device design following each trial. With minor adjustments to the current model and good results from upcoming acceptability studies in the USA and India, it could be in efficacy testing soon. PATH is also developing a new nonlatex female condom. Family Health International (Research Triangle Park, NC) is conducting studies on the feasibility of reuse of Reality® as a means of reducing its per-use cost.

Today® sponge

The Today® sponge was introduced in 1983 and became the largest selling over-the-counter female contraceptive in the USA. It is made of soft polyurethane foam and contains nonoxynol-9. After being moistened with water and inserted into the vagina, Today® sponge protects against pregnancy for 24 hours without additional spermicide, even with repeated acts of intercourse. It is meant for single use. In 1995, the sponge's manufacturer, American Home Products (Madison, NJ), decided that correction of certain manufacturing problems necessary to remain in compliance with FDA regulations would be too expensive, given the revenue from the product, and decided to withdraw it from the market. In early 1999, Allendale Pharmaceuticals (Allendale, NJ) bought the rights to the product, corrected the manufacturing problem, and applied for FDA approval.

New developments in female steroidal contraception

Advances in our understanding of reproductive physiology and steroid delivery and metabolism as well as feedback from users of contraception have led to advances in steroidal contraception. Innovations in oral contraceptives are aimed at higher effectiveness, fewer side-effects, and greater convenience of use. Delivery of contraceptive steroids by methods other than oral dosage has the advantage of reducing gastrointestinal side-effects and avoiding first-pass metabolism and the peaks and valleys of oral delivery, thereby allowing use of a lower dose. The subdermal implant Norplant® (Wyeth Ayerst, Philadelphia, PA) was the first non-oral steroidal contraceptive approved by the FDA in 1990, followed by the injectable Depo-Provera® (Pharmacia, Peapack, NJ), approved in 1992. Improved implants and injectables are in development as well as vaginal rings, progestin-delivering IUDs, and transdermal patches.

Oral contraceptives

The traditional regimen of "three-weeks-on and one-week-off" has been re-examined. This approach was originally taken in order to cause uterine bleeding every 28 days in simulation of a woman's normal cycle. However, there is no physiological reason why a woman must bleed every 28 days and, once this is understood, most women welcome less frequent bleeding (Loudon et al., 1977). Because of the epidemiological association between iron and cardiovascular disease (de Valk and Marx, 1999), some have proposed that a woman's lower risk of heart disease until after menopause is the result of her monthly shedding of blood and "excess" iron. This may represent a disadvantage to a pill regimen that causes less frequent bleeding for women in developed countries where iron deficiency anemia is not a major problem. In developing countries, however, reducing the frequency of bleeding would probably have a medical benefit in terms of reducing anemia.

Clinicians have long recommended to women wishing to avoid bleeding during a honeymoon or other special event that they take the active pills from more than one pack consecutively over, for example, six weeks. Researchers at the Jones Institute of the Eastern Virginia Medical School in Norfolk, Virginia, patented a "tricycling" regimen and signed the development and marketing rights to Barr Labs (Pomona, NY). Barr Labs is now sponsoring a large clinical trial of an oral contraceptive called Seasonale™, which contains 84 active pills (12 weeks) followed by seven placebo pills (one week). A woman taking this pill would theoretically bleed only four times per year instead of the 13 times she would if she took conventional oral contraceptives. Clinical trials have shown that women on this regimen tend to experience breakthrough bleeding in the early cycles (de Valk and Marx, 1999). However, bleeding decreases over time and the regimen may have advantages for certain women: for example, those who experience bothersome symptoms, such as nonfocal migraines, during the pill-free interval on traditional regimens (Sulak et al., 1997); those with very heavy menses; and women with endometriosis who may benefit from the continued suppression of follicular development.

The clinical trial of Seasonale™ will enroll 1350 women in 10 sites, who will be followed for one year. One-sixth of the participants will be randomized to an oral contraceptive containing 150 µg levonorgestrel and 30 µg ethinylestradiol (EE) (150/30), one-sixth to an oral contraceptive containing 100 µg levonorgestrel and 20 µg EE (100/20), one-third to Seasonale™ containing the 150/30 regimen and one-third to Seasonale™ containing the 100/20 regimen. Endpoints are pregnancy and bleeding; lipids, coagulation parameters, and endometrial biopsies will be studied in subsets of participants. The trial is expected to be completed in the beginning of 2002.

An approach aimed at improving effectiveness was the introduction in 1998 of Mircette™ by Organon Inc. (West Orange, NJ). This regimen consists of 21 days of pills containing 150 µg desogestrel and 20 µg EE, followed by two placebo pills and then five pills containing 10 µg/EE . In essence, each 21-day time span of desogestrel/EE pills is preceded by five days of pills containing only a low dose of EE. In theory, this should reduce the chance of an ovarian follicle developing during the "pill-free" interval and may make the regimen more forgiving for pills missed just prior to and after the "pill-free" interval, thus improving effectiveness. Comparative trials of

Mircette™ have not been carried out, but a noncomparative trial of 1250 women followed for 18 months yielded a Pearl rate of 1.02/100 women years (Mircette Study Group, 1998).

Missed pills are a leading cause of oral contraceptive failure. One study showed that 47% of women miss one or more pills per cycle and 22% miss two or more (Rosenberg and Waugh, 1999). In 1999, Ortho-McNeil (Raritan, NJ) introduced a new DialPak refillable dispenser for its oral contraceptives that has a more cosmetic, less medical appearance. It is hoped that this seemingly simple innovation will make carrying the dispenser in a woman's purse and accessing it in case of a forgotten pill significantly less embarrassing and more acceptable, thus improving compliance and effectiveness.

Subdermal implants

Norplant® is a highly effective contraceptive, but its initial promise has not been realized, partly because of poor training of providers in removal techniques and partly because of a combination of unfounded lawsuits and unfavorable media coverage (Boonstra et al., 2000). Recent data indicate that Norplant® is effective for seven years, two years longer than its current labeling (Sivin et al., 2000).

Norplant II®, which employs two rods instead of the six used in Norplant™, has received FDA approval but its manufacturer, Wyeth-Ayerst, has not yet launched it because of manufacturing issues. A clinical trial of a new inserter that prevents "too-deep" insertion and resulting removal problems is ongoing. The product, under the trade name Jadelle, has been marketed in Europe.

The Population Council (New York, NY), which originally developed Norplant®, is working on an implant that will deliver the new progestin Nesterone (16-methylene-17-acetoxy-19-norprogesterone), also called elcometrine and ST-1435. Nesterone is not active orally and, therefore, may be particularly suitable for lactating women whose babies may ingest small amounts of progestin contained in breast milk. In a study comparing it with the Paragard® T380A IUD in 135 breast-feeding women followed for one year postpartum, there were two pregnancies in the IUD group and none in the implant group (Coutinho et al., 1999). The single-rod implant is designed to last for two years although this will require some reformulation as luteal activity was seen in 27% and 35% of the sampling periods at months 18 and 24 of use in one trial of 60 volunteers followed for 24 months (Brache et al., 2000).

Organon Inc. is also developing a single-rod implant containing 68 mg etonogestrel (3-keto-desogestrel), the active metabolite of desogestrel, a progestin used in several marketed oral contraceptives. The implant, called Implanon, initially releases 67 µg etonogestrel per day, is designed to last for three years, and is marketed in the UK, Switzerland, other European countries, and Indonesia. In a four-year open-label, noncomparative, pilot efficacy study involving 200 women in Indonesia, there were no pregnancies (Affandi et al., 1999). The manufacturer is currently weighing the decision of whether it should submit to the FDA for approval of the implant. The history of Norplant® has created reluctance on the part of many manufacturers to introduce any new contraceptives to the US market, particularly new implants.

CONRAD in collaboration with FEI Technologies, Inc. (Tonowanda, NY) is developing a lower-cost alternative to currently available implants. A phase I pharmacokinetic study of a single-rod implant which releases levonorgestrel was recently completed.

Injectables

Cyclofem is an injectable contraceptive marketed outside the USA. Like Depo-Provera®, Cyclofem contains depot medroxyprogesterone acetate, but only 25 mg compared with the 150 mg in Depo-Provera®. It also contains 5 mg estradiol cypionate and is given monthly rather than four times per year. Advantages over Depo-Provera® include more regular bleeding and a more rapid return to fertility following discontinuation (Bahamondes et al., 1997a). In a clinical trial sponsored by World Health Organization, 10 969 women were randomized to receive Cyclofem and were followed for one year.

There were no pregnancies and fewer than 10% of participants discontinued for bleeding irregularities, including amenorrhea (World Health Organization, 1988). Cyclofem was submitted by Pharmacia to the FDA for approval under the trade name Lunelle™ in 1997. Approval was received in 2000. Pharmacia is also looking into subcutaneous delivery of both Depo-Provera® and Lunelle™ for possible self-administration, an approach that has proven to be feasible for developing countries (Bahamondes et al., 1997b).

Vaginal rings

A vaginal ring releasing 7.5 µg estradiol is available for treatment of urogenital symptoms in menopause (Estring®, Pharmacia). Vaginal rings for contraception are generally about the size of the smallest diaphragm and offer a woman a steroidal method that does not require daily attention but that, once prescribed, can be initiated and terminated without the involvement of a clinician. Rings are of two types: progestin combined with EE and progestin alone. The combined ring is used in a three-weeks-in/one-week-out regimen similar to oral contraceptives. The progestin-only ring is designed for continuous use. The combined ring has been shown to afford better cycle control than oral contraceptives containing a higher dose of steroids (Ballagh et al., 1994). The most common side-effect associated with rings is nausea from the initial release of steroids after the ring is first inserted.

The Population Council has done extensive work on a ring that releases 1 mg norethindrone acetate and 20 µg EE daily for one year. In a clinical trial involving 60 women who used the ring in a schedule of three-weeks-in/one-week out for one year, there were no pregnancies, although some luteal activity was seen, especially among heavier women (Weisberg et al., 1999). Current efforts are focused on developing rings delivering Nesterone, both alone and in combination with EE. Early trials have shown adequate safety, and large efficacy trials of the combined rings began in 2001 (Alvarez-Sanchez et al., 1992; Fraser et al., 2000b).

Organon is developing a ring that releases 150 µg etonorgestrel and 15 µg EE per day. An early trial showed acceptable bleeding patterns and no evidence of ovulation in 11 women who used the ring for three months (Olsson and Odlind, 1990). Other trials done outside the USA have been completed in support of the company's recent submission to the FDA for approval.

Investigators in Chile have developed a ring releasing 10 mg/day of progesterone for use by breast-feeding women. In a clinical trial enrolling 802 ring users and 734 T380A IUD users, the one year life table pregnancy rate was 1.5 per 100 among ring users, which did not differ significantly from that among IUD users (Chen et al., 1998). A CONRAD-sponsored study is underway that will determine whether each ring can provide sufficient hormone release for four months instead of three, thereby reducing the cost of the method to the woman by about 25%.

Earlier studies of vaginal rings suggested that their use could lead to patches of vaginal erythema of unknown clinical significance (Bounds et al., 1993). More recent data, however, generally refute this, showing the same incidence of significant colposcopic findings among historical controls and ring users (Fraser et al., 2000a). Results of a World Health Organization-sponsored study of the vaginal effects of a placebo ring should be published soon.

Transdermal patches

Ortho-McNeil Pharmaceuticals received approval in 2001 for a patch called Ortho-Evra™, which delivers 20 µg EE and 150 µg norelgestromin (formerly called 17–D-norgestimate, the active metabolite of the progestin norgestimate) daily. It is meant to be worn for seven days before being replaced by another patch. After patches have been worn for three weeks, no patch is worn for one week, inducing a menstrual-like bleed. It is hoped that having to remember to replace a patch once a week will make contraception easier than having to remember to take a pill every day. The Population Council is also working on transdermal patches and gels for delivery of Nesterone.

Intrauterine devices

The Population Council developed an IUD that releases 20 µg levonorgestrel per day and is marketed in Europe under the trade name Mirena®. Compared with copper-bearing IUDs, Mirena is at least as effective and is associated with less pain and bleeding. In a seven-year randomized comparison with the T380A copper-bearing IUD, cumulative pregnancy rates were not significantly different at 1.1 per 100 at seven years for the steroid-releasing IUD and 1.4 per 100 for the copper-releasing IUD (Sivin et al., 1991). The cumulative rate per 100 women for pain and menstrual problems other than amenorrhea were 20.4 and 30.0, respectively ($p < 0.01$), and rates for amenorrhea were 24.6 and 1.1, respectively ($p < 0.001$). Application for approval has been submitted to the FDA by Berlex Labs (Wayne, NJ) and approval was received in 2000.

The Population Council is also developing a Nesterone-releasing IUD. Current efforts are aimed at finding a dose that prevents implantation but not ovulation; such a low dose is likely to have few systemic side-effects.

New developments in male contraception

Millions of women have enjoyed the benefits of highly effective, readily reversible oral contraceptives since the 1960s; by comparison, men eager to participate in controlling their own fertility have been left with methods that have relatively high failure rates (e.g., condoms and coitus interruptus) or are not reliably reversible (vasectomy). Even though latex condoms are the primary method available to reduce sexual transmission of infectious disease(s), they have low acceptability in many parts of the world. Improved male contraception methods are greatly needed.

Hormonal approaches

The approaches most advanced in terms of clinical trials are based on administration of steroid hormones designed to inhibit the production and release of endogenous hormones that are critical for spermatogenesis. This same approach has been used successfully for oral contraceptives, injectables, and implants in women. Exogenous estrogen and/or progestin administration interferes with the hypothalamic–pituitary–gonadal axis, suppressing the production of gonadotropin-releasing hormone (GnRH) by the hypothalamus and the gonadotropins follicle-stimulating hormone (FSH) and luteinizing hormone (LH), by the pituitary. In females, low FSH and LH levels prevent the ovulation of a mature follicle.

In males, exogenous GnRH analogs or androgen and/or progestin administration also inhibits the release of FSH and LH. In the absence of normal FSH and LH levels in the testis, androgens and other factors produced by testicular cells are significantly inhibited, thereby preventing sperm production and differentiation.

Perhaps not surprisingly, complete suppression of 100 million sperm or more per day has proved to be challenging. Testicular sperm maturation in men takes approximately 70 days plus up to 12 additional days of processing in the epididymis (Cummins and Bremner, 1994). Inducing azoospermia (the absence of sperm in the ejaculate), therefore, typically requires two to three months or longer in most men. When exogenous hormone administration is terminated, sperm production reinitiates.

Numerous surveys in diverse cultures confirm the willingness of men and women to use male methods that will rely on hormonal induction of male infertility (Davidson et al., 1985; Ringheim, 1993; Martin et al., 2000a). Since no products are marketed or available for this purpose, the surveys and focus groups rely on hypothetical characterization of potential systemic methods. At a minimum, any systemic male contraceptive must be highly effective and produce minimal adverse effects to be acceptable.

Androgens alone

The feasibility of developing an effective hormone-based contraceptive for men was first clearly demonstrated by two multicenter trials sponsored by World Health Organization and CONRAD of a prototype androgen formulation (World Health Organization, 1990, 1996). In the first study, weekly injections of 200 mg testosterone enanthate induced azoospermia in only 60% (157 of 271) of the men. However, only one pregnancy occurred during the six-month contraceptive efficacy phase. The subsequent trial demonstrated that high contraceptive efficacy was possible among men rendered either azoospermic or severely oligozoospermic (defined as sperm counts <3 million/ml). A low pregnancy rate of 1.4 per 100 person-years was achieved. Though minimal and reversible, undesirable short-term side-effects occurred (e.g., weight gain, acne, and decreased high density lipoprotein (HDL) cholesterol) that were the result of the relatively high circulating testosterone concentrations. Chinese men in the study suppressed to a greater extent than Caucasian men, perhaps because of variation in the metabolism of testosterone within the testis. Development of more acceptable hormonal regimens with improved delivery systems and spermatogenic suppression and fewer side-effects has been a key objective of recent and ongoing studies.

Injectable formulations of testosterone esters such as in tea seed or castor oil provide prolonged androgen bioavailability (Behre et al., 1999). A recent study found that monthly injections of testosterone undecanoate induced azoospermia in a group of 25 Chinese men (Zhang et al., 1999). These promising results formed the basis for an ongoing multicenter contraceptive efficacy trial involving 300 men in China. However, the apparent increased susceptibility of Chinese men (compared with most Caucasian men) to spermatogenesis suppression by androgens alone may limit the widespread practicality of this approach.

The World Health Organization and US National Institutes of Health (NIH) are developing other long-acting testosterone esters (e.g., testosterone bucicclate). Once stable supplies of these formulated steroids become available, clinical testing in men focusing on bioavailability, dose-finding, and safety can begin.

Androgen/progestin combinations

In general, combinations of a progestin and an androgen induce azoospermia and severe oligozoospermia more rapidly and at a higher rate than androgens alone. The progestin acts additively, if not synergistically, with androgens to suppress the endogenous hormones, permitting the use of less testosterone, which in turn should result in fewer androgenic side-effects such as acne, weight gain, and adverse reductions of serum lipids, especially HDL-cholesterol (Cummins and Bremner, 1994).

A main goal of several ongoing clinical trials involving androgen/progestin combinations is to determine optimal dose combinations that induce high rates of azoospermia and severe oligozoospermia while maintaining normal serum lipid levels and other metabolic parameters. Unfortunately, the specific pharmacodynamic outcome of a given hormonal combination in a group of men is not completely predictable. As a result, different hormonal combinations and their formulations and delivery systems (e.g., transdermal patches, subdermal implants, orally active progestins, injectable androgens and progestins) have been and continue to be investigated to identify a regimen that provides high efficacy and acceptability with minimal adverse side-effects.

The synthetic progestin, levonorgestrel, widely used in oral contraceptives and available as a five-year implant system for women (Norplant®), has been combined with a variety of androgen formulations for testing in men (reviewed in Cummins and Bremner, 1994), although an optimal regimen has yet to be identified (Cummins and Bremner, 1994). Oral daily doses of levonorgestrel are being studied in combination with weekly testosterone enanthate injections to determine the lowest dose that suppresses spermatogenesis without adversely affecting serum lipids (Anawalt et al., 1999). This combination suppresses a very high percentage of men to severe oligozoospermia. Effects on serum lipids and weight gain appear to be dose related, in that the men who received the lowest tested levonorgestrel doses (125 µg per day) experienced less of a reduction in serum lipids than the men who received the highest dose. Although the clinical relevance of the HDL-cholesterol level reductions remains to be clearly established, the study has been extended to include two lower levonorgestrel dose groups in an attempt to minimize serum lipid reductions.

Several investigators are studying the efficacy of sustained release of levonorgestrel in combination with more physiological androgen replacement. For example, transdermal testosterone patches designed to release 6 mg testosterone per day have been combined with Norplant II rods (developed by the Population Council). Somewhat expectedly, administration of four levonorgestrel rods plus two testosterone-releasing patches did not suppress sperm adequately (Gonzalo et al., 2000). Continued studies by this research group are designed to assess the combination of four Norplant II rods plus weekly testosterone enanthate injections as well as daily treatment with oral levonorgestrel and testosterone patches in an effort to determine which component of the initial study provided inadequate hormonal suppression. As these studies involve the simultaneous use of multiple delivery routes, parallel studies will include subcutaneous implantation of both levonorgestrel (using Norplant II rods) and testosterone (using pellets manufactured by N.V. Organon) (C. Wang, personal communication, 2000). Four of these testosterone pellets provide adequate androgen for about four months in contraceptive regimens.

In women, oral contraceptives containing "third-generation" synthetic progestins, such as desogestrel, which are less androgenic than levonorgestrel, seem to have less of an adverse effect on lipids than those containing levonorgestrel (Kuusi et al., 1985). Oral desogestrel has been combined with different formulations of testosterone to determine whether lipids are less adversely affected in men as well. When oral desogestrel is combined with weekly injection of testosterone enanthate, sperm suppression to azoospermia or severe oligozoospermia was achieved in almost all men (Wu et al., 1999); nevertheless, HDL-cholesterol was still reduced. However, when oral desogestrel was combined with a more uniform delivery of testosterone (as pellets) profound suppression of sperm production occurred without adverse metabolic effects (Martin et al., 2000b). These promising outcomes are very encouraging and will be the basis for further studies.

The feasibility of achieving highly effective sperm suppression with minimal metabolic side-effects using testosterone pellets plus another well-characterized progestin, depot medroxyprogesterone acetate (DMPA), was established by Handelsman (Handelsman et al., 1996). Treatment with four 200 mg testosterone pellets plus a single injection of 300 mg DMPA induced azoospermia in 9 of 10 men and severe oligozoospermia in the tenth man. A multicenter contraceptive efficacy study based on DMPA injection every three months and testosterone pellet replacement every four months is now ongoing in Australia. Chinese investigators have recently initiated studies of DMPA in combination with testosterone undecanoate, both administered as bimonthly injections. A similar combination with testosterone undecanoate, though using different dosages and schedules, will be tested in Indonesian men.

Based on encouraging pilot studies in which the combination of cyproterone acetate (CPA, an anti-androgen with progestin activity) and testosterone enanthate produced complete azoospermia (Meriggiola et al., 1998), subsequent studies have focused on minimizing the dose of CPA required and utilizing the long-acting androgen testosterone undecanoate. If a regimen is identified that achieves azoospermia or severe oligozoospermia in all men, then an expanded multicenter study will be considered.

Norethindrone acetate serves as an effective progestin in oral contraceptives, vaginal rings, and monthly injectable contraceptives for women. Perceived advantages, such as lower androgenicity than levonorgestrel and the potential to formulate norethindrone acetate in a single combined injectable formulation with a long-acting androgen, such as testosterone undecanoate, has led to initial clinical testing of this progestin in men. Single injections of 200 mg norethindrone acetate in a limited number of men resulted in strong suppression of serum gonadotropins, serum testosterone, and spermatogenesis without significant effects on sexual function and serum lipids (Kamishcke et al., 2000). Continued studies of its use in combination with long-acting androgens to determine optimal doses and effects on serum lipids and other metabolic parameters are ongoing.

Some concern exists that long-term testosterone treatment for male hormonal contraception could have adverse effects on prostate growth. The Population Council is developing an androgen, 7α-methyl-19-nortestosterone (MENT™), that is not metabolized to dihydrotestosterone (which is more potent at stimulating prostate enlargement). Consequently, MENT™ is not expected to affect the prostate adversely when used for male contraception. In animal models, this drug is more potent for gonadotropin suppression than testosterone. Initial clinical trials in normal men have confirmed that implants releasing MENT™ acetate provide potent gonadotropin and androgen suppression (Noe, 1999). Developmental work continues on an implant that will deliver MENT™ for one year.

Analogs of gonadotropin-releasing hormone

High rates of azoospermia can be achieved by the administration of peptide analogs of GnRH. GnRH antagonists suppress FSH, LH, and testosterone more completely than GnRH agonists and have been the focus of numerous clinical studies (for review see Cummings and Bremner, 1994). However, most of the highly substituted peptide analogs studied in the clinical trials to-date are relatively expensive, have poor solubility, require frequent administration (typically daily injection), and can induce local skin irritation. An androgen, such as testosterone, must also be administered to maintain libido and sexual potency. More recent clinical studies of existing antagonists have concentrated on finding regimens that minimize the amount of antagonist needed.

New GnRH antagonists are being developed by private companies and public sector organizations with the hope of increasing drug potency (and thus lower the amount of drug needed) and decreasing side-effects and costs. For example, the National Institutes of Health is developing formulations of acyline, a promising new peptide antagonist, for pilot clinical studies (H. K. Kim, personal communication, 1999). Potent nonpeptide antagonists devoid of the drawbacks of peptide antagonists are actively being sought.

Other considerations for hormonal male contraception

The encouraging results from ongoing clinical studies of potential hormonal regimens support the expectation that a practical male contraceptive will be available in the not too distant future. It should be noted, though, that other issues will need to be resolved before systemic male methods can reach the marketplace. Well-designed studies are needed to verify that exogenous administration of androgens does not adversely affect behavior (e.g., increased irritability or aggressiveness) and that long-term use is safe and induces reversible infertility. Cross-cultural acceptability by men and women for any particular regimen will also depend on suitable service delivery, affordability, and current contraceptive usage. Since achieving infertility by induction of azoospermia may take three months or longer with these methods, other contraceptive methods must be used in the meantime. Because of this delay, development of a convenient and inexpensive home "test kit" for verification of male method-induced infertility might be helpful in marketing.

Some of the potential hormonal regimens may require daily oral administration and because the need to take a daily pill increases the potential for noncompliance, long-term studies will be needed to monitor the effect on fertility of missing pills. Needless to say, that concern underlies the focus on sustained-release delivery systems.

Complete development of a systemic male contraceptive will continue to require significant resources. Pharmaceutical companies such as Schering AG (Berlin, Germany) have taken up the challenge of bringing a practical male contraceptive

to the market and will be key to the success of these efforts (Bremner et al., 2000). Affordability to men in developing countries is an important objective for many of the public sector organizations intent on developing new male products. Productive collaborations between for-profit and not-for-profit development organizations will be essential to bring affordable male contraceptives to the private and public sectors.

Nonhormonal approaches

Reversible nonhormonal systemic approaches for men are much less advanced than hormonal approaches in terms of clinical testing or product development. Few compounds have been synthesized solely as potential nonhormonal antifertility agents; however, a variety of leads have originated from drugs exhibiting antifertility effects when taken orally for other purposes (reviewed by Cosentino and Matlin, 1997). In most cases, the agents inhibit specific testicular enzymes required for sperm development or fertilizing capacity, or inhibit other maturation steps that occur in the epididymis. Ornidazole, diaminopyrimidines, indenopyridine are examples of synthetic compounds studied extensively in preclinical animal models. Numerous antifertility compounds (e.g., gossypol, tryptolide, and embelin) have been extracted from medicinal plants and studied in animal models or clinically. However, almost all of the agents studied induce other undesirable side-effects or exert varying degrees of toxicity in human or animal models.

Although completely novel compounds will require significant preclinical toxicology testing, a few promising leads continue to be explored for mechanism of action, toxicity testing, and fertility trials. Previous research found that lonidamine, an anticancer drug developed in the 1970s, resulted in significant antispermatogenic activity (Floridi et al., 1981). Development of lonidamine as an antispermatogenic agent was abandoned in the 1980s because kidney damage was induced by high doses. More recent research has focused on identifying analogs of lonidamine that are equally effective but not toxic. Two orally active lonidamine derivatives appear very promising (Bremner et al., 2000; Cheng et al., 2001). In a small animal model, these compounds promote the release of sperm lacking fertilizing capacity, rendering the males infertile for up to eight weeks. While still in the early phase of development, the feasibility of this approach to disrupt fertility is evident.

Other nonhormonal approaches continue to be considered and will be developed as their feasibility is established. Immunocontraceptives targeting sperm or epididymal antigens, such as the lactate dehydrogenase antigen C4, SP-17, DE/AEG/CRISP, and fertilin, are being tested in small animal models and nonhuman primates (reviewed in Bremner et al., 2000). This approach has proceeded slowly, as generation of adequate immune responses in primate trials has proven difficult to achieve. Concerns about inducing irreversible immune responses in the testis have hindered research on male immunocontraception. However, an immunocontraceptive based on active immunization against GnRH is being tested for safety, efficacy, and reversibility in normal men (Population Council, 2000). A low dose of androgen supplementation will be needed to ensure that libido and secondary sex characteristics are not adversely affected. Development efforts are currently focused on improving the efficacy of the method by modifying the construct of the immunogen, adding adjuvants to increase its contraceptive effect, and developing biodegradable, controlled-release injection formulations.

Vasectomy and reversible vas occlusion

Besides the condom and coitus interruptus, the only currently available male contraceptive technique is permanent sterilization, i.e., vasectomy, the sectioning and removal of a portion of the vas deferens. Two basic vasectomy techniques are practiced: the "standard" technique and the "no-scalpel" method. The no-scalpel method is less traumatic than the standard technique and differs from it in that the vas deferens is first isolated under the skin surface with the thumb and forefinger and grabbed with forceps before a very small skin incision is made and the vas exposed. Depending on the experience of the surgeon, complications such as bleeding and pain tend to be less frequently associated with the no-scalpel method than with the standard technique (Hargreave, 1992). Sterilization success after vasectomy varies from 96 to 99.6%, depending on the skill of the surgeon. Antisperm antibodies develop in about 75% of men but these do not seem to be pathogenic, and reported increases in cardiovascular diseases and prostatic cancer were shown to be unfounded (Soonawalla, 1999).

Vasectomy reversal is accomplished by microsurgically reanastomosing the cut ends of the vas deferens. This is a complicated procedure that is time consuming (up to 5 hours) and costly (up to $7000) in the USA. Experienced surgeons can have reasonable reversal success with 80–90% of men recovering spermatozoa in their ejaculate and about half of men producing a pregnancy (Soonawalla, 1999).

Vasectomy is quite popular in only a small number of countries such as the USA, UK and some other European countries, China, and India. Even in these countries, a large number of men do not undergo this sterilization procedure, primarily because of its relative irreversibility and fear of loss of fertility and even of libido and virility. Potential surgical complications are also a deterrent. Much work was performed in the 1970s to develop a reversible vas deferens method. Techniques included extravasal clips or wires, extraluminal intravasal devices such as valves, and intraluminal intravasal methods such as injectables, plugs, threads, wires, or copper iontophoresis (Zaneveld et al., 1999; Guha, 1999). Although the reported success rate of vas occlusion and reversal varied tremendously, the data suggested overall that a reversible vas device is feasible.

Unfortunately, only few investigators have pursued this line of research since the 1970s, primarily because of a lack of funding. Presently, two general approaches are still being tested. The first approach is the injection of liquid material into the vas lumen, which subsequently hardens and forms a plug. Examples of such materials are polyurethane (Zhao, 1990; Chen et al., 1992; Zhao et al., 1992a), silicone (Zhao et al., 1992b; Soebadi et al., 1995; Soebadi, 1999), and styrene maleic anhydride (Guha et al., 1993, 1998; Guha, 1999). High contraceptive efficacy rates have been reported with all three methods. Advantages of injecting material is that the plug will adapt to the shape and size of the vas lumen and that the procedure can be done through the skin, making an incision unnecessary (although such percutaneous placement is more likely associated with device problems). However, the technique used for injection results in a short unanchored plug, potentially allowing migration to the abdominal area of the vas deferens from where the plug is difficult to remove if reversal is desired. To avoid this problem, enough material is injected into the vas lumen to produce a very thick plug, but this tends to cause rupture and/or necrosis of the vas wall (Soebadi et al., 1995; Chen et al., 1996). In contrast to polyurethane and silicone, styrene maleic anhydride may affect the sperm's fertilizing capacity so that spermatozoa that pass by the plug will be infertile, allowing use of a plug that does not completely obstruct the vas lumen (Guha, 1999).

The second approach is the insertion of a preformed silicone plug into the vas lumen (Zaneveld et al., 1999). Previously, this plug was called the SHUG ("soft hollow plug") but the name was changed to "intra vas device" (IVD) to indicate a similarity to its female equivalent, the IUD, i.e., the IVD aims at being a contraceptive method rather than a sterilization technique (vasectomy, tubal ligation). The optimal conformation of the IVD was selected after a series of phase I clinical studies (Zaneveld et al., 1999). The vas lumen is sized after exposure of the vas by a procedure modified from the no-scalpel vasectomy technique, and two IVDs with the appropriate diameter are placed in series into the lumen and anchored there, preventing migration. Spermatozoa that pass by the first IVD because of luminal enlargement through pressure exerted by accumulated fluids and sperm are trapped between the two plugs and cannot pass by the second IVD; if

some pass, they are damaged and infertile. A recently completed two-year clinical pilot study with 31 men confirmed the high contraceptive effectiveness of the IVD (L.J.D. Zaneveld, M.P. De Castro, G. Faria, and R. Ferraro, unpublished data). Reversal is accomplished by making a small incision in the vas wall and removing the IVDs. Reversal success has not yet been tested in the human. It is expected to be high because no permanent damage is caused to the vas. Two primate studies each showed a 100% reversal success (Zaneveld et al., 1988b). A small start-up company, Shepherd Medical (Minneapolis, MN), is presently pursuing further development of the IVD for commercial purposes.

Acknowledgement/Disclaimer

The views expressed by the authors do not necessarily reflect those of the CONRAD Program.

REFERENCES

Affandi, B., Korver, T., Geurts, T.B., and Coelingh Bennink, H.J. (1999). A pilot efficacy study with a single-rod contraceptive implant (Implanon) in 200 Indonesian women treated for ≤4 years. *Contraception*, **59**, 167–74.

Alliance for Microbicide Development (2000). *Research and Developmental Status of Microbicides*. Alliance for Microbicide Development, Silver Spring, MD.

Alvarez-Sanchez, F., Brache, V., Jackanicz, T., and Faundes, A. (1992). Evaluation of four different contraceptive vaginal rings: steroid serum levels, luteal activity, bleeding control and lipid profiles. *Contraception*, **46**, 387–98.

Amaral, E., Faundes, A., Zaneveld, L., Waller, D., and Garg, S. (1999). Study of the vaginal tolerance to Acidform, acid-buffering bioadhesive gel. *Contraception*, **60**, 361–6.

Anawalt, B.D., Bebb, R.A., Bremner, W.J., and Matsumoto, A.M. (1999). A lower dosage levonorgestrel and testosterone combination effectively suppresses spermatogenesis and circulating gonadotropin levels with fewer metabolic effects than higher dosage combinations. *Journal of Andrology*, **20**, 407–14.

Andersch, B., Forssman, L., Lincoln, K., and Torstennson, P. (1986). Treatment of bacterial vaginosis with an acid cream: a comparison between the effect of lactate-gel and metronidazole. *Gynecological and Obstetrical Investigations*, **21**, 19–25.

Anderson, D.J. and Quayle, A.J. (1996). Mucosal immunologic approaches. In: *Contraceptive Research and Development. Looking in the Future*, Harrison, P.F. and Rosenfield, A., eds. National Academic Press, Washington, DC, pp. 446–73.

Anderson, R.A. and Sharpe, R.M. (2000). Regulation of inhibin production in the human male and its clinical applications. *International Journal of Andrology*, **23**, 136–44.

Anderson, R.A., Feathergill, K., Diao, X., et al. (2000). Evaluation of poly(styrene-4-sulfonate) as a preventive agent for conception and sexually transmitted diseases. *Journal of Andrology*, **21**, 862–75.

Archer, D.F., Mauck, C.K., Viniegra-Sibal, A., and Anderson, F.D. (1995). Lea's Shield: a phase I postcoital study of a new contraceptive barrier device. *Contraception*, **52**, 167–73.

Bahamondes, L., Lavin, P., Ojeda, G., et al. (1997a). Return of fertility after discontinuation of the once-a-month injectable contraceptive Cyclofem. *Contraception*, **55**, 307–10.

Bahamondes, L., Marchi, N.M., Nakagava, H.M., et al. (1997b). Self-administration with UniJect of the once-a-month injectable contraceptive Cyclofem. *Contraception*, **56**, 301–4.

Baird, D.T. and Glasier, A.F. (1999). Contraception. *British Medical Journal*, **319**, 969–72.

Ballagh, S.A., Mishell, D.R., Jr., Jackanicz, T.M., Lacarra, M., and Eggena, P. (1994). Dose-finding study of a contraceptive ring releasing norethindrone acetate/ethinyl estradiol. *Contraception*, **50**, 535–49.

Behre, H.M., Abshagen, K., Oettel, M., Hubler, D., and Nieschlag, E. (1999). Intramuscular injection of testosterone undecanoate for the treatment of male hypogonadism: phase I studies. *European Journal of Endocrinology*, **140**, 414–19.

Bentley, M.E., Morrow, K.M., Fullem, A., Chesney, M.A., Horton, S.D., and Rosenberg, Z. (2000). Acceptability of a novel vaginal microbicide during a safety trial among low-risk women. *Family Planning Perspectives*, **32**, 1–10.

Bounds, W., Szarewski, A., Lowe, D., and Guillebaud, J. (1993). Preliminary report of unexpected local reactions to a progestogen-releasing contraceptive vaginal ring. *European Journal of Obstetrics, Gynecology and Reproductive Biology*, **48**, 123–5.

Boonstra, H., Duran, V., Northington, et al. (2000). The 'Boom and Bust phenomenon': the hopes, dreams, and broken promises of the contraceptive revolution. *Contraception*, **61**, 9–25.

Bourinbaiar, A.S. and Lee-Huang, S. (1994a). Comparative in vitro study of contraceptive agents with anti-HIV activity: gramicidin, nonoxynol-9 and gossypol. *Contraception*, **49**, 131–7.

Bourinbaiar, A.S. and Lee-Huang, S. (1994b). Acrosin inhibitor, 4′-acetamidophenyl 4-guanidinobenzoate, an experimental vaginal contraceptive with anti-HIV activity. *Contraception*, **51**, 319–22.

Bourne, N., Bernstein, D.I., Ireland, J., Sonderfan, A.J., Profy, A.T., and Stanberry, L.R. (1999). The topical microbicide PRO 2000 protects against genital herpes infection in a mouse model. *Journal of Infectious Diseases*, **180**, 203–5.

Brache, V., Massai, R., Mishell, D.R., et al. (2000). Ovarian function during use of Nestorone subdermal implants. *Contraception*, **61**, 199–204.

Bremner, W.J., Cheng, C.Y., Cuasnicu, P.S., Habenicht, U.F., Colvard, D.S., and Doncel, G.F. (2000). Current approaches to systemic male contraception: an update. In: *Current Knowledge in Reproduction*, Coutinho, E.M. and Spinola, P., eds. Elsevier Science, Amsterdam, the Netherlands, pp. 347–63.

Brode, G. (1998). Principles in microbicide formulations with emphasis on hydrophobe modified cationic polysaccharides. In: *Vaginal Microbicide Formulations Workshop*, Rencher, W.F., eds. Lippincott-Raven, Philadelphia, PA, pp. 38–50.

Brode, G., Doncel, G.F. and Kemnitzer, J.E. (2000) Hydrophobe modified cationic polysaccharides for topical microbicide delivery. In: *Polymeric Drugs and Drug Delivery Systems*, Attenbrite, R. and Kim, S.W., eds. Technomics Publishing, Lancester, PA, pp. 211–30.

Cachrimanidou, A.C., Hellberg, D. Nilsson, S., Waldenstrom, U., Olsson, S.E., and Sikstrom, B. (1993). Long-interval treatment regimen with a desogestrel-containing oral contraceptive. *Contraception*, **48**, 205–16.

Cates, W. (2000). Sexually transmitted diseases, HIV, and contraception. *Infertility and Reproductive Medicine Clinics of North America*, **11**, 687–704.

Chen, J.H., Wu, S.C., Shao, W.Q., et al. (1998). The comparative trial of TCu 380A IUD and progesterone-releasing vaginal ring used by lactating women. *Contraception*, **57**, 371–9.

Chen, Z., Gu, Y., Liang, X., Wu, Z., Yin, E., and Li, H. (1992). Safety and efficacy of percutaneous injection of polyurethane elastomer (MPU) plugs for vas occlusion in man. *International Journal of Andrology*, **15**, 468–72.

Chen, Z., Gu, Y., Liang, X., Shen, L., and Zou, W. (1996). Morphological observations of vas deferens occlusion by the percutaneous injection of medical polyurethane. *Contraception*, **53**, 275–9.

Cheng, C.Y., Silvestrini, B., Grima, J. et al. (2001). Two new male contraceptives exert their effects by depleting germ cells prematurely from the testis. *Biology of Reproduction*, **62**, 446–61.

Cohen, M.S., Weber, R.D., and Mardh, P.A. (1990). Genitourinary mucosal defenses. In: *Sexually Transmitted Diseases*, 2nd edn,

Holmes, K.K., Mardh, P.A., Sparling, P.F., et al., eds. New York, McGraw-Hill.

Cone, R.A. and Whaley, K.J. (1994). Monoclonal antibodies for reproductive health. Part I. Preventing sexual transmission of disease and pregnancy with topically applied antibodies. *American Journal of Reproductive Immunology*, **32**, 114–31.

Corner, A.M., Dolan, M.M., Yankell, S.L., and Malamud, D. (1998). C31G, a new agent for oral use with potent antimicrobial and antiadherence properties. *Antimicrobiol Agents and Chemotherapy*, **32**, 350–3.

Cosentino, M.J. and Matlin, S.A. (1997). Pharmacological developments in male contraception. *Experimental Opinions and Investigations in Drugs*, **6**, 635–53.

Coutinho, E.M, Athayde, C., Dantas, C., Hirsch, C., and Barbosa, I. (1999). Use of a single implant of elcometrine (ST-1435), a nonorally active progestin, as a long contraceptive for post-partum nursing women. *Contraception*, **59**, 115–22.

Cu-Uvin, S., Chapman, S., Mayer, K., Rodriguez, I., and Moench, T. (2000). Treatment of bacterial vaginosis with an acidic buffering gel (BufferGel): pilot study. In: *Microbiocides 2000 Conference*, 13–16 March. Washington, DC, p. 38.

Cummins, D.E. and Bremner, W.J. (1994). Prospects for new hormonal contraceptives. *Endocrinology and Metabolism Clinics of North America*, **22**, 893–922.

Davidson, A.R., Ahn K.C., Chandra S., et al. (1985). The acceptability of new contraceptive methods for men. In: *The 113 Annual Meeting of the American Public Health Association*. American Public Health Association, Washington, DC, p. 34.

D'Cruz, O.J., Zhu, Z., Yiv, S.H., Chen, C.L., Waurzyniak, B., and Uckun, F.M. (1999). WHI-05, a novel bromo-methoxy substituted phenyl phosphate derivative of zidovudine, is a dual-action spermicide with potent anti-HIV activity. *Contraception*, **59**, 319–31.

de Valk, B. and Marx, J.J. (1999). Iron, atherosclerosis, and ischemic heart disease. *Archives of Internal Medicine*, **26**, 1542–8.

Digenis, G.A., Nosek, D., Mohammadi, F., Darwazeh, N.B., Anwar, H.S., and Zavos, P.M. (1999). Novel vaginal controlled-delivery systems incorporating coprecipitates of nonoxynol-9. *Pharmaceutical Development and Technology*, **4**, 421–30.

Dzuik, P.J. (1998). Fertility and fecundity. In: *Encyclopedia of Reproduction*, Vol. 2, Knobil, E. and Neill, J.D., eds. Academic Press, San Diego, CA, pp. 252–6.

Edelstein, M.C., Gretz, J.E., and Bauer, T.J. (1991). Studies on the in vitro spermicidal activity of synthetic magainins. *Fertility and Sterility*, **92**, 974–82.

Elias, C.J. and Coggins, C. (1996). Female-controlled methods to prevent sexual transmission of HIV. *AIDS*, **10**(Suppl. 3), S43–51.

Evans, J.P. (2000). Getting sperm and egg together: things conserved and things diverged. *Biology of Reproduction*, **63**, 355–60.

Floridi, A., DeMartino, C., Marcante. M.L., Apollonj, C., Scorza Barcellona, P., and Silvestrini, B. (1981). Morphological and biochemical modifications of rat germ cell mitochondria induced by new antispermatogenic compounds: studies in vivo and in vitro. *Experimental Molecular Pathology*, **35**, 314–31.

Fraser, I.S, Lacarra, M., Mishell, D.R., Alvarez, F., et al. (2000a). Vaginal epithelial surface appearances in women using vaginal rings for contraception. *Contraception*, **61**, 131–8.

Fraser, I.S.,Weisberg, E., Minehan, E., and Johansson, E.D. (2000b). A detailed analysis of menstrual blood loss in women using Norplant and Nestorone progestogen-only contraceptive implants or vaginal rings. *Contraception*, **61**, 241–51.

Gagne, N., Cormier, H., Omar, R.F., et al. (1999). Protective effect of a thermoreversible gel against the tonicity of N-9. *Sexually Transmitted Diseases*, **26**, 177–83.

Ganz, T. and Lehrer, R.I. (1994). Defensins. *Current Opportunities in Immunology*, **6**, 584–9.

Gerbase, A.C., Rowley, J.T., Heymann, D.H.L., Berkley, S.F.B., and Piot, P. (1998). Global prevalence and incidence estimates of selected curable STDs. *Sexually Transmitted Infections*, **74**(Suppl. 1), S12–16.

Gonzalo, I.T.G., Serdloff, R.S., Nelson, A., et al. (2000). Comparison of the efficacy of combined progestagen implant and transdermal androgen versus androgen alone in the suppression of spermatogenesis in normal men. In: *The 82nd Annual Meeting of the Endocrine Society*, Toronto, Canada. Endocrine Society, abstract 2352.

Guha, S.K. (1999). Current status of development and clinical testing of male intravasal contraceptives. In: *Male Contraception: Present and Future*, Rajalakshmi, M. and Griffin, P.D., eds. New Age International, New Delhi, pp. 265–74.

Guha, S.K., Singh, G., Anand, S., Ansari, S., Kumar, S., and Koul, V. (1993). Phase I clinical trial of an injectable contraceptive for the male. *Contraception*, **48**, 376–85.

Guha, S.K., Singh, G., Srivastava, A., et al. (1998). Two-year clinical efficacy trial with dose variations of a vas deferens injectable contraceptive for the male. *Contraception*, **58**, 165–74.

Handelsman, D.J., Conway, A.J., Howe, C.J., Turner, L., and Mackey, M.A. (1996). Establishing the minimum effective dose and additive effects of depot progestin in suppression of human spermatogenesis by a testosterone depot. *Journal of Clinical Endocrinology and Metabolism*, **81**, 4113–21.

Hardy, E., De Padua, K.S., Jimenez, A.L., and Zaneveld, L.J.D.

(1998). Women's preferences for vaginal antimicrobial contraceptives. II. *Contraception*, **58**, 239–44.

Hargreave, T.B. (1992). Towards reversible vasectomy. *International Journal of Andrology*, **15**, 455–9.

Harrison, P.F. (2000). Microbicides: forging scientific and political alliances. *AIDS Patient Care and STDs*, **14**, 1–7.

Harrison, P.F. and Rosenfield, A. (1996). *Contraceptive Research and Development. Looking in the Future.* National Academic Press, Washington, DC.

Hatcher, R.A., Trussell, J., Stewart, F., et al. (1994). *Contraceptive Technology*, 16th revised edn. Irving, New York.

Herold, B.C., Siston, A., Bremer, J. et al. (1997). Sulfated carbohydrate compounds prevent microbial adherence by sexually transmitted disease pathogens. *Antimicrobial Agents in Chemotherapy*, **41**, 2776–80.

Herold, B.C., Bourne, N., Marcellino, D., et al. (2000). Poly(sodium 4-styrenesulfonate): an effective candidate topical anti-microbial for the prevention of sexually transmitted diseases. *Journal of Infectious Diseases*, **181**, 770–3.

Howett, M.K., Neely, E.B., Wigdahl, B., et al. (2000). Sodium dodecyl sulfate-a potent vaginal microbicide. In: *Microbiocides 2000 Conference*, 13–16 March, Washington, DC, p. 14.

Kamischke, A., Diebacker, J., and Nieschlag, E. (2000). Potential of norethisterone enanthate for male contraception: pharmacokinetics and suppression of pituitary and gonadal function. *Clinical Endocrinology (Oxford)*, **53**, 351–8.

Khanna, J., Van Look, P.F.A., and Griffin, P.D. (eds.) (1992). *Reproductive Health: A Key to a Brighter Future.* Biennial Report 1990–1991. World Health Organization, Geneva.

Kokuba, H., Aurelian, L., and Neurath, A.R. (1998). 3–Hydroxyphtaloyl β-lactoglobulin. IV. Antiviral activity in the mouse model of genital herpesvirus infection. *Antiviral Chemistry and Chemotherapy*, **9**, 353–7.

Kreiss, J., Ngugi, E., Holmes, K., et al. (1992). Efficacy of nonoxynol-9 contraceptive sponge use in preventing heterosexual acquisition of HIV in Nairobi prostitutes. *Journal of the American Medical Association*, **268**, 477–82.

Kuusi, T., Nikkila, E.A., Tikkanen, M.J., and Sipinen, S. (1985). Effects of two progestins with different androgenic properties on hepatic endothelial lipase and high density lipoprotein 2. *Atherosclerosis*, **54**, 251–62.

Ladipo, O.A., De Castro, M.P., Filho, L.C.C.T., et al. (2000). A new vaginal antimicrobial contraceptive formulation: phase I clinical pilot studies. *Contraception*, **62**, 91–7.

Laga, M., Diallo, M.O., and Buve, A. (1994). Inter-relationship of sexually transmitted diseases and HIV: where are we now? *AIDS*, **8**(suppl. 1), S119–24.

Loudon, N.B., Foxwell, M., Potts, D.M., Guild, A.L., and Short,

R.V. (1977). Acceptability of an oral contraceptive that reduces the frequency of menstruation: the tri-cycle pill regimen. *British Medical Journal*, **ii**, 487–90.

Mahmoud, E.A., Svensson, L.O., Olsson, S.E., and Mardh, P.A. (1995). Antichlamydial activity of vaginal secretion. *American Journal of Obstetrics and Gynecology*, **172**, 1268–72.

Maguire, R.A., Zacharopoulos, V.R., and Phillips, D.M. (1998). Carrageenan-based nonoxynol-9 spermicides for prevention of sexually transmitted infections. *Sexually Transmitted Diseases*, **25**, 494–500.

Martin, C.W., Anderson, R.A., Cheng, L., et al. (2000a). Potential impact of hormonal male contraception: cross-cultural implications for development of novel preparations. *Human Reproduction*, **15**, 637–45.

Martin, C.W., Riley, S.C., Everington, D., et al. (2000b). Dose-finding study of oral desogestrel with testosterone pellets for suppression of the pituitary-testicular axis in normal men. *Human Reproduction*, **15**, 1515–24.

Mauck, C.K. and Doncel, G.F. (2000). Spermicides. *Infertility and Reproductive Medicine Clinics of North America*, **11**, 657–67.

Mauck, C.K., Cordero, M., Gabelnick, H., Spieler, J.M., and Rivera, R. (1994). *Barrier Contraceptives; Current Status and Future Prospects.* John Wiley, New York.

Mauck, C., Glover, L.H., Miller, E., et al. (1996). Lea's Shield: a study of the safety and efficacy of a new vaginal barrier contraceptive used with and without spermicide. *Contraception*, **53**, 329–35.

Mauck, C., Callahan, M., Weiner, D.H., and Dominik, R. (1999). A comparative study of the safety and efficacy of FemCap, a new vaginal barrier contraceptive, and the Ortho All-Flex diaphragm. The FemCap Investigators' Group. *Contraception*, **60**, 71–80.

Mermillod, P., Oussaid, B., and Cognie, Y. (1999). Aspects of follicular and oocyte maturation that affect the development potential of embryos. *Journal of Reproduction and Fertility*, **54**(Suppl.), 449–60.

Meriggiola, M.C., Bremner, W.J., Costantino, A., Di Cintio, G., and Flamigni, C. (1998). Low dose of cyproterone acetate and testosterone enanthate for contraception in men. *Human Reproduction*, **13**, 1225–9.

Mircette Study Group (1998). An open label, multicenter, non-comparative safety and efficacy study of Mircette, a low dose estrogen progestin oral contraceptive. *American Journal of Obstetrics and Gynecology*, **179**, S2–8.

Mori, T., Gustafson, K.R., Pannell, L.K., et al. (1998). Recombinant production of cyanovirin-N, a potent human immunodeficiency virus-inactivating protein derived from a cultured cyanobacterium. *Protein Expression and Purification*, **12**, 151–8.

Neurath, A.R., Strick, N., Li, Y.-Y., Lin, K., and Jiang, S. (1999). Design of a "microbicide" for prevention of sexually transmitted diseases using "inactive" pharmaceutical excipients. *Biologicals*, **27**, 11–21.

Noe, G., Suvisaari, J., Martin, C., et al. (1999). Gonadotrophin and testosterone suppression by 7-alpha-methyl-19-nortestosterone acetate administered by subdermal implant to healthy men. *Human Reproduction*, **14**, 2200–6.

Olsson, S.E. and Odlind, V. (1990). Contraception with a vaginal ring releasing 3-keto desogestrel and ethinylestradiol. *Contraception*, **42**, 563–72.

Pauwels, R. and De Clercq, E. (1996). Development of vaginal microbicides for the prevention of heterosexual transmission of HIV. *Journal of Acquired Immune Deficiency Syndrome and Human Retrovirology*, **11**, 211–21.

Population Council on Male Contraceptive Development. http://www.popcouncil.org/biomed/malecontras.html. Updated April 3, 2000.

Reddy, K.V., Shahani, S.K., and Meherji, P.K. (1996). Spermicidal activity of magainins: in vitro and in vivo studies. *Contraception*, **53**, 205–10.

Rencher, W.F. (ed.) (1998). *Vaginal Microbicide Formulations Workshop*. Lippincott-Raven, Philadelphia, PA.

Rencher, W.F., Doncel, G., Anderson, R.A., et al. (2000). Development of a new contraceptive/antimicrobial agent. *Microbicides 2000 Conference*, 13–16 March, Washington, DC, p. 26.

Ringheim, K. (1993). Factors that determine prevalence of use of contraceptive methods for men. *Studies in Family Planning*, **24**, 87–99.

Roddy, R.E., Cordero, M., Cordero, C., and Fortney, J.A. (1993). A dosing study of nonoxynol-9 and genital irritation. *International Journal of STD and AIDS*, **4**, 165–70.

Roddy, R.E., Schulz, K.F., and Cates, W. (1998a). Microbicides, meta-analysis, and the N-9 question. *Sexually Transmitted Diseases*, **25**, 151–3.

Roddy, R.E., Zekeng, L., Ryan, K.A., Tamoufe, U., Weir, S.S., and Wong, E.L. (1998b). A controlled trial of nonoxynol-9 film to reduce male-to-female transmission of sexually transmitted diseases. *New England Journal of Medicine*, **339**, 504–10.

Rosenberg, M. and Waugh, M.S. (1999). Causes and consequences of oral contraceptive noncompliance. *American Journal of Obstetrics and Gynecology*, **180**, 276–9.

Savle, P.S., Doncel, G.F., and Bryant, S.D. (1999). Acylcarnitine analogues as topical microbicidal spermicides. *Boorg Medical and Chemical Letters*, **9**, 2545–48.

Schill, W.B. and Wolff, H.H. (1981). Ultrastructure of human spermatozoa in the presence of the spermicide nonoxynol-9 and a vaginal contraceptive containing nonoxynol-9. *Andrologia*, **13**, 42–9.

Senanayake, P. (1994). Contraception by the end of the 20th century – the role of voluntary organizations. (In: *New Concepts in Fertility Control*, Edwards, R.G. ed.) *Human Reproduction*, **9**(Suppl. 2), 133–44.

Shah, K., Tillman, W., Doncel, G., and Rencher, W. (2000). Long-acting microbicide delivery system. In: *Microbicides 2000 Conference*, 13–16 March. Washington, DC, p. 28.

Sivin, I., Stern J., Coutinho, E., et al. (1991). Prolonged intrauterine contraception: a seven-year randomized study of the levonorgestrel 20 mcg/day (LNg 20) and the Copper T380 Ag IUDS. *Contraception*, **44**, 473–80.

Sivin, I., Mishell, D.R., Jr., Diaz, S., et al. (2000). Prolonged effectiveness of Norplant capsule implants: a 7-year study. *Contraception*, **61**, 187–94.

Soebadi, D.M. (1999). Medical grade silicone rubber vasocclusion: an alternative method of male contraception. In: *Male Contraception: Present and Future*, Rajalakshmi, M. and Griffin, P.D., eds. New Age International, New Delhi, pp. 275–92.

Soebadi, D.M., Gardjito, W., and Mensink, H.J.A. (1995). Intravasal injection of formed-in-place medical grade silicone rubber for vas occlusion. *International Journal of Andrology*, **18**(Suppl. 1), 45–52.

Soonawalla, F.P. (1999). Vasectomy-safety and reversibility. In: *Male Contraception: Present and Future*. Rajalakshmi, M. and Griffin, P.D., eds. New Age International, New Delhi, pp. 251–64.

Stafford, M.K., Cain, D., Rosenstein, I., et al. (1997). A placebo-controlled, double-blind prospective study in healthy female volunteers of dextrin sulfate gel. *Journal of Acquired Immune Deficiency Syndrome and Human Retrovirology*, **14**, 213–18.

Stephenson, J. (2000). Widely used spermicide may increase, not decrease risk of HIV transmission. *Journal of the American Medical Association*, **284**, 949.

Sulak, P.J., Cressman, B.E., Waldrop, E., Holleman, S., and Kuehl, T.J. (1997). Extending the duration of active oral contraceptive pills to manage hormone withdrawal symptoms. *Obstetrics and Gynecology*, **89**, 179–83.

Talwar, G.P., Garg, S., Singh, R., et al. (1994). Praneem polyherbal cream and suppositories. In: *Barrier Contraceptives; Current Status and Future Prospects*, Mauck, C.K., Cordero, M., Gabelnick, H., Spieler, J.M., and Rivera, R., eds. John Wiley, New York, pp. 273–6.

Talwar, G.P., Raghuvanshi, P., Mishra, R., et al. (2000). Polyherbal formulations with wide spectrum antimicrobial activity against reproductive tract infections and sexually transmitted pathogens. *American Journal of Reproductive Immunology*, **43**, 144–51.

Tamamura, H., Murakami, T., Horiuchi, S., et al. (1995).

Synthesis of protegrin-related peptides and their antibacterial and anti-human immunodeficiency virus activity. *Chemical and Pharmaceutical Bulletin*, **43**, 853–8.

Visconti, P.E., Galantino-Homer, H., Moore, G.D., et al. (1998). The molecular basis of sperm capacitation. *Journal of Andrology*, **19**, 242–8.

Voeller, B. and Anderson, D.J. (1992). Heterosexual transmission of HIV. *Journal of the American Medical Association*, **267**, 1917–18.

Weinbauer, G.F. and Wessels, J. (1999). "Paracrine" control of spermatogenesis. *Andrologia*, **31**, 249–62.

Weisberg, E., Fraser, I.S., Lacarra, M., et al. (1999). Efficacy, bleeding patterns, and side effects of a 1-year contraceptive vaginal ring. C*ontraception*, **59**, 311–18.

World Health Organization Task Force on Long-Acting Systemic Agents for Fertility Regulation (1988). A multicenter phase III comparative study of two hormonal contraceptive preparations given once-a-month by intramuscular injection: I. Contraceptive efficacy and side effects. *Contraception*, **37**, 1–20.

World Health Organization Task Force on Methods for Regulation of Male Fertility (1990). Contraceptive efficacy of testosterone-induced azoospermia in normal men. *Lancet*, **336**, 955–9.

World Health Organization Task Force on Methods for Regulation of Male Fertility (1996). Contraceptive efficacy of testosterone-induced azoospermia and oligospermia in normal men. *Fertility and Sterility*, **65**, 821–9.

Wu, F.C., Balasubramanian, R., Mulders, T.M., and Coelingh-Bennink, H.J. (1999). Oral progestogen combined with testosterone as a potential male contraceptive: additive effects between desogestrel and testosterone enanthate in suppression of spermatogenesis, pituitary–testicular axis, and lipid metabolism. *Journal of Clinical Endocrinology and Metabolism*, **84**, 112–22.

Yeung, C.H., Sonnenberg-Riethmacher, E., and Cooper, T.G. (1998). Receptor tyrosine kinase c-*ros* knockout mice as a model for the study of epididymal regulation of sperm function. *Journal of Reproductive and Fertility*, **53**(Suppl.), 137–47.

Zaneveld, L.J.D. (1994). Vaginal contraception since 1984: chemical agents and barrier devices. In: *Contraceptive Research and Development 1984 to 1994*, Van Look, P.F.A. and Perez-Palacious, G., eds. Oxford University Press, Delhi, India, pp. 69–90.

Zaneveld, L.J.D., Kaminski, J.M., Waller, D.P., et al. (1988a). Aryl 4-guanidinobenzoates: potential vaginal contraceptives. In: *Female Contraception*, Runnebaum, B., Rabe, T., and Kiesel, L., eds. Springer-Verlag, Berlin, p. 286.

Zaneveld, L.J.D., Burns, J.W., Beyler S., Depel, W., and Shapiro, S. (1988b). Development of a potentially reversible vas deferens occlusion device and evaluation in primates. *Fertility and Sterility*, **49**, 527–33.

Zaneveld, L.J.D., Anderson, D.J., and Whaley, K.J. (1996). Barrier methods. In: *Contraceptive Research and Development. Looking in the Future*, Harrison, P.F. and Rosenfield, A., eds. National Academic Press, Washington, DC, pp. 430–45.

Zaneveld, L.J.D., De Castro, M.P., Faria, G., Derrick, F., and Ferraro, R. (1999). The soft, hollow plug ('Shug'): a potential reversible vas deferens occlusive device. In: *Male Contraception: Present and Future*, Rajalakshmi, M., and Griffin, P.D., eds. New Age International, Dehli, pp. 293–307.

Zeitlin, L., Olmstedt, S.S., Moench, T.R., et al. (1998). A humanized monoclonal antibody produced in transgenic plants for immunoprotection of the vagina against genital herpes. *Nature Biotechnology*, **16**, 1–5.

Zhang, G.Y., Gu, Y.Q., Wang, X.H., Cui, Y.G., and Bremner, W.J. (1999). A clinical trial of injectable testosterone undecanoate as a potential male contraceptive in normal Chinese men. *Journal of Clinical Endocrinology and Metabolism*, **84**, 3642–7.

Zhao, S. (1990). Vas deferens occlusion by percutaneous injection of polyurethane elastomer plugs: clinical experience and reversibility. *Contraception*, **41**, 453–9.

Zhao, S., Yu, R., and Zhang, S. (1992a). Recovery of fertility after removal of polyurethane plugs from the human vas deferens occluded for up to 5 years. *International Journal of Andrology*, **15**, 465–7.

Zhao, S., Zhang, S., and Yu, R. (1992b). Intravasal injection of formed-in-place silicone rubber as a method of vas occlusion. *International Journal of Andrology*, **15**, 460–4.

23

Developing immunocontraceptives

Eileen A. McLaughlin and Michael K. Holland

Pest Animal Control CRC, Canberra, Australia

Introduction

In mid-2000, the world human population reached 6.1 billion people, an increase of over 1 billion in a decade (Anon., 2001). While in the most developed nations birth rates are expected to fall below replacement levels in the next 50 years, those of the less developed nations are expected to increase or at best remain constant (Anon., 2001).

Since the advent of the oral contraceptive pill in the early 1960s, there have been no completely novel methods of contraception developed (Baird and Glasier, 1999). This is in part a consequence of the great efficacy and low side-effects associated with current versions of the pill and because of the substantial litigation that has accompanied other forms of contraception such as the intrauterine device. Nevertheless, there is a clear need for alternative forms of fertility control particularly in the developing world where much of the population growth is occurring. Consequently, some researchers in reproductive medicine have turned their attention to the development of new and safer methods of fertility control. One possibility is immunocontraception via a vaccine aimed at disrupting key processes in human reproduction (Gupta, 1998).

Many animal populations also require fertility control, particularly those that closely interact with humans. They include companion animals such as cats and dogs, livestock (e.g., cattle, sheep), and exotic animals being kept in captivity for conservation and educational purposes in zoos. The administration of a safe reversible vaccine, rather than more invasive current methods of contraception (such as operative or chemical castration), would be a significant alternative option. In addition, management of pest animals using an immunocontraceptive vaccine that results in permanent sterility is an attractive humane alternative to the current poisoning, shooting, and trapping practices of many farmers and government agencies (Holland, 1999). In this review, we do not seek to provide a comprehensive analysis of the considerable body of research in this area. Rather we concentrate on a brief analysis of the antigens that might be included in an immunocontraceptive vaccine, followed by a discussion of the nature of immune response required and recent advances in vaccine technology that might achieve these goals.

Prerequisites for a successful immunocontraception vaccine

Any candidate fertility vaccine must be safe for human use with minimal side-effects and, in order to match those contraceptive methods already available, be as near 100% effective as possible. Above all it must be reversible if it is to gain acceptability in both medical and patient communities. As development costs are a significant factor to pharmaceutical companies and the most likely future users are to be found amongst the young adults of developing nations, any immunocontraceptive vaccine must be financially viable by ultimately being affordable to the end-user (Alexander and Bialy, 1994).

Immunocontraceptive targets

Several points during the reproductive process, including gametogenesis, fertilization, implantation, and early fetal development, could be potential targets for an immunocontraceptive vaccine. In reality, any birth control method that causes the abortion or miscarriage of an implanted embryo is likely to meet with stiff resistance from social and religious groups and aid-giving organizations. In particular, the unauthorized and unethical use by unscrupulous regimens of such a vaccine has raised many concerns in the human rights movement about the development of this form of contraception. Consequently, researchers have largely, though not exclusively, confined their immunocontraceptive endeavors to the investigation of those reproductive processes occurring prior to implantation.

Hormone/hormone receptor antigens

To-date, the only completed phase II human trials using an immunocontraceptive vaccine rely on the female recipients producing antibodies to the β-subunit of human chorionic gonadotropin (β-hCG), a hormone produced by the developing embryo. Trials have shown that this vaccine is capable of offering a high degree of protection against pregnancy in the subgroup of women generating significant serum anti-β-hCG titers (Talwar, 1997). As some of the vaccinated women did not achieve a satisfactory response to the immunogen, further refinement of the vaccine by optimizing the immunogenic capability of the carrier peptide has been undertaken (Mandokhot et al., 2000). Surprisingly prior immunization of the woman with another vaccine containing a carrier such as diphtheria or tetanus toxoid, enhances antibody responses to hCG in recipients of the hCG conjugate vaccine (Shah et al., 1999). The mechanism of this effect remains unclear.

Potential hormone/hormone receptor-based male contraceptive vaccines such as luteinizing hormone-releasing hormone (LHRH) and follicle-stimulating hormone (FSH) have also met with problems such as incomplete efficacy and significant side-effects (e.g., loss of libido), in the limited trials conducted so far (Moudgal et al., 1997). Such hormone-based immunocontraceptive vaccines hold much promise but require modification and further primate and human trials before wide-scale use can be contemplated.

The zona pellucida proteins as target antigens

Alternative targets for immunocontraceptive vaccines include surface antigens present on oocytes and spermatozoa. Many groups have concentrated on the elucidation of the mechanisms involved in gametogenesis, gamete transport, and fertilization. Since the early 1980s, the use of molecular genetic techniques has contributed greatly to the identification and partial characterization of the many proteins that appear important in mammalian reproduction.

Work on ovarian antigens has concentrated largely on the family of glycoproteins that constitute the zona pellucida. In early studies in the mouse, zona proteins were classified into three groups (ZP1, ZP2, and ZP3) according to their perceived size (Wassarman, 1988). Zona pellucida proteins are heavily glycosylated and are synthesized and secreted by both granulosa cells and the oocyte in the mammalian ovary to form a unique acellular translucent matrix that surrounds the ovulated egg and early embryo. Studies with ZP1, ZP2, and ZP3 "knockout" mice (Rankin et al., 1996, 1999), confirm that the zona matrix is a prerequisite for normal follicular development and plays an essential role in both fertilization and preimplantation embryo transport and development.

Different researchers have adopted several nomenclature systems for zona proteins for different species, resulting in a great deal of confusion when comparing among species. Latterly, most zona proteins have been classified into one of three gene families (ZPA, ZPB, ZPC) based on their homology at the nucleic acid/amino acid level. In the mouse, the most well-characterized system, ZP3 (ZPC) appears to function as the primary sperm receptor molecule though alternative zona proteins such as ZP1 (ZPB) appear to fulfill this role in other species such as the rabbit (Prasad et al., 1996) and monkey (Govind et al., 2001).

The primary sperm receptor has obvious inherent attraction for the development of an immunocontraceptive vaccine intended to act by prevention of fertilization. Immunocontraceptive immunization studies have been carried out using both homologous and heterologous zona proteins in a number of animal species ranging from mouse, guinea pig, and rabbit to nonhuman primates, with somewhat conflicting results. In most cases where an adequate immune response was generated, infertility occurred but this was often associated with ovarian pathology (Kirkpatrick et al., 1996).

The easy accessibility of large numbers of pig ovaries from abattoirs allowed the collection and purification of substantial quantities of zona proteins. Intramuscular immunization using whole native porcine zona pellucida (pZP) as the immunogen has resulted in the induction of infertility in many mammalian species with the notable exception of the mouse. In almost all studies, the use of whole pZP has resulted in significant side-effects including disturbance of ovarian cyclicity, loss of primordial and antral follicles, abnormal follicular development, and significant ovarian pathology with oophoritis. While induction of permanent sterility would be welcomed in pest animal control (Jackson et al., 1998), the occurrence of these adverse side-effects would be unacceptable in a human immunocontraceptive vaccine.

Researchers have chosen to produce and investigate recombinant zona proteins as alternative immunogens. The range of expression systems employed (bacterial, baculovirus, and eukaryotic) has resulted in differing immunogenicity of these recombinant proteins and varying degrees of associated ovarian pathology depending on the animal model investigated (Sacco et al., 1981; Kerr et al., 1999). The pathogenicity of these zona proteins appears to be related primarily to the protein backbone as the use of deglycosylated recombinant and native protein in several studies resulted in ovarian

dysfunction (Keenan et al., 1991; Jones et al., 1992; Paterson et al., 1992). Characterization of the proteinaceous core of mouse ZP3 using overlapping peptides has identified two T cell epitopes linked to induction of oophoritis and leukocytic infiltration characteristic of autoimmune disease (Garza and Tung, 1995) and a single B cell epitope (Lou et al., 1995). The nature of this approach means only linear epitopes can be identified and that all conformational epitopes are excluded. The relative importance of linear and conformational epitopes remains to be defined.

Avoidance of ovarian pathogenesis has been achieved in the mouse, macaque, and marmoset (Bagavant et al., 1997; Paterson et al., 1999) using peptides incorporating a promiscuous foreign testosterone helper cell epitope with the ZP3 B cell epitope. While these chimeric peptides do not induce the unwanted ovarian pathology seen in some inbred mouse strains, in others they fail to have a substantial impact on fertility. This suggests that a single epitope is insufficient to block sperm–egg recognition and binding in all individuals in some species (Paterson et al., 1999). Based on knowledge gleaned from our experience with other vaccines, the variation in response in an outbred species to a single epitope might be unpredictable.

In summary, immunization against zona pellucida proteins does induce substantial infertility in the species tested so far. Targeting the zona pellucida can achieve sterility and shows great promise in the control of animal populations, but until researchers achieve the separation of the immunocontraceptive effect from the unwanted pathology induced by the immunodominant epitopes, these proteins remain unlikely target antigen candidates for a human immunocontraceptive vaccine.

Spermatozoa as immunocontraceptive target antigens

Approximately 5% of those couples consulting for failure to conceive are attributed to the presence in the sera of antisperm antibodies (Hull et al., 1985). The presence of antisperm antibodies in the sera and accessory gland fluids of 70% of vasectomized men indicated that spermatozoa or their breakdown products are powerful immunogens. The fact that many of the men who subsequently have their vasectomy reversed remain infertile means this immune response can often also be contraceptive. In fact, 70 years ago Baskin (1932) demonstrated (in an ethically unrepeatable experiment) that immunizing women using whole semen from their partners resulted in prolonged infertility and he even applied for a patent on this discovery. Given the high immunogenicity of sperm in both females and males, the development of an immunocontraceptive vaccine for use in both sexes seemed a feasible concept. A human vaccine would require a defined antigen rather than a crude mixture such as whole sperm. The search to identify a cell surface protein that has an essential role in reproduction and is found exclusively on spermatozoa has occupied much of the 1990s.

A plethora of sperm protein antigen candidates for a fertility vaccine have been investigated so far. Proteins characterized include SP-17 (O'Rand, 1981), PH-20 and PH30/fertilin (Primakoff et al., 1987, 1988), lactate dehydrogenase isozyme C4 (LDH-C4; Goldberg, 1990), SP-10 (Herr et al., 1990), sp-56 (Bleil and Wassarman, 1990), FA-1 (Naz and Wolf, 1994) SOB-2 (Lefevre et al., 1997), and most recently a novel form of CD52 (Diekman et al., 1999).

In most cases, the antibodies raised against these proteins are capable of preventing or inhibiting fertilization in vitro by either interfering with sperm–egg recognition and binding or causing sperm–sperm agglutination. However, only a few studies in animal models have convincingly demonstrated a loss of fertility in immunized animals. The most striking example is the active immunization of male and female guinea pigs with PH-20, a sperm membrane protein with hyaluronidase activity and a role in sperm–zona pellucida binding. A single, low-dose intramuscular injection resulted in 100% infertility in both males and females (Primakoff et al., 1987, 1988). Further investigation revealed that immunization had provoked experimental autoimmune orchitis in the males, with a complete absence

of spermatozoa in the epididymides (Tung et al., 1997). Both these effects were reversible, with males and females regaining fertility some months after immunization. So far, the ability of PH-20 to achieve a similar contraceptive effect in other species remains unproven (Holland et al., 1997) and the recent identification of the mouse homolog of PH-20 (Spam-1) in cells of the epididymis and kidney (Deng et al., 2000) and in human laryngeal cancer (Godin et al., 2000) would question selection of PH-20 as an ideal immunocontraceptive target antigen for human use.

Probably the most intensively studied sperm antigen is the testes-specific LDH-C4 (O'Hern et al., 1995, 1997). Unlike most somatic forms of the enzyme, LDH-C4 appears to be expressed on the cell surface and has been detected on the mid-piece and principal piece of the sperm tail in mouse and human. Immunization of several species, including nonhuman primates, has demonstrated reversible infertility in both males and females (Gupta and Malhotra, 1994; O'Hern et al., 1995). However, studies in hyperimmunized male mice have detected a substantial autoimmune reaction to LDH-C4, with lesions in the testis and epididymis akin to experimental autoimmune orchitis (Gupta and Malhotra, 1994). This may be overcome by the use of a chimeric peptide containing a LDH-C4 B cell epitope and a "promiscuous" T cell epitope from tetanus toxin. This construct gave reversible infertility in immunized female rabbits and baboons (O'Hern et al., 1997). Worryingly, a recent report suggests that immunochemically cross-reactive epitopes are exposed in sperm-specific LDH following glucosylation and interaction with gossypol and result in LDH-C4 antisera cross-reacting with somatic LDH in vivo (Gupta and Syal, 2000).

Another potential target antigen is sp56, the putative sperm receptor molecule for ZP3 in the mouse (Cheng et al., 1994). Antibodies to sp56 can inhibit sperm–egg interaction in vitro, suggesting that sp56 might induce an immunocontraceptive response in vivo. However, multiple immunizations of a recombinant form of sp56 proved necessary to achieve a suitable immunocontraceptive response (Hardy and

Mobbs, 1999). Why this is the case is unclear. Whether it will remain true for native sp56 remains to be investigated.

Problems have also been encountered with another candidate antigen, fertilin (or PH-30), a heterodimeric sperm membrane protein consisting of α- and β-subunits (Blobel et al., 1992). Fertilin, a member of the ADAM family, contains disintegrin-like and cysteine-rich domains (Wolfsberg et al., 1995; Frayne et al., 1997) and is postulated to be involved in sperm–oolemma binding and fusion (Myles et al., 1994; Evans et al., 1998). A small-scale immunocontraceptive trial in guinea pigs (Ramarao et al., 1996) resulted in subfertility in a proportion of the animals tested, indicating that this protein had possibilities as a target antigen. However, the failure to achieve a similar result in rabbits (Hardy et al., 1997), the discovery that the gene for the fertilin α-subunit is non-functional in the human (Jury et al., 1997), and the identification of a diverse range of effects in knockout mice for fertilin β-subunit (Cho et al., 2000) effectively rule fertilin out as a target antigen for a human immunocontraceptive.

To summarize, after more than a decade of research and even though sperm surface antigens look promising, no single protein fulfills all the criteria of complete infertility and long-lasting immunity with no significant side-effects, which are necessary for a human vaccine.

The role of the systemic versus mucosal immunity in immunocontraceptive vaccines

Depending on the nature and localization of the antigen being considered for inclusion in an immunocontraceptive vaccine, high titers might need to be achieved in serum or within the reproductive tract. Vaccines requiring high serum titers such as those based on zona pellucida antigens have been widely studied. The options for enhancing their efficacy for human use are limited. Alum remains the only adjuvant approved for use and while it is possible to see developments in this area, they are more likely to occur through the use of biologically active molecules such as cytokines or by direct modifications to the antigens themselves. However, mucosa-based immunocontraceptive vaccines present a number of novel options.

Route and timing of vaccine administration

The reproductive tract is part of the common mucosal immune system and as such most of the antibodies are produced locally in the mucosal tissue by subepithelial plasma cells (Brandtzaeg, 1985; Conley and Delacroix, 1987). Antibodies in the gastrointestinal tract and reproductive tract secretions are mainly polymeric IgA (pIgA) whereas those found in blood are usually of the IgG isotype. Therefore, systemic immunization may be of limited value in the production of an effective immunocontraceptive effect against a target antigen confined to the reproductive tract, as antibodies from the circulation do not always enter the reproductive tract (Mestecky et al., 1991). The ability of both bacterial and viral sexually transmitted diseases (such as *Chlamydia trachomatis* and the human immunodeficiency virus (HIV)) to infect mucosal surfaces has spurred vaccine immunologists to consider methods of inducing a specific immune response to such pathogens at the site of infection. Similar strategies could be employed to elicit a response to gamete antigens within the reproductive tract.

Despite repeated exposure to spermatozoa via natural intercourse, only a tiny minority of women develop detectable antisperm antibodies in reproductive tract fluids such as cervical mucus (Eggert-Kruse et al., 1993). Although it has been shown that intravaginal and intrarectal immunization can elicit an immune response in the reproductive tract (for review see Kutteh and Mestecky, 1996), these routes of administration are unlikely to prove popular with human patients. As the reproductive tract is part of the common mucosal immune system, this has led researchers to consider induction of a suitable immune response in the reproductive tract via another mucosal site. Immunization via the nasal-associated lymphoid tissue and, to a lesser extent, the gut-associated lymphoid tissue has been shown to induce antibody-secreting cells in the vagina and cervix in a number of model systems (Russell et al., 1996; Rosenthal and Gallichan, 1997). Consequently, the route of immunization is an important factor in optimizing the immunocontraceptive response.

In the rodent and human female reproductive tract, reproductive hormonal status heavily influences mucosal immunity. Increased levels of IgA are detected in cervical mucus just prior to ovulation when estradiol levels peak (Franklin and Kutteh, 1999). Cytokines (McGhee et al., 1989; Prabhala and Wira, 1991, 1995; Kutteh et al., 1998) including interleukins 1b and 10, which play a role in the maturation of B lymphocytes to immunoglobulin-producing plasma cells (Edwards et al., 1995), appear to be the mediators of this effect. Whether these hormone-induced responses are seen in the oviduct, where an immunocontraceptive vaccine targeting fertilization would need to produce peak antibody levels, is unclear.

Latterly transcutaneous immunization (Glenn et al., 1998, 1999) has been shown to be adept at producing a strong immune response in both the mucosal and the systemic immune system. Recent studies with mice using tetanus toxoid admixed with cholera toxin and administered via topical application to the skin of the lower back was able to induce a significant response within the female reproductive tract of mice (Gockel et al., 2000). Further studies demonstrating the feasibility and the safe application of a vaccine for humans via a skin patch (Glenn et al., 2000) raises the possibility that future human gamete antigen immunocontraceptive vaccines may be easily administered via a transcutaneous route.

Carrier proteins to maximize immune response

The immunostimulatory ability of small immunocontraceptive peptides is limited and research with the hormone-based vaccines has used either diphtheria toxoid or tetanus toxoid as carrier molecules conjugated to the specific antigen. The construction

of a heterospecies dimer vaccine (HSD), where the β-subunit of hCG was associated with the α-subunit of ovine luteinizing hormone, achieved maximum immunostimulation. In animal models, cholera toxin and Escherichia coli-derived heat-labile enterotoxin are traditionally used to induce mucosal immune responses, but these are both unsuitable as they are toxic in humans. Their β-subunits, however, are nontoxic and bind to the mucosa; these are very promising and conjugation of a test antigen (human gammaglobulin) to either β-subunit resulted in a dramatic increase in their potential to induce mucosal immune responses (Rask et al., 2000) following either oral or intranasal administration.

Administration of adjuvants with antigens to improve immune response

Since the 1920s, human vaccines have largely been delivered using aluminum salts as adjuvants. Although these are potent stimulators of the systemic immune system via release of cytokines (Ulanova et al., 2001), they are not ideal for producing a local mucosal response. Subsequently, research has concentrated on the use of other more immunostimulatory adjuvants, though alum salts remain the only widespread products licensed for human use.

Traditional adjuvants used in animal studies, such as Freunds, cholera toxin and heat-labile enterotoxin, are not suitable for use in humans because of their toxicity, and research has concentrated on identification of new and more potent adjuvants. One possibility is modification of existing adjuvants. LTR72 is a genetically modified molecule derived from heat-labile enterotoxin but with less residual toxicity. When it is administered intranasally to mice with a genital form of human papilloma virus (HPV-6b), it was able to provoke a substantial immune response compared with that achieved by parenteral immunization (Greer et al., 2000).

Recently, QS-21, a saponin derived from the soap-bark tree and known to have good immunostimulatory properties in animals, was combined with a recombinant soluble form of the HIV-1 membrane protein gp120 and shown to produce a suitable immune response safely in human HIV-negative volunteers (Evans et al., 2001). In a trial of a cancer vaccine in mice, QS-21 was shown to be the most potent adjuvant compared with several others including bacterial nucleotide CpG, monophosphoryl lipid A, and granulocyte macrophage-colony stimulating factor (GM-CSF) Fc fusion peptide (Kim et al., 2000).

Most promisingly, the use of cytokines (such as interleukin 12) and bacterial CpG oligonucleotides in mice has been shown to enhance the efficiency of coadministered antigens such as the mycobacterium bovine BCG (bacille Calmette-Guérin) vaccine (Freidag et al., 2000) by increasing the magnitude of the T helper type 1 response. Interleukin 12, stimulating the production of interferon gamma, also enhances murine antibody responses to bacterial infection (Buchanan et al., 2001). However as interleukin 12 has been shown to be toxic in high doses, it may be preferable to administer low-dose recombinant interleukin 12 in combination with another potent adjuvant such as QS-21 (Hancock et al., 2000) to achieve optimal mucosal immune stimulation.

DNA vaccines

Vaccination using plasmid DNA encoding the antigen of choice is capable of inducing a specific immune response (Shedlock and Weiner, 2000). Delivery to host cells can be via intramuscular injection, with various adjuvants, or through biolistic immunization by gene gun delivery of DNA-coated gold particles to the epidermis (Donnelly and Ulmer, 1999). However, despite early promise, the DNA vaccines have largely proved incapable of inducing sufficient immunity to provide protection against challenge from pathogenic organisms (Ramshaw and Ramsay, 2000). It is suggested that this results from failure to induce an amnestic response. One way to overcome this is to fuse the ligand CTLA-4 (cytotoxic T lymphocyte antigen 4), which targets

antigen-presenting cells, to the immunogen of choice (Deliyannis et al., 2000). CTLA-4 binds specifically to B7 molecules on antigen-presenting cells and thus strongly increases the immunogenicity of the target antigen (Huang et al., 2000). An alternative ligand, L-selectin, has a similar effect by increasing lymphocyte proliferation through binding to endothelial cells in the lymph nodes (Lew et al., 2000).

Rodriguez and colleagues have pioneered another approach. They showed that ubiquitation of a viral protein upregulates its intracellular degradation, thus leading to enhanced antigen presentation and, consequently, to improved induction of cytotoxic T lymphocytes (Rodriguez et al., 1997).

The latest strategy is to employ DNA vaccines for the initial immunization or priming and to follow this with immunization with an attenuated recombinant viral vector such as modified recombinant vaccinia virus to boost the immune response (Ramshaw and Ramsay, 2000).

Immunocontraceptive target antigens may be amenable to delivery via DNA vaccines but the safety of these vaccines has yet to be fully evaluated. A number of different DNA-based vaccines against HIV are currently under clinical tests. These should provide important data for those developing immunocontraceptive vaccines.

Possibilities for the future

With the publication of the human genome sequence (Lander et al., 2001) and the implementation of proteonomics in reproductive biology, additional ovarian/oogonia-specific and spermatozoa-specific antigens may be identified. Vaccine design and molecular technology advances rapidly, and the use of genetically modified organisms such as recombinant replication-deficient avian poxviruses expressing GM-CSF as biological adjuvants to enhance antigen-specific immunity (Kass et al., 2001) now appears to be a viable option. Such recombinant viruses will require careful monitoring, as animals studies have shown that, while viral-vectored immunocontraceptive recombinant viruses containing ovarian antigens can induce infertility (Jackson et al., 1998), inclusion of adjuvants such as the cytokine interleukin 4 can result in unwanted side-effects (Jackson et al., 2001), which would be totally unacceptable in a human vaccine.

REFERENCES

Alexander, N.J. and Bialy, G. (1994). Contraceptive vaccine development. *Reproduction, Fertility and Development*, **6**, 273–80.

Anon. (2001). *World Population Prospects: The 2000 Revision.* Population Division of the UN Department of Economic and Social Affairs New York, p. 34.

Bagavant, H., Fusi, F.M., Baisch, J., et al. (1997). Immunogenicity and contraceptive potential of a human zona pellucida 3 peptide vaccine. *Biology of Reproduction*, **56**, 764–70.

Baird, D.T. and Glasier, A.F. (1999). Science, medicine, and the future. Contraception. *British Medical Journal*, **319**, 969–72.

Baskin, M.J. (1932). Temporary sterilization by the injection of human spermatozoa. A preliminary report. *American Journal of Obstetrics and Gynecology*, **24**, 892–7.

Bleil, J.D. and Wassarman, P.M. (1990). Identification of a ZP3-binding protein on acrosome-intact mouse sperm by photo-affinity crosslinking. *Proceedings of the National Academy of Sciences USA*, **87**, 5563–7.

Blobel, C.P., Wolfsberg, T.G., Turck, C.W., et al. (1992). A potential fusion peptide and an integrin ligand domain in a protein active in sperm–egg fusion. *Nature*, **356**, 248–52.

Brandtzaeg, P. (1985). The oral immune system under normal and pathological conditions. *Pathology Research Practices*, **179**, 619–21.

Buchanan, R.M., Briles, D.E., Arulanandam, B.P., et al. (2001). IL-12-mediated increases in protection elicited by pneumococcal and meningococcal conjugate vaccines. *Vaccine*, **19**, 2020–8.

Cheng, A., Le, T., Palacios, M., et al. (1994). Sperm–egg recognition in the mouse: characterization of sp56, a sperm protein having specific affinity for ZP3. *Journal of Cell Biology*, **125**, 867–78.

Cho, C., Ge, H., Branciforte, D., et al. (2000). Analysis of mouse fertilin in wild-type and fertilin beta(−/−) sperm: evidence for C-terminal modification, alpha/beta dimerization, and lack of essential role of fertilin alpha in sperm-egg fusion. *Developmental Biology*, **222**, 289–95.

Conley, M.E. and Delacroix, D.L. (1987). Intravascular and mucosal immunoglobulin A: two separate but related systems of immune defense? *Annals of Internal Medicine*, **106**, 892–9.

Deliyannis, G., Boyle, J.S., Brady, J.L., et al. (2000). A fusion DNA vaccine that targets antigen-presenting cells increases protection from viral challenge. *Proceedings of the National Academy of Sciences USA*, **97**, 6676–80.

Deng, X., He, Y., Martin-Deleon, P.A., et al. (2000). Mouse Spam1 (PH-20): evidence for its expression in the epididymis and for a new category of spermatogenic-expressed genes. *Journal of Andrology*, **21**, 822–32.

Diekman, A.B., Norton, E.J., Klotz, K.L., et al. (1999). Evidence for a unique N-linked glycan associated with human infertility on sperm CD52: a candidate contraceptive vaccinogen. *Immunological Reviews*, **171**, 203–11.

Donnelly, J.J. and Ulmer, J.B. (1999). DNA vaccines for viral diseases. *Brazilian Journal of Medicine and Biological Research*, **32**, 215–22.

Edwards, R.P., Kuykendall, K., Crowley-Nowick, P., et al. (1995). T lymphocytes infiltrating advanced grades of cervical neoplasia. CD8-positive cells are recruited to invasion. *Cancer*, **76**, 1411–15.

Eggert-Kruse, W., Bockem-Hellwig, S., Doll, A., et al. (1993). Antisperm antibodies in cervical mucus in an unselected subfertile population. *Human Reproduction*, **8**, 1025–31.

Evans, J.P., Schultz, R.M., Kopf, G.S., et al. (1998). Roles of the disintegrin domains of mouse fertilins alpha and beta in fertilization. *Biology of Reproduction*, **59**, 145–52.

Evans, T.G., McElrath, M.J., Matthews, T., et al. (2001). QS-21 promotes an adjuvant effect allowing for reduced antigen dose during HIV-1 envelope subunit immunization in humans. *Vaccine*, **19**, 2080–91.

Franklin, R.D. and Kutteh, W.H. (1999). Characterization of immunoglobulins and cytokines in human cervical mucus: influence of exogenous and endogenous hormones. *Journal of Reproductive Immunology*, **42**, 93–106.

Frayne, J., Jury, J.A., Barker, H.L., et al. (1997). Rat MDC family of proteins: sequence analysis, tissue distribution, and expression in prepubertal and adult rat testis. *Molecular Reproduction and Development*, **48**, 159–67.

Freidag, B.L., Melton, G.B., Collins, F., et al. (2000). CpG oligodeoxynucleotides and interleukin-12 improve the efficacy of *Mycobacterium bovis* BCG vaccination in mice challenged with *M. tuberculosis*. *Infection and Immunity*, **68**, 2948–53.

Garza, K.M. and Tung, K.S. (1995). Frequency of molecular mimicry among T cell peptides as the basis for autoimmune disease and autoantibody induction. *Journal of Immunology*, **155**, 5444–8.

Glenn, G.M., Scharton-Kersten, T., Vassell, R., et al. (1998). Transcutaneous immunization with cholera toxin protects mice against lethal mucosal toxin challenge. *Journal of Immunology*, **161**, 3211–14.

Glenn, G.M., Scharton-Kersten, T., Vassell, R., et al. (1999). Transcutaneous immunization with bacterial ADP-ribosylating exotoxins as antigens and adjuvants. *Infection and Immunity*, **67**, 1100–6.

Glenn, G.M., Taylor, D.N., Li, X., et al. (2000). Transcutaneous immunization: a human vaccine delivery strategy using a patch. *Nature Medicine*, **6**, 1403–6.

Gockel, C.M., Bao, S., Beagley, K.W., et al. (2000). Transcutaneous immunization induces mucosal and systemic immunity: a potent method for targeting immunity to the female reproductive tract. *Molecular Immunology*, **37**, 537–44.

Godin, D.A., Fitzpatrick, P.C., Scandurro, A.B., et al. (2000). PH20: a novel tumor marker for laryngeal cancer. *Archives of Otolaryngology – Head and Neck Surgery*, **126**, 402–4.

Goldberg, E. (1990). Developmental expression of lactate dehydrogenase isozymes during spermatogenesis. *Progress in Clinical Biology Research*, **344**, 49–52.

Govind, C.K., Gahlay, G.K., Choudhury, S., et al. (2001). Purified and refolded recombinant bonnet monkey (*Macaca radiata*) zona pellucida glycoprotein-B expressed in *Escherichia coli* binds to spermatozoa. *Biology of Reproduction*, **64**, 1147–52.

Greer, C.E., Petracca, R., Buonamassa, D.T., et al. (2000). The comparison of the effect of LTR72 and MF59 adjuvants on mouse humoral response to intranasal immunisation with human papillomavirus type 6b (HPV-6b) virus-like particles. *Vaccine*, **19**, 1008–12.

Gupta, S.K. (1998). The immunology of reproduction: update 1998. *Immunology Today*, **19**, 433–4.

Gupta, G.S. and Malhotra, R. (1994). Autoimmune-like activity of sperm specific LDH: a pathophysiological and electron microscopic study of atrophied testis and epididymis. *Indian Journal of Biochemistry and Biophysics*, **31**, 480–5.

Gupta, G.S. and Syal, N. (2000). Newly exposed immunochemically cross-reactive epitopes in sperm-specific LDH after glucosylation and gossypol interaction. *American Journal of Reproductive Immunology*, **44**, 303–9.

Hancock, G.E., Heers, K.M., Smith, J.D., et al. (2000). QS-21 synergizes with recombinant interleukin-12 to create a potent adjuvant formulation for the fusion protein of respiratory syncytial virus. *Viral Immunology*, **13**, 503–9.

Hardy, C.M. and Mobbs, K.J. (1999). Expression of recombinant mouse sperm protein sp56 and assessment of its potential for use as an antigen in an immunocontraceptive vaccine. *Molecular Reproduction and Development*, **52**, 216–24.

Hardy, C.M., Clarke, H.G., Nixon, B., et al. (1997). Examination of the immunocontraceptive potential of recombinant rabbit fertilin subunits in rabbit. *Biology of Reproduction*, **57**, 879–86.

Herr, J.C., Flickinger, C.J., Homyk, M., et al. (1990). Biochemical and morphological characterization of the intra-acrosomal antigen SP-10 from human sperm. *Biology of Reproduction*, **42**, 181–93.

Holland, M.K. (1999). Fertility control in wild populations of animals. *Journal of Andrology*, **20**, 579–85.

Holland, M.K., Andrews, J., Clarke, H., et al. (1997). Selection of antigens for use in a virus-vectored immunocontraceptive vaccine: PH-20 as a case study. *Reproduction, Fertility and Development*, **9**, 117–24.

Huang, T.H., Wu, P.Y., Lee, C.N., et al. (2000). Enhanced antitumor immunity by fusion of CTLA-4 to a self tumor antigen. *Blood*, **96**, 3663–70.

Hull, M.G., Glazener, C.M., Kelly, N.J., et al. (1985). Population study of causes, treatment, and outcome of infertility. *British Medical Journal (Clinical Research Education)*, **291**, 1693–7.

Jackson, R.J., Maguire, D.J., Hinds, L.A., et al. (1998). Infertility in mice induced by a recombinant ectromelia virus expressing mouse zona pellucida glycoprotein 3. *Biology of Reproduction*, **58**, 152–9.

Jackson, R.J., Ramsay, A.J., Christensen, C.D., et al. (2001). Expression of mouse interleukin-4 by a recombinant ectromelia virus suppresses cytolytic lymphocyte responses and overcomes genetic resistance to mousepox. *Journal of Virology*, **75**, 1205–10.

Jones, G.R., Sacco, A.G., Subramanian, M.G., et al. (1992). Histology of ovaries of female rabbits immunized with deglycosylated zona pellucida macromolecules of pigs. *Journal of Reproduction and Fertility*, **95**, 513–25.

Jury, J.A., Frayne, J., Hall, L., et al. (1997). The human fertilin alpha gene is non-functional: implications for its proposed role in fertilization. *Biochemical Journal*, **321**, 577–81.

Kass, E., Panicali, D.L., Mazzara, G., et al. (2001). Granulocyte/macrophage-colony stimulating factor produced by recombinant avian poxviruses enriches the regional lymph nodes with antigen-presenting cells and acts as an immunoadjuvant. *Cancer Research*, **61**, 206–14.

Keenan, J.A., Sacco, A.G., Subramanian, M.G., et al. (1991). Endocrine response in rabbits immunized with native versus deglycosylated porcine zona pellucida antigens. *Biology of Reproduction*, **44**, 150–6.

Kerr, P.J., Jackson, R.J., Robinson, A.J., et al. (1999). Infertility in female rabbits (*Oryctolagus cuniculus*) alloimmunized with the rabbit zona pellucida protein ZPB either as a purified recombinant protein or expressed by recombinant myxoma virus. *Biology of Reproduction*, **61**, 606–13.

Kim, S.K., Ragupathi, G., Cappello, S., et al. (2000). Effect of immunological adjuvant combinations on the antibody and T-cell response to vaccination with MUC1–KLH and GD3–KLH conjugates. *Vaccine*, **19**, 530–7.

Kirkpatrick, J.F., Turner, J.W.J., Liv, I.K., et al. (1996). Applications of pig zona pellucida immunocontraception to wildlife fertility control. *Journal of Reproduction and Fertility*, **50**(Suppl), 183–9.

Kutteh, W.H. and Mestecky, J. (1996). The concept of mucosal immunology. In: *Reproductive Immunology*, Bronson, R., Alexander, N.J., Anderson, D.J., Branch, D.W., and Kutteh, W.H., eds. Blackwell Science, Oxford, pp. 28–51.

Kutteh, W.H., Moldoveanu, Z., Mestecky, J., et al. (1998). Mucosal immunity in the female reproductive tract: correlation of immunoglobulins, cytokines, and reproductive hormones in human cervical mucus around the time of ovulation. *AIDS Research and Human Retroviruses*, **14**(Suppl. 1), S51–5.

Lander, E.S., Linton, L.M., Birren, B., et al. (2001). Initial sequencing and analysis of the human genome. *Nature*, **409**, 860–921.

Lefevre, A., Martin Ruiz, C., Chokomian, S., et al. (1997). Characterization and isolation of SOB2, a human sperm protein with a potential role in oocyte membrane binding. *Molecular Human Reproduction*, **3**, 507–16.

Lew, A.M., Brady, B.J., Boyle, B.L., et al. (2000). Site-directed immune responses in DNA vaccines encoding ligand-antigen fusions. *Vaccine*, **18**, 1681–5.

Lou, Y., Ang, J., Thai, H., et al. (1995). A zona pellucida 3 peptide vaccine induces antibodies and reversible infertility without ovarian pathology. *Journal of Immunology*, **155**, 2715–20.

Mandokhot, A., Pal, R., Nagpal, S., et al. (2000). Humoral hyporesponsiveness to a conjugate contraceptive vaccine and its bypass by diverse carriers using permissible adjuvant. *Clinical and Experimental Immunology*, **122**, 101–8.

McGhee, J.R., Mestecky, J., Elson, C.O., et al. (1989). Regulation of IgA synthesis and immune response by T cells and interleukins. *Journal of Clinical Immunology*, **9**, 175–99.

Mestecky, J., Lue, C., Russell, M.W., et al. (1991). Selective transport of IgA. Cellular and molecular aspects. *Gastroenterology Clinics of North America*, **20**, 441–71.

Moudgal, N.R., Murthy, G.S., Prasanna Kumar, K.M., et al. (1997). Responsiveness of human male volunteers to immunization with ovine follicle stimulating hormone vaccine: results of a pilot study. *Human Reproduction*, **12**, 457–63.

Myles, D.G., Kimmel, L.H., Blobel, C.P., et al. (1994). Identification of a binding site in the disintegrin domain of fertilin required for sperm-egg fusion. *Proceedings of the National Academy of Sciences USA*, **91**, 4195–8.

Naz, R.K. and Wolf, D.P. (1994). Antibodies to sperm-specific human FA-1 inhibit in vitro fertilization in rhesus monkeys: development of a simian model for testing of anti-FA-1 contraceptive vaccine. *Journal of Reproductive Immunology*, **27**, 111–21.

O'Hern, P.A., Bambra, C.S., Isahakra, M., et al. (1995). Reversible contraception in female baboons immunized with a synthetic epitope of sperm-specific lactate dehydrogenase. *Biology of Reproduction*, **52**, 331–9.

O'Hern, P.A., Liang, Z.G., Bambra, C.S., et al. (1997). Colinear synthesis of an antigen-specific B-cell epitope with a 'promiscuous' tetanus toxin T-cell epitope: a synthetic peptide immunocontraceptive. *Vaccine*, **15**, 1761–6.

O'Rand, M.G. (1981). Inhibition of fertility and sperm-zona binding by antiserum to the rabbit sperm membrane autoantigen RSA-1. *Biology of Reproduction*, **25**, 621–8.

Paterson, M., Koothan, P.T., Morris, K.D., et al. (1992). Analysis of the contraceptive potential of antibodies against native and deglycosylated porcine ZP3 in vivo and in vitro. *Biology of Reproduction*, **46**, 523–34.

Paterson, M., Wilson, M.R., Jennings, Z.A., et al. (1999). Design and evaluation of a ZP3 peptide vaccine in a homologous primate model. *Molecular Human Reproduction*, **5**, 342–52.

Prabhala, R.H. and Wira, C.R. (1991). Cytokine regulation of the mucosal immune system: in vivo stimulation by interferongamma of secretory component and immunoglobulin A in uterine secretions and proliferation of lymphocytes from spleen. *Endocrinology*, **129**, 2915–23.

Prabhala, R.H. and Wira, C.R. (1995). Influence of estrous cycle and estradiol on mitogenic responses of splenic T- and B-lymphocytes. *Advances in Experimental Medicine and Biology*, **371**, 379–81.

Prasad, S.V., Wilkins, B., Hyatt, H., et al. (1996). Evaluating zona pellucida structure and function using antibodies to rabbit 55 kDa ZP protein expressed in baculovirus expression system. *Molecular Reproduction and Development*, **43**, 519–29.

Primakoff, P., Hyatt, H., Tredick-Kline, J., et al. (1987). Identification and purification of a sperm surface protein with a potential role in sperm–egg membrane fusion. *Journal of Cell Biology*, **104**, 141–9.

Primakoff, P., Cowan, A., Hyatt, H., et al. (1988). Purification of the guinea pig sperm PH-20 antigen and detection of a site-specific endoproteolytic activity in sperm preparations that cleaves PH-20 into two disulfide-linked fragments. *Biology of Reproduction*, **38**, 921–34.

Ramarao, C.S., Myles, D.G., White, J.M., et al. (1996). Initial evaluation of fertilin as an immunocontraceptive antigen and molecular cloning of the cynomolgus monkey fertilin beta subunit. *Molecular Reproduction and Development*, **43**, 70–5.

Ramshaw, I.A. and Ramsay, A.J. (2000). The prime-boost strategy: exciting prospects for improved vaccination. *Immunology Today*, **21**, 163–5.

Rankin, T., Familari, M., Lee, E., et al. (1996). Mice homozygous for an insertional mutation in the Zp3 gene lack a zona pellucida and are infertile. *Development*, **122**, 2903–10.

Rankin, T., Talbot, P., Lee, E., et al. (1999). Abnormal zonae pellucidae in mice lacking ZP1 result in early embryonic loss. *Development*, **126**, 3847–55.

Rankin, T.L., O'Brien, M., Lee, E., et al. (2001). Defective zonae pellucidae in Zp2-null mice disrupt folliculogenesis, fertility and development. *Development*, **128**, 1119–26.

Rask, C., Fredriksson, M., Lindblad, M., et al. (2000). Mucosal and systemic antibody responses after peroral or intranasal immunization: effects of conjugation to enterotoxin B subunits and/or of co-administration with free toxin as adjuvant. *Acta Pathologica, Microbiologica, et Immunologica Scandinavica*, **108**, 178–86.

Rodriguez, F., Zhang, J., Whitton, J.L., et al. (1997). DNA immunization: ubiquitination of a viral protein enhances cytotoxic T-lymphocyte induction and antiviral protection but abrogates antibody induction. *Journal of Virology*, **71**, 8497–503.

Rosenthal, K.L. and Gallichan, W.S. (1997). Challenges for vaccination against sexually-transmitted diseases: induction and long-term maintenance of mucosal immune responses in the female genital tract. *Seminars in Immunology*, **9**, 303–14.

Russell, M.W., Moldoveanu, Z., White, P.L., Sibert, G.J., Mestecky, J., and Michalek, S.M. (1996). Salivary, nasal, genital, and systemic antibody responses in monkeys immunized intranasally with a bacterial protein antigen and the cholera toxin B subunit. *Infection and Immunity*, **64**, 1272–83.

Sacco, A.G., Subramanian, M.G., Yurewicz, E.C., et al. (1981). Active immunization of mice with porcine zonae pellucidae: immune response and effect on fertility. *Journal of Experimental Zoology*, **218**, 405–18.

Shah, S., Raghupathy, R., Singh, O., et al. (1999). Prior immunity to a carrier enhances antibody responses to hCG in recipients of an hCG-carrier conjugate vaccine. *Vaccine*, **17**, 3116–23.

Shedlock, D.J. and Weiner, D.B. (2000). DNA vaccination: antigen presentation and the induction of immunity. *Journal of Leukocyte Biology*, **68**, 793–806.

Talwar, G.P. (1997). Fertility regulating and immunotherapeutic vaccines reaching human trials stage. *Human Reproduction Update*, **3**, 301–10.

Tung, K.S., Primakoff, P., Woolman-Gamer, L., et al. (1997). Mechanism of infertility in male guinea pigs immunized with sperm PH-20. *Biology of Reproduction*, **56**, 1133–41.

Ulanova, M., Tarkowski, A., Hahn-Zoric, M., et al. (2001). The common vaccine adjuvant aluminum hydroxide up-regulates accessory properties of human monocytes via an interleukin-4-dependent mechanism. *Infection and Immunity*, **69**, 1151–9.

Wassarman, P.M. (1988). Zona pellucida glycoproteins. *Annual Review of Biochemistry*, **57**, 415–42.

Wolfsberg, T.G., Straight, P.D., Myles, D.G., et al. (1995). ADAM, a widely distributed and developmentally regulated gene family encoding membrane proteins with a disintegrin and metalloprotease domain. *Developmental Biology*, **169**, 378–83.

24

ARTistic licence: should assisted reproductive technologies be regulated?

Nanette R. Elster

Institute for Bioethics, Health Policy and Law, University of Louisville, Louisville, USA

Introduction

Since the first in vitro fertilization (IVF) birth in 1978, the field of assisted reproductive technology (ART) has expanded and triumphed, allowing hundreds of thousands of infertile individuals to build their families. Despite this enormous success, the new technologies have not been without conflict and controversy: eggs and embryos have been misappropriated (Weber and Marquis, 1995); couples have engaged in disputes over custody and control of frozen embryos (*J.B.* v. *M.B.* 2000); websites have paraded supermodels as potential egg donors (McKenna and Lore, 1999); couples have offered US$100000 to an under-30, athletic egg donor (Enge, 2000); a Virginia physician inseminated over 70 of his patients with his own sperm (*U.S.* v. *Jacobson* 1992); a couple in their sixties sought a surrogate to carry their dead daughter's embryo (Masciola, 1997); wives, parents, and girlfriends have requested that sperm be extracted from their recently deceased or comatose loved one (Kerr et al., 1997); an Iowa woman gave birth to the first known set of surviving septuplets following treatment with fertility drugs (Klotzko, 1998); and a child born with the assistance of an egg donor, sperm donor, and surrogate was found by a trial court to have no legal parents (*Buzzanca* v. *Buzzanca* 1998). These are but a few examples of the legal and ethical quandaries raised by ART since 1978, but they illustrate the range of new issues confronting individuals and society that must be addressed.

In light of the myriad legal and ethical questions posed by current fertility treatments and the contin-ued growth and development of ART, it is surprising that little regulation or oversight of this field or these practices exists. Practitioners have argued that this area of medicine should not be regulated in a different manner than other areas of medical practice (Institute for Science, Law, and Technology Working Group, 1998). Unlike other medical technologies, however, ART does not restore or extend life; it creates life. This is one of the fundamental ways in which ART differs from any other area of medicine and this would seem to justify enhanced regulation.

Background

In 1998, a survey was conducted by the International Federation of Fertility Societies (IFFS) reviewing guidelines and legislation of IVF and ART in 38 nations (Jones and Cohen, 1999). The survey indicated that only 20 of those nations surveyed had established legislation regarding IVF–ART. Conspicuously absent from that list was the USA. This is particularly notable given that IVF–ART is "big business" in the USA, generating approximately $4 billion annually (Andrews, 1999) and costing individual consumers anywhere between $7000 and $11000 per treatment cycle (Fidler and Bernstein, 1999).

Approximately 10% of the US population of reproductive age is affected by infertility (Patient-FAQ, 2000), and in 1998 alone – the latest year for which data are available – 360 fertility clinics reported that nearly 81000 ART cycles were performed, resulting in the birth of over 28 000 babies (Centers for Disease Control and Prevention (CDC), 2000). This is in addition to approximately 60 000 births through artificial insemination (Institute for Science, Law, and Technology Working Group, 1998). Considering the prevalence of infertility in the USA, the number of treatment cycles, and the amount of money expended on and generated by this field, the lack of a national, comprehensive regulatory scheme is striking, especially when compared with adoption. Each year, only about 30 000 healthy infants are available for adoption (Institute for Science, Law, and Technology Working Group, 1998), which does not come close to the number of children conceived through gamete donation and other ARTs. Nevertheless, every state has comprehensive adoption legislation regulating such issues as data collection, payment, and parentage (Andrews and Elster, 1998).

What current regulation of ART that does exist in the USA is an amalgamation of varied state laws, limited case law, merely one federal law of limited applicability, and voluntary professional society guidelines. Consistency, uniformity, and enforceability are sorely lacking in this patchwork quilt of regulation. Why is it that the USA has taken such a *laissez-faire* approach to regulating ARTs? Several factors may serve as explanation. First, the law is typically reactive, responding to disputes or dilemmas once they arise. One commentator phrased it this way, "a 'cause celebre' which culminated in litigation is often the forerunner of legislation" (Lorio, 1999). Second, the politics surrounding the abortion debate are closely intertwined with the issues inherent in ART of creating and inevitably destroying embryos. This political undertow has caused every administration since the late 1970s to reject requests for federal funding of most embryo and fetal research (Institute for Science, Law, and Technology Working Group, 1998). Legislators are loathe to fan the flame of this heated controversy further. Yet another explanation stems from the fact that, in the USA, reproductive choice is considered to be a fundamental right protected by the Constitution (*Griswold* v. *Connecticut* 1965; *Eisenstadt* v. *Baird*

1972; *Planned Parenthood* v. *Casey* 1992). In the 1992 US Supreme Court case, *Planned Parenthood* v. *Casey* (1992), the Court reaffirmed the "recognized protection accorded to liberty relating to intimate relationships, the family, and decisions about whether to bear and beget a child." Against this backdrop, the slow pace at which regulation is evolving is not surprising; nevertheless, the dramatic and rapid social impact of ART necessitates a reconsideration of this current lax regulatory structure.

Current state laws

State laws relating to ART have begun to evolve through both the courts and the legislatures.

Case law

While the outcome of court cases is often instructive, the precedential value of the judgments is limited in that what one state court decides does not have to be followed in any other state. Because of the lack of legislative guidance with respect to ART, courts confronted with an issue of first impression will often look to other jurisdictions for guidance where a similar matter may have been decided. As such, some trends have begun to emerge with regard to resolution of certain issues raised by ART. For example, a pattern seems to be developing in those cases deciding disputes between couples over the care and control of frozen embryos. The first case to examine this issue, *Davis* v. *Davis* (1992), occurred in 1992 in Tennessee. In that case, a divorcing couple sought a determination of who would have control over embryos that had been frozen following prior attempts at IVF. Mary Sue Davis wanted to donate the excess embryos to another infertile couple, while Junior Davis wanted them destroyed. The court, holding the status of embryos to fall somewhere between person and property, ultimately determined that the party seeking to avoid procreation should prevail and thus ruled in favor of Junior Davis (*Davis* v. *Davis* 1992). Six years later in New York, the court in *Kass* v. *Kass* (1998) was faced with a similar dilemma. When the Kasses divorced, seven embryos remained frozen. The wife sought sole custody over the embryos so that she could utilize them in her continued attempt to have a child. The husband objected, asserting that he did not want to parent a child with his ex-wife. The trial court ruled in favor of Mrs Kass reasoning that the man's role in procreation ends with ejaculation (NY Supreme Court 1995). This line of reasoning is sensible when a termination of a pregnancy is at issue. However, unlike termination of a pregnancy, which is clearly the sole right of the woman as her bodily integrity is at issue, no pregnancy had occurred here: the embryos were extracorporeal. Not attempting to grapple with this distinction, the higher court did nevertheless reverse the decision. The higher court enforced a written directive issued by the couple at the time the embryos had been created. The directive indicated that, in the event the couple could not reach a mutual decision regarding disposition of the embryos, they wanted the embryos to be donated for scientific research. While this decision was rendered on different grounds than the decision in *Davis* v. *Davis* (1992), in that a prior agreement controlled, the outcome was the same.

In yet another similar case, decided in 2000, a Massachusetts court refused to enforce a prior written dispositional agreement where one of the parties later reconsidered his earlier decision. The court in *A.Z.* v. *B.Z.* 2000 held (as in *Davis* v. *Davis* 1992) that "individuals shall not be compelled to enter into intimate family relationships." In June 2000, a New Jersey court resolving a dispute between divorcing spouses over embryo control held that forced procreation is not amenable to judicial enforcement (*J.B.* v. *M.B.* 2000).

These four cases illustrate a trend in embryo disputes between couples, favoring the party who wishes to avoid procreation. However, the rationale of the courts differed. In *Davis* v. *Davis* (1992), the couple did not have an advanced directive indicating their wishes for disposition of excess embryos. In *Kass* v. *Kass* (1998), such an agreement existed, and the court opted to enforce the agreement; however, in *A.Z.* v. *B.Z.* (2000), the court ignored the advanced

directive ruling in favor of the party seeking to avoid procreation. Therefore, while one might infer a trend based on the outcome of these cases, the varied rationales applied by the courts suggests that this is not so. Amidst resolution of *Kass* v. *Kass* (1998), Senate Bill 1120 was introduced in the New York legislature, which, if adopted, would have required that couples indicate, in advance of treatment, their desired disposition of stored embryos under various circumstances including dissolution of marriage (N.Y.S.B. 1120 (1999)). If this bill is adopted, it is possible that a decision might result wherein the individual seeking to utilize the embryos would prevail. This is an example of a legislative response to a litigated dispute. Another example is found in California, where legislation was enacted in response to the alleged misappropriation of eggs and embryos at University of California at Irvine (UCI). In reaction to the UCI scandal, Senator Tom Hayden proposed a bill that would criminalize utilizing gametes or embryos without the written informed consent of the progenitors. The bill was enacted in 1996 (Cal. Bus. and Prof. Code sec. 2260 (2000)).

State laws

The lack of predictability and certainty of case law offers little guidance to couples and practitioners and provides little protection for the children created through ART. Legislation is the mechanism by which to set quality control standards, delineate the rights and obligations of participants in ART – especially collaborative arrangements in which an egg donor, sperm donor, and/or surrogate is involved – and determine the parentage of resulting children. Nevertheless, such guidance has yet to appear in many states. Additionally, as with case law, the law in one state does not apply to practices in any other state.

Presently, at least 35 states have laws regarding artificial insemination by donor (Andrews and Elster, 2000). In general, these laws deem the intended father, with his consent to the insemination, to be the legal father of any child born of the arrangement. These statutes also impose safety measures such as requiring the procedure to be performed under the supervision of a physician and requiring written informed consent of the intended father. In stark contrast, only about five states have laws specifically addressing egg donation (Florida, North Dakota, Oklahoma, Texas, and Virginia). All of these laws are quite similar in that they are very brief and focus particularly on the issue of parental rights and obligations. Each recognizes the intended parents as the legal parents of any child born through such an arrangement and all confer no rights or obligations upon the donor of the eggs.

State laws pertaining to surrogacy, while also sparse, are not nearly as consistent or uniform as the egg and sperm donor laws. Currently, at least 23 states have laws that directly address the practice of surrogacy, yet there is little similarity between those states (Andrews and Elster, 2000). Even such a critical issue as determining parentage in disputed arrangements differs among the states. For example, in Arizona, North Dakota, and Utah, the presumption is that the surrogate and her husband are the legal parents of the child (Ariz. Rev. Stat. Ann. Sec. 25-218 (1996); N.D. Cent. Code sec. 14-18-05 (1991); Utah code Ann. Sec 76-7-204 (1997)). In contrast, in New Hampshire and Virginia, the contracting couple are presumed to be the legal parents if the surrogate does not change her mind within a limited period of time specified by the statutes (N.H. Rev. Stat. Ann. Sec. 168-B:23;25 (1996); Va. Code Ann. Secs. 20-158; 20-161 (Michie 1996)).

Dispute resolution in surrogacy arrangements is complex enough when statutory guidance is available, but a 1998 California case clearly illustrates just how chaotic, if not absurd, resolution of disputes can be when no legislation exists. In *Buzzanca* v. *Buzzanca* (1998), a couple selected an egg donor and a sperm donor and contracted with a gestational surrogate to carry the resultant embryo. Prior to the birth of the child, John and LuAnne Buzzanca divorced, with John claiming no issue of the marriage and, therefore, no child support obligations. LuAnne contested, and at the trial court level, a determination was made that the child, Jaycee, had

no legal parents since neither John nor LuAnne had a genetic or biologic link to the child nor had they adopted her. This was an ironic twist given that five potential parents were involved in Jaycee's conception and birth: John and LuAnne, the egg donor, the sperm donor, and the surrogate. On appeal, though, the court reversed the decision without relying on biology or genetics – the traditional determinants of parentage. The court held that, but for the actions of the Buzzancas (selecting gamete donors and contracting with a surrogate), Jaycee would never have been born (*Buzzanca* v. *Buzzanca* 1998); therefore, John and LuAnne were deemed the legal parents of the child.

Codifying this intent-based approach to resolving parentage would be one mechanism for avoiding "legal orphans" in the future. Another approach might be a requirement that at least one of the intended parents be genetically related to the child in any collaborative reproductive arrangement. Such is the case in New Hampshire, where the surrogacy law requires that "the intended mother or the intended father shall provide a gamete to be used to impregnate the surrogate" (N.H. RSA sec. 168-B:17 (2000)).

Questions of parentage are not the only issues that legislation might help to resolve. Legislation might also be enacted to protect and promote consumer safety through the setting of minimum standards of practice. Even in the controversial practice of abortion, states have adopted legislation setting out particular health and safety requirements (A.R.S. sec. 36-449.03 (2000); La. R.S. sec. 40:1299.35.2 (2000)).

Recognizing the need to protect the health and safety of consumers of ART, some states have set forth some basic protective standards with particular screening requirements for donated semen. For example, in California and Indiana, screening must be done for human immunodeficiency virus (HIV) and other communicable diseases (Cal. Health and Safety Code sec. 1644.5 (2000); Burns Ind. Code Ann. Sec. 16-41-14-1 et. seq.). In Illinois, intentionally, knowingly, or negligently performing artificial insemination using semen of an untested donor or a donor who has tested positive for HIV may result in criminal liability (20 ILCS 2310/2310-325 2000).

Other consumer protection standards set by state statutes include Pennsylvania's requirement that those who perform IVF must file quarterly reports with the state Department of Health that include information about the number of eggs fertilized, number of eggs discarded or destroyed, and the number of women implanted with fertilized eggs (18 Pa.C.S.sec. 3213 (1999)). This report must be made available to the public. Along these lines of public disclosure, Virginia law requires that, before treating patients for infertility by ART, a disclosure form must be signed by the patient which includes program success rates for the particular procedure to be performed (Va. Code Ann. Sec. 54-1-2971.1 (2000)). Other information that must be disclosed to patients includes donor HIV-screening protocols, the number of livebirths achieved by the program, and rates of pregnancy and delivery bracketed by age group (Va. Code Ann. Sec. 54-1-2971.1. (2000)). A recently proposed bill in California would take this disclosure requirement one step further by requiring the state Department of Health to develop a standard, written summary of ART and egg donation procedures that physicians and surgeons would be mandated to provide to patients (1999 CA S.B. 1630 (2000)). Failure to comply with this requirement would constitute unprofessional conduct under the state Medical Practice Act and thus a crime (1999 CA S.B. 1630 (2000)). Additionally, the Act would require that the medical director of a licensed facility be certified in an approved specialty or subspecialty (1999 CA S.B. 1630 (2000)). This Bill, proposed by Senator Tom Hayden, would be one of the first pieces of legislation specifically to recognize the practice of egg donation and address related health and safety concerns.

States also attempt to set quality control standards through another mechanism: insurance regulations. Currently, at least a dozen states mandate coverage or the offer of coverage for fertility treatment (National Conference of State Legislatures, 2000). In several of those states, coverage is predicated on the requirement that facilities meet standards set by the American College of Obstetricians and Gynecologists (ACOG) or the American Society of Reproductive Medicine (ASRM) (Ark. Stat. Ann. Sec.

23-85-137 (1999); Hawaii Rev. Stat. Sec. 431-10A-116.5 (2000)). While insurance coverage is an important step in consumer safety, it is important to note that state laws in insurance do not apply to self-funded plans. These plans are exempt from state laws under the federal Employee Retirement Income Security Act. About 40% of people in the USA with private employer-based health insurance are covered by self-funded plans; therefore, the protection provided by these laws is of limited applicability (Government Accounting Office, 1997).

Other state laws have also attempted to codify the voluntary standards set by professional organizations such as ASRM and ACOG. In Louisiana, for example, no person shall perform IVF unless s/he has met the standards established by ASRM and ACOG. (La. R.S. sec. 9:128 (2000)). What this overview of state laws illustrates is the diversity and scarcity of oversight and regulation of ART across the nation. Important issues such as parentage and consumer safety are unaddressed in a majority of states, leaving resolution of such matters to be determined on a case-by-case basis through the judicial system, which may yield inconsistent results.

Self-regulation

State laws requiring adherence to guidelines developed by medical professional groups are essentially a codified recognition of the self-regulation that defines the practice of medicine. Self-regulation of medical professionals takes several forms. One is state licensing requirements. All states require licensing of physicians, but the majority of licensing schemes "assume that adequate professional and industry standards exist, and that the tasks of quality assurance under licensure is to identify and deal with relatively rare cases of individual provider deviation from those norms" (Annas et al., 1990). Another type of self-regulation takes the form of membership in professional organizations, which set standards and provide guidelines on particular treatments or procedures for their members. Membership in professional organizations, however, is purely voluntary and, therefore, any group guidelines are merely suggestive rather than authoritative. That does not mean that these guidelines are meaningless; they may serve as evidence of the standard of care in a medical malpractice action, and they may, in fact, strongly influence physician practice. Additionally, membership in a particular professional society may influence consumer preference in selecting a particular physician.

Three professional groups are particularly influential in setting the standards for the practice of ART: ACOG, ASRM, and the American Association of Tissue Banks (AATB). ACOG, for example, has issued guidelines for the genetic screening of gamete donors (ACOG, 1997). In response to the dramatic increase in multiple births, the ACOG Committee on Ethics issued a statement on multifetal reduction recognizing that "nonselective embryo reduction should be viewed as a response to an unforseen and unavoidable contingency, not a routinely accepted treatment for an iatrogenic problem" (ACOG Committee on Ethics, 1999). AATB has established elaborate standards for semen banking which "represent the current accepted standard practice for donor screening and testing and for retrieval, processing, storage, disease screening, and distribution of semen" (Linden and Centola, 1997). Additionally, the ASRM Ethics Committee has been quite prolific in issuing guidelines on a range of practices in ART from screening of gamete donors (Ethics Committee of the American Society for Reproductive Medicine, 1994) to posthumous reproduction and postmenopausal maternity (Ethics Committee of the American Society for Reproductive Medicine, 1997). Most recently, ASRM issued guidelines addressing the payment of oocyte donors finding that "monetary compensation should reflect the time, inconvenience, and physical and emotional demands associated with the oocyte donation process . . . at this time sums of $5,000 or more require justification and sums above $10,000 go beyond what is appropriate" (Ethics Committee of the American Society for Reproductive Medicine, 2000).

While all of these guidelines or standards are extensive, informative to professionals and protective of consumers, they lack teeth. No mechanism exists for enforcing these standards. Compliance with them is strictly voluntary and no penalty exists for failure to comply, nor is there any formal oversight structure by which to assess if professionals are, in fact, following the guidelines. Therefore, violation of or failure to comply with these standards leaves a harmed consumer with only an after-the-fact remedy – a tort action in malpractice. At that point, the harm has been done and compensation for that harm is the remedy made available through a tort action. As attorney Keith Byers observes, "a deceived consumer might have a tort remedy, but the idea behind quality control regulation is to be pro-active and prevent problems or deception before they occur" (Byers, 1997).

Enforceable quality control standards are the best way to prevent consumer harms and to protect the interests of participants in ART as well as the children conceived. Professional guidelines often set forth what those standards should be based on the expertise and experience of practitioners. Without enforcement or disincentives for noncompliance, however, such guidelines provide little more than an ideal.

Federal laws

While state laws are scarce and lacking in uniformity and professional guidelines are strictly voluntary, the federal government has been nearly inert with respect to questions raised by ART. To date, only one law specific to ART exists at the federal level, the Fertility Clinic Success Rate and Certification Act of 1992 (42 USCS sec. 263a-1 through 263a-7 (2000)). The purpose of the Act was to provide consumers with information that they could use to compare the effectiveness of fertility programs and ensure the quality of provided services by certifying embryo laboratories (64 F.R. 39374 (1999)). The Act requires that ART programs report pregnancy success rates for each ART procedure performed to the Secretary of Health and Human Services through the CDC. A wide range of information is required to be reported about both the clinic and the patients. Information about the clinic includes whether the clinic is a member of the Society for Assisted Reproductive Technologies (SART), whether services provided include surrogacy, and the total number of ART cycles performed during a year. Information about patients includes demographic details, the patient's history, medical reasons for the ART, source of oocyte, any ART complications, and information about the outcome of the procedure (65 F.R. 53310 (2000)). All of the data is made publicly available and is published in four components: a national overview, a clinic-specific component which lays out the specifics for each reporting clinic, a section explaining the medial and statistical terms in lay language to facilitate consumer understanding and an appendix listing those clinics reporting and those not reporting (65 F.R. 53310 (2000)).

The Act also requires that the CDC develop a model program for the certification of embryo laboratories by individual states (42 USCS sec. 263a-2 (2000)). In November of 1998, the CDC did set up a model program. The CDC proposal, however, would not mandate compliance with the model program; compliance is voluntary by interested states. The model sets forth Embryo Laboratory Standards which include: Personnel Qualifications and Responsibilities, Facilities and Safety, Quality Management, and Maintenance of Records (64 F.R. 39374 (1999)). Despite the comprehensive approach to quality management articulated in the CDC proposal, adherence to its terms by states is voluntary.

The Act does much to inform consumers about the success of particular technologies and attempts to protect consumers through its proposed laboratory guidelines, but it does not go far enough to protect participants in ART. For now, though, this is the only federal regulation of ART that exists.

In 1997 the Food and Drug and Administration (FDA) also contributed to the subject. The "proposed approach" takes a necessary first step in regulation by requiring registration of all tissue-processing facilities. Registration is important for collecting information about which organizations exist and are involved in tissue processing, and it then provides a baseline from which oversight is possible. As another step in this process of regulation, in September 1999, the FDA issued a proposal requiring manufacturers of human cellular and tissue-based products "to screen and test the donors of cells and tissues used in those products for risk factors for and clinical evidence of relevant communicable disease agents and diseases" (64 F.R. 52696 (1999)). Under the proposal, reproductive materials are subject to the least amount of oversight especially between sexually intimate partners.

If adopted, this FDA regulation would provide a uniform, authoritative standard for donor screening rather than the current voluntary guidelines provided by ACOG and ASRM and the varied requirements of existing state laws. This is one small step in providing some form of comprehensive, authoritative regulation – setting a national standard – eliminating variance in approach from state to state and from clinic to clinic. The regulation would set the minimum standards, leaving open the option for states and individual practitioners to require even more rigorous screening.

Regulatory gaps

Having briefly reviewed the current regulatory framework for ARTs at the federal, state, and professional society levels, it is clear that many gaps and inconsistencies exist. For example, an issue of paramount importance – the determination of parentage in collaborative arrangements – is left unanswered by many states. In addition, those states with laws may yield completely opposite results from one state to the next. This uncertainty leaves the status of the parent–child relationship in doubt when third parties are involved in the reproductive process, illustrating how the interests of the children created through ART are oftentimes an afterthought. The rights and obligations of all parties in a collaborative arrangement should be delineated in advance of a child's birth in order to protect the interests of the child.

Another regulatory gap is that no process has been developed for approving the safety and efficacy of new procedures before they are applied to humans. Unlike research involving new drugs and new medical devices, which must comply with FDA requirements, no such review of new ART procedures is currently mandated (Institute for Science, Law and Technology Working Group, 1998). With little or no federal funding available for research involving human embryos, a vast amount of ART research occurs in the private sector where no requirement exists for institutional review and approval before conducting research on human subjects.

Yet another gap in regulation of ARTs pertains to recordkeeping. There are no requirements detailing the type of information that must be collected and maintained in collaborative arrangements involving gamete donors and/or surrogates. As a result, many children conceived through donated gametes may never gain access to medical or health information from one of their progenitors. This is contrary to the practice in adoption, where a range of non-identifying information must be collected and maintained and is accessible to the child when he or she reaches adulthood (Andrews and Elster, 1998). One way to accomplish data collection for children of collaborative arrangements would be to establish a donor registry. A registry would enable children conceived with donor gametes to gain access to medical and genetic information of the donor in order to assess their own health and reproductive needs. In a survey done in 1979, the majority of physicians surveyed felt that keeping records of donors and children would interfere with maintaining participant privacy (Currie-Cohen et al., 1979), which could compromise the number of donors willing to participate in donor insemination. A study of donor attitudes conducted five years later, however, indicated that most donors were actually willing to provide non-identifying information such as medical and social histories (Swanson, 1993). In 1985, Sweden enacted a law requiring collection of donor information to be maintained for 70 years (Swanson, 1993). Physicians were initially skeptical and indicated some decline in donation, but by 1986 the number of donors had returned to the previous

level (Swanson, 1993). This suggests that, while collection and maintenance of the information might be time consuming, donors are willing to provide the information and there are clear benefits to the children of having such information available.

Another problem with minimal recordkeeping is that there is little information about how ART impacts the growth and development of children. Currently, little longitudinal research has been done in the USA to determine whether children born through ART suffer any long-term physical or psychological harms as a result of their technological conceptions.

Finally, informed consent in ARTs appears to be woefully inadequate (New York State Task Force on Life and the Law, 1998). For example, couples are often informed of the risk of conceiving multiples but are not informed of the myriad health, financial, and psychological risks for the children and the family (Elster, 2000). As mentioned previously, a few states such as Virginia and California are attempting to remedy this deficit by requiring particular basic information be disclosed, but this clearly does not address the majority of ART participants.

Conclusions

Coordinated and complimentary regulation at the federal, state, and professional society level is imperative to address these and other questions raised by ART. The prospect of regulation often causes a negative reaction across the board. The fear of regulation stems from the perception that regulation equals prohibition. At times, however, regulation might actually promote an activity. Given the number of people availing themselves of fertility services and benefiting from their use, prohibition of ARTs does not seem reasonable or desirable. However, oversight is essential because of the multitude of interests at stake: professionals; consumers, including gamete donors, surrogates, and intended parents; children born; society; and the life-creating nature of ART itself.

Now that the technology has been discovered, it will continue to develop. Stopping its progress is not the solution. The novel scientific, legal, ethical, and social issues raised by ART demand innovative policies. Setting national minimal standards, allowing states to refine and expand such standards, would be progress toward protecting the interests of all participants in ART. In view of the rapid changes in ART, involving professional societies such as ASRM, AATB, and ACOG, consumers, and other interested parties in defining these minimum standards will improve research and practice as well as provide flexibility and fluidity while ensuring participant protection. Regulation and oversight of ARTs will promote such practices rather than prevent them.

REFERENCES

ACOG (American College of Obstetricians and Gynecologists) (1997). *Genetic Screening of Gamete Donors*. Committee Opinion No. 192, ACOG, Washington, DC.

ACOG (American College of Obstetricians and Gynecologists) Committee on Ethics (1999). *Nonselective Embryo Reduction: Ethical Guidance for the Obstetrician–gynecologist*. ACOG Committee Opinion No. 214, ACOG, Washington, DC.

Andrews, L.B. (1999). Eighteenth annual health law symposium: reproductive technology comes of age. *Whittier Law Review*, **21**, 375.

Andrews, L.B. and Elster, N. (1998). Adoption, reproductive technologies, and genetic information. *Health Matrix*, **8**, 125–51.

Andrews, L.B. and Elster, N. (2000). Regulating reproductive technologies. *Journal of Legal Medicine*, **21**, 35–65.

Annas, G., Law, S., Rosenblatt, R., and Wing, K. (1990). *American Health Law*, Ch. 5, *Quality of Care and the Law*. Little, Brown, Boston, MA, p. 505.

Byers, K.A. (1997). Infertility and in vitro fertilization: a growing need for consumer-oriented regulation of the in vitro fertilization industry. *Journal of Legal Medicine*, **18**, 265–313.

Centers for Disease Control and Prevention (CDC) (2000). *1998 Assisted Reproductive Technology Success Rates; National Summary and Fertility Clinic Reports*. CDC, Atlanta, GA, http://www.cdc.gov/nccdphp/drh/art.htm

Currie-Cohen, M., Luttrell, L., and Shapiro, S. (1979). Current practices of artificial insemination by donor in the United States. *New England Journal of Medicine*, **300**, 585–90.

Elster, N. (2000). Less is more: the risks of multiple births. *Fertility and Sterility*, **74**, 617–23.

Enge, M. (2000). Couple offers $100 000 for egg donor: infertile pair's solicitation may be highest price yet. *The Denver Post*, 10th February, A-02.

Ethics Committee of the American Society for Reproductive Medicine (1994). Ethical considerations of assisted reproductive technologies. *Fertility and Sterility*, **62**, 1S.

Ethics Committee of the American Society for Reproductive Medicine (1997). Ethical considerations of assisted reproductive technologies. *Fertility and Sterility*, **67**, 1S.

Ethics Committee of the American Society for Reproductive Medicine (2000). Financial incentives in recruitment of oocyte donors. *Fertility and Sterility*, **74**, 216–19.

Fidler, A.T. and Bernstein, J. (1999). Infertility from a personal to a public health problem. *Public Health Reports*, **114**, 494–511.

Government Accounting Office (1997). *Private Health Insurance – Continued Erosion of Coverage Linked to Cost Pressures*. 24 July. US Government Printing Office, Washington, DC.

Institute for Science, Law, and Technology Working Group (1998). ART into science: regulation of fertility techniques. *Science*, **281**, 651.

Jones, H.W., Jr. and Cohen, J. (1999). Surveillance 1998. *Fertility and Sterility*, **71**, 796–7.

Kerr, S., Caplan, A., Polin, G., Smugar, S., O'Neill, K., and Urowitz, S. (1997). Postmortem sperm procurement. *Journal of Urology*, **157**, 2154–8.

Klotzko, A.J. (1998). Medical miracle or medical mischief? The saga of the McCaughey septuplets. *Hastings Center Report*, **28**, 5–8.

Linden, J. and Centola, G. (1997). New American Association of Tissue Banks standards for semen banking. *Fertility and Sterility*, **68**, 597–600.

Lorio, K.V. (1999). The process of regulating assisted reproductive technologies: what we can learn from our neighbors – what translates and what does not. *Loyola Law Review*, **45**, 247, 153, n. 31.

Masciola, C. (1997). Surrogate to carry dead woman's baby. *Orange County Register*, 23 May, A1.

McKenna, M.A.J. and Lore, D. (1999). Hatching hype off the net: highly publicized offer of human eggs highlights issues of commercial ethics. *Atlanta Journal and Constitution*, 6 November, 1A.

National Conference of State Legislatures (2000). *Women's Health Insurance Converage for Infertility Therapy*. Available from http://www.ncsl.org/programs/health/Infert.html [Accessed 25 July 2000].

New York State Task Force on Life and the Law (1998). *Assisted Reproductive Technologies: Analysis and Recommendations for Public Policy*. New York State Printing Office, New York.

Patient-FAQ (2000). *Quick Facts about Infertility*. Available from: http://www.asrm.org/patients/faqs.html [accessed 17 September 2000].

Swanson, H. (1993). Donor anonymity in artificial insemination: is it still necessary? *Columbia Journal of Law and Social Problems*, **27**, 151, 171–3.

Weber, T. and Marquis, J. (1995). In quest for miracles, did fertility clinic go too far? *L.A. Times*, 4 June, A1.

LEGAL CASES, STATUTES AND CODES

Ark. Stat. Ann. Sec. 23-85-137 (1999)

Ariz. Rev. Stat. Ann. Sec. 25-218 (1996)

A.R.S. Sec. 36-449.03 (2000)

A.Z. v. *B.Z.* 725 N.E.2d 1051 (2000)

Burns Ind. Code Ann. Sec. 16-41-14-1 et. seq.

Buzzanca v. *Buzzanca*, 61 Cal. App. 4th 1410 (1998)

Cal. Bus. and Prof. Code sec. 2260 (2000)

Cal. Health and Safety Code sec. 1644.5 (2000)

Davis v. *Davis* (1992) 842 S. W. 2d 588 (Tenn. 1992) remand on reh'g and reh'g denied in part, Nov 1992, Tenn. LEXIS 622 (Tenn. Nov. 23, 1992), later proceeding sub nom. *Stowe* v. *Davis*, 113 S. Ct. 1259 (1993)

Eisenstadt v. *Baird*, 405 U.S. (1972)

Griswold v. *Connecticut*, 381 U.S. 379 (1965)

Hawaii Rev. Stat. Sec. 431-10A-116.5 (2000)

J.B. v. *M.B.*, 751 A.2d 613 (2000)

Kass v. *Kass* 273 N.Y. S2d. 350 (1998)

La. R.S. sec. 9:128 (2000)

La. R.S. sec. 40:1299.35.2 (2000)

N.D. Cent. Code sec. 14-18-05 (1991)

N.H. Rev. Stat. Ann. Sec. 168-B:23;25 (1996)

N.H. RSA sec. 168-B:17 (2000)

N.Y.S.B. 1120 (1999)

N.Y. Supreme Court 1995, Nassau County (Jan. 23, 1995)

Planned Parenthood v. *Casey*, 505 U.S. 833 (1992)

U.S. v. *Jacobson*, 785 F. Supp. 563 (E.D. Va. 1992)

Utah code Ann. Sec. 76-7-204 (1997)

Va. Code Ann. Sec. 54-1-2971.1 (2000)

Va. Code Ann. Secs. 20-158; 20-161 (Michie 1996)

18 Pa.C.S. sec. 3213 (1999)

1999 CA S.B. 1630 (2000)

20 ILCS 2310/2310–325 (2000)

42 USCS sec. 263a-1 through 263a-7 (2000)

42 USCS sec. 263a-2 (2000)

64 F.R. 39374 (July 21, 1999)

64 F.R. 52696 (Sept. 30, 1999)

65 F.R. 53310 (Sept. 1, 2000).

25

Finances and access to assisted reproductive technologies: justice and publication of results

Francoise Shenfield

University College Hospital and Royal Free and University College Hospitals Medical School, London, UK

Introduction

There are numerous ethical issues in assisted reproductive technologies (ART), some of which are discussed in this chapter. Some issues can be described as microethical, that is particular problems that are specifically linked to the techniques of ART: for example, cryopreservation of embryos and the decisions involved in determining their ultimate fate, or the application of preimplantation genetic diagnosis for sex selection. This chapter, however, will discuss the macroethical issue of *justice* (as represented by access and disclosure of information), an issue present in all fields of health care and perhaps most infamously illustrated by the unmet therapeutic needs of patients with human immunodeficiency virus infection in many African countries.

This chapter will also analyse the access our patients have to ART and then discuss how well informed they might be about the success rate of these treatments.

Justice, access, and assisted reproductive technology

The gap between the theoretical access to health care and the needs of patients, as expressed in the tactful terms of priority setting (Klein, 1998), is not always publicized at large. It is likely that the gap between access and need is more prevalent in the affluent economy of ART than in many other health care specialities. Access to necessary (in)fertility

treatment is far from equitable worldwide, sometimes varying even within different parts of one country, and it often follows (or not) a political decision. We know this partly because of the intense public and often statutory scrutiny our field receives as a result of the enormous value that most societies place on the embryo: that entity which represents our future. This is ironic because if the embryo is worthy of respect because of what it represents (Warnock, 1984), then it follows logically that a child can be assumed to be even more valuable, representing, as it does, the *actual* and not just the *potential* future of any society. Therefore, logically, it could be assumed that society in general would feel compelled to provide the appropriate (medical) help to patients suffering from the disease "infertility". This line of reasoning represents one example of a "just" health care system, for which many analyses and definitions have been offered.

The characteristics of justice as applied to delivery of health care have been described by Benatar (1996) as: "universal access, access to an adequate level of care, access without excessive burdens, fair distribution of the financial costs of ensuring universal access to an adequate level of care and capacity for improvement towards a more just system." These criteria can be applied equally to any medical field, whether they are more or less specialized. In addition, Milliez (1999) states: "any reflection on the issue of the ethical aspects of inequality in access to health care relies on indisputable but debatable premises, that all men are created equal, all human life are equally valuable, and any human being is entitled, physically, mentally and socially to a healthy condition. These requisites are inscribed in the Universal Declaration of Human Rights, in the Constitution of many nations and in the charter of the World Health Organisation." Paradoxically, there is indeed inequality, which is reflected by the wide discrepancy with regard to both ease of access and equity in access to ART amongst European and other health systems.

Access is neither universal nor without heavy cost, inflicting an excessive burden of financial sacrifice for many couples. This financial burden too often results in high-order pregnancies, especially of triplets and more. As a consequence, the burden is imposed not only on the previously infertile couple (Garel et al., 1997) and society in general, but also on the vulnerable third party, the child(ren) to be, who too often is afflicted by the serious and significant side-effects associated with high-order births. For instance, the incidence of cerebral palsy in triplets is 47 times the incidence in a singleton pregnancy (Petterson et al., 1993). The approach that gives rise to these consequences is criticized by Pennings (2000): "somehow the establishment of a pregnancy became separated from the general goal of well being of the patient and her future children." This statement might be appropriately rephrased by stressing instead that a responsible attitude takes into account first the interest of the vulnerable and then that of the cognizant adult.

The essential interaction between economic choice and "duty" to the patient raises similar problems (as for justice) for all health care fields. Providers should give information to patients so that they can make an informed decision and give proper consent for treatment. As part of this process, safety and cost-effectiveness must be considered. The safety aspect is paramount, in all fields, often described in ethical terms as the balance between beneficence (that being beneficial) and nonmalefi-cence (that being not harmful). In our speciality, we consider the birth of a person as an indicator of success. Because of their vulnerability, we (ART providers) have a responsibility to the future child(ren); a responsibility that has been argued to be even stronger than that we accord to the prospective parents. Since one of the main complications of ART, in personal and public health terms, is the creation of multiple pregnancies with all the associated consequences for children and their parents, it is essential that this information be taken into account when success rates of ART are published. Accurate facts as to the results per attempted cycle of in vitro fertilization (IVF), including the multiple pregnancy rate, should allow all parties concerned to make appropriate decisions, both at individual and societal level. One may wonder, however, how educated and informed our vulnerable patients truly are before they embark on the (often) final attempt to accomplish their desire for parenthood.

Access to assisted reproductive technology in different countries

The first part of this section will compare the provisions for IVF made in different countries where figures are available. The second part of this section will discuss the information that is made available to patients so they can make autonomous decisions concerning their fertility treatments; it will also cover the sensitive subject of advertising and its ethical implications.

It is beyond the scope of this chapter to compare access to all fertility treatments (ovulation induction, surgery, intrauterine insemination, gamete donation, IVF), but some idea of the disparity of access and availability can be obtained by comparing the number of cycles of IVF performed relative to a country's population.

In France, access to IVF and other fertility treatments is only permitted to couples married or living together for 2 years whereas, in the UK, the law will not prevent access to single women, for instance, provided the "welfare of the child" is taken into account (Human Fertilization and Embryology Act, 1990). Indeed, in general, two main factors limit access: first there are criteria selection based upon legislation (as in France) or codes of practice (age, marriage, etc.); second, there are the modalities of reimbursement (often based on criteria that serve as a major obstacle for funding) for those who qualify for access to IVF. In spite of the steady improvement in success rates of ART, the "poor success rate" of IVF is often fallaciously used in order to justify the lack of public funding. It is rare to find a lay article pointing out that the success rate per cycle is not far removed from that expected from a cycle of natural conception.

The inequality that results from the lack of national policy for infertility funding is seen particularly in the UK and USA, where many techniques of assisted reproduction are confined to the private sector. Three-quarters of IVF cycles are not subsidized by the National Health Service (NHS) in the UK and most in the USA are performed in the private sector. Therefore, there is a dearth of state-subsidized resources in the face of demand. To restate this, it means that health care providers are unable to perform the duty of care they owe their patients because the most appropriate treatment for the patient's plight is not available to those who cannot afford it. This UK treatment by "post code", or area of residence, where the local health authorities provide (or not as is more often the case) ART without national policy guidance (with the notable exception of Scotland) is such a bane of the system that it has become integrated in journalistic parlance and it affects our speciality in a "double pronged iniquity" (Shenfield, 1997).

The collated figures for the European Society for Human Reproduction and Embryology (ESHRE) collaborative IVF data collection program for European countries, where 18 countries took part (11 with complete figures), were recently published (Nygren and Anderson, 2001). In Europe in 1997, a total of 203893 IVF cycles were recorded for 482 clinics. The US Society for Assisted Reproductive Techniques (SART) report of 1997 details 71826 cycles, i.e., there were almost three times as many cycles in Europe as in the USA. Over half the IVF cycles in Europe occurred in just three countries: France with 45697 cycles, the UK with 34398 cycles, and Germany with 27923 cycles. If, however, the number of cycles are compared with the total population, these figures

change drastically. Finland, Denmark, and Iceland have the highest number of cycles/million (C/M) population with 1538, 1448, and 1422 C/M, respectively; then comes Sweden with 952 C/M; the Netherlands with 897 C/M; Norway with 811 C/M; France and the Czech Republic practically equal with 780 and 771 C/M, respectively; followed by the UK with 583 C/M, Switzerland 472 C/M, and Portugal 330 C/M. All this compares with about 200 C/M in the USA.

National public policy appears to have an important impact on these figures; for example, in Denmark the social security system pays three cycles of ART, including drugs, in public clinics (Consumers' Forum, 1998; Nygren and Andersen, 2001). In Sweden there is a mixture of private and public funded treatment, while in France there is reimbursement for up to four cycles to the patients in a system that is a mixture of public and private health care. Finally, the UK falls far below, where it is estimated that only about 20% of patients obtain IVF through the (free) NHS. In the UK, the only alternative to the NHS is private treatment, since insurance does not typically cover fertility treatment. It is also interesting to mention that in Germany insurance companies pay 70% of costs of up to four IVF cycles but refuse to refund donor insemination. If, for instance, access in Germany is theoretically more "just" than in the UK, then the lower incidence of cycles per million population in Germany must be a result of the restrictions, both implied and applied, imposed by the strict regulation of the German Embryo Protection Act (Beier and Beckman, 1991).

Although the differences between European countries in terms of patient access to ART may be striking, they all have much higher access than that in the USA, a wealthy country in terms of world economy but where there is practically no state subsidy for IVF treatment. The availability/lack of financial support can lead to inherent problems with "justice" of access. This is especially evident when one evaluates the differences, in the context of access, between Europe and the USA (where private is more common than state-subsidized treatment) in terms of the availability of information, including but not solely represented by the publication of results and advertizing in ART. The question that immediately arises is whether the health care market can apply ethical rules of fair and accurate information in the face of the mechanisms of free market economics. In a time when governments and ministerial authorities scrutinize more and more how they will spend public money, with some justification on economic and moral grounds, basing their decisions either in the public's global best interest (the optimistic view) or in the direction that will win them most votes (the cynical view), anyone fighting for resources, whether patients' group or health care providers, must be able to put forward arguments concerning the monetary value or appropriateness of any treatment. Public pressure is part of the democratic process, but the public has to be well informed in order for such pressure to be effective. Therefore, responsibility for dissemination of proper information still falls on the shoulders of those who are best able to gather this information, often the profession itself and/or epidemiologists.

Proper information, what does it mean?

Once it is established that fair access should be offered to our patients, how do we inform them? Respecting the autonomy of our patients implies conveying proper information as to the balance between the risks and benefits of treatment, including those to the potential mother and the future children, as well as the success rate appropriate to their case. For the couple undergoing treatment, the long sought for benefit is the future parenting of a (hopefully healthy) child. This does not mean that all risks to the offspring may be excluded, but that the outlook for the future child should not be widely different to that of the child born through natural (unassisted) conception. Recent evidence indicates that the majority of the risks to children born from ART occur as a result of the complications from multiple pregnancies and the ensuing prematurity of the offspring (Nisand and Shenfield, 1997).

Success rates are often presented in terms of live-birth rate per treatment cycle, without being qualified by such dangers to the offspring as the sequelae from high-order gestation. Particularly, but not exclusively, in the free market environment, advertising of "best" success rates is used to attract couples that are seen as clients rather than patients. This arguably is not compatible with our "duty of care" to the patients, nor does it give proper information to enable and empower them to make an autonomous decision as to the most appropriate number of embryos for replacement per cycle.

It is interesting to analyze the way pregnancy rates are reported in different models before one tries to fathom the optimum and most patient friendly way of explaining the success rates of IVF, including which elements should be included in the publications. With regards to the duty of care we have to all concerned (potential parents and their children), the livebirth rate is certainly a good index of the common goal of health care providers and patients. However, in order to increase our patients' autonomous decision by giving relevant information, this should be appreciated as a function of multiple or single birth and whether there was embryo reduction. The incidence of prematurity and of its specific complications for the children born from multiple pregnancies is information that should be at the forefront of national and international reports.

In practice, there are several ways of reporting success rates, including clinical pregnancy or live delivery, both on the basis per cycle started, per oocyte retrieval, or per embryo transfer. Success rates may also be published as a function of age of the female partner, of the etiology of infertility, the duration of infertility, or the previous number of cycles attempted (Templeton et al., 1996).

There follows three examples of the ways in which information is given to prospective IVF patients. The first, from the UK, is a statutory one and utilizes a publication to announce both national average and center-by-center results; this report is available to all prospective patients by statutory duty of the health care providers. It is also important to mention the Australian model, and particularly that in the State of Victoria, where the Infertility Treatment Act of 1995

(Section 137) established the Infertility Treatment Authority and required it to report yearly to the Minister (Infertility Treatment Authority Annual Report, available on-line). The second, FIVNAT from France, is a voluntary system and uses a publication announcing a national compendium of results, excluding center-by-center data. Access to IVF is generally subsidized for three to four cycles by the national health system until the (female) age of 40. The third approach is a legislated one and occurs in the USA. SART has an annual publication that arose from legislation entitled The Fertility Clinic Success Rate and Certification Act of 1992. This legislative act required the Secretary of Health, the Department of Health and Human Services, and the Center for Disease Control and Prevention (CDC) to develop a model program for the certification of embryo laboratories to be carried out voluntarily by interested states. Currently SART and the CDC collaborate to produce the mandatory publication of ART results in national and center-by-center format (Centers for Disease Control and Prevention, 1999). There is neither national healthcare policy for subsidy nor is there consistent insurance coverage in the USA.

Statutory example

In the UK, public transparency has been at the forefront of the annual patient's guide that was first published as part of the establishment of the Human Fertilization and Embryology Authority (HFEA) by the 1990 Human Fertilization and Embryology Act. The first guides used a complex statistical formula to take account of various factors that can affect success rates, e.g., demographics, etiology of infertility, women's age, and duration of infertility. A paper in the *British Medical Journal* showed that only the very best and worst results were statistically different in their success rate, but the press reported the results of all centers as a league table (Marshall and Spiegelhalter, 1998). The most recent HFEA report (Human Fertilization and Embryology Authority Patients' Guide, 1999) sought to include at least one important factor in the results of the patient's guide: the age of the female going through IVF.

This publication reported livebirth rates for females under 38 years of age and for all cycles; these, respectively, are 21.2 and 19.0% per egg collection, 23.6 and 21.1% per embryo transfer, and 13.4 and 12.3% per frozen embryo transfer. IVF results were given per embryo transfer (23 and 20.6% for age <38 years and all cycles, respectively) and intracytoplasmic sperm injection as 24.4 and 22.0% per embryo transfer for age <38 years and all cycles, respectively. Multiple gestations were also given: from 5755 deliveries, 1441 were twins (or 25% of all deliveries) and 176 triplet (3.3% of all deliveries).

The second example (Victoria, Australia) in this statutory model (Infertility Treatment Authority Annual Report) can be looked up on its website and interestingly states "the complexity of reporting data related to assisted reproduction," stressing that centers may have different treatment (and recruitment) policies. A final outcome of treatment procedures reported for 1998 showed the number of cycles per clinic, clinical pregnancies, confinements, and total numbers of babies born. From this it is necessary to calculate center by center the proportion of multiple pregnancies. The total for the year with 565 confinements and 707 babies born (for IVF) indicates the rate of multiple pregnancies in Victoria that year (1999). An interesting table gives also the actual number of multiple births per licensed place, with an aggregated total of 479 confinements and 577 babies born: 387 singletons, 86 sets of twins, 6 sets of triplets, and none of quads or more.

The voluntary model

The voluntary model, FIVNAT, reported in France pregnancies per egg collection as 19 and 20.5% in 1996 and 1997, respectively; pregnancies per embryo transfer as 24.3 and 26.0% for 1996 and 1997, respectively; and a livebirth rate (at least one living) of 14.2% in 1997.

The legislated model

Finally, for the legislated model in the US (Society for Assisted Reproductive Technology and the

American Society for Reproductive Medicine, 1999), outcome measures were clinical pregnancy (fetal heart beat) rates, ectopic pregnancy, abortion, still-births, term delivery, and congenital abnormality rates. The data for this national report come from the 360 fertility clinics in operation in 1998, which provided and verified data on the outcomes of all ART cycles started in their clinics (Centers for Disease Control and Prevention, 1999). ART cycles performed at the reporting clinics in 1998 resulted in 19 891 deliveries of one or more living infants (livebirths) and 28 500 babies. Most of these cycles (68.9%) did not produce a pregnancy, while a very small proportion (0.6%) resulted in an ectopic pregnancy. Clinical pregnancy was achieved in 30.5% of these ART cycles, for which 18.7% resulted in a single-fetus pregnancy and 11.8% resulted in a multiple-fetus pregnancy. Approximately 82% of the pregnancies resulted in a livebirth (50.9% in a singleton birth and 30.9% in multiple-infant births). Approximately 18% of pregnancies resulted in an adverse outcome (miscarriage, induced abortion, or stillbirth). For 18 800 pregnancies that resulted from ART cycles using fresh, nondonor eggs or embryos, 61% were singleton pregnancies, 28% were twin pregnancies, and 11% were triplet or greater pregnancies. Therefore, overall, approximately 39% of the pregnancies included more than one fetus. Of the pregnancies that culminated in livebirth, 38% of these livebirths produced more than one infant (32% twins and 6% triplets or more).

Comparison of information sources

Evaluation of the four examples shows that comparison of results between different methods of reporting data is not easy, especially with regards to the objective of a live healthy (enough) birth, which necessarily entails the preference of a singleton birth. Of note is the fact that in no system is the rate of embryo reduction in multiple pregnancies easily matched to the published success rate per cycle. As an aside, the data from the USA can be compared with some of the European figures recently published (Nygren and Andersen, 2001): in Spain, 45% of pregnancies

were multiple with 11.9% triplets, while in Sweden, 25.8% were multiple with only 0.4% triplets. This stems from a national policy implemented in 1998 in Sweden for a maximum transfer of two embryos per cycle.

"Shared risks" programs, mostly occurring in the USA, illustrate the dangers resulting from the pressures (coercion) felt by patients who cannot afford a treatment that is not considered worthy of subsidy by the health system they live under (Andereck et al., 1998). These shared risk or refund programs in ART were the subject of an article and a report by the Ethics Committee of the American Society for Reproductive Medicine (ASRM) (1998). (In this scheme, patients are initially charged more for a given number of fresh ART cycles but if the treatment fails (no term pregnancy) they are refunded 90–100% of the cost.) The Ethics Committee of the ASRM warns that: "there may be incentives to providers to take risks to assure success." The nature of the endpoint, the "success", being either delivery of a child or a pregnancy of specified duration, is clearly underlined. Although this ignores the therapeutic value of having tried all possibilities before coming to terms with one's sterility, accepting gamete donation, or adopting, the Ethics Committee nevertheless recognizes the "dangers of increasing the risks to the woman's health by a powerful stimulation protocol, or transferring a large number of embryos, and stresses the importance of consent and full information in such programme." This statement represents no more or less than what is expected of any patient/doctor relationship that strives to enhance patients' autonomy by complete and accurate information. However, the further statement that: "there may be a potential conflict of interest" between the caring team and the patients makes uneasy reading. Indeed in the Assisted Fertilization Society Practice committee report (Assisted Fertilization Society, 1998) several points are made that are worthy of analysis. The "right to know" of patients and referring physicians is stressed, which reminds us that in the USA the political language of rights is still very much used in common parlance even if less so in philosophical circles. Accurate reporting (of the results) is aptly described as promoting and reinforcing patients' confidence in the integrity of their healthcare providers. This appeal to the notion of integrity is in the spirit of the language of virtues used by Chervenak and McCullough (1999) in their ethical analysis of dilemmas in obstetrics and is essential to our professional ethos.

Conclusions

A health care approach that considers "justice" should provide for the needs of our patients with equity of access at a national level. The value of international comparisons lies in contrasting the different ways in which similar circumstances, in this case the treatments of infertility, are viewed by different societies. After comparisons are made and their values identified (less bias achieved by using different angles of appraisal), accurate information can be provided to our patients to enhance their autonomy. In terms of obtaining informed consent from our patients, information provided to them should be unbiased, clear, and tailored to the recipient.

The *prima facie* factual information is "what is the success rate?" The answer to the question, "Does publication of results increase patients' autonomy?", is yes, as long as information is given regarding how the results are published and how they relate to the different characteristics of the couple (age, diagnosis, duration of infertility). The information should take into account the major element of risk to future progeny, especially multiple pregnancies. This action addresses duty of care to the vulnerable party (child to be), a statutory duty in English law. There should be none of the apparent conflict between duty to the couple and duty to the children of ART if the future parents are well informed and able to make a responsible decision on behalf of their future child(ren).

Although reproductive choice is a value often quoted in a libertarian system, professional duty, both in the singular health care provider/patient relationship and in the larger exchange at societal level, must also be considered. The consequences of multiple pregnancy are also a matter of public health, explanations should be given to governments who do not provide multiple access to IVF cycles as to the cost-effectiveness of singleton versus high-order birth in terms of public expenditure as well as private suffering. The ultimate solution may be in informing our patients of the chances of singleton pregnancy through a reasonable number (three or four) of attempts at IVF (Engman et al., 1999), giving them the professional guidance that is an element of their autonomous informed consent. As long as their options are severely limited by poorly subsidized access to fertility treatments, including IVF, this is going to be difficult to implement.

REFERENCES

Andereck, W.S., Thomasma, D.C., Goldworth, A., and Kushner, T. (1998). The ethics of guaranteeing patient outcome. *Fertility and Sterility*, **70**, 416–21.

Assisted Fertilization Society (1998). *Guidelines for Advertising by ART Programs*. AFS Practice Committee Report.

Beier, H.M. and Beckman, J.O. (1991). Implications and consequences of the German Embryo Protection Act. *Human Reproduction*, **6**, 607–8.

Benatar, S. (1996). What makes a just health care system. *British Medical Journal*, **313**, 1567–68.

Centers for Disease Control and Prevention (1999). 1997 Assisted Reproductive Technology Success Rates; National Summary and Fertility Clinic Reports. CDC, Atlanta, GA, on-line at http://www.cdc.gov/nccdphp/drh/art.htm

Chervenak, F.A. and McCullough, L.B. (1999). Ethics in fetal medicine. *Baillière's Best Practice and Research in Clinical Obstetrics and Gynaecology*, **13**, 491–502.

Consumers' Forum (1998). *EHRE Annual Meeting on the Legislation and Regulations of ART*, Edinburgh.

Engman, L., Machochie, N., Bekir, J.S., Jacobs, H.S., and Tan Seang Lin (1999). Cumulative probability of clinical pregnancy and livebirth rate after a multiple cycle IVF package: a more realistic assessment of overall and age specific success rates? *British Journal of Obstetrics and Gynaecology*, **106**, 165–70.

Ethics Committee of the American Society for Reproductive Medicine (1998). Shared-risk or refund programs in assisted reproduction. *Fertility and Sterility*, **70**, 414–15.

Garel, M., Salobir, C., and Blondel, B. (1997). Psychological consequences of having triplets: a 4-year follow-up study. *Fertility and Sterility*, **67**, 1162–5.

Human Fertilization and Embryology Act (1990). HMSO, London.

Human Fertilization and Embryology Authority Patients' Guide (1999). Patients' Guide to DI and IVF clinics. HFEA, London, www.hfea.gov.uk

Infertility Treatment Authority Annual Report, www.ita.org.au

Klein, R. (1998). Puzzling out priorities. *British Medical Journal*, **317**, 959–60.

Marshall, E.C. and Spiegelhalter, D.J. (1998). Reliability of league tables of IVF clinics: retrospective analysis of livebirth rates. *British Medical Journal*, **316**, 1701–3.

Milliez, J. (1999). Economics and justice: the ethical aspects of inequity or inequality in health care. *Baillière's Best Practice and Research Clinical Obstetrics and Gynaecology*, **13**, 543–53.

Nisand, I. and Shenfield, F. (1997). Multiple pregnancies and embryo reduction: ethical and legal issues. In: *Studies in Profertility Series*, Vol. 7, *Ethical Dilemmas on Assisted Reproduction*, Shenfield, F. and Sureau, C., eds. Parthenon Press, London, pp. 67–75.

Nygren, K.G. and Andersen, A.N. (2001). Assisted reproductive technologies in Europe, 1997. Results generated from European registers by ESHRE. *Human Reproduction*, **16**, 384–91.

Pennings, G. (2000). Multiple pregnancies: a test case for the moral quality of medically assisted reproduction (Human Reprod Website)

Petterson, B., Nelson, K.B., Watson, L., and Stanley, F. (1993). Twins, triplets, and cerebral palsy in births in Western Australia in the 1980s. *British Medical Journal*, **307**, 1239–43.

Shenfield, F. (1997). Justice and access to fertility treatments. In: *Studies in Profertility Series*, Vol. 7, *Ethical Dilemmas in Assisted Reproduction*, Shenfield, F. and Sureau, C., eds. Parthenon Press, London, pp. 7–14.

Society for Assisted Reproductive Technology and the American Society for Reproductive Medicine (1999). Assisted reproductive technology in the United States: 1996 results generated from the American Society for Reproductive Medicine/Society for Assisted Reproductive Technology Registry. *Fertility and Sterility*, **71**, 798–807.

Templeton, A., Morris, J., and Parslow, B. (1996). Factors that affect outcome of IVF treatment. *Lancet*, **348**, 1402–6.

Warnock, M. (1984). *Report of the Committee of Enquiry into Fertilisation and Embryology*. HMSO, London.

26

Sex selection

Joe Leigh Simpson and Sandra Ann Carson

Baylor College of Medicine, Houston, USA

Introduction

The sex ratio (given throughout as male/female) at birth has been calculated as 1.05 (Chahazarian, 1988; Ruegsegger and Jewelewicz, 1988) or 1.06 (MacMahon and Pugh, 1954). Predicting or influencing the sex ratio before conception has long been of clinical interest and cultural significance. Allusions to influencing the sex of a child have been made throughout history, and modern authors frequently cite Biblical references and other classical allusions. Yet until recently, it has not been clear whether or not the sex ratio at birth can actually be altered. Despite equal numbers of X- and Y-bearing sperm theoretically existing as a result of meiosis I, the sex ratio is not precisely 1.0. This alone offers support for the sex ratio being subject to influence. That is, some factor must be responsible for the deviation from 1.0: genetic, demographic, or environmental. If such a factor could be identified, it could be exploited clinically.

In addition to interest in balancing gender within a given family, there exist situations in which determining the sex of an embryo is desirable for medical reasons. The prime example is a couple at risk for an X-linked recessive trait, a situation in which it is obviously desirable for females to be born. In X-linked dominant traits the converse may arise.

In this chapter, we shall first review the demographic factors most frequently claimed to influence sex ratio. In vitro biological methods of sperm separation will be explored, specifically density gradient and flow sorting methods to enrich for X or Y sperm.

Sexing embryos by single-cell embryo biopsy and molecular analysis will also be discussed. Finally, the propriety of offering sex selection will be discussed, specifically whether current proscriptions against family balancing are truly necessary.

Demographic variables influencing sex ratio

Innumerable studies have considered the relationship between various demographic factors and the sex ratio. Citations are provided by James (1987), Carson (1988), and Zarutskie et al. (1989). Variables most likely to be associated with perturbations in sex ratio appear to be parental ages and coital frequency. However, any observed alteration is only slight (1–2%), virtually without clinical significance.

Advanced paternal age has been associated with decreased sex ratio (Robertson and Sheard, 1973; James and Rostron, 1985; Ruder, 1985; Spira et al., 1993), although not all studies agree (see Zarutskie et al., 1989). The study of James and Rostron (1985) comprised of all births in England and Wales, 1968–1977. Maternal age shows a more variable effect on sex ratio, although James and Rostron (1985) found a peak sex ratio in the third decade; thereafter, the ratio is said either to plateau or to decrease, depending upon the report (Hytten, 1982). In other studies, there is no effect (Robertson and Sheard, 1973; Ruder, 1985; Spira et al., 1993). Coital frequency could also be positively correlated with sex ratio. It has been said that all three variables discussed above exert an independent effect. However, advanced paternal age and decreased coital frequency are correlated, both associated with decreased male births. In a study by one of us, prolonged abstinence was found to be associated with a 3% increase in Y-bearing sperm; however, that order of magnitude is of arguable biological significance (Hilsenrath et al., 1997). Increased coital frequency could help to explain observations that more male births occur postwar, compared with immediate prewar years. After World War I, the sex ratio in Europe increased from 1.035–1.039 (prewar) to 1.047 to 1.051 (postwar) (Russell, 1936). MacMahon and Pugh (1954) found a small but similarly increased ratio in the USA after the World War II, although such a change was not observed after World War I: sex ratio for the years 1942–1946 was 1.061 compared with 1.053 in the 10-year prewar period.

Other social and environmental factors claimed to influence sex ratio include maternal class, birth order, sex of prior siblings, maternal illness like hepatitis B or multiple sclerosis, dizygotic twinning, and ethnic background (for references see James, 1987; Zarutskie et al., 1989). Given that sex ratio is more consistently correlated with parental ages and coital frequencies than with these factors they could merely be surrogate markers for parental age or coital frequency. The same might explain certain data suggesting an altered sex ratio in men who have testicular cancer (Jacobsen et al., 2000a), where other studies showed no effect (Swerdlow et al., 1989; Heimdal et al., 1996). It has also been claimed (Møller, 1996, 1998) that sex ratio is decreasing temporally in many populations. Low sex ratio has been proposed as a marker for reproductive hazards (James, 1996, 1997b) but not for subfertility (Jacobsen et al., 2000b). There is also no relationship between semen analysis and sex ratio (Jacobsen et al., 2000b).

In conclusion, correlation between sex ratio and either parental age or coital frequency is minimal, little more than 1–2%. Decreased sex ratio with increased paternal age is more consistently observed. Altering demographic variables to affect sex ratio is not only impractical but would have only minimal effect.

Timing of intercourse and conception relative to ovulation

Timing of intercourse in relationship to ovulation has long been claimed to affect sex ratio. This was the primary basis for the well-publicized ideas of Shettles (1970). The study of Guerrero (1975) has been cited in support, although this particular study has long been a puzzle because the outcome in natural insemination cycles was inexplicably different from that in artificial insemination cycles. In a larger study, Spira et al. (1993) found no change in sex ratio with timed intercourse, based on prospective studies of more than 5000 women. This study involved couples not desiring a child of a particular gender; the experimental design is, therefore, preferable to smaller studies involving couples desiring a particular gender (Guerrero, 1974, 1975). In the general population, timing of intercourse alone seems unlikely to result in a large alteration of the sex ratio.

Analysis of certain population subsets has sometimes shown perturbations of sex ratio of minimal to modest degree. In particular, women using natural family planning (NFP) have been used to correlate sex ratio with date of conception in relation to ovulation. In this population, several studies suggested that the sex ratio might vary with timing of conception relative to the day of ovulation (Perez et al., 1985). Sex ratio has generally shown a U-shaped association: fewer male conceptions around the time of ovulation than in conceptions pre- and postovulatory (Guerrero, 1974, 1975; Harlap, 1979; Perez et al., 1985; France et al., 1992). However, this has not been a universal finding (World Health Organization, 1984; Gray, 1991; Weinberg et al., 1995).

To address this issue, a cohort study was carried out with NFP users identified in centers in Chile, Colombia, Italy, and Washington. Pregnancies among these users were generally identified in the fifth week of gestation (third week of embryogenesis) and followed systematically through delivery. The estimated day of conception relative to ovulation, the length of the follicular phase of the conception cycle, and the planned/unplanned status of all

Table 26.1. Effect of timing of insemination relative to ovulation and planning status of the pregnancy on the sex ratio

Timing of insemination[a] (days)	Unplanned pregnancies		Planned pregnancies		Total pregnancies	
	M/F	Sex ratio[b]	M/F	Sex ratio[b]	M/F	Sex ratio[b]
≤5	89/87	102.3	12/8	150.0	101/95	106.3
−2 to −4	52/67	77.6	41/45	91.1	93/112	83.0
−1	26/16	162.5	66/58	113.8	92/74	124.3
0	23/16	143.8	87/104	83.7	110/120	91.7
+1	17/12	141.7	15/18	83.3	32/30	106.7
≥2	40/29	137.9	6/7	85.7	46/36	127.8
Total	247/227	108.9	227/240	94.6	474/467	101.5

Notes:

M/F, male/female.

[a] The number of days from the most probable insemination intercourse to probable day of ovulation (day 0).

[b] Sex ratio, M/F × 100.

Source: Reproduced with permission from Gray et al. (1998). *Human Reproduction,* **13**, 1397–400.

pregnancies were determined. The act of intercourse most probably leading to conception was determined from NFP charts in which were recorded acts of intercourse and physical signs (e.g., mucus changes and peak mucus day) enabling the date of ovulation to be deduced. Chart reviewers were blinded with respect to pregnancy outcome (Simpson et al., 1988; Gray et al., 1995). In 947 single-ton births, there were 477 boys and 470 girls, yielding a sex ratio of 1.015 (101.5 males per 100 females). This was not significantly different from the expected sex ratio of 1.05 ($\chi^2 = 1.37$; $p = 0.24$). Overall, these results did not agree with the studies reporting an overall excess of male births (Guerrero, 1975; Perez et al., 1985; France et al., 1992), nor with those showing significant association between timing of insemination and sex ratio (Guerrero, 1975; Harlap, 1979; Perez et al., 1985; France et al., 1992). Neither was there evidence for the hypothesis that pregnancies conceived around the time of ovulation result in a predominance of female births (James, 1987, 1995, 1997a). These findings were consistent with those of Weinberg et al. (1995), who conducted a prospective study of 221 women planning a pregnancy. They are also consistent with a 1984 study of women who experienced method failures

during NFP; no correlation was detected between the timing of insemination intercourse on sex ratio (World Health Organization, 1984).

When the NFP users were stratified by intent, deviations in sex ratio were observed (Gray et al., 1998). The sex ratio was 1.088 among 474 unplanned pregnancies, but 0.946 in 467 planned pregnancies. Among unplanned pregnancies, the sex ratio was lower (fewer males) in preovulatory conceptions (those estimated to have occurred two or more days before ovulation) compared with conceptions occurring around the time of ovulation or during the postovulatory period. Among planned pregnancies, no difference was observed in sex ratio associated with timing of conception (Table 26.1). No biological explanation readily explains differences in sex ratio between couples using NFP for conception (planned pregnancies) and those using NFP for contraception (unplanned pregnancies). Nonetheless, if these observations prove true, they could explain discrepant findings in various NFP populations.

It has been claimed that a short follicular phase is associated with an excess of male births and longer phases with an excess of female births (Weinberg et al., 1995). This was based on data that showed no association between sex ratio and the timing of intercourse (Weinberg et al., 1995; Wilcox et al., 1995). Conclusions were reached by analysis of a cohort of young women discontinuing contraception and attempting to become pregnant; hormonal status during the conception cycles was determined using daily urinary radioimmunoassays of steroid and gonadotropin hormones (Wilcox et al., 1995). Within our South American and Italian NFP sample described above, there was no significant association between estimated follicular phase length and sex ratio in NFP users (Gray et al., 1998). Given that all pregnancies studied by Weinberg et al. (1995) were planned, Gray et al. (1998) further examined the sex ratio only for planned births; again no association was observed between follicular phase length and sex ratio. Among the subset of women with unplanned pregnancies, sex ratio was highest in those with a short follicular phase; however, this difference was not significant. In contrast to Weinberg et al. (1995), Gray et al. (1998) failed to find an association between follicular phase length and sex ratio, nor a differential in the mean length of the follicular phase preceding male or female conceptions. These results are compatible with data from Japan (James, 1997a), where no difference was found in mean cycle length between women who conceived male or female infants. However, aggregate data were used in the latter study; therefore, it was not possible to examine the conception cycle per se.

Related to timing per se are the popularized proposals of Shettles (1960), who recommended using coital timing with other techniques in hopes of optimizing conditions for either X- or Y-bearing sperm to reach the egg first. Conceiving a male child is said to be favored by an alkaline douche before intercourse, female orgasm before or simultaneous with male orgasm, and rear-entry intercourse to maximize deep penetration on the day of ovulation. A female child is said to be favored by an acidic douche, no female orgasm, face-to-face intercourse, and ejaculation nearer the introitus two or three days before ovulation. Using these approaches, Shettles (1970) reported 19 of 22 boys and 16 of 19 girls successfully conceived (Shettles, 1970). However, later studies

have not confirmed Shettles' observation (Williamson et al., 1978; Simcock, 1985). One study not only failed to observe more males at ovulation but found that males were more common when conceived from intercourse several days prior to ovulation (France et al., 1984). A major problem that has made it difficult to assess Shettle's method is that rigorous follow-up never seemed to have been achieved. Successful couples are surely more likely to report favorable results, whereas unsuccessful couples might be less likely. Furthermore, validation of compliance with Shettle's recommendations is difficult if not impossible. The method asks that, after a period of abstinence and with libido at its highest near ovulation, the woman about to have intercourse must first douche. Then, she must have orgasm before or with her partner if she desires a boy. If a girl is desired, ejaculation must be directed shallow in the vagina and the woman cannot have orgasm. It seems unlikely that couples can follow these instructions faithfully.

Another variable related to the issue of timing of conception is presence or absence of ovulation induction regimens. Zarutskie et al. (1989) concluded from a dozen reports of ovulation induction that a significant female skew in the sex ratio existed in four reports. However, in these reports few potential confounding variables were taken into account; little information was provided concerning source of sperm, status of sperm cryopreservation, and insemination technique.

Overall, there is no clinically meaningful relationship between sex ratio and conception timing. A small increase in sex ratio may occur in postovulatory conception in unplanned pregnancies, but this is not clinically useful.

Sperm separation

Density gradients

Given frustration at using environmental or demographic factors to alter sex ratio to a meaningful extent, attempts have turned to biological methods of sperm selection. Could the proportion of X- or Y-bearing sperm be enriched to improve odds of having a male or female? Attempts have involved sperm separation based upon density gradients, specifically albumin gradients, Percoll or Ficoll gradients, or Sephadex columns. Briefly, sperm is first placed on the top of the gradient, after which centrifugation is thought to result in X- and Y-bearing sperm being enriched at different points along the gradient.

Differential separation of X and Y sperm is presumed to depend on cell surface or nuclear differences between X- and Y-bearing sperm. X-bearing sperm contain 2.8% more DNA than Y-bearing sperm (Johnson and Welch, 1999). Theoretically, this should result in Y-bearing sperm being lighter and having greater swimming ability. The X sperm can be calculated as having a 1% larger head radius (Krzanowski, 1970; Rohde et al., 1975; Goodall and Roberts, 1976; Sumner and Robinson, 1976; Cui, 1997). Differences in swimming and sedimentation velocities exist (Sarkar, 1984; Sofikitis et al., 1993). The higher negative charge of X-bearing sperm could also influence interaction with Percoll gradients.

Despite the theoretical appeal of density gradient techniques, results have been inconsistent. Work in this area was initially popularized by Ericsson and coworkers (1973), who reported approximately 85% enrichments of Y-bearing sperm using an albumin gradient. Several investigators reported varying degrees of success using Ericsson's methodology (Dmowski et al., 1979; Beernink and Ericsson, 1982; Corson et al., 1983, 1984; Ericsson and Beernick, 1987; Jaffe et al., 1991; Beernink et al., 1993), but in general it has not proved possible to confirm Ericsson's results (Ross et al., 1975; Schilling et al., 1978; Sofikitis et al., 1993; Windsor et al., 1993). Ericsson (1994) would answer that his methodological details must be followed exactly. Yet when Chen et al. (1997) seemed to follow Ericsson's two- and three-layer albumin separation precisely, little X enrichment (1.4 to 3.5%) was found, based on fluorescence in situ hybridization (FISH) with chromosome-specific probes. Likewise, Claassens

et al. (1995) reported only a 3% increase in Y spermatozoa. Vidal et al. (1993), Wang et al. (1994a) and Flaherty et al. (1997) found no enrichment. We conclude that the technique is not efficacious in most hands.

The same lack of success seems to hold for separation using Percoll (Kaneko et al., 1983, 1984), Ficoll (Rohde et al., 1975) and Sephadex gradients (Shastry et al., 1977). Steeno et al. (1975) did find some success for X enrichment using Sephadex, and Kaneko et al. (1983, 1984) enjoyed modest success. A few clinical trials have shown a difference. For example, Beernink et al. (1993) had a 72% success rate among 1034 couples desiring males; however, simultaneous control groups were not assessed using similar ovulation detection methods and sperm treatment. Studies based on molecular identification of X- and Y-bearing sperm (chromosome-specific DNA probes) have likewise failed to show meaningful alterations in the Y- to X-bearing sperm ratio in Percoll or Sephadex colums (Beckett et al., 1989; Lobel et al., 1993; Vidal et al., 1993; Wang et al., 1994b).

A newer variation of these techniques is the "swim-up" procedure. After multiple centrifugations and recentrifugation in media, the final sperm pellet is gently layered with a small amount of culture media. The sperm from the pellet is allowed to "swim-up" into the media, which after 30–60 minutes is decanted and used for insemination. For six years, Khatamee et al. (1999) used a modified "swim-up" technique in couples desiring a child of particular sex. Eleven patients experiencing a subsequent miscarriage were excluded; there remained 15 desiring a female and 37 a male. In a "control" group of 162 pregnancies conceived spontaneously and not undergoing sperm separation, 80 desired a female and 82 desired a male. Using "swim-up," the success rate was 13 of 15 (86.7%) for those desiring females and 33 of 37 (89.2%) for those desiring males; control "successes" were 42.5% for females and 50% for males. Rawlins et al. (1988) reported 10 of 11 pregnancies for those couples desiring a male, whereas Check et al. (2000) reported 86% success at achieving males. Few sperm remain after processing and all three studies cited above required intra-uterine insemination (IUI) or in vitro fertilization (IVF). These results are encouraging, but sample sizes are still very small, confounding variables not addressed, and proper controls lacking. Moreover, De Jonge et al. (1997) and Flaherty et al. (1997) failed to find "swim-up" efficacious; Lobel et al. (1993) and Han et al. (1993) found no X or Y enrichment based on FISH with X or Y probes.

In conclusion, density gradient techniques have not been proved to be able to separate X- or Y-bearing sperm to a clinically meaningful extent. After review, Reubinoff and Schenker (1996), Flaherty et al. (1997), Hossain et al. (1998), and Seidel (1999) all concluded that albumin, Sephadex, Ficoll and Percoll gradients are ineffective, whereas flow sorting is (see below). The "swim-up" technique may or may not be more effective than traditional gradient separations.

Immunological and electrophoretic techniques

If the cell surface differed in X- and Y-bearing spermatozoa, electrophoretic or immunological techniques could be exploited. Sarkar (1984), Blottner et al. (1994), and Windsor et al. (1993) discuss alterations in the cell surface charges that could plausibly serve as the basis for electrophoretic separation. Unfortunately, immunological and electrophoretic approaches have not yet been successful, based upon in vitro studies. Sills et al. (1998) immunomagnetically separated sperm into groups positive and negative for anti-H-Y antigen, presumably reflecting the presence of the Y-directed H-Y antigen. FISH analysis revealed the antigen expression to be only minimally more prevalent among Y-bearing sperm (54%). A large proportion of Y-bearing sperm failed to express H-Y, indicating that immunological separation for H-Y is unlikely to separate human sperm in Y and X into components.

Flow cytometry

In flow sorting, individual cells are separated based upon one or more characteristics. Such characteristics could include size, shape, cell surface antigens, or nuclear content. In order for flow sorting to take advantage of nuclear characteristics like DNA content, cells may need to be stained with DNA-specific fluorochromes, which can then be excited by ultraviolet light. The 2.8% difference in DNA between X- and Y-bearing human sperm can be recognized and used to separate X and Y sperm. Van Munster et al. (1999) and Welch and Johnson (1999) discuss at length the basis for flow sorting into X and Y sperm. Figure 26.1 shows the approach of Johnson (1997).

Flow sorting sperm is well established in many nonhuman mammals. In some, enrichments of 80% for X or Y sperm can be expected (Johnson, 1997; Johnson and Welch, 1999). Enrichment has been validated by polymerase chain reaction (PCR) for X and Y sequences, FISH, and embryonic sex. One potential problem in humans is that X and Y sperm DNA content differs less (2.8%) than in other mammalian species (Fig. 26.2). Therefore, separation into X- and Y-bearing sperm might be expected to be lower in humans than in many nonhuman mammals.

Efforts to partition human sperm into X- and Y-bearing fractions by flow sorting were reported in 1993 by Johnson et al. Separating X- and Y-bearing sperm by flow cytometry has been reported to result in at least 80% purity for X spermatozoa and 70–75% purity for Y spermatozoa (Johnson et al., 1993; Edward and Beard, 1995; Johnson, 1995, 1997; Cran and Johnson, 1996). In 1998, Fugger et al. published results of their initial clinical experience and in 1999 updated these results (Fugger, 1999).

In the initial report (Fugger et al., 1998), 13 out of 14 (92.9%) pregnancies based on flow sorting with "known fetal or birth gender" had only female concepti. This ratio was consistent with expectations based on the observed proportion of X-bearing spermatozoa (84.5%) using Y-specific FISH probes. In their 1999 update, sperm enrichment was stated to be 88% for X-bearing sperm and 69% for Y-bearing sperm. The IVF rate was 50% (96/192). The low number of sperm recovered requires IUI or intracytoplasmic sperm injection (ICSI). The average number of motile sperm required is 170×10^3 for IUI and 79.4×10^3 for IVF/ICSI. Pregnancy rate was

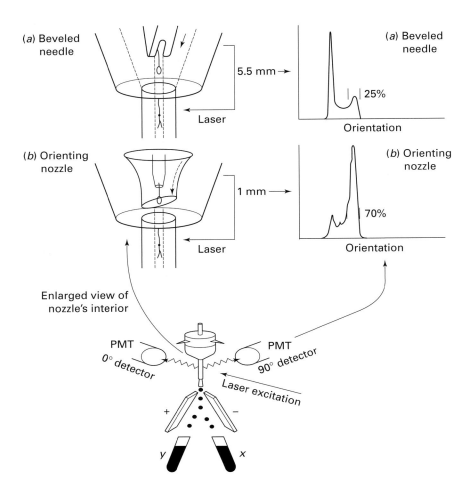

Fig. 26.1. Schematic diagram of basic cell sorter modified for use in enriching sperm for fractions carrying the X and Y chromosomes. (Adapted from *Theriogenology* 52, Johnson, L.A. and Welch, G.R. Sex preselection: high speed flow cytometric sorting of X and Y sperm for maximum efficiency, 1323, copyright (1999), with permission from Excerpta Medica Inc.)

11.8% (61/518) in IUI and 24.1% (35/145) for IVF/ICSI. Nonetheless, correct sex was achieved in 94.4% (37/39) desiring daughters and 73% (11/15) desiring sons. During this same initial period, an unaffected daughter was born to a couple at risk for X-linked hydrocephaly (Levinson et al., 1995).

There are obvious problems with this method. First, sperm separation to enrich for a given sex is not yet 100% successful and may never be. This may not be acceptable for all patients. Second, pregnancy rates are relatively low: approximately 10% for IUI and 25% for IVF/ICSI. Given low pregnancy rates, sperm separation might be most attractive to young highly fertile couples willing to undergo sperm separation in repeated IUI cycles, or couples willing to undertake the expense and exertion of ICSI/IVF.

Safety is also a potential concern, but we do not believe the problem is insurmountable. The theoretical concern is that the ultraviolet light and the bis-

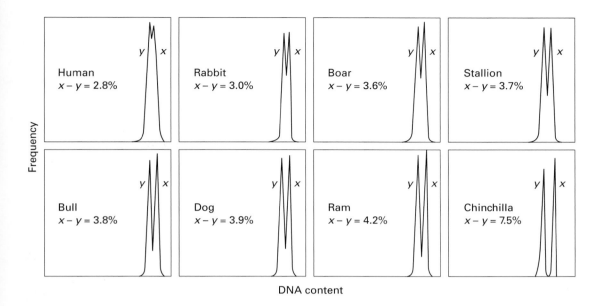

Fig. 26.2. Flow cytometric histograms produced from ejaculated sperm semen from eight common species illustrating the differences in relative DNA content between sperms bearing the X and Y chromosomes. Difference ranges from the 2.8% in humans to 7.5% in *Chincilla langier*. (Reprinted from *Theriogenology* **52**, Johnson, L.A. and Welch, G.R. Sex preselection: high speed flow cytometric sorting of X and Y sperm for maximum efficiency, 1323, copyright (1999), with permission from Excerpta Medica Inc.)

benzimide dye (Hoechst 33342) used for fluorescent-based sperm separation could be deleterious. Bisbenzimide supposedly does not intercalate with DNA, rather binding to AT base pairs in the minor helical groove; therefore, binding should be reversible (Catt et al., 1996). Bisbenzimide also absorbs UV light at a different wave length spectrum than DNA, presumably further mitigating against a mutagenic effect. Extensive animal studies are reassuring, for example the report of Abeydeera et al. (1998) of triplet pigs. There are also favorable reports involving cattle (Cran et al., 1995), rabbits (Johnson et al., 1989), and other species. Extant human data are limited but are, to-date, reassuring.

Overall, there seems every reason to proceed clinically (Simpson and Carson, 1999). Of course, categorical reassurance can never be given because the total sample size does not yet confer the requisite power. For example, analysis of 244 neonates would provide a power of only 0.8 $(1 - \beta)$ to detect a three-fold increase $(\alpha = 0.05)$ in anomalies over a background rate of 3%. Almost 1000 cases would be necessary to exclude a twofold increase above a background rate of 2%. Excluding a specific anomaly would require a larger sample. Yet this situation is no different to that than when many other procedures were introduced (e.g., amniocentesis in 1968 or IVF in 1978). At the onset, these now widely accepted procedures had their naysayers. Moreover, our obligation as critical investigators is not to place roadblocks impeding technology transfer but rather to assure reasonable likelihood of benefit, objective collection of data allowing evaluation of success and complications, and publication of outcomes. Recommendations made regarding verifying safety of preimplantation genetic diagnosis apply here as well (Simpson and Liebaers, 1996).

In conclusion, limited data are encouraging that flow sorting can safely enrich for X and Y sperm, even though yielding low pregnancy rates.

Sex determination following embryo biopsy

Preimplantation genetic diagnosis (PGD) has been discussed in depth elsewhere by ourselves and others (Ch. 12). Suffice it to state that embryonic sex can be determined readily following embryo biopsy aspiration of a single blastomere, which contains only 6 pg DNA. Discussing the molecular basis of single-cell (gamete) diagnosis is beyond the topic of this brief chapter. Methods widely utilized to determine sex (XX versus XY embryos) include FISH analysis with chromosome-specific X and Y probes or PCR-based assessment for X and Y sequences that differ slightly but discernibly (e.g., the gene for amelogenin or *ZFY/ZFX*). Either method readily distinguishes male from female embryos. Both approaches are widely used in PGD for evaluating X-linked recessive and X-linked dominant traits, and both could be used to distinguish between X and Y sequences for nongenetic reasons. In our own laboratory we utilize both FISH and PCR techniques but, like most PGD units, are now almost exclusively using FISH analysis with chromosome-specific probes.

In PGD, accuracy approximates 100% reliability for determining embryos of a given sex, which could then be transferred. There is no serious argument against performing PGD for genetic indications, but using this technology for family balancing is more arguable. The Ethics Committee of the American Society of Reproductive Medicine (ASRM) (1999) believes that embryo biopsy for nongenetic sex selection is inappropriate. Reasons were said to be that sex selection would "identify gender as a reason to value one person over another," "reinforce gender bias in society," place "unreasonable" demands on women for they alone must undergo IVF, and result in "inappropriate use and allocation of medical resources." Not all agree with such reasoning (Savulescu and Dahl, 2000). We, too, believe that flexibility is appropriate and, in fact, we are in substantial agreement with the point-by point refutation by Savulescu (1999) of the ASRM Ethics Committee Report (1999). We favor a more liberal approach. We even believe widespread availability of noninvasive sperm separation would not affect the sex ratio overall (Simpson and Carson, 1999). In Western cultures, we doubt noninvasive sex selection separation would be abused. In cultures favoring only a single child, imbalance might occur temporarily but surely would soon be only temporary; the "rarer" sex in liveborns would become relatively more valuable. Thus, ephemeral alterations in sex ratio in any given 5- or 10-year interval would likely be counterbalanced by the converse in the next temporal cycle. Offering family balancing only after the first child would further minimize any societal effect in Western venues, blunting any educational advantage incurred by the firstborn child (Simpson and Carson, 1999). Consequently, we do not fear societal or personal consequences of sex selection for family balancing. Naturally, the above is our personal belief about a topic for which society must have considerable dialog before consensus evolves.

Summary and conclusions

Various approaches to altering sex ratios have been proposed. Some are fanciful, but others have been pursued seriously. Most noninvasive techniques are not effective.

Sex ratio has been said to be correlated with certain sociodemographic variables, but effects are minimal. Variables most consistently correlated are advanced parental age (decreased sex ratio at advanced age), and perhaps also maternal age (increased sex ratio at advanced ages, peaking in the third decade) and coital frequency (positively correlated with increased sex ratio). However, the magnitude of any change is too small (1–2%) to be clinically meaningful.

In the general population, sex ratio does not seem to be affected greatly by conception day in relation to date of ovulation. In some studies of NFP populations, U-shaped sex ratios are observed; conceptions of male births are higher when intercourse occurs before and after ovulation than at ovulation. Such observations have, in particular, been made in unplanned pregnancies in NFP users. Some studies show 5–10% increase in male births from conceptions occurring two to three days after ovulation. Alterations of the sex ratio of this magnitude are of little use clinically.

Altering sex ratio by fertilization after sperm are separated into X or Y fractions by density gradients has been popularized by many. Density gradients involving albumin (Ericcson), Percoll, Ficoll, and Sephadex columns have been used. Most studies show little effect, based upon both liveborn pregnancy outcome and molecular studies performed on separated sperm (FISH using chromosome-specific probes). In particular, the well-publicized albumin gradient method of Ericsson has not received confirmation. The more recent "swim-up" technique may be more promising.

A more recent approach involves flow sorting sperm into X and Y fractions on the basis of DNA content (2.8% greater in females than males). Sperm nuclei can be stained with fluorochromes and are said to be enriched by sorting to 80–90% and 70–75% for X- and Y-bearing sperm, respectively, based on initial livebirth data and FISH studies of the separated sperm. A major pitfall is the low fertilization rate, only 10% with IUI and 25% with ICSI/IVF. Questions of safety have been raised, based on the necessity of using fluorophores that must be excited with ultraviolet light; animal and human experience are reassuring to date.

Molecular analyses readily permit embryonic sex to be determined following single-cell biopsy. This technique is widely used in PGD for X-linked recessive and dominant traits, and it could be used in other circumstances. In PGD, accuracy approximates 100% for determining embryos of a given sex.

There is no serious discussion against sexing embryos for genetic indications, but using this technology for family balancing is more arguable. The Ethics Committee of the ASRM (1999) believes that embryo biopsy for nongenetic sexing is inappropriate. We favor a more liberal approach. We even believe that widespread availability of noninvasive sperm separation would not affect the sex ratio overall. In Western cultures, we doubt whether noninvasive sex selection would be abused. Indeed,

responsible couples should be congratulated for utilizing such techniques for family balancing rather than practicing unlimited propagation.

REFERENCES

Abeydeera, L.R., Johnson, L.A., Welch, G.R., et al. (1998). Birth of piglets preselected for gender following in vitro fertilization of in vitro matured pig oocytes by X and Y chromosome bearing spermatozoa sorted by high speed flow cytometry. *Theriogenology*, **50**, 981–8.

Beckett, T.A., Martin, R.H., and Hoar, D.I. (1989). Assessment of the sephadex technique for selection of X-bearing human sperm by analysis of sperm chromosomes, deoxyribonucleic acid, and Y-bodies. *Fertility and Sterility*, **52**, 829–35.

Beernink, F.J. and Ericsson, R.J. (1982). Male sex preselection through sperm isolation. *Fertility and Sterility*, **38**, 493–5.

Beernink, F.J., Dmowski, W.P., and Ericsson, R.J. (1993). Sex preselection through albumin separation of sperm. *Fertility and Sterility*, **59**, 382–6.

Blottner, S., Bostedt, H., Mewes, K., and Pitra, C. (1994). Enrichment of bovine X and Y spermatozoa by free-flow electrophoresis. *Zentralblatt für Veterinarmedizin A*, **41**, 466–74.

Carson, S.A. (1988). Sex selection: the ultimate in family planning. *Fertility and Sterility*, **50**, 16–9.

Catt, S.L., Catt, J.W., Gomez, M.C., Maxwell, W.M., and Evans, G. (1996). The birth of a male lamb derived from an in vitro matured oocyte fertilized by intracytoplasmic injection of a single presumptive "male" sperm. *Veterinary Records*, **139**, 494–5.

Chahazarian, A. (1988). Determinants of the sex ratio at birth: review of recent literature. *Social Biology*, **35**, 214–35.

Check, M.L., Bollendorf, A., Check, J.H., Hourani, W., Long, R., and McMonagle, K. (2000). Separation of sperm through a 12-layer Percoll column decreases the percentage of sperm staining with quinacrine. *Archives of Andrology*, **44**, 47–50.

Chen, M.J., Guu, H.F., and Ho, E.S. (1997). Efficiency of sex preselection of spermatozoa by albumin separation method evaluated by double-labelled fluorescence in-situ hybridization. *Human Reproduction*, **12**, 1920–6.

Claassens, O.E., Franken, D.R., Oosthuizen, C.J.J., Franken, D.R., and Kruger, T.F. (1995). Fluorescent *in situ* hybridization evaluation of human Y-bearing spermatozoa separated by albumin density gradients. *Fertility and Sterility*, **63**, 417–18.

Corson, S.L., Batzer, F.R., and Schlaff, S. (1983). Preconceptual female gender selection. *Fertility and Sterility*, **40**, 384–85.

Corson, S.L., Batzer, F.R., Alexander, N.J., Schlaff, S., and Otis, C.

(1984). Sex selection by sperm separation and insemination. *Fertility and Sterility*, **42**, 756–60.

Cran, D.G. and Johnson, L.A. (1996). The predetermination of embryonic sex, using flow cytometrically separated X and Y spermatozoa. *Human Reproduction Update*, **2**, 355–63.

Cran, D.G., Johnson, L.A., and Polge, C. (1995). Sex preselection in cattle: a field trial. *Veterinary Records*, **136**, 495–6.

Cui, K.H. (1997). Size differences between human X and Y spermatozoa and prefertilization diagnosis. *Molecular Human Reproduction*, **3**, 61–7.

De Jonge, C.J., Flaherty, S.P., Barnes, A.M., Swann, N.J., and Matthews, C.D. (1997). Failure of multitube sperm swim-up for sex preselection. *Fertility and Sterility*, **67**, 1109–14.

Dmowski, W.P., Gaynor, L., Rao, R., Lawrence, M., and Scommegna, A. (1979). Use of albumin gradients for X and Y sperm separation and clinical experience with male sex preselection. *Fertility and Sterility*, **31**, 52–7.

Edward, R.G. and Beard, H.K. (1995). Sexing human spermatozoa to control sex ratios at birth is now a reality. *Human Reproduction*, **10**, 977–8.

Ericsson, R.J., Langevin, C.N., and Nishino, M. (1973). Isolation of fractions rich in human Y sperm. *Nature*, **246**, 421.

Ericsson, R.J. (1994). Validity of X and Y sperm separation techniques. *Fertility and Sterility*, **62**, 1286–8.

Ericsson, R.J. and Beernink, F. (1987). Sex chromosome ratios in human sperm [letter]. *Fertility and Sterility*, **47**, 531–2.

Ethics Committee of the American Society of Reproductive Medicine (1999). Sex selection and preimplantation genetic diagnosis. *Fertility and Sterility*, **72**, 595–8.

Flaherty, S.P., Michalowska, J., Swann, N.J., Dmowski, W.P., Matthews, C.D., and Aitken, R.J. (1997). Albumin gradients do not enrich Y-bearing human spermatozoa. *Human Reproduction*, **12**, 938–42.

France, J.T., Graham, F.M., Gosling, L., and Hair, P.I. (1984). A prospective study of the preselection of the sex of offspring by timing intercourse relative to ovulation. *Fertility and Sterility*, **41**, 894–900.

France, J.T., Graham, F.M., Gosling, L., Hair, P., and Knox, B.S. (1992). Characteristics of natural conceptual cycles occurring in a prospective study of sex preselection; fertility awareness symptoms, hormone levels, sperm survival, and pregnancy outcome. *International Journal of Fertility*, **37**, 244–55.

Fugger, E.F. (1999). Clinical experience with flow cytometric separation of human X- and Y-chromosome bearing sperm. *Theriogenology*, **52**, 1435–40.

Fugger, E.F., Black, S.H., Keyvanfar, K., and Schulman, J.D. (1998). Births of normal daughters after MicroSort sperm separation and intrauterine insemination, in-vitro fertilization, or intracytoplasmic sperm injection. *Human Reproduction*, **13**, 2367–70.

Goodall, H. and Roberts, A.M. (1976). Differences in motility of human X- and Y-bearing spermatozoa. *Journal of Reproductive Fertility*, **48**, 433–6.

Gray, R.H. (1991). Natural family planning and sex selection: fact or fiction? *American Journal of Obstetrics and Gynecology*, **165**(Suppl. Part 2), 1982–4.

Gray, R.H., Simpson, J.L., Kambic, R.T., et al. (1995). Timing of conception and the risk of spontaneous abortion among pregnancies occurring during the use of natural family planning. *American Journal of Obstetrics and Gynecology*, **172**, 1567–72.

Gray, R.H., Simpson, J.L., Bitto, A.C., et al. (1998). Sex ratio associated with timing of insemination and length of the follicular phase in planned and unplanned pregnancies during use of natural family planning. *Human Reproduction*, **13**, 1397–1400.

Guerrero, R. (1974). Association of the type and time of insemination within the menstrual cycle with the human sex ratio at birth. *New England Journal of Medicine*, **291**, 1056–9.

Guerrero, R. (1975). Type and time of insemination within the menstrual cycle and the human sex ratio at birth. *Studies in Family Planning*, **6**, 367–71.

Han, T.L., Flaherty, S.P., Ford, J.H., and Matthews, C.D. (1993). Detection of X- and Y-bearing human spermatozoa after motile sperm isolation by swim-up. *Fertility and Sterility*, **60**, 1046–51.

Harlap, S. (1979). Gender of infants conceived on different days of the menstrual cycle. *New England Journal of Medicine*, **300**, 1445–48.

Heimdal, K., Olsson, H., Tretli, S., Flodgren, P., Borresen, A.L., and Fossa, S.D. (1996). Risk of cancer in relatives of testicular cancer patients. *British Journal of Cancer*, **73**, 970–3.

Hilsenrath, R.E., Swarup, M., Bischoff, F.Z., Buster, J.E., and Carson, S.A. (1997). Effect of sexual abstinence on the proportion of X-bearing sperm as assessed by multicolor fluorescent in situ hybridization. *Fertility and Sterility*, **68**, 510–13.

Hossain, A.M., Barik, S., Rizk, B., and Thorneycroft, I.H. (1998). Preconceptional sex selection: past, present, and future. *Archives of Andrology*, **40**, 3–14.

Hytten, F.E. (1982). Boys and girls. *British Journal of Obstetrics and Gynaecology*, **89**, 97–9.

Jacobsen, R., Bostofte, E., Engholm, G., Hansen, J., Skakkebaek, N.E., and Møller, H. (2000a). Fertility and offspring sex ratio of men who develop testicular cancer: a record linkage study. *Human Reproduction*, **15**, 1958–61.

Jacobsen, R., Bostofte, E., Skakkebaek, N.E., Hansen, J., and

Møller, H. (2000b). Offspring sex ratio of subfertile men and men with abnormal sperm characteristics. *Human Reproduction*, **15**, 2369–70.

Jaffe, S.B., Jewelewicz, R., Wahl, E., and Khatamee, M.A. (1991). A controlled study for gender selection. *Fertility and Sterility*, **56**, 254–8.

James, W.H. (1987). The human sex ratio. Part 1: a review of the literature. *Human Biology*, **59**, 721–52.

James, W.H. (1995). Clomiphene citrate, gonadotrophins and sex ratio of offspring. *Human Reproduction*, **10**, 2465–6.

James, W.H. (1996). Male reproductive hazards and occupation. *Lancet*, **347**, 773.

James, W.H. (1997a). Follicular phase length, time of insemination, mean cycle length, season of mother's birth and sex ratio of offspring. *Human Reproduction*, **12**, 398–9.

James, W.H. (1997b). Secular trends in monitors of reproductive hazard. *Human Reproduction*, **12**, 417–21.

James, W.H. and Rostron, J. (1985). Parental age, parity and sex ratio in births in England and Wales, 1968–1977. *Journal of Biosocial Science*, **17**, 47–56.

Johnson, L.A. (1995). Sex preselection by flow cytometric separation of X- and Y-chromosome bearing sperm based on DNA difference: a review. *Reproduction, Fertility and Development*, **7**, 893–903.

Johnson, L.A. (1997). Advances in gender preselection in swine. *Journal of Reproduction and Fertilility Suppl.*, **52**, 255–66.

Johnson, L.A. and Welch, G.R. (1999). Sex preselection: high speed flow cytometric sorting of X and Y sperm for maximum efficiency. *Theriogenology*, **52**, 1323–41.

Johnson, L.A., Flook, J.P., and Hawk, H.W. (1989). Sex preselection in rabbits: live birth from X and Y sperm separated by DNA and cell sorting. *Biology of Reproduction*, **41**, 199–203.

Johnson, L.A., Welch, G.R., Keyvanfar, K., Dorfmann, A., Fugger, E.F., and Schulman, J.D. (1993). Gender preselection in humans? Flow cytometric separation of X and Y spermatozoa for the prevention of X-linked diseases. *Human Reproduction*, **8**, 1733–39.

Kaneko, S., Yamaguchi, J., Kobayashi, T., and Iizuka, R. (1983). Separation of X- and Y-bearing sperm using Percoll density gradient centrifugation. *Fertility and Sterility*, **40**, 661–9.

Kaneko, S., Oshio, S., Kobayashi, T., Iizuka, R., and Mohri, H. (1984). Human X- and Y-bearing sperm differ in cell surface sialic acid content. *Biochemical and Biophysical Research Communications*, **124**, 950–5.

Khatamee, M.A., Horn, S.R., Weseley, A., Farooq, T., Jaffe, S.B., and Jewelewicz, R. (1999). A controlled study for gender selection using swim-up separation. *Gynecologic and Obstetric Investigation*, **48**, 7–13.

Krzanowski, M. (1970). Dependence of primary and secondary sex ratio on the rapidity of sedimentation of bull semen. *Journal of Reproduction and Fertility*, **23**, 11–20.

Levinson, G., Keyvanfar, K., Wu, J.C., et al. (1995). DNA-based X-enriched sperm separation as an adjunct to preimplantation genetic testing for the prevention of X-linked disease. *Human Reproduction*, **10**, 979–82.

Lobel, S.M., Pomponio, R.J., and Mutter, G.L. (1993). The sex ratio of normal and manipulated human sperm quantitated by the polymerase chain reaction. *Fertility and Sterility*, **59**, 387–92.

MacMahon, B. and Pugh, T. (1954). Sex ratio of white births in the United States during the Second World War. *American Journal of Human Genetics*, **6**, 284.

Møller, H. (1996). Change in male:female ratio among newborn infants in Denmark. *Lancet*, **348**, 828–9.

Møller, H. (1998). Trends in sex-ratio, testicular cancer and male reproductive hazards: are they connected? *Acta Pathologica, Microbiologica et Immunologica Scandinavica*, **106**, 232–8.

Perez, A., Eger, R., Domenichini, V., Kambic, R., and Gray, R.H. (1985). Sex ratio associated with natural family planning. *Fertility and Sterility*, **43**, 152–3.

Rawlins, R.G., Sachdeva, S., Radwenska, E., Binor, Z., Rana, N., and Dmowski, W.P. (1988). Human sex preselection and in vitro fertilization (IVF): fraction separation of sperm enhances probability of conceiving male offspring. *35th Annual Meeting Society for Gynecologic Investigation*, Baltimore 1988, abstract 156.

Reubinoff, B.E. and Schenker, J.G. (1996). New advances in sex preselection. *Fertility and Sterility*, **66**, 343–50.

Robertson, J.S. and Sheard, A.V. (1973). Altered sex ratios after an outbreak of hepatitis. *Lancet*, **i**, 532–4.

Rohde, W., Porstmann, T., Prehn, S., and Dorner, G. (1975). Gravitational pattern of the Y-bearing human spermatozoa in density gradient centrifugation. *Journal of Reproduction and Fertility*, **42**, 587–91.

Ross, A., Robinson, J.A., and Evans, H.J. (1975). Failure to confirm separation of X- and Y-bearing human sperm using BSA gradients. *Nature*, **253**, 354–5.

Ruder, A. (1985). Paternal age and birth order effect on the human secondary sex ratio. *American Journal of Human Genetics*, **37**, 362–72.

Ruegsegger, V.E.I.T. and Jewelewicz, R. (1988). Gender preselection: facts and myths. *Fertility and Sterility*, **49**, 937–40.

Russell, W.T. (1936). Statistical study of the sex ratio at birth. *Journal of Hygiene*, **36**, 25.

Sarkar, S. (1984). Motility, expression of surface antigen, and X and Y human sperm separation in in vitro fertilization medium. *Fertility and Sterility*, **42**, 899–905.

Savulescu, J. (1999). Sex selection – the case for. *Medical Journal of Australia*, **171**, 373–5.

Savulescu, J. and Dahl, E. (2000). Sex selection and preimplantation diagnosis; a response to the Ethics Committee of the American Society of Reproductive Medicine. *Human Reproduction*, **15**, 1879–80.

Schilling, E., Lafrenz, R., and Klobasa, F. (1978). Failure to separate human X and Y chromosome bearing spermatozoa by Sephadex gel-filtration. *Andrologia*, **10**, 215–19.

Seidel, G.R. Jr. (1999). Sexing mammalian spermatozoa and embryos – state of the art. *Journal of Reproduction and Fertility Suppl.*, **54**, 477–87.

Shastry, P.R., Hegle, U.C., and Roa, S.S. (1977). Use of Ficoll-sodium metrizoate density gradient to separate human X- and Y-bearing sperm. *Nature*, **269**, 58–60.

Shettles, L.B. (1960). Nuclear morphology of human spermatozoa. *Nature*, **186**, 648.

Shettles, L.B. (1970). Factors influencing sex ratios. *International Journal of Gynaecology and Obstetrics*, **8**, 643.

Sills, E.S., Kirman, I., Colombero, L.T., Hariprashad, J., Rosenwaks, Z., and Palermo, G.D. (1998). H-Y antigen expression patterns in human X-and Y-chromosome-bearing spermatozoa. *American Journal of Reproduction and Immunology*, **40**, 43–7.

Simcock, B.W. (1985). Sons and daughters – a sex preselection study. *Medical Journal of Australia*, **142**, 541–2.

Simpson, J.L. and Carson, S.A. (1999). The reproductive option of sex selection. *Human Reproduction* **14**, 870–2.

Simpson, J.L. and Liebaers, I. (1996). Assessing congenital anomalies after preimplantation genetic diagnosis. *Journal of Assisted Reproductive Genetics* **13**, 170–6.

Simpson, J.L., Gray, R.H., Queenan, J.T., et al. (1988). Pregnancy outcome associated with natural family planning (NFP): scientific basis and experimental design for an international cohort study. *Advances in Contraception*, **4**, 247–64.

Sofikitis, N., Miyagawa, I., and Zavos, P.M. (1993). Selection of single-stranded DNA spermatozoa via the spermprep filtration column. *Fertility and Sterility*, **59**, 690–2.

Spira, A., Ducot, B., Guihard-Moscato, M.-L., et al. (1993). Conception probability and pregnancy outcome in relation to age, cycle regularity, and timing of intercourse. In: *International Studies in Demography, Biomedical and Demographic Determinants of Reproduction*, Gray, R., Leridon, H., and Spira, A., eds. Clarendon Press, Oxford, p. 271.

Steeno, O., Adimoelja, A., and Steeno, J. (1975). Separation of X and Y bearing human spermatozoa with the Sephadex gel-filtration method. *Andrologia* **7**, 95–8.

Sumner, A.T. and Robinson, J.A. (1976). A difference in dry mass between the heads of X- and Y-bearing human spermatozoa. *Journal of Reproduction and Fertility*, **48**, 9–15.

Swerdlow, A.J., Huttly, S.R., and Smith, P.G. (1989). Testis cancer: post-natal hormonal factors, sexual behaviour and fertility. *International Journal of Cancer*, **43**, 549–53.

van Munster, E.B., Stap, J., Hoebe, R.A., te Meerman, G.J., and Aten, J.A. (1999). Difference in sperm head volume as a theoretical basis for sorting X- and Y-bearing spermatozoa: potentials and limitations. *Theriogenology*, **52**, 1281–93.

Vidal, F., Moragas, M., Catala, V., et al. (1993). Sephadex filtration and human serum albumin gradients do not select spermatozoa by sex chromosome: a fluorescent in situ hybridization study. *Human Reproduction*, **8**, 1740–3.

Wang, H.X., Flaherty, S.P., Swann, N.J., and Matthews, C.D. (1994a). Assessment of the separation of X- and Y-bearing sperm on albumin gradients using double label fluorescence in situ hybridization. *Fertility and Sterility*, **61**, 720–6.

Wang, H.X., Flaherty, S.P., Swann, N.J., and Matthews, C.D. (1994b). Discontinuous Percoll gradients enrich X-bearing human spermatozoa: a study using double-label fluorescence in situ hybridization. *Human Reproduction*, **9**, 1265–70.

Weinberg, C.R., Baird, D.D., and Wilcox, A.J. (1995). The sex of the baby may be related to the length of the follicular phase in the conception cycle. *Human Reproduction*, **10**, 304–7.

Welch, G.R. and Johnson, L.A. (1999). Sex preselection: laboratory validation of the sperm sex ratio of flow sorted X- and Y-sperm by sort reanalysis of DNA. *Theriogenology*, **52**, 1343–52.

Wilcox, A.J., Weinberg, C.R., and Baird, D.D. (1995). Timing of sexual intercourse in relation to ovulation. Effects on probability of conception, survival of the pregnancy, and sex of the baby. *New England Journal of Medicine*, **333**, 1517–21.

Williamson, N.E., Lean, T.H., and Vengadasalam. D. (1978) Evaluation of an unsuccessful sex preselection clinic in Singapore. *Journal of Biosocial Sciences*, **10**, 375–88.

Windsor, D.P., Evans, G., and White, I.G. (1993). Sex predetermination by separation of X and Y chromosome-bearing sperm: a review. *Reproductive Fertility and Development*, **5**, 155–71.

World Health Organization (1984). A prospective multicentre study of the ovulation method of natural family planning. IV. The outcome of pregnancy. Task Force on Methods for the Determination of the Fertile Period, Special Programme of Research, Development and Research Training in Human Reproduction. *Fertility and Sterility*, **41**, 593–8.

Zarutskie, P.W., Muller, C.H., Magone, M., and Soules, M.R. (1989). The clinical relevance of sex selection techniques. *Fertility and Sterility*, **52**, 891–905.

27

Intracytoplasmic sperm injection: a time bomb?

Herman J. Tournaye and André C. Van Steirteghem

Center for Reproductive Medicine, Dutch-speaking Brussels Free University, Brussels, Belgium

Introduction

The rapid introduction of intracytoplasmic sperm injection (ICSI) in daily clinical practice has given rise to much concern about the possible risks involved. These possible risks are related mainly to the mechanical perforation of the oocyte and the possible transmission of foreign genetic material, the use of immature or senescent germ cells, and the association between genetic disorders and some forms of male infertility. So far, evaluation studies on a substantial sample of children born after ICSI have failed to show any increased rate of congenital malformations when a uniformly consistent ICSI technique is applied.

However, sex chromosome abnormalities have been reported in approximately 1% of the offspring of ICSI. The risk of aneuploidy in ICSI progeny merely reflects the higher aneuploidy rate in the fathers and the production of a higher proportion of aneuploidic germ cells in subfertile men with normal karyotypes. Rigorous genetic screening and, possibly, new sperm selection procedures may lower this aneuploidy rate substantially.

Since, at present, the inheritance pattern of male infertility is unknown, it is far from clear whether ICSI will eventually perpetuate infertility. We recommend that all ICSI candidates should be thoroughly screened and counseled. Ultimately, they themselves should judge whether the concerns outweigh the benefits. To-date, the data available indicate that ICSI is a safe procedure provided it is performed in clinics with the highest standards of expertise and having an organized continuous follow-up program for the offspring.

The introduction of a powerful technique

For years, the use of donor sperm was the only means to motherhood for the partners of most men with extreme oligozoospermia or azoospermia. Since its introduction (Palermo et al., 1992; Van Steirteghem et al., 1993), ICSI has been the subject of a continuing debate, particularly with regards to its safety. When ICSI was first shown to produce viable pregnancies (Palermo et al., 1992), only a few reports existed in the literature with regard to its efficacy. Fertilization was obtained by ICSI in the hamster (Uehara and Yanagimachi, 1976) and live offspring were born in the rabbit (Iritani et al., 1988) and the cow (Goto et al., 1990). Although the first applications in the human were not that successful, normal fertilization was obtained in a few oocytes (Lanzendorf et al., 1988). Before the birth of the first child from ICSI, no safety studies were available and only casuistic (case) reports existed on the technique.

Since the report by Palermo et al. (1992) on a more refined micromanipulation technique, ICSI has become more reproducible, with associated high success rates in terms of both fertilization and implantation. Fertilization after ICSI with ejaculated sperm fails in less than 3% of cycles (Liu et al., 1995). This technique, therefore, represents the most powerful tool available to the reproductive andrologist in treating severe idiopathic male infertility. Over a few years, ICSI has become a routine assisted reproductive technique (SART, 2000; Tarlatzis and Bili, 2000). However, our basic understanding of both the fertilization processes after ICSI and the andrological problems that are being treated is still limited. For ICSI, the clinical phase is far ahead of the research phase.

To resolve this problem, animal models are currently being developed, but the question remains whether these models will answer all the safety issues regarding ICSI in the human. In many animal research models, the ICSI technique has important technical differences from human ICSI, for example piezo-driven microinjection, cooling of the oocytes, or use of acrosome-reacted spermatozoa. Furthermore, species-specific differences limit the extrapolation of results from animal models to humans, for example differences in polyspermia block, differences in in vitro development, differences in inheritance of the centrosome, and, of course, the differences in the pathophysiological background of the spermatozoa used. Rodent models are among the most popular models (Yanagimachi, 1998) but are probably not the best models to extrapolate events occurring during assisted fertilization in the human situation because there is maternal rather than paternal inheritance of the centrosome. Guinea pigs are an exception to this, but the current experience with this model is limited and furthermore the embryos show a block in vitro at the 4-cell stage (Ogura et al., 2000). Many primates or even domestic mammals (e.g., rabbits, cows, sheep, pigs) do have cytoskeletal dynamics at fertilization that are homologous to those in humans (Schatten, 1994). Thanks to the successful development of primate ICSI models, a better evaluation of the safety of the ICSI technique will become possible in the near future (Hewitson et al., 1998). These models are, however, very expensive and are currently being applied to completely fertile animals. So the question remains whether these models will enable us to assess all the safety aspects regarding ICSI in the human.

Currently, the vast amount of data available for analysis and interpretation in order to assess the emerging physical and mental health concern issues related to the clinical application of ICSI is derived from retrospective case series and surveys on human ICSI.

The fuse and the detonator: technical concerns relating to ICSI

Two aspects of ICSI, the piercing of the oocyte and the deposition of a germ cell that had not been selected in a natural way, immediately gave rise to much concern regarding the safety of the technique, and there has been continuous debate on possible adverse effects. It has even been argued that ICSI represents the "ultimate rape of the oocyte."

The piercing of the oocyte by the injection pipette may cause damage to the second meiotic spindle of the oocyte. The meiotic spindle apparatus has been studied in hamster oocytes undergoing ICSI with human sperm (Asada et al., 1995). After immunofluorescent staining of the spindle, no significant differences were observed in either the spindle appearance or the chromosome alignments between test and control human oocytes, provided ICSI was performed away from the polar body. However, recent studies in the hamster (Silva et al., 1999) and a primate model (Hewitson et al., 1999, Luetjens et al., 1999) have demonstrated that even with correct positioning (i.e., first polar body at a right angles to the site of injection) spindle damage remains a theoretical risk since the localization of the first polar body does not indicate the exact localization of the spindle. These findings were confirmed in human oocytes (Hewitson et al., 1999).

Another possible hazard results from the dislocation of cytoplasm during sperm injection. The chromosome breakage rate in uncleaved oocytes after failed ICSI was reported to be higher than after failed conventional in vitro insemination (Bergère et al., 1995; Edirisinghe et al., 1997). However, another study comparing chromosome breakage rate after failed ICSI or in vitro fertilization (IVF) found a higher breakage rate after conventional IVF than after ICSI (Plachot, 1996).

A more important, but yet unproven, concern is the introduction of contaminating foreign material into the oocyte's cytoplasm during ICSI. The use of polyvinylpyrrolidone to slow down sperm movement may constitute a toxic risk because it can contain endotoxins. Although sound evidence is as yet unavailable to support this risk, this compound has been withdrawn from the market by its manufacturer and replaced by products controlled for endotoxin contamination.

Microbiological contamination of semen is frequent. Whether microorganisms may act as vectors is unknown. Washing and further semen preparation eliminates most microbiological contaminants. On the basis of the current literature, this hazard is assumed to be minimal or even nonexistent for bacteria (Michelmann, 1998), but the issue is less clear for viruses (e.g., human papillomavirus; Brossfield et al., 1999). Theoretically, prions too may be introduced during an ICSI procedure (Lacey and Dealler, 1994). Although the technique used was of debatable reproducibility, it has been shown that exogenous DNA could be integrated during ICSI in the mouse, producing transgenic offspring (Perry et al., 1999). More recently, foreign DNA was successfully introduced into nonhuman primate oocytes during ICSI; however, this did not produce transgenic offspring (Chan et al., 2000). All these hazards may constitute highly sensitive but yet unknown detonators. Some authors, therefore, propose to subject human spermatozoa to a sequence of sanitizing treatments before ICSI (Chan et al., 2000).

A powerful payload: concerns relating to the male germ cells used

The major parameter for successful ICSI is the injection of a spermatozoon with DNA that can decondense within the oocyte's cytoplasm. In practice, this means that motile or live sperm can be recovered from any point in the male reproductive tract in order to perform ICSI. The ultimate selection of the sperm to be injected is made subjectively through the light microscope, selecting a "good-looking"

motile spermatozoon on sight. Although no adverse effects in terms of outcome have been reported after microinjection of spermatozoa from patients with morphologically abnormal spermatozoa (Nagy et al., 1995; Svalander et al., 1996; Kupker et al., 1998), most of these studies do not correlate the morphology of the spermatozoon that is eventually injected with the ICSI outcome.

Only few studies, involving a limited number of cases, report on the outcome after injection of morphologically abnormal sperm. Both Mansour et al. (1995) and Tasdemir et al. (1997) showed a reduced fertilization rate when abnormal sperm was used for ICSI. These findings are not surprising: in mouse–ICSI models, an increase in sperm chromosome aberration rate was observed after injection of human spermatozoa with gross head abnormalities (Yanagimachi, 1998). An increase in chromosomal aberrations has been observed in spermatozoa from oligozoospermic individuals using fluorescence in situ hybridization (FISH) (Miharu et al., 1994; Bernardini et al., 1997; Egozcue et al., 1997; McInnes et al., 1998; Pang et al., 1999). Furthermore, up to 3% of patients with oligozoospermia are reported to have autosomal karyotype abnormalities, while the incidence of sex chromosome abnormalities in azoospermic men is reported to be 14% (Van Assche et al., 1996; Yoshida et al., 1996). The incidence of karyotype abnormalities is inversely related to the number of spermatozoa in the ejaculate. In patients with moderate oligozoospermia (10×10^6 to 20×10^6 spermatozoa/ml), karyotype abnormalities were observed in about 3%, while in patients with extreme oligozoospermia ($<5 \times 10^6$ spermatozoa/ml), this figure is about 7% (Yoshida et al., 1996). Both azoospermic and oligozoospermic patients must, therefore, be karyotyped before any ICSI treatment in order to prevent possible transmission of aneuploidy to the offspring.

This increase in aneuploidy rate in subfertile men will probably at least partly explain the increase in sex chromosome abnormalities in the offspring of ICSI patients. In a study of 1082 ICSI children, the sex chromosome aneuploidy rate was 0.83% (95% confidence interval (CI): 0.3–1.6) (Bonduelle et al.,

1999). In the general population, the sex chromosome aneuploidy rate reported is only 0.20% (95% CI: 0.19–0.23) (Nielsen and Wohlert, 1991). These sex chromosome abnormalities may be associated with extreme oligozoospermia. The above FISH studies on spermatozoa showed that the incidence of aneuploidy is inversely correlated with sperm numbers. Abnormal sperm decondensation after ICSI may also contribute to this problem of increased de novo sex chromosome aneuploidy (Hewitson et al., 1999). The current methods of sperm selection for ICSI are clearly unable in themselves to prevent injection of disomic sperm, thus leading to an increased risk of sex chromosome aneuploidy. Since at present this is the only well-documented adverse outcome affect demonstrated in offspring after ICSI, more reliable methods should be developed in order to avoid sex chromosome aneuploidy in the offspring. Current semen preparation techniques do not select against aneuploid spermatozoa (Samura et al., 1997).

In the future, perhaps aneuploid sperm may be excluded from the sperm preparations used for ICSI on the basis of zona-binding assays or even flow cytometric separation techniques. A recent study showed that zona-bound spermatozoa had a significantly lower frequency of aneuploidy than the spermatozoa from the swim-up motile fraction or the pellet fraction (Van Dyk et al., 2000).

With ICSI, pregnancies can be obtained using epididymal spermatozoa or testicular spermatozoa irrespective of whether spermatogenesis is histologically normal (Tournaye, 1999). Pregnancies have even been reported after the use of elongated spermatids and round spermatids from testicular biopsies or from ejaculates (Sousa et al., 1999). The use of these immature haploid germ cells gives rise to much concern: it is difficult to distinguish these haploid germ cells from diploid germ cells by their morphological appearance (Verheyen et al., 1998) and there are concerns relating to genomic imprinting (Tesarik and Mendoza, 1996). However, it has been shown that genomic imprinting is completed at the spermatid stage in a mouse model (Shamanski et al., 1999) and that normal viable young with normal behavior up to the fifth generation can be

obtained after round spermatid injection (Tamashiro et al., 1999). Since mouse offspring obtained after injection of secondary spermatocytes were found to be fertile, it was concluded that imprinting may be completed by the second meiotic division or may even be completed within the oocyte's cytoplasm (Kimura and Yanagimachi, 1995). Therefore, the results from animal models in which ICSI is performed with immature germ cells do not raise any concerns. Again, it must be asked if these results can be extrapolated to the human model.

Pregnancies can also ensue after ICSI with senescent spermatozoa. These spermatozoa, however, may have DNA strand breakage because of aging and generation of reactive-oxygen species, especially during extended epididymal storage. In patients with only senescent or dead sperm in their ejaculates, testicular spermatozoa may be used for ICSI (Tournaye et al., 1996). Using viable testicular sperm may be preferable because even senesent ejaculated spermatozoa with DNA damage may fertilize successfully after ICSI (Twigg et al., 1998).

Finally, a distinct subpopulation of men can benefit from ICSI treatment to alleviate infertility that may have a genetic background related to or causing their fertility problem (for review, see Tournaye et al., 1997). In recent years, microdeletions in the long arm of the Y chromosome have been intensively studied (for review, see Simoni et al., 1999). These Yq deletions will be passed to the next male generation by ICSI (Kent-First et al., 1996; Page et al., 1999). Autosomal Y homologs or other unknown recessive gene defects may exist, and many genes related to spermatogenesis may be interlinked in gene networks. Apart from Yq deletions, mutations in the androgen receptors (i.e., an increased number of CAG repeats in the androgen receptor gene) have been reported to cause male infertility (Tut et al., 1997; Dowsing et al., 1999). However, this may only represent "the tip of the iceberg".

At present, all the inheritance patterns of male infertility have not been elucidated, but more evidence is arising that hereditary traits may be involved in the problems leading to the presentation of many candidates for ICSI (Meschede et al., 2000a).

Globozoospermia and immotile cilia syndromes are now increasingly assumed to be hereditary disorders. Apart from reproductive disorders, ICSI candidates may also have a slightly higher prevalence of potentially heritable nonreproductive disorders (Meschede et al., 2000b). Notwithstanding genetic counseling, many patients may still prefer to use their own gametes and, thus, take the risk of passing male infertility to their sons.

Defusing the time bomb: should there be a moratorium on ICSI?

So far, all the concerns relating to possible oocyte damage described above do not translate into an increased risk of pregnancy wastage in ICSI pregnancies compared with IVF pregnancies (Wennerholm et al., 1996; Wisanto et al., 1996; Bonduelle et al., 1998; Van Golde et al., 1999). However, low birthweight and perinatal mortality were reported to be slightly more frequent after ICSI than after natural conception (Aytoz et al., 1998).

To-date, in our large prospective follow-up study, the risk of a major congenital malformation in children conceived in our program was 3.4% (96/2840) after ICSI and 3.8% (113/2955) after IVF (unpublished data from a press release by the Center for Reproductive Medicine of the Brussels Dutch-speaking Free University, June 2000). For ICSI, where a prospective follow-up program was organized from its start, this figure includes malformations in stillbirths, fetal deaths and induced abortion, and the malformations were diagnosed with a follow-up of at least 2 months. The recorded major congenital malformations involved different organ systems. Most frequent are cardiac malformations (heart septum defects), genitourinary defects (i.e., mainly undescended testis in ICSI and hypospadias in IVF), and musculoskeletal defects (i.e., mainly hip instability) (Bonduelle et al., 1999). A higher incidence of hypospadias was also reported earlier for IVF offspring (Silver et al., 1999).

Although there has been debate on the definition of major congenital malformation (Bonduelle et al.,

1997; Kurinczuk and Bower, 1997) with regard to the scrutiny of the follow-up protocol in ICSI babies, the above figure compares well with congenital malformation rates in the general population (Bonduelle et al., 1999). Furthermore, these data compare well with those from other large follow-up programs (Palermo et al., 1996; Loft et al., 1999). Although at present, few data exist on the subgroups where epididymal or testicular sperm were used, some reports mention even lower figures in these patients (Bonduelle et al., 1999).

There has also been an as yet inconclusive debate as to whether children conceived through ICSI have slower mental and psychological development. In an Australian study, the mental development of ICSI children seemed to be significantly lower than that of children conceived after IVF and natural conception, with the development of boys being significantly more retarded than that of girls (Bowen et al., 1998). This was not the case in our larger study, which indicated no difference in mental development compared with that of the general population (Bonduelle et al., 1998). Moreover, the ICSI group in the Australian study included a significantly greater number of couples from lower socioeconomic groupings, older fathers, somewhat less tertiary education, and a higher likelihood of coming from a non-English-speaking background. These factors may have introduced bias into the Australian study and the conclusions drawn.

In spite of all the theoretical risks mentioned above, so far ICSI seems to have been remarkably safe. Maybe the introduction of a spermatozoon into the oocyte's cytoplasm may not bypass all steps of the fertilization process and early embryonic development. There may be many subsequent checkpoints that filter out deficiencies at these levels. In some couples, repeated fertilization failures after ICSI do occur and it has been argued that this phenomenon may be associated with this natural filtering process (Ludwig et al., 1999). A recent report has showed that centrosome deficiencies will cause implantation failure after ICSI (Obasaju et al., 1999).

Although the inheritance patterns of male infertility are far from elucidated, it is often stated that ICSI will eventually perpetuate forms of male infertility that can be cured only by ICSI itself. But in this respect, we may not forget that the same is true for some conventional therapies too. One of the golden examples of conventional andrological treatment is the induction of spermatogenesis by gonadotropins in azoospermic men with Kallmann's disease. Kallmann's disease is known to be caused by a *KALIG-1* mutation (Bick et al., 1992). In other words, conventional treatments may also perpetuate hereditary forms of male infertility.

The main concern raised has been with regard to the Yq deletions in oligozoospermic and azoospermic men and the propagation of these deletions to offspring by ICSI. However, in a mathematical model, it has been estimated that the incidence of Yq deletions will stabilize rapidly over the next generations even if ICSI treatment becomes very successful (Kremer et al., 1998).

There has also been some fear that some DNA mutations may be amplified in the next generations by ICSI. An increase in CAG repeats in the androgen receptor gene may cause male infertility, but increasing numbers of CAG repeats may also translate into Kennedy's disease. However, preliminary studies in ICSI offspring do not show any increase in these CAG repeats (Cram et al., 2000). In the coming years, it is anticipated that many other deficiencies at the DNA level will become associated with male infertility.

How long will the clock tick? ICSI may not be considered to be a safe treatment

Although no other technique of assisted reproduction has been scrutinized so much for outcome and so far no hazards have been observed, we may not conclude that ICSI is a safe procedure. Further research on the safety of the technique is certainly needed along with continuous follow-up of the offspring produced.

One of the lowest incidences of major congenital anomalies ever reported in the general population is 2.1% by Leppig et al. (1987). At present, the sample size of our series has enough power to pick up an increase of 1.5% (i.e., to 3.6%), which we did not. If an increase by 0.5% would be anticipated by ICSI, at least 20000 ICSI offspring should be evaluated. However, according to world surveys, probably even more babies have already been born after ICSI. We only lack the valuable information on each ICSI baby born.

There is emerging evidence that implantation rates of embryos derived from ICSI with testicular spermatozoa retrieved from men with nonobstructive azoospermia are decreased compared with those of men with normal spermatogenesis (Tournaye, 1999). This finding may simply be associated with higher sperm aneuploidy rates in these men (Bernardini et al., 2000). However, the number of children reported born from patients with well-defined nonobstructive azoospermia is very limited, and no reliable data on their outcome are available. Furthermore, we lack information on the outcome after ICSI using immature germ cells. These techniques are far from successful and have an ill-defined target group (Vanderzwalmen et al. 1998; Prapas et al., 1999). ICSI using immature testicular germ cells should be considered as experimental, and preimplantation aneuploidy screening of embryos obtained after ICSI should be part of the ICSI treatment cycle.

ICSI treatment follow-up programs should not be installed only for scientific reasons. Follow-up may also serve as a quality control for the ICSI technique used. As long as follow-up studies have limited power to detect small increases in malformations and as long as no information is available on long-term and next-generation cohorts, ICSI must be applied with caution and only when no other treatment option is available. It is our feeling that all candidates for ICSI should be rigorously screened and thoroughly informed of the limitations of current screening methods and our knowledge of the genetic background to male infertility. Specifically, we require that all ICSI candidates have a male and female karyotype and Yq deletion screening if the sperm count is less than 5×10^6 sperm. We establish, through extensive history evaluation of the patients, if there is any history of a possible genetic disorder. If any of the above results are abnormal then a geneticist sees the patients.

Ultimately, patients themselves have to judge whether the concerns outweigh the benefits of ICSI. In practice, it has been shown that counseling may be valuable for patients when making their final decision (Nap et al., 1999). It has also been shown that parents may opt for ICSI even when a clear hereditary risk is present (Giltay et al., 1999).

REFERENCES

Asada, Y., Baka, S.G., Hodgen, G.D. and Lanzendorf, S.E. (1995). Evaluation of the meiotic spindle apparatus in oocytes undergoing intracytoplasmic sperm injection. *Fertility and Sterility*, **64**, 376–81.

Aytoz, A., Camus, M., Tournaye, H., Bonduelle, M., Van Steirteghem, A. and Devroey, P. (1998). Outcome of pregnancies after intracytoplasmic sperm injection and the effect of sperm origin and quality on this outcome. *Fertility and Sterility*, **70**, 500–5.

Bergère, M., Selva, J., Volante, M., et al. (1995). Cytogenetic analysis of uncleaved oocytes after intracytoplasmic sperm injection. *Journal of Assisted Reproduction and Genetics*, **12**, 322–5.

Bernardini, L., Martini, E., Geraedts, J., et al. (1997). Comparison of gonosomal aneuploidy in spermatozoa of normal fertile men and those with severe male factor detected by in-situ hybridization. *Molecular Human Reproduction*, **3**, 431–8.

Bernardini, L., Gianaolli, L., Fortini, D., et al. (2000). Frequency of hyper-, hypoploidy and diploidy in ejaculate, epididymal and testicular germ cells of infertile patients. *Human Reproduction*, **15**, 2165–72.

Bick, D., Franco, B., Sherins, R.J., et al. (1992). Brief report: intragenic deletion of the *KALIG-1* gene in Kallmann"s syndrome. *New England Journal of Medicine*, **326**, 1752–5.

Bonduelle, M., Devroey, P., Liebaers I. and Van Steirteghem, A. (1997). Major birth defects are overestimated. *British Medicine Journal*, **7118**, 1265–6.

Bonduelle, M., Joris, H., Hofmans, K., Liebaers, I. and Van Steirteghem, A.C. (1998). Mental development of 201 children at 2 years of age. *Lancet*, ii, 1535.

Bonduelle, M., Camus, M., De Vos, A., et al. (1999). Seven years of intracytoplasmic sperm injection and follow-up of 1987 children. *Human Reproduction* **14**(Suppl.), 243–64.

Bowen, J.R., Gibson, F.L., Leslie, G.I. and Saunders, D.M. (1998). Medical and developmental outcome at 1 year for children conceived by intracytoplasmic sperm injection. *Lancet*, ii, 1529–34.

Brossfield, J.E., Chan, P.J., Patton, W.C. and King, A. (1999). Tenacity of exogenous human papillomavirus DNA in sperm washing. *Journal of Assisted Reproduction and Genetics*, **16**, 325–8.

Chan, A.W., Luetjens, C.M., Dominko, T., et al. (2000). TransgenICSI reviewed: foreign DNA transmission by intracytoplasmic sperm injection in rhesus monkey. *Molecular Reproduction and Development*, **56**, 325–8.

Cram, D.S., Song, B., McLachlan, R.I. and Trounson, A.O. (2000). CAG trinucleotide repeats in the androgen receptor gene of infertile men exhibit stable inheritance in female offspring conceived after ICSI. *Molecular Human Reproduction*, **6**, 861–6.

Dowsing, A.T., Yong, E.L., Clark, M., McLachlan, R., de Kretser, D.M. and Trounson, A.O. (1999). Linkage between male infertility and trinucleotide repeat expansion in the androgen-receptor gene. *Lancet*, **354**, 640–3.

Edirisinghe, W.R., Murch, A., Junk, S. and Yovich, J.L. (1997). Cytogenetic abnormalities of unfertilized oocytes generated from in-vitro fertilization and intracytoplasmic sperm injection: a double-blind study. *Human Reproduction*, **12**, 2784–91.

Egozcue, J., Blanco, J. and Vidal, F. (1997). Chromosome studies in human sperm nuclei using fluorescence in-situ hybridization (FISH). *Human Reproduction Update*, **3**, 441–52.

Giltay, J.C., Kastrop, P.M., Tuerlings, J.H., et al. (1999). Subfertile men with constitutive chromosome abnormalities do not necessarily refrain from intracytoplasmic sperm injection treatment: a follow-up study on 75 Dutch patients. *Human Reproduction*, **14**, 318–20.

Goto, K., Kinoshita, A., Takuma, Y. and Ogawa, K. (1990). Fertilisation of bovine oocytes by the injection of immobilised, killed spermatozoa. *Veterinary Records*, **24**, 517–20.

Hewitson, L., Takahashi, D., Dominko, T., Simerly, C. and Schatten, G. (1998). Fertilization and embryo development to blastocysts by intracytoplasmic sperm injection in the rhesus monkey. *Human Reproduction*, **13**, 2786–90.

Hewitson, L., Dominko, T., Takahashi, D., et al. (1999). Unique checkpoints during the first cell cycle of fertilization after intracytoplasmic sperm injection in rhesus monkeys. *Nature Medicine*, **5**, 431–3.

Iritani, A., Utsumi, K., Miyake, M., Hosoi, Y. and Saeki, K. (1988). In vitro fertilization by a routine method and by micromanipulation. *Annals of the New York Academy of Sciences*, **541**, 583–90.

Kent-First, M.G., Kol, S., Muallem, A., et al. (1996). The incidence and possible relevance of Y-linked microdeletions in babies born after intracytoplasmic sperm injection and their infertile fathers. *Molecular Human Reproduction*, 2, 943–50.

Kimura, Y. and Yanagimachi, R. (1995). Development of normal mice from oocytes injected with secondary spermatocyte nuclei. *Biology of Reproduction*, 53, 855–62.

Kremer, J.A., Tuerlings, J.H., Borm, G., et al. (1998). Does intracytoplasmic sperm injection lead to a rise in the frequency of microdeletions in the AZFc region of the Y chromosome in future generations? *Human Reproduction*, 13, 2808–11.

Kupker, W., Schulze, W. and Diedrich K. (1998). Ultrastructure of gametes and intracytoplasmic sperm injection: the significance of sperm morphology. *Human Reproduction*, 13(Suppl.), 99–106.

Kurinczuk, J.J. and Bower, C. (1997). Birth defects in infants conceived by intracytoplasmic sperm injection – an alternative interpretation. *British Medical Journal*, 315, 1260–5.

Lacey, R.W. and Dealler, S.F. (1994). Vertical transfer of prion disease. *Human Reproduction*, 9, 1792–1800.

Lanzendorf, S.E., Mahoney, M.K., Veeck, L.L., Slusser, J., Hodgen, G.D. and Rosenwaks, Z. (1988). A preclinical evaluation of pronuclear formation by microinjection of human spermatozoa into human oocytes. *Fertility and Sterility*, 49, 835–42.

Leppig, K.A., Werler, M.M., Cann, C.I., et al. (1987). Predictive value of minor anomalies, association with major anomalies. *Journal of Pediatrics*, 110, 531–7.

Liu, J., Nagy, Z, Joris, H., et al. (1995). Analysis of 76 total fertilization failure cycles out of 2732 intracytoplasmic sperm injection cycles. *Human Reproduction*, 10, 2630–6.

Loft, A., Petersen, K., Erb, K., et al. (1999). A Danish national cohort of 730 infants born after intracytoplasmic sperm injection (ICSI) 1994–1997. *Human Reproduction*, 14, 2143–8.

Ludwig, M., Strik, D., Al-Hasani, S. and Diedrich, K. (1999). No transfer in a planned ICSI cycle: we cannot overcome some basic rules of human reproduction. *European Journal of Obstetrics, Gynaecology, and Reproductive Biology*, 87, 3–11.

Luetjens, C.M., Payne, C. and Schatten, G. (1999). Non-random chromosome positioning in human sperm and sex chromosome anomalies following intracytoplasmic sperm injection. *Lancet*, 353, 1240.

Mansour, R.T., Aboulghar, M.A., Serour, G.I., Amin, Y.M. and Ramzi, A.M. (1995). The effect of sperm parameters on the outcome of intracytoplasmic sperm injection. *Fertility and Sterility*, 64, 982–6.

McInnes, B., Rademaker, A., Greene, C.A., Ko, E., Barclay, L. and Martin, R.H. (1998). Abnormalities for chromosomes 13 and 21 detected in spermatozoa from infertile men. *Human Reproduction*, 13, 2787–90.

Meschede, D., Lemcke, B., Behre, H.M., De Geyter, C., Nieschlag, E. and Horst, J. (2000a). Clustering of male infertility in the families of couples treated with intracytoplasmic sperm injection. *Human Reproduction*, 15, 1604–8.

Meschede, D., Lemcke, B., Behre, H.M., Geyter, C.D., Nieschlag, E. and Horst, J. (2000b). Non-reproductive heritable disorders in infertile couples and their first degree relatives. *Human Reproduction*, 15, 1609–12.

Michelmann, H.W. (1998). Influence of bacteria and leukocytes on the outcome of in vitro fertilization (IVF) or intracytoplasmic sperm injection (ICSI). *Andrologia*, 30(Suppl. 1), 99–101.

Miharu, N., Best, R.G. and Young S.R. (1994). Numerical chromosome abnormalities in spermatozoa of fertile and infertile men detected by fluorescence in situ hybridization. *Human Genetics*, 93, 502–6.

Nagy, Z., Liu, J., Joris, H., et al. (1995). The result of intracytoplasmic sperm injection is not related to any of the three basic sperm parameters. *Human Reproduction*, 10, 1123–9.

Nap, A.W., Van Golde, R.J., Tuerlings, J.H., et al. (1999). Reproductive decisions of men with microdeletions of the Y chromosome: the role of genetic counseling. *Human Reproduction*, 14, 2166–9.

Nielsen, J. and Wohlert, M. (1991). Chromosome abnormalities found among 34 910 newborn children: results from a 13-year incidence study in Arthus, Denmark. *Human Genetics*, 22, 81–3.

Obasaju, M., Kadam, A., Sultan, K., Fateh, M. and Munne, S. (1999). Sperm quality may adversely affect the chromosome constitution of embryos that result from intracytoplasmic sperm injection. *Fertility and Sterility*, 72, 1113–15.

Ogura, A., Inoue, K., Ogonuki, N., et al. (2000). Recent advances in the microinsemination of laboratory animals. *International Journal of Andrology*, 23(Suppl. 2), 60–2.

Page, D.C., Silber, S. and Brown, L.G. (1999). Men with infertility caused by AZFc deletion can produce sons by intracytoplasmic sperm injection but are likely to transmit the deletion and infertility. *Human Reproduction*, 14, 1722–6.

Palermo, G.D., Colombero, L.T., Schattman, G.L., Davis, O.K. and Rosenwaks, Z. (1996). Evolution of pregnancies and initial follow-up of newborns delivered after intracytoplasmic sperm injection. *Journal of the American Medical Association*, 276, 1893–7.

Palermo, G.P., Joris, H., Devroey, P. and Van Steirteghem, A.C. (1992). Pregnancies after intracytoplasmic injection of single spermatozoon into an oocyte [letter]. *Lancet*, 340, 826–35.

Pang, M.G., Hoegerman, S.F., Cuticchia, A.J., et al. (1999). Detection of aneuploidy for chromosomes 4, 6, 7, 8, 9, 10, 11, 12, 13, 17, 18, 21, X and Y by fluorescence in-situ hybridization in spermatozoa from nine patients with oligoasthenoteratozoospermia undergoing intracytoplasmic sperm injection. *Human Reproduction*, 14, 1266–73.

Perry, A.C.F., Wakayama, T., Kishikawa, H., et al. (1999).

Mammalian transgenesis by intracytoplasmic sperm injection. *Science*, **284**, 1180–3.

Plachot, M. (1996). Les risques génétiques spécifiques de l'ICSI. *Contraception, Fertility and Sexuality*, **24**, 577–80.

Prapas, Y., Chatziparasidou, A., Vanderzwalmen, P., et al. (1999). Reconsidering spermatid injection. *Human Reproduction*, **14**, 2186–7.

Samura, O., Miharu, N., He, H., Okamoto, E. and Ohama, K. (1997). Assessment of sex chromosome ratio and aneuploidy rate in motile spermatozoa selected by three different methods. *Human Reproduction*, **12**, 2437–42.

SART (2000). Assisted reproductive technology in the United States: 1997 results generated from the American Society for Reproductive Medicine/Society for Assisted Reproductive Technology Registry. *Fertility and Sterility*, **74**, 641–53.

Schatten, G. (1994). The centrosome and its mode of inheritance: the reduction of the centrosome during gametogenesis and its restoration during fertilisation. *Developmental Biology*, **165**, 299–325.

Shamanski, F.L., Kimura, Y., Lavoir, M.C., Pedersen, R.A. and Yanagimachi, R. (1999). Status of genomic imprinting in mouse spermatids. *Human Reproduction*, **14**, 1050–6.

Silva, C.P., Kommineni, K., Oldenbourg, R. and Keefe, D.L. (1999). The first polar body does not predict accurately the location of the metaphase II meiotic spindle in mammalian oocytes. *Fertility and Sterility*, **71**, 719–21.

Silver, R.I., Rodriguez, R., Chang, T.S. and Gearhart, J.P. (1999). In vitro fertilization is associated with an increased risk of hypospadias. *Journal of Urology*, **161**, 1954–7.

Simoni, M., Bakker, E., Eurlings, M.C.M., et al. (1999). Laboratory guidelines for molecular diagnosis of Y-chromosomal microdeletions. *International Journal of Andrology*, **22**, 292–9.

Sousa, M., Barros, A., Takahashi, K., Oliveira, C., Silva, J. and Tesarik, J. (1999). Clinical efficacy of spermatid conception: analysis using a new spermatid classification scheme. *Human Reproduction*, **14**, 1279–86.

Svalander, P., Jakobson, A.H., Forsberg, A.S., Bengtsson, A. C. and Wikland, M. (1996). The outcome of intracytoplasmic sperm injection is unrelated to "strict criteria" morphology. *Human Reproduction*, **11**, 1019–22.

Tamashiro, K.L.K., Kimura, Y., Blanchard, R.J., Blanchard, D.C. and Yanagimachi, R. (1999). Bypassing spermiogenesis for several generations does not have detrimental consequences on the fertility and neurobehavior of offspring: a study using the mouse. *Journal of Assisted Reproduction and Genetics*, **16**, 315–24.

Tarlatzis, B.C. and Bili, H. (2000). Intracytoplasmic sperm injection: survey of world results. *Annals of the New York Academy of Sciences*, **900**, 336–44.

Tasdemir, I., Tasdemir, M., Tavukcuoglu, S., Kahraman, S. and Biberoglu, K. (1997). Effect of abnormal sperm head morphology on the outcome of intracytoplasmic sperm injection in humans. *Human Reproduction*, **12**, 1214–17.

Tesarik, J. and Mendoza, C. (1996). Genomic imprinting abnormalities: a new potential risk of assisted reproduction. *Molecular Human Reproduction*, **2**, 295–8.

Tournaye, H. (1999). Surgical sperm recovery for intracytoplasmic sperm injection: which method is to be preferred? *Human Reproduction*, **14**(Suppl. 1), 71–81.

Tournaye, H., Liu, J., Nagy, Z., Verheyen, G., Van Steirteghem, A.C. and Devroey, P. (1996). The use of testicular sperm for intracytoplasmic sperm injection in patients with necrozoospermia. *Fertility and Sterility*, **66**, 331–4.

Tournaye, H., Lissens, W., Liebaers, I., et al. (1997). Heritability of sterility: clinical implications. In: *Genetics of Human Male Fertility*, Barratt, C., De Jonge, C., Mortimer, D. and Parinaud, J., eds. Editions EDK, Paris, pp. 123–44.

Tut, T.G., Ghadessy, F.J., Trifiro, M.A., Pinsky, L. and Yong, E.L. (1997). Long polyglutamine tracts in the androgen receptor are associated with reduced *trans*-activation, impaired sperm production, and male infertility. *Journal of Clinical Endocrinology and Metabolism*, **82**, 3777–82.

Twigg, J.P., Irvine, D.S. and Aitken, R.J. (1998). Oxidative damage to DNA in human spermatozoa does not preclude pronucleus formation at intracytoplasmic sperm injection. *Human Reproduction*, **13**, 1864–71.

Uehara, T. and Yanagimachi, R. (1976). Microsurgical injection of spermatozoa into hamster eggs with subsequent transformation of sperm nuclei into male pronuclei. *Biology of Reproduction*, **15**, 467–70.

Van Assche, E., Bonduelle, M., Tournaye, H., et al. (1996). Cytogenetics of infertile men. *Human Reproduction*, **11**(Suppl. 4), 1–24.

Vanderzwalmen, P., Nijs, M., Stecher, A., et al. (1998). Is there a future for spermatid injections? *Human Reproduction*, **13**(Suppl. 4), 71–84.

Van Dyk, Q., Lanzendorf, S., Kolm, P., Hodgen, G.D. and Mahony, M.C. (2000). Incidence of aneuploid spermatozoa from subfertile men: selected with motility versus hemizonabound. *Human Reproduction*, **15**, 1529–36.

Van Golde, R., Boada, M., Veiga, A., Evers, J., Geraedts, J. and Barri, P. (1999). A retrospective follow-up study on intracytoplasmic sperm injection. *Journal of Assisted Reproduction and Genetics*, **16**, 227–32.

Van Steirteghem, A.C., Nagy, Z., Joris, H., et al. (1993). High fertilization and implantation rates after intracytoplasmic sperm injection. *Human Reproduction*, **8**, 1061–6.

Verheyen, G., Crabbe, E., Joris, H. and Van Steirteghem, A. (1998). Simple and reliable identification of the human round spermatid by inverted phase-contrast microscopy. *Human Reproduction*, **13**, 1570–7.

Wennerholm, U.B., Bergh, C., Hamberger, L., et al. (1996). Obstetric and perinatal outcome of pregnancies following intracytoplasmic sperm injection. *Human Reproduction*, **11**, 1113–19.

Wisanto, A., Bonduelle, M., Camus, M., et al. (1996). Obstetric outcome of 904 pregnancies after intracytoplasmic sperm injection. *Human Reproduction*, **11**, 121–9.

Yanagimachi, R. (1998). Intracytoplasmic sperm injection experiments using the mouse as a model. *Human Reproduction*, **13**(Suppl.), 87–98.

Yoshida, A., Miura, K. and Shirai, M. (1996). Chromosome abnormalities and male infertility. *Assisted Reproduction Reviews*, **6**, 93–9

28

Cryopreservation of gametes and embryos: legal and ethical aspects

Susan M. Avery and Peter R. Brinsden

Bourn Hall Clinic, Bourn, UK

Introduction

The practice of gamete and embryo cryopreservation is widespread in human in vitro fertilization (IVF) programs. In a survey of 37 countries worldwide (Jones and Cohen, 1999), all permitted embryo cryopreservation, 34 actively stated that they permitted or carried out sperm cryopreservation, while 23 permitted oocyte freezing. There are local variations in the detail of what is and is not permitted, and sensitivity to moral and ethical concerns may also vary. However, there is no doubt that cryopreservation of gametes and embryos has opened up a number of possibilities for greater flexibility in reproductive choices and is now an important adjunct to fertility treatment.

Gamete cryopreservation

The concept of storing human gametes was first entertained by Spallanzani (1776), who experimented with sperm of a number of species and suggested that there might be a practical application for freezing human sperm. The first births following insemination with cryopreserved human semen were reported in 1953 (Bunge and Sherman, 1953). Sperm may be frozen to conserve fertility, prior to treatment for cancer or surgery, to assist in conception where the male partner is consistently absent, to limit the need for further surgery following surgical sperm retrieval, or for the purposes of quarantining and maintaining the availability of donated sperm.

There has been very little argument against the storage of semen to preserve fertility. Perhaps the biggest problems arise when minors are involved. Sperm can be stored from boys as young as 12 or 13 years. The law in England and Wales allows valid consent to be given if the child is considered "Gillick competent" (*Gillick* v. *West Norfolk and Wisbech Health Authority*, 1985). It might be argued that is unfair to expect children to make choices about their reproductive future, particularly when they are under stress because of cancer therapy, and that sperm storage is just an additional pressure. However, in Europe, the Human Rights Act 1998 maintains an individual's right to marry and found a family; denying the opportunity to store sperm, thereby potentially removing this choice at a later date, could be considered an infringement of this fundamental right. Another problem that can arise in this situation is the possibility that parents may view this as the only opportunity to continue their germline, and they may bring pressure to bear on their offspring. Even if the child was clearly competent to make his own decisions and to understand the process, it would be difficult to ascertain whether he is making his own choice or following his parents' wishes.

Oocyte cryopreservation is a more recent development. The first pregnancy resulting from cryopreserved oocytes was reported in 1986 (Chen, 1986). Since then several groups have reported successes (Fabbri et al., 1998). The use of frozen oocytes has so far been inefficient, with only 1% of oocytes likely to result in a baby. There is some question as to whether it is ethically acceptable to offer oocyte cryopreservation when the success rate is currently so low, and when there have been so few births on which to assess the safety of the technique, particularly since the initial work on oocyte cooling showed that the meiotic spindle is vulnerable to damage by cooling (Pickering et al., 1990). However, there is no evidence to-date that the techniques in current use do give rise to abnormalities (Fabbri et al., 1998).

Oocyte cryopreservation remains an option for women who do not have a partner and whose fertility is likely to become permanently impaired. Oocyte cryopreservation also has the potential to give women greater control over their reproductive lives. It is well recognized that female fertility declines markedly from the mid-thirties, and the chances of natural conception and healthy pregnancy for women in their forties is small. Demographic and social changes have led an increasing number of women to delay starting their families until they have achieved their career or financial goals (Lockwood, 1999). In addition, marriage is more likely to be delayed and the increased rate of divorce leads to a greater likelihood of their wishing to embark on second families. It is possible to store oocytes at a young age, with the idea of delaying starting a family but preserving high-quality oocytes to circumvent age-related infertility or subfertility, thus avoiding the increased risk of abnormality associated with aged oocytes. This has caused some consternation amongst those groups who are against artificial interference in the reproductive process, and it has been suggested that this increases the risk of children being treated as commodities or accessories. However, it might also be argued that this process may reduce the risk of abnormal children being born to women who choose to have their family later when they may be better able to support their children. This may represent the ultimate form of family planning, by not only reducing the pressure on women to choose reproduction over career options but also allowing them greater choice of partners. They would have the freedom to wait for "Mr Right," rather than settling for a less than ideal partner in fear of missing out on their opportunity to reproduce.

In fact this approach could be considered a highly responsible one, rather than an avoidance of responsibility. It has been possible for men to store their gametes for many years and it would, therefore, be difficult to deny this possibility to women. The question remains open as to whether this should, or will, be used to take the process a step further, so that postmenopausal women conceive using their own gametes, in the way that currently they can using donated gametes.

Storage of gametes necessarily involves the consent of the gamete provider. In the UK, no gametes may be stored without the written consent of the provider and storage can only be continued while this consent is in place. Under the Human Fertilisation and Embryology Act 1990, gametes can only be stored for 10 years unless it can be argued that the provider is permanently infertile, in which case storage can be extended until the provider reaches the age of 55. Clearly, problems of storage and responsibility arise if there is no limit on storage time, and the providers die or become untraceable. The existence of consent simply permits storage but places no obligation on the service provider. Storage centres have their own contracts with patients, clarifying circumstances under which storage may or should be terminated, such as lack of contact or failure to pay fees.

Embryo cryopreservation

The first pregnancy from cryopreserved human embryos was reported in 1983 (Trounson and Mohr, 1983), and embryo cryopreservation is now an established adjunct to assisted reproductive therapy (Avery, 1999). The use of superovulation in IVF treatment often results in more embryos than is safe, desirable, or legal to transfer, and surplus embryos may be frozen. Cryopreservation of embryos helps to optimize the pregnancy potential of each IVF cycle and reduces the number of stimulation cycles necessary to produce a pregnancy. This has benefits in terms of cost and, more importantly, in terms of patient safety.

The legal, ethical and religious aspects associated with embryo freezing have been discussed extensively, and in some countries legislation has been passed to regulate the practice. It has been argued that cryopreservation of embryos threatens their dignity as human beings, or potential human beings. However, the alternative is usually disposal, and thus the embryo is denied any opportunity for implantation. Survival rates for frozen embryos can be in excess of 75%, and the use of frozen embryos significantly enhances the birth rate from IVF (Jones and Cohen, 1999); implantation rates per thawed embryo should be similar to those of fresh embryos in the best programs. Previously, many IVF programs did not offer embryo freezing; but many consider it unethical not to offer embryo freezing in terms of the possible waste of embryos.

In all European countries, couples must give their consent to storage and use of embryos. In some countries, frozen embryos may be donated to other couples or used in research projects, with the couple's consent. The legal status of the cryopreserved embryo is difficult to establish if it is considered to be a person, or even a potential person. In most countries it has no legal status. There is some suggestion that the embryo may be property, but this is inconsistent with the concept of personhood. Consequently, there remains the legal question of the right to use, dispose of, sell or purchase embryos.

In the UK the issue is, as with gametes, one of consent rather than ownership. Embryos can only be stored with the consent of both parties and can only continue in storage as long as that consent remains valid. If either party withdraws consent, the embryo(s) must be removed from storage regardless of the wishes of the other party. Therefore, if a couple disagree, separate, or divorce and one partner wishes the embryo(s) to be destroyed, then this wish will take precedence over those of the partner who wishes to keep the embryos. This is enshrined in the Human Fertilisation and Embryology Act 1990. This is also the case if donated gametes were involved in the creation of the embryo(s). Legislation in some countries, including

the UK, and regulations in others gives gamete donors the right to decide the fate of the embryo(s). Gamete donors have the same right to withdraw their consent at any time, up to the point at which embryos are transferred, disposed of, or used in research. From a UK perspective, the law is clear, and in theory should limit legal disputes over the use of embryos. Since embryos cannot be considered as property they cannot be given, sold, bought, or willed to or by another party. The providers of the gametes can only consent to use by others, but this does not convey any rights of ownership or place any obligation on treatment providers.

In many countries, a maximum storage period has been determined by legislation. In those European countries where the length of time embryos can be stored is limited, the storage periods range from 1 to 10 years (Schenker, 1997). One year (Austria and Denmark) makes it extremely difficult for couples who have achieved a pregnancy with fresh embryos to try for a sibling with frozen embryos within that time period. A maximum storage period of 10 years has been set in Finland, Israel, Spain and the UK. In the UK, the basic storage term is 5 years, which can be extended to 10 for medical reasons and beyond this in exceptional circumstances, for example where radiotherapy has rendered one partner permanently infertile. In Israel, the initial period is also 5 years with the possibility of a second 5 years at the end of this period.

While there is little evidence that long-term storage increases the risk of abnormalities (Wada et al., 1994; Avery et al., 1995), the advantage of limiting storage periods lies in preventing the legal and ethical complications that may arise if couples die, separate, or cannot be contacted. At the end of the storage period, embryos that have not been used must be allowed to perish.

There has been some concern expressed about the waste of embryos that occurs when they are disposed of at the end of the legal storage period (Ashwood-Smith, 1995; Brinsden et al., 1995; Saunders et al., 1995), particularly because of the shortage of embryos for donation or research. However, it might be considered that couples could have consented to research or donation within the legal storage period, and that no other use could be allowed at the end of the storage period if couples are denied them for their own use. Many units face the problem of abandoned embryos when the parents, either deliberately or through oversight, fail to make contact and become untraceable. The question then arises of whether to dispose of them before the consent period expires. The issue of tracing couples at the end of an initial storage period can result in distress for practitioners as well as couples, since inability to trace couples may result in disposal of their embryos when the couple might have chosen to continue storage. It is not unreasonable to expect couples to take responsibility for the fate of their embryos, if only in terms of keeping clinics informed of their whereabouts.

Disposal of embryos and the means of disposal are of great concern to pro-life and some religious groups who oppose embryo cryopreservation. Some feel that embryos should be afforded the same respect as adult humans in terms of funeral rituals. However, this type of choice must remain with couples, and many clinics allow them to collect and dispose of their deceased embryos in a manner they feel comfortable with.

Ovarian and testicular tissue preservation

Preservation of fertility for patients undergoing anticancer therapies is becoming increasingly important as recovery rates increase. It is estimated that 1 in 1000 20 year olds are long-term survivors of childhood malignancies (Birch et al., 1988). High-dose chemotherapy and total body irradiation result in gonadal toxicity and reduced fecundity rates (Apperley and Reddy, 1995). While men can preserve sperm, and women may have the option to freeze eggs or embryos, the only option for pre-pubertal boys and girls is the storage of gonadal tissue. At the time of writing, the technology does not exist to reimplant testicular or ovarian tissue successfully, such that conception occurs, although some success has been achieved in mice and sheep

(Rutherford and Gosden, 1999; Gosden, 2000; Shaw et al., 2000).

For postpubertal males, cryopreservation of sperm is a simple and safe technique and, with enough time, sufficient semen can be frozen to give a high chance of conception in the future. For females, ovarian tissue preservation may ultimately be a far safer and more efficient option than oocyte or embryo cryopreservation. While autografting may have the greatest potential for success, there are concerns about the reintroduction of malignant cells. Such risks cannot currently be quantified and, therefore, there is difficulty in obtaining fully informed consent. There are also the risks involved in surgical tissue collection, where the health of the individual is already compromised by disease. This is a particular concern in relation to small children, and the motivation for such a procedure must be clear. While it might be argued that failure to carry out surgery may be denying the chance of and right to attempt to achieve a family in the future, we must be concerned that parental ambition and desires are not the primary driving force. It is not always possible to define whose best interests are being served by such a procedure. In addition, the experimental nature of this work should make us think twice before opting for such a procedure where the patient is not capable of being fully appraised of the risks and potential outcome.

Storage of ovarian tissue might, in the long term, be the option of choice for women, since it avoids the need for ovarian stimulation and reduces the time scale, an important factor in relation to cancer therapies. The numbers of oocytes that might be obtained from ovarian tissue are also likely to be vastly in excess of those that could be achieved using safe levels of ovarian stimulation. In addition, it provides an option for those with estrogen-sensitive tumors, for whom ovarian stimulation would carry additional risks. However, the need to preserve fertility should always be weighed against any additional risks and discomfort. Consent and motivation must be clear and patients should always be aware of the limitations of any technique in order to avoid unreasonable expectations.

Posthumous conception

It is now possible for women to conceive their dead partner's children using frozen embryos or cryopreserved sperm. It has been and should be questioned whether this is acceptable or appropriate. Where embryos are concerned, UK law requires specific consent for posthumous use. In France, embryos are viewed as a "project" that ceases to have a purpose when one partner is deceased (Englert, 1998). Israeli law allows the transfer of frozen embryos to the wife even in the absence of consent, but only after a year has elapsed from the time of her husband's death. By imposing a time lag, the female partner is forced to take time to consider her decision and, should she choose to proceed, it is less likely to be on the basis of a grief-induced reflex.

In the USA, the Uniform Anatomical Gift Act gives the next of kin the right to make material gifts of the body without limiting the uses that can be made of the gift. Robertson (1998) proposes that it is both plausible and reasonable to interpret this act as including embryos.

The use of cryopreserved sperm from a deceased partner to impregnate their surviving spouse is similarly contentious. In the UK, while it is possible for a widow to use her late husband's sperm in treatment, provided the required consents for storage and use are in place, the father's name cannot currently appear on the birth certificate, although the government in 2002 supports a change in this regulation. However, the situation at present implies a perceived distinction in status between children conceived before death, even if it were only days before, and those conceived after death using stored gametes.

The Warnock Report of 1984, which gave rise to the Human Fertilisation and Embryology Act, considered the posthumous use of gametes and expressed "grave misgivings" because such use might give rise to "profound psychological problems for the child and the mother". However, the report made no direct recommendation for action, stating instead that "posthumous use of gametes is a practice we feel should be discouraged". Consequently, the use of posthumous gametes is not forbidden but requires specific consent from the gamete provider for both posthumous storage and use.

Posthumous use of cryopreserved gametes is not limited to use of sperm stored well before death. Gametes can be obtained at the point of or immediately after death, for storage and later use by a spouse. In the highly publicized case of Diane Blood, sperm was taken and stored at the point of death without the consent of Mr Blood. Mrs Blood was finally allowed to take the stored sperm out of the UK to be used in treatment. Since the Bloods were undergoing infertility treatment together prior to Mr Blood's death, his desire to have children was clearly indicated. However, he had not given his consent to attempt conception posthumously, nor had he given consent to sperm storage, a clear violation of the law. There is a major difference between a couple conceiving and bringing up a child together, and the conception of a child after the death of one partner. It is possible that an individual who is keen to proceed with the first may have serious moral and ethical objections to the second, i.e., consent to the first option does not infer consent to the second.

This issue of posthumous gamete use can also be considered in terms of the next of kin and the usual rights that they may have over other organs of the body. Under UK law, extraction of sperm at the point of, or after, death is regarded quite differently to other body tissues and organs. One good reason for this is the potential for next of kin who are not spouses or partners to make some claim on the gametes. Sperm can be obtained by electroejaculation or surgically retrieved even when a patient is considered brain-dead, even dead, if the procedure is carried out immediately. This raises a number of ethical issues. First, there is the issue of consent. Where death has not been anticipated, and the individual has had no opportunity to discuss or consent to the procedure, should their partner have a right to demand extraction of sperm in order to fulfill their own right to found a family? Alternatively, could the extraction of sperm without consent be considered assault? There is also the question of the patient's right to dignity, and whether he should be subject to such a procedure without consent at the point of, or after, death at the behest of another.

Ohl et al. (1996) cite seven cases where the authors were requested to retrieve sperm from individuals who were neurologically dead. In one case, hypogonadal state was diagnosed, and no retrieval attempted. In a second, the wife decided not to proceed with retrieval when she discovered that it involved electroejaculation, as her husband's death had been caused by an electrical storm. In a third case, the wife made tentative enquiries but did not follow them up, and no retrieval was performed. One man, whose death was caused by a brain tumor, had put elaborate plans in place to ensure the conception of an heir after his death. However, the authors felt that, despite being legally competent, his thinking may have been affected by the tumor and/or by his radiotherapy treatment, and retrieval was not carried out. The fifth case involved the victim of a road accident, whose wife wished to have sperm retrieved. However, the victim had repeatedly expressed his wish not to have further children, and retrieval was not performed.

In the first of the two cases where sperm was retrieved, it was the father of an accident victim who made enquiries about obtaining sperm from his son, who was in a persistent vegetative state, in order to inseminate the son's fiancée The authors have no knowledge as to whether insemination was ever carried out.

In the final case, the family of an assault victim and his wife gave evidence that the couple had been planning to start a family within months of his death. There was evidence that the family would assist in the care of any resulting child to allow the mother to continue working to support the family. Sperm were retrieved by electroejaculation. At the time of writing, the authors reported that the wife had not yet decided to use the frozen sperm. Ohl et al. (1996) raise two questions on which US law gives little guidance. Are the express or reasonably implied wishes of the sperm donor legally binding if he is mentally incompetent at the time of potential retrieval? Does anyone other than the potential or actual donor have the legal or moral right to request retrieval and use of the sperm in the absence of any expressed intent from the donor?

Recent case law suggests that the wishes of the donor should play a major part in the decision as to whether to retrieve sperm. In the case of *Hecht* v. *Kane*, a man bequeathed his frozen sperm to his girlfriend for the purposes of conceiving a child. His existing adult children convinced a court to order destruction of the sperm, but this was overruled by a higher court based on the evidence that both gamete providers had clearly expressed their wishes.

In Canada, France, Germany and Sweden, posthumous conception is forbidden by legislation (Aziza-Shuster, 1994). In the UK, there is not only the need for consent to be considered, but the Human Fertilisation and Embryology Act 1990 demands that the welfare of any potential child be taken into account, including the need of that child for a father. In the case of *Mme Claire G.* v. *CECOS* (1991), Claire G. contested the refusal to allow her to use her deceased husband's sperm on the basis that she had a right to procreate (Aziza-Shuster, 1994; Benshushan and Schenker, 1998). However, the court ruled that the desire to have a child does not create an indefensible right to have a child.

Conclusions

The ability to cryopreserve gametes and embryos successfully has had an impact well beyond the treatment of fertility problems and maximizing the potential of IVF cycles. Preservation of fertility is an increasingly important role for clinics providing cryopreservation and it is likely that it will be used more and more frequently for reasons other than as a precaution against anticancer treatment. Women may wish to safeguard against the decline of gamete quality with age for social reasons and men may wish to do the same as there is increasing awareness of risks of congenital abnormalities associated with paternal age (Thepot et al., 1993, 1996; Crow, 1997; Tolarova et al., 1997; Tellier et al., 1998; Plas et al., 2000).

Cryopreservation of ovarian tissue may eventually negate the need for oocyte freezing, as it has the potential to preserve larger numbers of oocytes and does not require ovarian stimulation. Many problems still need to be overcome, and whether the most efficient approach is transplantation or in vitro maturation of oocytes remains to be seen.

The potential for posthumous use of gametes and embryos could be viewed as the most sinister aspect of cryopreservation. However, as society becomes used to the increases in reproductive choices, even this may become more acceptable.

There is little doubt that cryopreservation of gametes and embryos has greatly increased our reproductive options. Both legislation and public education need to evolve in parallel. Banking of gametes and embryos also requires efficient and accurate administration. Regulation and legislation are necessary to protect the providers from exploitation but not to restrict their choices too much. However, consideration of the welfare of the potential child must remain paramount and should never be overlooked in favor of lifestyle choices.

REFERENCES

Apperley, J.F. and Reddy, N. (1995). Mechanisms and management of treatment related gonadal failure in recipients of high dose chemoradiotherapy. *Blood Reviews*, 9, 93–116.

Ashwood-Smith, M.J. (1995). Frozen Canadian embryos. *Human Reproduction*, 10, 3082.

Avery, S. (1999). Embryo cryopreservation. In: *A Textbook of in vitro Fertilisation and Assisted Reproduction*, Brinsden, P.R., ed. Parthenon, London, pp. 211–1217.

Avery, S., Marcus, S., Spillane, S., Macnamee, M.C. and Brinsden, P.R. (1995). Does the length of storage time affect the outcome of frozen embryo replacement? *Journal of Assisted Reproduction and Genetics*, 12(Suppl.), 76S.

Aziza-Shuster, E. (1994). A child at all costs: posthumous conception and the meaning of parenthood. *Human Reproduction*, 9, 2182–5.

Benshushan, A. and Schenker, J.G. (1998). The right to an heir in the era of assisted reproduction. *Human Reproduction*, 13, 1407–10.

Birch, J.M., Marsden, H.B., Morris-Jones, P.H., Pearson, D. and Blair, V. (1988). Improvements in survival from childhood cancer: results of a population based survey over 30 years. *British Medical Journal*, 286, 1372–6.

Brinsden, P.R., Avery, S.M., Marcus, S.F. and Macnamee, M.C. (1995). Frozen embryos: decision time in the UK. *Human Reproduction*, 10, 3083–4.

Bunge, R.G. and Sherman, J.K. (1953). Fertilizing capacity of frozen human spermatozoa. *Nature*, 172, 767.

Chen, C. (1986). Pregnancy after human oocyte preservation. *Lancet*, i, 884–6.

Crow, J.F. (1997). The high spontaneous mutation rate: is it a health risk? *Proceedings of the National Academy of Sciences USA*, 94, 8380–6.

Englert, Y. (1998). Gamete donation: current ethics in the European Union. *Human Reproduction*, 13(Suppl. 2), 108–19.

Fabbri, R., Porcu, E., Marsella, T., et al. (1998). Oocyte cryopreservation. *Human Reproduction*, 13(Suppl. 4), 98–108.

Gillick v. *West Norfolk and Wisbech Health Authority and another* (1985) 3 All ER 402.

Gosden, R.G. (2000). Low temperature storage and grafting of human ovarian tissue. *Molecular and Cellular Endocrinology*, 163, 125–9.

Jones, H.W. and Cohen, J. (1999). Surveillance 1998. *Fertility and Sterility*, 71, 1S–34S.

Human Fertilisation and Embryology Act 1990. Her Majesty's Stationary Office, London.

Lockwood, G.M. (1999) Ethical dilemmas arising from cryopreservation of gametes. *Human Fertility*, 2, 115–17.

Mme Claire G. c. *CECOS* (1992). Tribunal de Grande Instance de Toulouse, 4 Ch. Civ., March 26, 1991. Jurisprudence 21807, La Semaine Juridique, (JCP) ed. No. 11. Paris, pp. 65–70.

Ohl, D.A., Goodman, K., Park, J., Menge, A.C. and Cohen, C. (1996). Procreation after death or mental incompetence: medical advance or technology gone awry? *Fertility and Sterility*, 66, 889–95.

Pickering, S.J., Braude, P.R., Johnson, M.H., et al. (1990). Transient cooling to room temperature can cause irreversible damage to the meiotic spindle in the human oocyte. *Fertility and Sterility*, 54, 102–8.

Plas, E., Berger, P., Hermann, M. and Pfluger, H. (2000). Effects of aging on male fertility? *Experimental Gerontology*, 35, 543–51.

Robertson, J.A. (1998). Posthumous reproduction. In: *Fertility and Reproductive Medicine*, Kempers, R.D., Cohen, J., Haney, A.F. and Younger, J.B., eds. Elsevier Science, Amsterdam, pp. 255–9.

Rutherford, A.J. and Gosden, R.G. (1999). Ovarian tissue cryopreservation: a practical option? *Acta Paediatrica*, 88(Suppl.), 13–18.

Saunders, D.M., Bowman, M.C., Grierson, A. and Garner, F. (1995). Frozen embryos: too cold to touch? *Human Reproduction*, 10, 3081–2.

Schenker, J. (1997). Assisted reproduction practice in Europe: legal and ethical aspects. *Human Reproduction Update*, **3**, 173–84.

Shaw, J.M., Cox, S.L., Trounson, A.O. and Jenkin, G. (2000). Evaluation of the long-term function of cryopreserved ovarian grafts in the mouse, implications for human applications. *Molecular and Cellular Endocrinology*, **161**, 103–10.

Spallanzani, L. (1776). *Opusculi di fisca. Animale e vegetabili, opusculi. II. Observatzioni e spermienze intorno ai vermicelli spermatici dell'uomo e degli animale.* Modena, Italy.

Tellier, A.L., Cormier-Daire, V., Abadue, V., et al. (1998). CHARGE syndrome: a report of 47 cases and review. *American Journal of Medical Genetics*, **76**, 402–9.

Thepot, F., Wack, T., Selva, J., et al. (1993). Paternal age and pregnancy issues. The CECOS experience. *Contraceptive, Fertility and Sexuality*, **21**, 388–90.

Thepot, F., Mayaux, M.J., Czyglick, F., et al. (1996). Incidence of birth defects after artificial insemination with frozen donor spermatozoa: a collaborative study of the French CECOS Federation on 11535 pregnancies. *Human Reproduction*, **11**, 2319–23.

Tolarova, M.M., Harris, J.A., Ordway, D.E. and Vargervik, K. (1997). Birth prevalence, mutation rate, sex ratio, parent's age and ethnicity in Apert syndrome. *American Journal of Medical Genetics*, **72**, 394–8.

Trounson, A. and Mohr, L. (1983). Human pregnancy following cryopreservation, thawing and transfer of an eight-cell embryo. *Nature*, **305**, 707–9.

Wada, I., Macnamee, M.C., Wick, K., Bradfield, J. and Brinsden, P.R. (1994). Birth characteristics and perinatal outcome of babies conceived from cryopreserved embryos. *Human Reproduction*, **9**, 543–6.

Warnock et al. (1984). *Report of the Committee of Inquiry into Human Fertilisation and Embryology.* HMSO, London.

Index

Numbers in italics indicate *tables* or *figures*; *cp* denotes color plate